MW00844664

NUTRITIONAL MODULATORS OF PAIN IN THE AGING POPULATION

NUTRITIONAL MODULATORS OF PAIN IN THE AGING POPULATION

Edited by

RONALD ROSS WATSON

University of Arizona, Tucson, AZ, United States

SHERMA ZIBADI

University of South Florida Medical School, Tampa, FL, United States

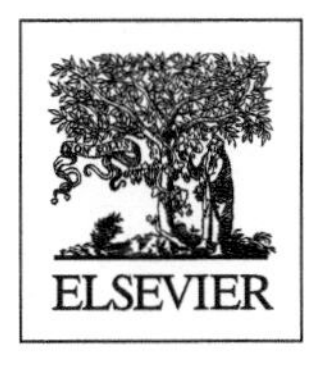

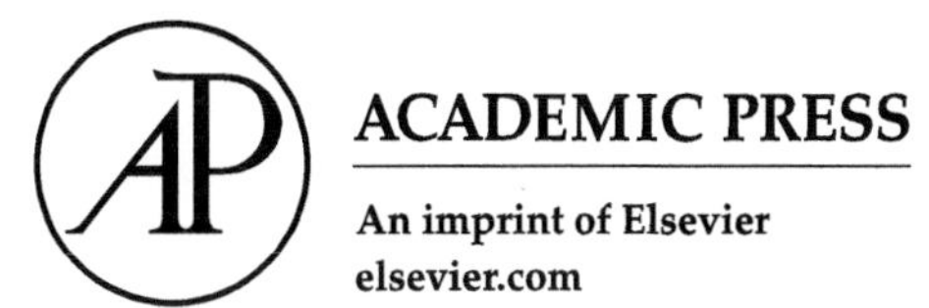

Academic Press is an imprint of Elsevier
125 London Wall, London EC2Y 5AS, United Kingdom
525 B Street, Suite 1800, San Diego, CA 92101-4495, United States
50 Hampshire Street, 5th Floor, Cambridge, MA 02139, United States
The Boulevard, Langford Lane, Kidlington, Oxford OX5 1GB, United Kingdom

Copyright © 2017 Elsevier Inc. All rights reserved.

No part of this publication may be reproduced or transmitted in any form or by any means, electronic or mechanical, including photocopying, recording, or any information storage and retrieval system, without permission in writing from the publisher. Details on how to seek permission, further information about the Publisher's permissions policies and our arrangements with organizations such as the Copyright Clearance Center and the Copyright Licensing Agency, can be found at our website: www.elsevier.com/permissions.

This book and the individual contributions contained in it are protected under copyright by the Publisher (other than as may be noted herein).

Notices

Knowledge and best practice in this field are constantly changing. As new research and experience broaden our understanding, changes in research methods, professional practices, or medical treatment may become necessary.

Practitioners and researchers must always rely on their own experience and knowledge in evaluating and using any information, methods, compounds, or experiments described herein. In using such information or methods they should be mindful of their own safety and the safety of others, including parties for whom they have a professional responsibility.

To the fullest extent of the law, neither the Publisher nor the authors, contributors, or editors, assume any liability for any injury and/or damage to persons or property as a matter of products liability, negligence or otherwise, or from any use or operation of any methods, products, instructions, or ideas contained in the material herein.

Library of Congress Cataloging-in-Publication Data
A catalog record for this book is available from the Library of Congress

British Library Cataloguing-in-Publication Data
A catalogue record for this book is available from the British Library

ISBN: 978-0-12-805186-3

For information on all Academic Press publications visit our website at https://www.elsevier.com/books-and-journals

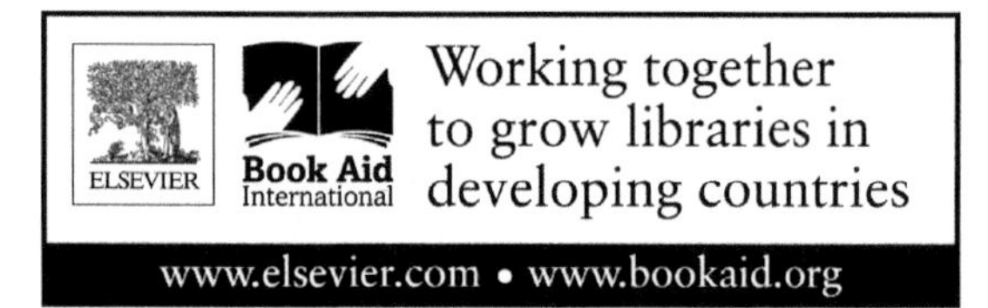

Publisher: Mara Conner
Acquisitions Editor: Melanie Tucker
Editorial Project Manager: Kathy Padilla
Production Project Manager: Chris Wortley
Designer: Christian Bilbow

Typeset by Thomson Digital

Contents

B
HERBS AND EXTRACTS IN PAIN MANAGEMENT

5. Getting to the Root of Chronic Inflammation: Ginger's Antiinflammatory Properties

P. INSERRA, A. BROOKS

6. Illegal Adulterations of (Traditional) Herbal Medicines and Dietary Supplements for the Treatment of Pain

E. DECONINCK

7. Diabetic Neuropathy Modulation by Zinc and/or Polyphenol Administration

L. BĂDESCU, M. CIOCOIU, C. BĂDESCU, M. BĂDESCU

8. Natural Remedies for Treatment of Cancer Pain

M.S. GARUD, M.J. OZA, A.B. GAIKWAD, Y.A. KULKARNI

9. *Capsicum*: A Natural Pain Modulator

Y.A. KULKARNI, S.V. SURYAVANSHI, S.T. AUTI, A.B. GAIKWAD

C
ROLE OF PAIN: DIET, FOOD AND NUTRITION IN PREVENTION AND TREATMENT

10. Honey—A Natural Remedy for Pain Relief

N.M. LAZIM, A. BAHARUDIN

11. Probiotics and Synbiotics for Management of Infantile Colic

H. AHANCHIAN, A. JAVID

D

OBESITY AND MACRONUTRIENTS IN PAIN

12. The Interrelationship of Obesity, Pain, and Diet/Nutrition

H.M. RODGERS

13. Effects of Obesity on Function and Quality of Life in Chronic Pain

L.I. ARRANZ

14. Postoperative Analgesia in Morbid Obesity: An Overview of Multimodal Analgesia and Complimentary Therapies

M.M. AMAN, A. MAHMOUD, A.C. SINHA

E

NUTRIENTS IN PAIN IN PREVENTION AND TREATMENT

15. Vitamin D Deficiency in Joint Pain: Effects of Vitamin D Supplementation

B. ANTONY, C. DING

16. Nutritional Modulators of Pain in the Aging Population

J. SMITHSON, K.A. KELLICK, K. MERGENHAGEN

17. Trace Elements Alleviate Pain in Mice and Humans

B.I. TAMBA, T. ALEXA-STRATULAT

18. Vitamin B_{12} for Relieving Pain in Aphthous Ulcers

H.-L. LIU

19. Vitamin K, Osteoarthritis, and Joint Pain

M.K. SHEA, S.L. BOOTH

20. Conservative and Postoperative Coanalgesic Therapy for Upper Limb Tendinopathy Using Dietary Supplements

GIOVANNI MEROLLA, S. CERCIELLO

21. Folic Acid in Pain: An Epigenetic Link

N. SHARMA, A.B. GAIKWAD, Y.A. KULKARNI

F

ANIMAL MODELS FOR PAIN: FOOD AND PLANT EXTRACT

22. Analgesic and Neuroprotective Effects of B Vitamins

X.-J. SONG

23. Pain Relief in Chronic Pancreatitis—Role of Nutritional Antioxidants

P. BHARDWAJ, R.K. YADAV, P.K. GARG

Contributors

H. Ahanchian Children's Health and Environment Program, Queensland Children's Medical Research Institute, University of Queensland, Brisbane, QLD, Australia; Department of Allergy and Immunology, Mashhad University of Medical Sciences, Mashhad, Iran

I.D. Alexa Centre for the Study and Therapy of Pain, Grigore T. Popa University of Medicine and Pharmacy, Iasi, Romania

T. Alexa-Stratulat Centre for the Study and Therapy of Pain, Grigore T. Popa University of Medicine and Pharmacy, Iasi, Romania

M.M. Aman Department of Anesthesiology, Drexel University College of Medicine, Philadelphia, PA, United States

B. Antony Menzies Institute for Medical Research, University of Tasmania, Hobart, TAS, Australia

L.I. Arranz Department of Nutrition and Food Sciences, Faculty of Pharmacy, University of Barcelona, Barcelona, Spain

S.T. Awati Shobhaben Pratapbhai Patel School of Pharmacy & Technology Management, SVKM's NMIMS, Vile Parle (West), Mumbai, Maharashtra, India

C. Bădescu Internal Medicine Clinic, St. Spiridon Hospital, University of Medicine and Pharmacy "Grigore T. Popa", Iasi, Romania

L. Bădescu Department of Cell and Molecular Biology, St. Spiridon Hospital, University of Medicine and Pharmacy "Grigore T. Popa", Iasi, Romania

M. Bădescu Department of Pathophysiology, St. Spiridon Hospital, University of Medicine and Pharmacy "Grigore T. Popa", Iasi, Romania

A. Baharudin Department of Otorhinolaryngology, Head and Neck Surgery, School of Medical Sciences, Universiti Sains Malaysia, Kubang Kerian, Kelantan, Malaysia

A. Bhanudas Gaikwad Department of Pharmacy, Birla Institute of Technology and Science, Pilani Campus, Pilani, Rajasthan, India

P. Bhardwaj Department of Gastroenterology, All India Institute of Medical Sciences, New Delhi; Tata Consultancy Services, Noida, Uttar Pradesh, India

C.-R. Bohotin Centre for the Study and Therapy of Pain, University of Medicine and Pharmacy Gr. T. Popa, Iasi, Romania

S.L. Booth Jean Mayer Human Nutrition Research Center on Aging, Tufts University, Boston, MA, United States

N.N. Bray Broward Health Medical Center, Fort Lauderdale, FL, United States

A. Brooks Virginia State University College of Agriculture, Petersburg, VA, United States

S. Cerciello Casa di cura Villa Betania, Rome; Marrelli Hospital, Crotone, Italy

S. Chakraborty Animal Resources Development Department, Agartala, Tripura, India

J. Chen Institute for Biomedical Sciences of Pain, Tangdu Hospital, The Fourth Military Medical University, Xi'an; Key Laboratory of Brain Stress and Behavior, PLA, Xi'an; Beijing Institute for Brain Disorders, Beijing, People's Republic of China

M. Ciocoiu Department of Pathophysiology, St. Spiridon Hospital, University of Medicine and Pharmacy "Grigore T. Popa", Iasi, Romania

R. Deb ICAR, Central Institute for Research on Cattle, Meerut, Uttar Pradesh, India

E. Deconinck Division of Food, Medicines and Consumer Safety, Section Medicinal Products, Scientific Institute of Public Health (WIV-ISP), Brussels, Belgium

C. Ding Menzies Institute for Medical Research, University of Tasmania, Hobart, TAS, Australia; Translational Research Centre, Academy of Orthopaedics, Southern Medical University, Guangzhou, Guangdong Province, China

A.B. Gaikwad Department of Pharmacy, Birla Institute of Technology and Science, Pilani Campus, Pilani, Rajasthan, India

P.K. Garg Department of Gastroenterology, All India Institute of Medical Sciences, New Delhi, India

M.S. Garud Shobhaben Pratapbhai Patel School of Pharmacy & Technology Management, SVKM's NMIMS, Mumbai, Maharashtra, India

S.-M. Guan School of Stomatology, The Fourth Military Medical University, Xi'an, People's Republic of China

P. Inserra John Tyler Community College, Chester, VA, United States

A. Javid Department of Pediatrics, Mashhad University of Medical Science, Mashhad, Iran

H. Katz Broward Health Medical Center, Fort Lauderdale, FL, United States

K.A. Kellick VA Western New York Healthcare System, Buffalo, NY, United States

Y.A. Kulkarni Shobhaben Pratapbhai Patel School of Pharmacy & Technology Management, SVKM's NMIMS, Vile Parle (West), Mumbai, Maharashtra, India

N.M. Lazim Department of Otorhinolaryngology, Head and Neck Surgery, School of Medical Sciences, Universiti Sains Malaysia, Kubang Kerian, Kelantan, Malaysia

H.-L. Liu Department of Nursing, Central Taiwan University of Science and Technology, Beitun District, Taichung City, Taiwan

A. Luca Centre for the Study and Therapy of Pain, University of Medicine and Pharmacy Gr. T. Popa, Iasi, Romania

A. Mahmoud Department of Anesthesiology, John H. Stroger, Jr. Hospital of Cook County, Chicago, IL, United States

K. Mandal West Bengal Agricultural University, Krishnagar, West Bengal, India

K. Mergenhagen VA Western New York Healthcare System, Buffalo, NY, United States

Giovanni Merolla Shoulder and Elbow Surgery Unit, "D. Cervesi" Hospital, Cattolica, AUSL della Romagna Ambito Territoriale di Rimini, Cattolica Rimini; "Marco Simoncelli" Biomechanics Laboratory, "D. Cervesi" Hospital, Cattolica, AUSL della Romagna AmbitoTerritoriale di Rimini, Cattolica, Rimini, Italy

M. Moreau Research Group in Animal Pharmacology of Quebec (GREPAQ), Department of Veterinary Biomedical Sciences, Faculty of Veterinary Medicine, Université de Montréal, Saint-Hyacinthe, QC; Osteoarthritis Research Unit, University of Montreal Hospital Research Centre (CRCHUM), Montreal, QC, Canada

M.J. Oza Shobhaben Pratapbhai Patel School of Pharmacy & Technology Management, SVKM's NMIMS, Vile Parle (West); SVKM's Dr. Bhanuben Nanavati College of Pharmacy, Mumbai, Maharashtra, India

H.M. Rodgers West Virginia University School of Medicine, Morgantown, WV, United States

M. Sedighi Shiraz Medical School, Shiraz University of Medical Sciences (Shiraz Branch), Shiraz, Iran

G. Sengar ICAR, Central Institute for Research on Cattle, Meerut, Uttar Pradesh, India

N. Sharma Department of Pharmacy, Birla Institute of Technology and Science, Pilani Campus, Pilani, Rajasthan, India

M.K. Shea Jean Mayer Human Nutrition Research Center on Aging, Tufts University, Boston, MA, United States

U. Singh ICAR, Central Institute for Research on Cattle, Meerut, Uttar Pradesh, India

A.C. Sinha Department of Anesthesiology, Drexel University College of Medicine, Philadelphia, PA, United States

J. Smithson VA Western New York Healthcare System, Buffalo, NY, United States

X.-J. Song Section of Basic Science Research, Parker University Research Institute, Dallas, TX, United States

S.V. Suryavanshi Shobhaben Pratapbhai Patel School of Pharmacy & Technology Management, SVKM's NMIMS, Vile Parle (West), Mumbai, Maharashtra, India

B.I. Tamba Centre for the Study and Therapy of Pain, Grigore T. Popa University of Medicine and Pharmacy, Iasi, Romania

E. Troncy Research Group in Animal Pharmacology of Quebec (GREPAQ), Department of Veterinary Biomedical Sciences, Faculty of Veterinary Medicine, Université de Montréal, Saint-Hyacinthe, QC; Osteoarthritis Research Unit, University of Montreal Hospital Research Centre (CRCHUM), Montreal, QC, Canada

B. Venkatasan ICAR, Central Institute for Research on Cattle, Meerut, Uttar Pradesh, India

R.K. Yadav Department of Physiology, All India Institute of Medical Sciences, New Delhi, India

Preface

Treatment with opioid like painkiller with powerful new drugs (OxyContin) is a major cause of their dramatic rise in use and abuse, as well as the related compound, heroin. This strengthens the already present interest in alternatives to pain medicines, such as dietary materials, the focus of this book.

Section A: Overview of Pain: Mechanisms of Causation and Treatment by Foods Pain involves an unpleasant feeling often caused by intense or damaging stimuli. The International Association for the Study of Pain states: "pain is an unpleasant sensory and emotional experience associated with actual or potential tissue damage, or described in terms of such damage." Chronic pain can persist despite removal of the stimulus and apparent healing of the body. While most pain is momentary, continuing until the stimulus is removed, chronic pain caused by rheumatoid arthritis, peripheral neuropathy, obesity, cancer, and idiopathic pain can last for a lifetime. Pain is the most common reason for physician consultation and a major component of many disease states. Deb et al. review the mechanisms of pain. Alexa's group describing nutritional modulation of chemotherapy induced neuropathic pain. Bray discusses a major pain, migraine. Finally Chen's group describes myelinodegeneration as influenced by age, diet, and genetic dysregulation.

Section B: Herbs and Extracts in Pain Management Inserra and Brooks investigate the uses of ginger via inflammation modulation. There are groups, who do not use the best practices and have adulterations. Deconinck reviews illegal adulterations of traditional herbs for pain treatment. Then Bădescu and coauthors describe diabetic neuropathy, which is difficult to treat and describe zinc and polyphenol's role. Many chronic diseases and cancers are found with higher frequency in the aged. Garud et al. further discuss cancer pain and natural remedies. Finally capsicum, a natural pain modulation by Kulkarni and coworkers.

Section C: Role of Pain: Diet, Food and Nutrition in Prevention and Treatment Lazim discusses honey, a historic therapy for a variety of pain for relief. Not unexpectedly, there are many reports of probiotics for pain especially in youth by Ahanchian.

Section D: Obesity and Macronutrients in Pain. Rodgers does an excellent review describing obesity, which plays many roles in disease promotion. She describes the interactions between obesity and pain and ultimately the effects of nutritional changes. Then Arranz Inglesis discusses obesity as an adverse promoter of pain, lifestyle, and physiological functions. Finally, Sinha describes the roles of diet and supplements in postoperative analgesia after this therapy to reduce morbid obesity. This book helps to understand the usefulness and to change the way we think about pain and functional foods and nutrition in treatment of chronic pain with less pharmaceutical drugs. While someday in the not too distant future chronic pain and its causative conditions may be cured by genetics or bioengineering, prevention, and treatment with nutrition and lifestyle is critical for reducing health care costs and promoting healthy aging.

Section E: Nutrients in Pain in Prevention and Treatment. Ding describes the negative effects in pain production that comes by vitamin D inadequacy. Nutrient requirements for optimum health and function of aging physiological systems often are quite distinct from those required for young people. Recognition and understanding of the special nutrition problems of the aged are being intensively researched and tested, especially due to the increases in the elderly as a percentage of the population. Then Smithson's group *discusses* other nutrients, which modulate pain in the aging adult. Tamba and Alexa review nonvitamins, trace elements in both animal models and humans in pain therapy. Liu reviews a major vitamin, vitamin B12 in the specific aphthous ulcer induced pain. Shea et al. describe vitamin K, a major supplement in seniors in relieving arthritic pain, osteoarthritis, and joint pain. Cerciello and Merolla review dietary supplements to limit postoperative pain using coanalgesic upper tendoninopathy. Sharma reviews another vitamin folic acid in pain as an epigenetic link.

Section F: Animal Models for Pain: Food and Plant Extracts. Song evaluates the family of B vitamins in neuroprotection and pain therapy. Bhardwaj et al. review nutrients as antioxidants in chronic pain due to pancreatitis. Many elderly are using foods and nutrients well above the recommended daily allowance, which may not always be needed for optimal health. The major objective of this book is to review in detail the health problems producing or resulting from pain as modified by functional and normal food, nutrition and dietary supplements to help treat them.

Acknowledgments

The work of Dr. Watson's editorial assistant, Bethany L. Stevens, in communicating with authors and working on the manuscripts was critical to the successful completion of *Nutritional Modulators of Pain in the Aging Population*. The support of Kathy Padilla, Development Editor, is also very much appreciated. Support for Ms. Stevens' and Dr. Watson's work was graciously provided by Natural Health Research Institute www.naturalhealthresearch.org. It is an independent, nonprofit organization that supports science-based research on natural health and wellness. It is committed to informing about scientific evidence on the usefulness and cost-effectiveness of diet, supplements, and a healthy lifestyle to improve health and wellness, and reduce disease. Finally, the work of librarian Mari Stoddard, of the Arizona Health Science Library, was vital and very helpful in identifying key researchers who participated in the book.

SECTION A

OVERVIEW OF PAIN: MECHANISMS OF CAUSATION AND TREATMENT BY FOODS

CHAPTER

1

Overview of Pain in Livestock: Mechanism to Nutritional Control

G.S. Sengar, R. Deb*, S. Chakraborty**, K. Mondal*[†], B. Venkatasan*, U. Singh**

***ICAR, Central Institute for Research on Cattle, Meerut, Uttar Pradesh, India; **Animal Resources Development Department, Agartala, Tripura, India; [†]West Bengal Agricultural University, Krishnagar, West Bengal, India**

INTRODUCTION

There are certain problems in measuring and evaluating animal welfare and pain and at the same time it is subjective in nature as there is no measurable parameter, which can be specifically indicative of pain. Pain in animal is aversive sensory, as well as emotional experience that represents an awareness of damage or threat to the tissue integrity by the animal. Therefore, a painful experience results in changes in physiology, behavioral output, which is designed for minimizing or avoiding further damage; thereby reducing the likelihood of repeating the experience, as well as for ensuring recovery from any kind of damage or injury incurred upon. It is not possible to directly measure subjective experiences or emotions in case of animals for which measurement of potentially painful stimulus is required. It is required to analyze information on the normal behavior that is pain free in nature for comparing with any abnormal behavior. There is activation of the sympathetic nervous system due to acute pain thereby changing the heart rate, diameter of pupils, tone of the skin, peripheral blood flow, and in releasing corticosteroids. Analgesics namely, opioids (like morphine); a2 agonists (like xylazine), and NSAIDs (like aspirin) have got a minor impact on many procedures but xylazine has been found to actually reduce the physiological and behavioral effects of tail docking. In order to monitor pain in animals recording of electrical activity from the nervous system is found to be a more direct approach. During castration and docking of tail there is increase in the neural activity significantly, particularly in the case of lamb. There is no way to directly measure pain but by investigation of a wide variety of behavioral and physiological parameters in response to a noxious event an informed judgment can be made as to whether an animal experiences pain and thereby attempts for minimizing suffering and improving welfare. This chapter deals with an overview of pain in livestock and mechanism of cure nutritionally (Alban, Agger, & Lawson, 1996; Barnett et al., 1999; Bateson, 1991; Bath, 1998; Calavas, Bugnard, Ducrot, & Sulpice, 1998; Corr, 1999; Cottrell & Molony, 1995; Danbury, Weeks, Chambers, Waterman-Pearson, & Kestin, 2000; Duncan, Beaty, Hocking, & Duff, 1991; Fraser & Duncan, 1998).

ACUTE PAIN

For a few hours or days, acute or short-term pain lasts and thereby should not outleast the process of healing. There is development of acute pain due to many procedures to which we subject animals to. Such procedures include mutilations namely, castration, tail docking, disbudding or horn bud destruction, dehorning, branding, debarking, and so also procedures of management namely, shackling, transport, milking, and housing which can result in acute painful states (Gentle, Hunter, & Corr, 1997; Gentle, Hunter, & Waddington, 1991; Gentle & Tilston, 2000; Gonyou, 1994; Graf & Senn, 1999; Hassall, Ward, & Murray, 1993; Haussmann, Lay, Buchanan, & Hopper, 1999; Hemsworth, Barnett, Beveridge, & Matthews, 1995).

Nutritional Modulators of Pain in the Aging Population. http://dx.doi.org/10.1016/B978-0-12-805186-3.00001-1
Copyright © 2017 Elsevier Inc. All rights reserved.

CHRONIC PAIN

There is increase in the occurrence of long-term painful conditions due to intensive farming practiced currently that lasts for weeks to months beyond the time of expected healing; thereby there is deterioration in welfare of animals and reduction in production, as well as financial gain. A collection of diseases is lameness, a common chronic condition that affects dairy cows, chickens, and sheep and is a major health problem not only because of the difficulty in animal in walking but also based on the problems in association with lameness namely, pain, reduction in intake of feed, and loss in body condition. There is pain for long duration substantially and also there is increased costs to the farmer due to increase in requirement of labor, cost of treatment, reduction in milk production, and fertility, and involuntary culling as well as decreased value of slaughter. The welfare implications of lameness include reduction in mobility and detrimental effects on physiology and behavior that include increase in susceptibility to disease, pain, and discomfort. The cows that are acutely affected have got reluctancy in getting up or to move and to walk with great tenderness due to pain in the digits. Papillomatous digital dermatitis and laminitis are both major causes of pain and lameness which cause lesions, foul in the foot, there is also separation of sole at the heel, exudate leakage, necrotic dermatitis, alopecia, and hyperkeratosis of the tail. There is also lameness in case of sheep due to foot rot causing chronic pain and impairing gait that gets reflected in increased level of cortisol in plasma that can get elevated for 3 months. In case of broilers and chicken's meat and turkeys there is lameness resulting in pain. It has been found that there is a selection of bird's meat for rapid growth, which results in too heavy weight thereby producing difficulties in carrying their bodies. This causes distortion of their skeleton. It has been found through studies that a normal chicken takes 11 s on an average for walking a set of distance whereas a lame chicken takes 34 s. Especially, in broiler chickens lameness have been detected to cause abnormal gait that becomes detectable in 90% of the birds. Such fast-growing birds have got more muscles in breast and legs that are shorter and wider with bones which, are immature. Thereby, leading to a typical short step feet that are positioned wide apart and turned out which result in abnormally large mediolateral force that are required to move to the center of gravity of the bird over the stance leg. Skeletal disease also gives rise to possible pain that has been investigated by use of analgesics with certain evidence of pain in association with lameness. Among young calves, infectious arthritis and osteomyelitis are common and in case of chronic infectious arthritis, there may not be effective antibodies since there are difficulties in treating the infections. As a last effort, amputation of the limb may remain as the sole solution but there may be problems in the rest of the limbs. Bone grafts have been used for replacement of the damaged tissues, however, problem with this type of major surgical intervention is that the financial cost involvement is more to the farmer. So the more efficacious is, the problem that is prevented or at least if the animal is treated effectively at an early stage of the disease (Jacobsen, 1996; Kent, Jackson, Molony, & Hosie, 2000; Kestin, Knowles, Tinch, & Gregory, 1992; Lay, Friend, Grissom, Bowers, & Mal, 1992; Ley, Livingston, & Waterman, 1991; Ley, Waterman, Livingston, & Parkinson, 1994; McGeown, Danbury, Waterman-Pearson, & Kestin, 1999; McGlone, Nicholson, Hellman, & Herzog, 1993; Molony & Kent, 1997; Molony, Kent, Fleetwood-Walker, Munro, & Parker, 1993; Ong et al., 1997; Riley & Farrow, 1998; Rushen, Foxcroft, & DePassille, 1993; Shearer & Hernandez, 2000; Schwartzkopf-Genswein & Stookey, 1997; Schwartzkopf-Genswein, Stookey, Crowe, & Genswein, 1998; Schwartzkopf-Genswein, Stookey, dePassille, & Rushen, 1997; Sparrey & Kettlewell, 1994; Thornton & Waterman-Pearson, 1999; Weary, Braithwaite, & Fraser, 1998; Weary & Fraser, 1995; Whay, 1997; Wood, Molony, Fleetwood-Walker, Hodgson, & Mellor, 1991; Yeruham et al., 1999; Zanella, Broom, Hunter, & Mendl, 1996).

NUTRITIONAL CURE

The only path to relief of pain may not be pharmaceutical drugs. An increasingly popular way for managing pain is the natural treatment of pain namely, herbal medicines, wherein a part of a plant is used for the treatment of health problems. Researches on herbal remedies are still in its infancy but several herbs are thought to provide management of pain and thereby decrease inflammation. However, to exercise caution is mandatory. Herbals or other neutraceuticals that may help in certain ways (and those which may not help actually) have got the potential of harming through side effects that are unwanted with allergic reactions, and undesirable interactions with other substances and medicines. The Duke Integrative Medicine (a division of Duke University Medical Center in Durham) has carried out researches on the basis of which it can be said that, against such likely effectiveness safety must be very carefully balanced (Wanzala et al., 2005; Toyang, Wanyama, Nuwanyakpa, & Django, 2007; Rigat, Bonet, Garcia, Garnatje, & Vallés, 2009; Ghosh & Das, 2007; Pieroni, 2010; Kumar, Vijayakumar, Govindarajan, & Pushpangadan, 2007; Roberts, Black, Santamauro, & Zaloga, 1998; Arun, Satish, & Anima, 2013; Biswas & Mukherjee, 2003; Tiwari, Kumar, Singh, & Gangwar, 2012; Gantwerker & Hom, 2011).

There are certain common herbal remedies that are used for natural relief to pain. They are: (1) *Capsaicin*: it is derived from hot chilli peppers. It has been found that capsaicin topically may be beneficial in certain instances. It works by depletion of substance P that conveys the sensation of pain from the periphery to the central nervous system. (2) *Ginger*: extracts of ginger are helpful in case of joint, as well as muscle pain as it contains phytochemicals that help in reducing inflammation. In small doses if taken, few side effects have been linked with. (3) *Feverfew*: for centuries, it has been used for treating stomachaches, as well as toothaches. It is nowadays used for rheumatoid arthritis. The herb is interestingly not associated with any serious side effects. There are however, mild side effects, such as canker sores, irritation on tongue and lips. (4) *Turmeric*: this spice has been used particularly for relieving arthritic pain and heartburn and also for reducing inflammation. Its activity may be due to a chemical known as curcumin that has got antiinflammatory characteristics. It is usually safe to use turmeric but it has been found that high doses or long-term use may result in indigestion. (5) *Devil's claw*: there are certain scientific evidences that this particular South African herb may become effective for management of arthritis and lower back pain but more researches are however, required. There are rare side effects if used at therapeutic dose that also for short term but is not advised in case of pregnancy. There are several other herbal remedies for natural relief of pain that include boswellia and willow bark. The American Pain Foundation has listed the following herbs for management of pain: ginseng (for fibromyalgia), kava-kava (for neuropathic pain), St. John's Wort (for sciatica, arthritis, and neuropathic pain), and valerian root (for spasms and muscle cramps) (Toyang et al., 2007; Rigat et al., 2009; Ghosh & Das, 2007; Pieroni, 2010; Kumar et al., 2007; Roberts et al., 1998; Arun et al., 2013; Biswas & Mukherjee, 2003; Tiwari et al., 2012; Gantwerker & Hom, 2011; Farnsworth, Akerele, Bingel, Soejarto, & Guo, 1985; Krishnan, 2006; Dhama et al., 2013a; Stephan & Landis, 2008; Adetutu, Morgan, & Corcoran, 2011; Hoffman & Pfaller, 2001; Mishra et al., 2007; Abd-Rabou, Zoheir, & Ahmed, 2012; Hasler, 2005).

It is however must be remembered that herbal therapies for management of pain is required to be thoroughly studied, so one needs to be careful while embarking on this treatment path. The herbs are not benign which must be remembered. There are still limitations in research for their safety and efficacy and above all the government does not regulate products of herbs for quality. So before testing out a herbal remedy the best care is to talk to a health care professional for precise use of the plants (Wanzala et al., 2005; Adetutu et al., 2011; Mishra et al., 2007; Abd-Rabou et al., 2012).

MINERALS AND VITAMINS IN THE CURE OF PAIN

In case of Plantar fasciitis or if there is pain in heel, the primary option for healing will revolve around rest, icing the heels, doing heel stretching exercises, and so on. However, one must remember that certain minerals and vitamins also play crucial role in heeling pain (Abd-Rabou et al., 2012; Hasler, 2005; Hoffman & Pfaller, 2001; Hayden & Ghosh, 2008; Hemarajata & Versalovic, 2013; Hemilä, Kaprio, Pietinen, Albanes, & Heinonen, 1999; Hemilä, 2006; Hess & Greenberg, 2012; Hesta et al., 2009; Hidiroglou, 1979; Bachiega, Sousa, Bastos, & Sforcin, 2012). Such minerals and vitamins are discussed under the following subheadings:

1. *Calcium*:

   Daily intake of calcium in adequate quantity may help prevent spur development (bony, calcium protrusions that are formed on the heel as a result of Plantar fasciitis). A daily calcium supplement can be taken or direct inclusion of calcium in the diet may also help. Almonds, sesame seeds, kale, turnip greens, black-eyed peas, and oranges are good sources of calcium (Central Institute for Research on Cattle (ICAR), Meerut, Uttar Pradesh, India).
2. *Magnesium*:
   While calcium is taken in the diet or in the form of supplement it must be remembered that certain form of magnesium must also be accessed. In order to absorb calcium properly the body required magnesium. If there is intake of large quantity of calcium without magnesium, as an individual may develop calcium deficiency. A balanced calcium–magnesium supplement may be taken or good source of magnesium may be accessed through the following foods: spinach, pumpkin seeds, black-eyed peas, garbanzos, lentils, and pinto beans, brown rice and millet, avocados, bananas, and dried figs.
3. *Vitamin C with bioflavonoids*:
   Studies currently indicate that individuals or animals with good levels of bioflavonoids in their bodies have lower concentration of C-reactive proteins (the culprit linked with several inflammatory diseases, cancers, and other illnesses). There are abundant concentration of vitamin C in citrus fruits, broccoli, Brussels sprouts, tomatoes, green peppers, melons, kiwis, strawberries, alfalfa sprouts, and the skins of potatoes. It is to be importantly noted that bioflavonoids are antioxidants that have got antiallergic, antiinflammatory, antimicrobial, and anticarcinogenic characteristics. They are found in the citrus fruits' rinds, green peppers, broccoli, tomatoes, purple grapes and berries, and certain herbal teas.

4. *Methylsulfonylmethane (MSM):*
MSM (a sulfur compound) is found in fresh fruits and vegetables, milk, fish, and grains. Overcooking and industrial processing can lead to destruction of MSM; therefore to eat least-cooked and raw foods are advised. MSM causes decrease in inflammation and pain.

The aforementioned minerals and vitamins along with plant like arnica and turmeric help in proper management of pain (Bhaskaram, 2002; Cavalcante et al., 2012; Dhama et al., 2011; Dhur, Galan, & Hercberg, 1991; Ding, Zhub, & Gaoa, 2012; Dinh, 2002; Dobson & Carter, 1996; Gershoff, 1993; Gianotti, Alexander, Pyles, & Fukushima, 1993; Gill & Prasad, 2008; Bumgarner, Scheerens, & Kleinhenz, 2012; Buncombe, 2010; Byron & Patton, 2009).

References

Abd-Rabou, A. A., Zoheir, K. M., & Ahmed, H. H. (2012). Potential impact of curcumin and taurine on human hepatoma cells using Huh-7 cell line. *Clinical Biochemistry, 45*(16–17), 1519–1521.

Adetutu, A., Morgan, W. A., & Corcoran, O. (2011). Ethnopharmacological survey and in vitro evaluation of wound-healing plants used in South-Western Nigeria. *Journal of Ethnopharmacology, 137*, 50–56.

Alban, L., Agger, J. F., & Lawson, L. G. (1996). Lameness in tied Danish dairy cattle: the possible influence of housing systems, management, milk yield and prior incidents of lameness. *Preventive Veterinary Medicine, 29*(2), 135–149.

Arun, M., Satish, S., & Anima, P. (2013). Herbal boon for wounds. *International Journal of Pharmacy and Pharmaceutical Sciences, 5*(2), 1–12.

Bachiega, T. F., Sousa, J. B., Bastos, J. K., & Sforcin, J. M. (2012). Clove and eugenol in noncytotoxic concentrations exert immunomodulatory/anti-inflammatory action on cytokine production by murine macrophages. *Journal of Pharmacy and Pharmacology, 64*(4), 610–616.

Barnett, J. L., Coleman, G. J., Hemsworth, P. H., Newman, E. A., Fewings Hall, S., & Ziini, C. (1999). Tail docking and beliefs about the practice in the Victorian dairy industry. *Australian Veterinary Journal, 77*(11), 742–747.

Bateson, P. (1991). Assessment of pain in animals. *Animal Behaviour, 42*(5), 147–156.

Bath, G. F. (1998). Management of pain in production animals. *Applied Animal Behaviour Science, 59*(1–3), 147–156.

Bhaskaram, P. (2002). Micronutrient malnutrition, infection, and immunity: an overview. *Nutrition Reviews, 60*, 40–45.

Biswas, T. K., & Mukherjee, B. (2003). Plant medicines of Indian origin for wound healing activity: a review. *International Journal of Low Extreme Wounds, 2*(1), 25–39.

Bumgarner, R., Scheerens, J. C., & Kleinhenz, M. D. (2012). Nutritional yield: a proposed index for fresh food improvement illustrated with leafy vegetable data. *Plant Foods Human Nutrition, 67*, 215–222.

Buncombe, A. (2010). A cure for cancer–or just a very political animal? *The Independent*, Retrieved 21 March 2011.

Byron, P. R., & Patton, J. S. (2009). Drug delivery via the respiratory tract. *Journal of Aerosol Medicine, 7*, 49–75.

Calavas, D., Bugnard, F., Ducrot, C., & Sulpice, P. (1998). Classification of the clinical types of udder disease affecting nursing ewes. *Small Ruminant Research, 29*, 21–31.

Cavalcante, A. A., Campelo, M. W., de Vasconcelos, M. P., Ferreira, C. M., Guimarães, S. B., Garcia, J. H., & de Vasconcelos, P. R. (2012). Enteral nutrition supplemented with L-glutamine in patients with systemic inflammatory response syndrome due to pulmonary infection. *Nutrition, 28*(4), 397–402.

Corr, S. A. (1999). *Avian gait analysis* (p. 269). PhD Thesis, University of Glasgow, Glasgow.

Cottrell, D. F., & Molony, V. (1995). Afferent activity in the superior spermatic nerve of lambs: the effects of application of rubber castration rings. *Veterinary Research Communications, 19*, 503–515.

Danbury, T. C., Weeks, C. A., Chambers, J. P., Waterman-Pearson, A. E., & Kestin, S. C. (2000). Self-selection of the analgesic drug carprofen by lame broiler chickens. *Veterinary Record, 146*, 307–311.

Dhama, K., Verma, V., Sawant, P. M., Tiwari, R., Vaid, R. K., & Chauhan, R. S. (2011). Applications of probiotics in poultry enhancing immunity and beneficial effects on production performances and health—a review. *Journal of Immunology and Immunopathology, 13*(1), 1–19.

Dhama, K., Chakraborty, S., Mahima Wani, M. Y., Verma, A. K., Deb, R., Tiwari, R., & Kapoor, S. (2013a). Novel and emerging therapies safeguarding health of humans and their companion animals: a review. *Pakistan Journal of Biological Science, 16*(3), 101–111.

Dhur, A., Galan, P., & Hercberg, S. (1991). Folate status and the immune system. *Progress in Food and Nutrition Science, 15*(1–2), 43–60.

Ding, X., Zhub, F., & Gaoa, S. (2012). Purification, antitumour and immunomodulatory activity of water-extractable and alkali-extractable polysaccharides from *Solanum nigrum* L. *Food Chemistry, 131*(2), 677–684.

Dinh, V. K. (2002). *Process development for chelated minerals and their effect on growing kids*. PhD Thesis, National Dairy Research Institute, Karnal, Haryana.

Dobson, A. P., & Carter, E. R. (1996). Infectious diseases and human population history. *Bioscience, 46*(2), 12.

Duncan, I. J. H., Beaty, E. R., Hocking, P. M., & Duff, S. R. I. (1991). Assessment of pain associated with degenerative hip disorders in adult male turkeys. *Research in Veterinary Science, 50*, 200–203.

Farnsworth, N. R., Akerele, O., Bingel, A. S., Soejarto, D. D., & Guo, Z. (1985). Medicinal plants in therapy. *Bulletin of WHO, 63*(6), 965–981.

Fraser, D., & Duncan, I. J. H. (1998). "Pleasures", "pains" and animal welfare: toward a neutral history of effect. *Animal Welfare, 7*(4), 383–396.

Gantwerker, E. A., & Hom, D. B. (2011). Skin: histology and physiology of wound healing. *Facial Plastic Surgery Clinic of North America, 19*(3), 441–453.

Gentle, M. J., & Tilston, V. L. (2000). Nociceptors in the legs of poultry: implications for potential pain in pre-slaughter shackling. *Animal Welfare, 9*(3), 227–236.

Gentle, M. J., Hunter, L. N., & Waddington, D. (1991). The onset of pain related behaviours following partial beak amputation in the chicken. *Neuroscience Letter, 128*(1), 113–116.

Gentle, M. J., Hunter, L. N., & Corr, S. A. (1997). Effects of caudolateral neostriatal ablations on pain-related behaviour in the chicken. *Physiology and Behavior, 61*(4), 493–498.

Gershoff, S. N. (1993). Vitamin C (ascorbic acid): new roles, new requirements? *Nutrition Reviews, 51*, 313.

Ghosh, C., & Das, A. P. (2007). Plants of ethno botanical significance for the tea garden workers in Teral and Duars of Darjeeling in West Bengal, India. In: A. P. Das & A. K. Pandey (Eds.), Advances in Ethno botany (pp. 133–147). Dehra Dun, India.

Gianotti, L., Alexander, J. W., Pyles, T., & Fukushima, R. (1993). Arginine-supplemented diets improve survival in gut-derived sepsis and peritonitis by modulating bacterial clearance: the role of nitric oxide. *Annals of Surgery, 217*, 644–653.

Gill, H., & Prasad, J. (2008). Probiotics, immunomodulation, and health benefits. *Advances in Experimental Medicine and Biology, 606*, 423–454.

Gonyou, H. W. (1994). Why the study of animal behaviour is associated with the animal welfare issue. *Journal of Animal Science, 72*(8), 2171–2177.

Graf, B., & Senn, M. (1999). Behavioural and physiological responses of calves to dehorning by heat cauterization with or without local anaesthesia. *Applied Animal Behaviour Science, 62*(2–3), 153–171.

Hasler, C. M. (2005). *Regulation of functional foods and nutraceuticals: A global perspective* (1st ed., 432 p.). Wiley-Blackwell, USA.

Hassall, S. A., Ward, W. R., & Murray, R. D. (1993). Effects of lameness on the behaviour of cows during the summer. *Veterinary Record, 132*(23), 578–580.

Haussmann, M. F., Lay, D. C., Buchanan, H. S., & Hopper, J. G. (1999). Butorphanol tartrate acts to decrease sow activity, which could lead to reduced pig crushing. *Journal of Animal Science, 77*(8), 2054–2059.

Hayden, M. S., & Ghosh, S. (2008). Shared principles in NF-κB signaling. *Cell, 132*, 344–362.

Hemarajata, P., & Versalovic, J. (2013). Effects of probiotics on gut microbiota: mechanisms of intestinal immunomodulation and neuromodulation. *Therapeutic Advances in Gastroenterology, 6*(1), 39–51.

Hemilä, H. (2006). Do vitamins C and E affect respiratory infections? PhD Thesis, University of Helsinki, Finland.

Hemilä, H., Kaprio, J., Pietinen, P., Albanes, D., & Heinonen, O. P. (1999). Vitamin C and other compounds in vitamin C rich food in relation to risk of tuberculosis in male smokers. *American Journal of Epidemiology, 150*, 632–641.

Hemsworth, P. H., Barnett, J. L., Beveridge, L., & Matthews, L. R. (1995). The welfare of extensively managed dairy cattle—a review. *Applied Animal Behaviour Science, 42*(3), 161–182.

Hess, J. R., & Greenberg, N. A. (2012). The role of nucleotides in the immune and gastrointestinal systems: potential clinical applications. *Nutrition in Clinical Practice, 27*(2), 281–294.

Hesta, M., Ottermans, C., Krammer-Lukas, S., Zentek, J., Hellweg, P., Buyse, J., & Janssens, G. P. (2009). The effect of vitamin C supplementation in healthy dogs on antioxidative capacity and immune parameters. *Journal of Animal Physiology and Animal Nutrition, 93*(1), 26–34.

Hidiroglou, M. (1979). Trace element deficiencies and fertility in ruminants: a review. *Journal of Dairy Science, 62*, 1195–1206.

Hoffman, H. L., & Pfaller, M. A. (2001). *In vitro* antifungal susceptibility testing. *Pharmacother, 21*(8), 111S–123S.

Jacobsen, K. L. (1996). The well-being of dairy cows in hot and humid climates. 2. Reducing stress. *Compendium on Continuing Education for the Practising of Veterinarian, 18*(9), s242–s250.

Kent, J. E., Jackson, R. E., Molony, V., & Hosie, B. D. (2000). Effects of acute pain reduction methods on the chronic inflammatory lesions and behaviour of lambs castrated and tail docked with rubber rings at less than two days of age. *Veterinary Journal, 160*(1), 33–41.

Kestin, S. C., Knowles, T. G., Tinch, A. E., & Gregory, N. G. (1992). Prevalence of leg weakness in broiler chickens and its relationship with genotype. *Veterinary Record, 131*, 190–194.

Krishnan, P. (2006). The scientific study of herbal wound healing therapies: current state of play. *Current Anaesthesia and Critical Care, 17*, 21–27.

Kumar, B., Vijayakumar, M., Govindarajan, R., & Pushpangadan, P. (2007). Ethnopharmacological approaches to wound healing—exploring medicinal plants of India. *Journal of Ethnopharmacology, 114*, 103–113.

Lay, D. C., Friend, T. H., Grissom, K. K., Bowers, C. L., & Mal, M. E. (1992). Effects of freeze or hot-iron branding of Angus calves on some physiological and behavioral indicators of stress. *Applied Animal Behaviour Science, 33*(2–3), 137–147.

Ley, S . J., Livingston, A., & Waterman, A. E. (1991). Effects of chronic lameness on the concentrations of cortisol, prolactin and vasopressin in the plasma of sheep. *Veterinary Record, 129*(3), 45–47.

Ley, S. J., Waterman, A. E., Livingston, A., & Parkinson, T. J. (1994). Effect of chronic pain associated with lameness on plasma cortisol concentrations in sheep—a field study. *Research in Veterinary Science, 57*(3), 332–335.

McGeown, D., Danbury, T. C., Waterman-Pearson, A. E., & Kestin, S. C. (1999). Effect of carprofen on lameness in broiler chickens. *Veterinary Record, 144*(24), 668–671.

McGlone, J. J., Nicholson, R. I., Hellman, J. M., & Herzog, D. N. (1993). The development of pain in young pigs associated with castration and attempts to prevent castration induced behavioral changes. *Journal of Animal Science, 71*(6), 1441–1446.

Mishra, N. N., Prasad, T., Sharma, N., Payasi, A., Prasad, R., Gupta, D. K., & Singh, R. (2007). Pathogenicity and drug resistance in *Candida albicans* and other yeast species. *Acta Microbiologica et Immunologica Hungarica, 54*(3), 201–235.

Molony, V., & Kent, J. E. (1997). Assessment of acute pain in farm animals using behavioral and physiological measurements. *Jornal of Animal Science, 75*(1), 266–272.

Molony, V., Kent, J. E., Fleetwood-Walker, S. M., Munro F., Parker, R. M. C. (1993). Effects of xylazine and L659874 on behaviour of lambs after tail docking. *Proceedings of the 7th IASP World Congress on Pain* (p. 80). Paris.

Ong, R. M., Morris, J. P., O'Dwyer, J. K., Barnett, J. L., Hemsworth, P. H., & Clarke, I. J. (1997). Behavioural and EEG changes in sheep in response to painful acute electrical stimuli. *Australian Veterinary Jornal, 75*(3), 189–193.

Pieroni, A. (2010). People and plants in Lëpushë: traditional medicine, local foods and post-communism in a northern Albanian village. In M. Pardo-de-Santayana, A. Pieroni, & R. K. Puri (Eds.), *Ethno botany in the new Europe, people, health and wild plant resources* (pp. 16–50). Oxford, UK: Berghahn Books.

Rigat, M., Bonet, M. A., Garcia, S., Garnatje, T., & Vallés, J. (2009). Ethnobotany of food plants in the high river Ter valley (Pyrenees, Catalonia, Iberian Peninsula): non-crop food vascular plants and crop food plants with medicinal properties. *Ecology of Food and Nutrition, 48*(4), 303–326.

Riley, C. B., & Farrow, C. S. (1998). Partial carpal arthrodesis in a calf with chronic infectious arthritis of the corpus and osteomyelitis of the carpel and metacarpel bones. *Canadian Veterinary Journal, 39*(7), 438–441.

Roberts, P. R., Black, K. W., Santamauro, J. T., & Zaloga, G. P. (1998). Dietary peptides improve wound healing following surgery. *Nutrition, 14*, 266–269.

Rushen, J., Foxcroft, G., & DePassille, A. M. (1993). Nursing-induced changes in pain sensitivity, prolactin and somatotropin in the pig. *Physiological Behaviour, 53*(2), 265–270.

Schwartzkopf-Genswein, K. S., & Stookey, J. M. (1997). The use of infrared thermography to assess inflammation associated with hot-iron and freeze branding in cattle. *Canadian Journal of Animal Sciences, 77*(4), 577–583.

Schwartzkopf-Genswein, K. S., Stookey, J. M., dePassille, A. M., & Rushen, J. (1997). Comparison of hot-iron and freeze branding on cortisol levels and pain sensitivity in beef cattle. *Canadian Journal of Animal Sciences, 77*, 369–374.

Schwartzkopf-Genswein, K. S., Stookey, J. M., Crowe, T. G., & Genswein, B. M. A. (1998). Comparison of image analysis, exertion force and behaviour measurements for use in the assessment of beef cattle responses to hot-iron and freeze branding. *Jornal of Animal Science, 76*(4), 972–979.

Shearer, J. K., & Hernandez, J. (2000). Efficacy of two modified non-antibiotic formulations (Victory) for treatment of papillomatous digital dermatitis in dairy cows. *Jornal of Dairy Science, 83*(4), 741–745.

Sparrey, J. M., & Kettlewell, P. J. (1994). Shackling of poultry—is it a welfare problem? *World's Poultry Science Journal, 50*(2), 167–176.

Stephan, J., & Landis, M. D. (2008). Chronic wound infection and antimicrobial use. *Advances in Skin and Wound Care, 21*(11), 531–540.

Thornton, P. D., & Waterman-Pearson, A. E. (1999). Quantification of the pain and distress responses to castration in young lambs. *Research in Veterinary Science, 66*(2), 107–118.

Tiwari, R., Kumar, A., Singh, S. K., & Gangwar, N. K. (2012). Skin and wound infections of animals: an overview. *Livestock Technology*, *2*(3), 16–18.

Toyang, N. J., Wanyama, J., Nuwanyakpa, M., & Django, S. (2007). *Ethno-veterinary medicine: a practical approach for the treatment of cattle diseases in sub-Saharan Africa*, 87.

Wanzala, W., Zessin, K. H., Kyule, N. M., Baumann, M. P. O., Mathias, E., & Hassanali, A. (2005). Ethnoveterinary medicine: a critical review of its evolution, perception, understanding and the way forward. *Livestock Research on Rural Development*, *17*(11), 55–78.

Weary, D. M., & Fraser, D. (1995). Signalling need—costly signals and animal welfare assessment. *Applied Animal Behaviour Science*, *44*(2–4), 159–169.

Weary, D. M., Braithwaite, L. A., & Fraser, D. (1998). Vocal responses to pain in piglets. *Applied Animal Behaviour Science*, *56*(2–4), 161–172.

Whay, H. R. (1997). Pain in the lame cow. *Veterinary Record*, *50*(10), 603–609.

Wood, G. N., Molony, V., Fleetwood-Walker, S. M., Hodgson, J. C., & Mellor, D. J. (1991). Effects of local anaesthesia and intravenous naloxone on the changes in behaviour and plasma concentrations of cortisol produced by castration and tail docking with tight rubber rings in young lambs. *Research in Veterinary Science*, *51*, 193–199.

Yeruham, I., Avidar, Y., Bargai, U., Adin, G., Frank, D., Perl, S., & Bogin, E. (1999). Laminitis and dermatitis in heifers associated with excessive carbohydrate intake: skin lesions and biochemical findings. *Journal of the South African Veterinary Association*, *70*(4), 167–171.

Zanella, A. J., Broom, D. M., Hunter, J. C., & Mendl, M. T. (1996). Brain opioid receptors in relation to stereotypies, inactivity, and housing in sows. *Physiological Behaviour*, *59*(4–5), 769–775.

C H A P T E R

2

Nutritional Modulators in Chemotherapy-Induced Neuropathic Pain

T. Alexa-Stratulat, A. Luca*, M. Bădescu**, C.-R. Bohotin*, I.D. Alexa*[†]

*Centre for the Study and Therapy of Pain, University of Medicine and Pharmacy Gr. T. Popa, Iasi, Romania; **Physiopathology, University of Medicine and Pharmacy Gr. T. Popa, Iasi, Romania; [†]Internal Medicine, University of Medicine and Pharmacy Gr. T. Popa, Iasi, Romania

INTRODUCTION

As cancer survival has significantly increased in the past 20 years, the focus in research is shifting toward the quality of life and the well-being of cancer patients (Fig. 2.1).

Chemotherapy-induced peripheral neuropathy (CIPN) is an iatrogenic condition that occurs during or after anticancer treatment. It is mainly a sensory neuropathy that may sometimes be accompanied by motor and autonomic modifications (Perry, 2012). CIPN is a major limiting factor in cancer treatment because some of the most effective chemotherapy drugs are neurotoxic. CIPN may lead to changes in dose or schedule of drug administration or even to drug discontinuation, which may in turn impact the patient's response to chemotherapy and ultimately impacting the morbidity and mortality rates. Current guidelines indicate a 20% dose reduction for all subsequent cycles in patients that develop severe peripheral neuropathy. In cases of intolerable or disabling CIPN, discontinuation is recommended (Rivera & Cianfrocca, 2015).

As an important percentage of patients will experience chronic sensory and/or motor neuropathy after chemotherapy, CIPN is also a major issue for cancer survivors. Neuropathy significantly decreases the quality of life and may decrease an individual's physical ability (Schloss et al., 2013). In some cases, neuropathy can appear or worsen after chemotherapy completion, a phenomenon called "coasting."

Epidemiology

Estimates show that one in three cancer patients will experience neuropathic symptoms (Schloss et al., 2013). A recent systematic review that included 31 studies and reported data from over 4000 patients treated with neurotoxic chemotherapy agents (oxaliplatin, cisplatin, paclitaxel, vincristine, thalidomide, and bortezomib) concluded that the incidence of CIPN is 48% during chemotherapy and the prevalence is 68.1% at 1 month after chemotherapy completion, 60% at 3 months, and 30% at 6 months (Seretny et al., 2014).

Signs and Symptoms

Symptoms vary from burning pain, tingling, and sensitivity to cold or touch, including numbness, loss of proprioception and sensitivity to vibrioception and a decrease in deep tendon reflexes (Fehrenbacher, 2015). In very severe cases, CIPN can manifest as paralysis, permanent sensory loss, and respiratory dysfunction secondary to weakness.

CIPN is widely underrecognized and underreported. On the one hand, patients will not report the intensity of their symptoms due to fear of treatment discontinuation and on the other hand, doctors will tend to ignore the more mild complaints due to lack of objective diagnostic tools and their focus on the oncological benefit of the drug. There

Nutritional Modulators of Pain in the Aging Population. http://dx.doi.org/10.1016/B978-0-12-805186-3.00002-3
Copyright © 2017 Elsevier Inc. All rights reserved.

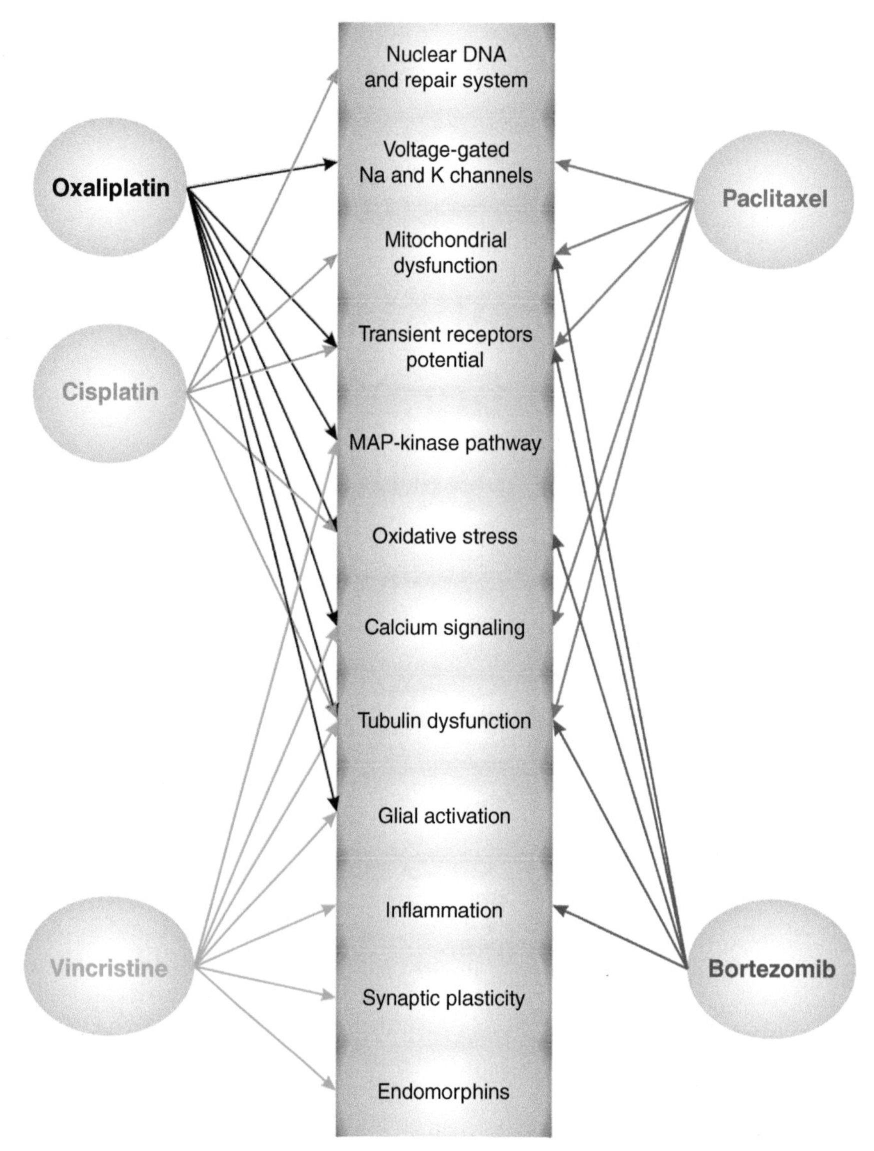

FIGURE 2.1 **Summary of the most important mechanisms believed to be involved in different types of CIPN.**

are still no accurate predictors to identify which patients will develop CIPN throughout or after chemotherapy.

Treatment

There are no approved drugs for preventing CIPN and there is only one pharmacological agent, duloxetine, which has been approved for CIPN treatment (Hershman et al., 2014). However, since duloxetine is a selective serotonin/norepinephrine reuptake inhibitor, used in the treatment for depression, this treatment has important side effects which have led to a very low compliance rate; thus, the drug has been shown to have modest results (Box 2.1).

In this setting, research has been increasingly focused on identifying the mechanisms responsible for CIPN and testing new methods of preventing and/or alleviating neuropathic pain in cancer patients. As CIPN is a chronic condition and chemotherapy alone is very toxic, an ideal prophylactic or therapeutic agent needs to have as few side effects as possible to be used during chemotherapy or in the chronic setting after cancer treatment completion.

In 2003, the World Health Organization identified nutrition as a major modifiable determinant of chronic disease (WHO, 2003). Essential fatty acids and micronutrients (such as, vitamin B12 or folate) are required for an adequate functioning nervous system. Some nutritional supplements, such as flavonoids, alpha-lipoic acid and vitamin E have antiinflammatory, antihyperalgesic, and antioxidant effects through which they can influence pain transmission (Bell, Borzan, Kalso, & Simonnet, 2012). This evidence, together with certain imbalances in micronutrients, proteins, vitamins, or enzymes found in patients receiving chemotherapy, generated the hypothesis that preventive and therapeutic

BOX 2.1

TAKE-HOME MESSAGES: VITAMINS AND CIPN

- There are currently no vitamins recommended in the prophylaxis or treatment of CIPN.
- Vitamin E has been investigated in OIPN and PIPN without demonstrating clinical benefit. CisIPN could be improved by vitamin E, as assessed by several clinical trials.
- Vitamin A's metabolite, ATRA, showed modest benefit in patients treated with cisplatin and paclitaxel. However, it was shown to reduce only symptoms by approximately 20% in the only trial published so far.
- Data regarding the effect of vitamin B complex on CIPN is scattered and outdated. In case of CIPN, decreased B vitamin plasma levels could suggest that supplementation with these vitamins would be beneficial.

strategies can be derived from the diet and from dietary supplements. The goal of this chapter is to assess relevant available information regarding the nutraceuticals most commonly investigated until now and to identify *new potential research areas.*

PHYSIOPATHOLOGY OF CIPN

In the peripheral nervous system, nerve fibers are divided into small fibers (unmyelinated, responsible for sensing pain and temperature) and large fibers (myelinated, responsible for motor control, position, and vibrioception). Chemotherapy drugs target both types of fibers, with a varying affinity, thus platinum compounds seem to target mostly large fibers, while taxanes and vinca alkaloids mainly target small fibers (Schloss et al., 2013). While some authors believe there is a common pathway for all types of CIPN (such as tubulin dysfunction suggested by Perry and coworker), others have tried to individualize each neurotoxic drug and identify specific mechanisms (Box 2.2). The most important theories and hypothesis in CIPN pathogenesis and the classes of drugs most often responsible for this side-effect can be summarized as follows.

Taxanes

Taxanes exert their anticancer effect by inhibiting the mitotic spindle—they bind to the microtubules and prevent their depolymerization, thus inhibiting mitosis and inducing apoptosis in cells undergoing the division process. The drugs are cell-cycle specific in the M-phase (Perry, 2012). Taxanes are used in a wide variety of solid tumors, including breast, lung, and ovarian cancer and Kaposi sarcoma. All taxanes induce CIPN, but paclitaxel has been the focus of preclinical and clinical research due to large-scale use and increased incidence and prevalence of CIPN secondary to this taxane. Mechanisms underlying their neurotoxicity are still controversial and several hypotheses have been suggested:

1. Mitochondrial dysfunction secondary to axonal degeneration plays an essential role. Several authors (Argyriou, Bruna, Marmiroli, & Cavaletti, 2012; Flatters & Bennett, 2006; Flatters, Xiao, & Bennett, 2006) have linked paclitaxel treatment with

BOX 2.2

DIETARY SUPPLEMENTS AND CIPN

- There are currently no dietary supplements recommended in the prophylaxis or treatment of CIPN.
- Acetyl-L-carnitine prophylactic supplementation was shown to increase chronic PIPN incidence.
- Omega-3 fatty acids seem to be effective in preventing PIPN.
- Alpha-lipoic acid is not effective as a prophylactic agent in cancer patients; however, it may benefit patients with already-established CIPN.
- Glutathione is not effective in protecting against neuropathy secondary to carboplatin-paclitaxel chemotherapy; however, it might be effective in OIPN and CisIPN.
- Glutamate and glutamine have shown some benefit in different types of CIPN. There is insufficient data available to demonstrate their neuroprotective effect.

BOX 2.3

TAKE-HOME MESSAGES: MINERALS, TRACE ELEMENTS, AND CIPN

- There are currently no minerals or trace elements recommended in the prophylaxis or treatment of CIPN.
- There is an important body of evidence against using Ca/Mg infusions for OIPN prophylaxis.
- Selenium could prove beneficial in improving chemotherapy tolerance.
- Lithium could prove beneficial in PIPN and VIPN.

mitochondrial swelling, probably secondary to the opening of the mitochondrial transition pore (MTP), which leads to a loss of mitochondrial membrane potential. It seems that paclitaxel acts directly on the mitochondria and the MTP (André et al., 2000) and induces significant mitochondrial structural changes as assessed by electron microscopy (Xiao & Bennett, 2008).

2. Disturbances in the calcium signaling and on sodium and potassium voltage-gated channels (Boehmerle et al., 2007).
3. TRPs dysfunction, especially TRPV1, TRPA1, and TPV4 could also play a role in the development of clinical neuropathy (Alessandri-Haber, Dina, Joseph, Reichling, & Levine, 2008).
4. Proinflammatory effect—the drug stimulates Langerhans cells and macrophages and also upregulates proinflammatory cytokine expression in the DRG (Cata, Weng, Lee, Reuben, & Dougherty, 2006; Peters et al., 2007).

Platinum Compounds

Platinum compounds have shown remarkable anticancer activity, which is why they are used in several types of solid tumors including, but not limited to, testicular, colorectal, gastric, head and neck, lung, bladder, ovary, and endometrium (Perry, 2012). These drugs enter the cell, where they undergo hydrolysis and form a molecule with a positive charge which then binds to the cell's DNA. Intra- and interstrand DNA cross-linkage with both nuclear and mitochondrial DNA ultimately leads to either apoptosis or necrosis of the cell (Fehrenbacher, 2015; McWhinney, Goldberg, & McLeod, 2009; Perry, 2012). The central nervous system is somewhat protected against platinum's neurotoxicity due to the presence of the blood–brain barrier (BBB). In the peripheral nervous system, however, these drugs largely accumulate in the dorsal root ganglia (DRG) and peripheral neurons; drug levels at these sites have been shown to correlate with the severity of CIPN (Argyriou et al., 2012). As platinum drugs are not specific to cells undergoing active division, the same DNA adducts will form in neurons which will lead to alterations in cell-cycle kinetics, eventually lead to apoptosis.

Preclinical data indicate that DRGs and neurons exposed to platinum-based drugs express nuclear condensation, fragmentation, cell shrinkage, tubulin dysfunction, disrupted vesicular axonal transport, and disrupted axonal microtubule assembly (Perry, 2012). These drugs affect several neuronal structures—axons, the myelin sheath, the neuronal cell body, and the glial component of the neurons (McWhinney et al., 2009). Furthermore, treatment with platinum compounds has been shown to increase mRNA expression of transient receptor potential (TRP), which play an important role in pain and inflammation secondary to toxins (Ta et al., 2010).

Another suggested mechanism for platinum-induced peripheral neuropathy involves oxidative stress and mitochondrial dysfunction secondary to the drugs entering the cell, triggering a series of intracellular events that ultimately induce apoptosis or necrosis (Argyriou et al., 2012). In time, due to repeated chemotherapy administration, the quantity of platinum drugs inside the neural cells increases, thus leading to chronic malfunction and symptomatic neuropathy (Ewertz, Qvortrup, & Eckhoff, 2015).

All the platinum-derived chemotherapy drugs induce neuropathy, but *cisplatin and oxaliplatin* are best-studied in the clinical and preclinical models, most likely sharing similar mechanisms of neurotoxicity (Box 2.3), but differ somewhat in clinical symptomatology and CIPN incidence due to different intermediary products of metabolization.

Oxaliplatin is unique among platinum compounds in the sense that it is the only drug that induces a form of acute neuropathy that appears during or shortly after the infusion and is characterized by peripheral nerve hyperexcitability. Most often, it is self-limited. It manifests as paresthesia in the extremities or in the mouth and throat, muscle cramps, and jaw tightness; its incidence is over 85% and it is triggered by exposure to cold (Ewertz et al., 2015).

The additional acute neuropathic symptoms induced by oxaliplatin, which sets it apart from the other platinum-based drugs, are most likely the result of an intermediary compound of oxaliplatin–oxalate. Oxalate induces a rapid chelation of calcium which affects different ion channels (especially sodium) resulting in nerve hyperexcitability which may be responsible for acute neuropathy (Ewertz et al., 2015). MAP kinase and glial activation are also suggested mechanisms for oxaliplatin-induced peripheral neuropathy (OIPN) (Carozzi, Canta, & Chiorazzi, 2015).

Vinca Alkaloids

Vinca alkaloids are a class of organic compounds derived from the Madagascar Periwinkle plant. Due to their cytotoxic effect, they are used as anticancer agents in the treatment of several adult and pediatric malignancies, such as germ cell tumors, Hodgkin lymphoma, non-Hodgkin lymphoma, choriocarcinoma, neuroblastoma, and lung cancer (Perry, 2012). Vinca alkaloids are cell-cycle specific in the M phase. They exert their antitumor effect by binding to microtubular proteins and inhibiting the polymerization of tubulin, which leads to the disruption of the microtubule assembly during mitosis and to the metaphase arrest of the cell (Moudi, Go, Yien, & Nazre, 2013). Currently, there are four vinca alkaloids used in the clinical setting. Among them, vincristine is the best-known and its neurotoxicity is the model mostly used to assess the efficacy of neuroprotective drugs for this class of cytotoxic agents. The mechanisms responsible for VIPN are still unknown and are believed to be similar to the ones responsible for taxane-induced neuropathy (due to similar anticancer mechanisms). However, the vinca alkaloid treatment is more often associated with autonomic and motor neuropathy in comparison with taxane-induced neuropathy (Fehrenbacher, 2015). Regarding VIPN (CIPN?), several mechanisms have been suggested:

1. In nondividing cells, vinca alkaloids are thought to alter the axonal transport along the microtubules, which may lead to neural dysfunction in both small and large nerve fibers.
2. Vincristine induces oxidative stress and (Box 2.4) glial activation. This in turn leads to the release of inflammatory mediators, such as NO, prostaglandins, interleukins, and TNF-α (Greeshma, Prasanth, & Balaji, 2015), which can lead to a decrease in nerve conduction velocity and axonal degeneration.
3. Vincristine treatment leads to infiltration of immune cells, such as macrophages and lymphocytes in the nervous system which increases neuroinflammation (Scholz & Woolf, 2007)
4. Vincristine induces a decrease in spinal endomorphins, changes in synaptic connections, MAP-kinase modulation and calcium homeostasis dysregulation (Carozzi et al., 2015).

Proteasome Inhibitors

Proteasome inhibitors are a class of cytotoxic drugs that exert their anticancer effect through reversibly inhibiting the chymotrypsin-like catalytic activity of the proteasome which is involved in intracellular protein degradation (Crawford, Walker, & Irvine, 2011). Bortezomib was the first proteasome inhibitor to enter clinical practice and it is currently approved for the treatment of multiple myeloma and some types of lymphoma (Perry, 2012). This drug specifically binds to the 26S proteasome subunit, leading to an increase in apoptosis and the inhibition of the cell cycle (Carozzi et al., 2015). Several hypothesis have been suggested for explaining bortezomib-induced peripheral neuropathy (BIPN), among which tubulin polymerization, mitochondrial dysfunction, increased oxidative stress, activation of TRPs, and neuroinflammation, are the most popular (Areti, Yerra, Naidu, & Kumar, 2014; Broyl et al., 2010; Papa & Rockwell, 2008).

VITAMINS AND CIPN

Vitamin E

Theoretical Background—Why it Should Work

Building on the oxidative stress hypothesis, vitamin E, a potent antioxidant, was proposed as a potential neuroprotective agent in CIPN. Two studies had reported a decrease of plasma vitamin E after cisplatin-based treatment (44.4% after four cycles when compared with the baseline) and one of the studies even suggested a

BOX 2.4

TAKE-HOME MESSAGES: SPECIFIC TYPES OF DIET AND CIPN

- There are currently no diets recommended in the prophylaxis or treatment of CIPN.
- A polyamine-deficient diet could decrease CIPN incidence and is currently being investigated in OIPN.
- Prolonged fasting should be further investigated by dedicated RCTs as a neuroprotective measure in CIPN.

cause-effect relationship between vitamin E levels and the development of CIPN (Bove, Picardo, Maresca, Jandolo, & Pace, 2001) (Ananth, Shetty, & Vasudevan, 2003). Also, a clinical similarity between the neuropathic symptoms induced by cisplatin and those induced by vitamin E deficiency was observed—both induce a peripheral sensory neuropathy with a stock and glove distribution, proprioceptive loss, muscle weakness, and loss of reflexes (Argyriou et al., 2006a; Pace et al., 2003). Last, but not least, vitamin E had shown promising results in the management of diabetic neuropathy in small clinical studies (Rajanandh, Kosey, & Prathiksha, 2014; Tütüncü, Bayraktar, & Varli, 1998).

Fundamental Studies

In mice, vitamin E supplementation was shown to protect against the toxic effects of cisplatin [20 mg/kg body weight (b.w.)] in terms of survival (30% in the control group versus 70% in the vitamin E group after 2 weeks of cisplatin treatment), weight loss, and neurotoxicity without influencing chemotherapy's efficacy. During chemotherapy, vitamin E supplementation was associated with fewer morphological changes in the peripheral nerve sheaths, DRG, spinal cords, and skin nerves and with decreased oxidative stress markers (Leonetti et al., 2003) when compared with the control group. Systemic and intrathecal vitamin E administration dose-dependently reduced pain behavior and neuronal electrophysiological changes in a spinal nerve ligation model of neuropathic (Kim et al., 2006).

Clinical Studies

Pace et al., assessed the potential neuroprotective effects of oral vitamin E (300 mg/day during chemotherapy and 3 months after) in a prospective study that enrolled patients that were about to initiate *cisplatin*-based chemotherapy. The results showed that neurotoxicity was 2 times more severe and almost 3 times more frequent in patients that received cisplatin alone when compared with those supplemented with vitamin E (Pace et al., 2003). Shortly after, another team of researchers published the results of a pilot study that included cancer patients undergoing different types of chemotherapy: *paclitaxel*-based, *cisplatin*-based, or a combination of the two. It included 31 patients randomized to receive either vitamin E (600 mg/day during chemotherapy and continued up to 3 months after) or placebo; the results were encouraging—25% of the patients in the vitamin E group developed neuropathy as compared with 73.3% of patients in the placebo group (Argyriou et al., 2005). Subsequently, the same group designed two other trials (that enrolled approximately 30 patients each) that were published shortly after: one of the trials included only patients that were about to receive *cisplatin* and the other only patients about to receive *paclitaxel*; both trials administered vitamin E 600 mg/day during chemotherapy and 3 months thereafter; the results were consistent with the ones obtained in the previous trial—vitamin E supplementation was associated with a three times lower incidence of neuropathy and lower peripheral neuropathy scores (Argyriou et al., 2006a, 2006b).

In 2010, the results from a second study performed by Pace et al., became available. Of the 108 patients enrolled, only 41 received an adeqaute Cisplatin dose to be eligible for data analysis. Despite the small number of patients, the results indicated a sevenfold decrease in the incidence of neurotoxicity in the vitamin E supplementation group (Pace et al., 2010).

Due to the encouraging results available in literature, a large phase III trial was designed—it enrolled patients with different types of solid malignancies that required different types of chemotherapy and distributed them randomly into two groups: group one that received vitamin E oral supplementation 300 mg twice a day and group two that received matching placebo. The data collected from almost 200 patients showed no statistically significant difference between the two groups as assessed by questionnaires, patient diaries and the common toxicity criteria (Kottschade et al., 2011). However, only 8 of the 189 patients received cisplatin chemotherapy, the rest received either paclitaxel, oxaliplatin, carboplatin, or combination therapy. Due to current evidence that supports different neuropathy-inducing mechanisms for all these drugs, the small number of patients receiving cisplatin may be a possible explanation for its negative results.

Aside from cisplatin- and paclitaxel-induced neuropathy, vitamin E has also been assessed as a potential neuroprotector against oxaliplatin toxicity. The results of a small prospective phase two trial were published in 2013—the authors enrolled cancer patients about to begin an oxaliplatin-based first-line anticancer regimen and assigned them either to the study group that received oral vitamin E supplementation (400 mg/day) or to the control group. The results showed no significant difference between the patients that received the actual treatment or the placebo (Afonseca et al., 2013). Similar results were obtained in a slightly larger prospective trial published 2 years later—vitamin E supplementation (400 mg/day) had no effect on oxaliplatin-induced neuropathy (Salehi & Roayaei, 2015).

Conclusions

The question regarding vitamin E's neuroprotective effect is far from answered, especially since it has been investigated in several types of CIPN. It is clear it has little to no effect in OIPN, although preclinical in vitro studies hypothesized that oxaliplatin and cisplatin have similar biological effects. Similarly, evidence that vitamin E has no effect on paclitaxel-induced peripheral neuropathy (PIPN) is convincing, despite the positive results obtained by two small trials performed by the same team that enrolled 45 patients in total. It is to be expected that vitamin E does not significantly alleviate PIPN, since more and more researchers believe the main mechanism responsible is mitochondrial dysfunction and not oxidative stress in this particular drug-induced neuropathy. Cisplatin, however, seems to have a different neuropathic mechanism than oxaliplatin and paclitaxel and there is no convincing data available against vitamin E's benefit in CisIPN. In light of available data, current American guidelines for CIPN state that clinicians should not offer vitamin E for the prevention of CIPN (Hershman et al., 2014).

Vitamin A and Related Compounds

Theoretical Background—Why it Should Work

Vitamin A has been proposed as a potential neuroprotective agent for the same reasons as vitamin E. It was believed that its antioxidant effect will protect against cisplatin-induced neuropathic pain (CisIPN) (characterized, among other changes, by decreased antioxidant levels). All-*trans* retinoic acid (ATRA)—the active metabolite of retinol is present in the developing spinal cord (Reiner et al., 2014) and increases neural growth factor concentration (Palencia et al., 2014). Due to the role of retinoids in cell growth, differentiation, and cell death, ATRA is currently used in the clinical setting in the treatment of acute promyelocytic leukemia.

Studies investigating other types of neuropathies have shown that ATRA prevents neuronal cell death in settings, such as beta-amyloid exposure (Sahin, Karauzum, Perry, Smith, & Aliciguzel, 2005), *N*-methyl-D-aspartate (NMDA) injections (Sakamoto et al., 2010) or oxygen–glucose deprivation (Shinozaki et al., 2007). Investigating ATRA's effect on other types of neuronal impairment indicated promising results in the prevention and the treatment of diabetic neuropathy (Hernández-Pedro et al., 2014) and solvent-induced neuropathy (Palencia et al., 2014).

However, ATRA and other retinoids have been reported as neurotoxic agents. In the clinical setting, oral therapy with acitretin (a second-generation retinoid) induced sensory nerve dysfunction in 69% of the patients after 3 months of daily administration (Chroni, Georgiou, Monastirli, Paschalis, & Tsambaos, 2001). Several other individual cases of acitretin-induced neuropathy are reported in the literature (Chroni et al., 2014; Tsambaos et al., 2003).

Fundamental Studies

An aqueous extract of *Pittosporum tobira*, a medicinal plant that contains four types of carotenoids, was shown to protect cortical cells against glutamate-induced neurotoxicity (Moon & Park, 2010). A biologically active derivative of vitamin A, 9-*cis* retinoic acid protected against methamphetamine-induced neurodegeneration both in vitro and in an animal study (Reiner et al., 2014)

The first published animal studies investigating the effect of vitamin A on neuropathy had modest results—a mild protective effect of retinoic acid administration was identified by Tredici et al., in cisplatin-induced neuropathic pain. In this study, vitamin A protected against behavioral changes, but failed to protect against morphometric, electrophysiological, and functional changes induced by cisplatin treatment in rats (Tredici, Tredici, Fabbrica, Minoia, & Cavaletti, 1998). More than 10 years later, one other animal study showed that a vitamin A metabolite (ATRA) can have protective effects in CIPN. The effects were evaluated in both cisplatin-induced and PIPN. The assessments were performed by means of behavioral tests, assessment of nerve growth factor (NGF) levels and ultrastructural evaluation of the sciatic nerve and results indicated a significant neuroprotective effect of oral ATRA (20 mg/kg b.w.) administration in both cisplatin-treated and paclitaxel-treated rats (Arrieta et al., 2011).

Clinical Studies

To date, the only data available from clinical studies comes from the trial published by Arrieta et al. (2011). Lung cancer patients (92 patients), scheduled to receive cisplatin and paclitaxel combination therapy, were randomized as follows: group 1 received ATRA daily (20 mg/m^2) starting 1 week prior to treatment until the completion of two courses and the second group received a matched placebo. Patients were assessed before the study at a baseline and later, after two chemotherapy cycles by means of toxicity criteria, serum NGF, and electrophysiological tests. ATRA treatment was associated with a 20% decrease in the incidence of grade 2 and 3 neuropathy, but no difference in NGF levels and NCV-assessed latency times were identified when compared with placebo (Arrieta et al., 2011).

Conclusions

There is not enough information available for deciding on ATRA's efficacy as a neuroprotective agent. Although the results of the only clinical study available showed a modest benefit derived from ATRA treatment, the study was performed on patients treated with two neurotoxic drugs, follow-up was performed for a very short period of time and ATRA had no benefit on structural changes associated with CIPN. More studies are required to evaluate if vitamin A derivatives and/or metabolites can play a therapeutic role in CIPN. Current American guidelines for CIPN state that clinicians should not offer ATRA for the prevention of CIPN (Hershman et al., 2014).

B Vitamins

Theoretical Background—Why it Should Work

The B complex consists of eight hydrosoluble vitamins essential for the functional and structural integrity of the nervous system. Of these, three—thiamin, pyridoxine, and cyanocobalamin—have been so far investigated in the prevention and/or treatment of CIPN.

Thiamin (vitamin B1) is essential to several metabolic processes, especially in the mitochondrial respiratory chain and in glucose metabolism. The nervous system needs thiamin for myelin production and neurotransmitter synthesis; B1 deficiency is associated with oxidative stress and neuropathic conditions, such as Wernicke–Korsakoff syndrome and nutritional polyneuropathy. Furthermore, thiamine supplementation increases NADP levels and antioxidant formation, which is why it was hypothesized it would be effective in preventing cisplatin-induced neuropathy (Turan et al., 2014).

Pyridoxine (vitamin B6) is involved in the synthesis of neurotransmitters, in the amino acid and glucose metabolism and acts as a cofactor for over 100 enzymes (Chawla & Kvarnberg, 2014). In cells, vitamin B6 has antioxidant effects, inhibiting superoxide formation and reducing lipid peroxidation (Jain & Lim, 2001). Micronutrient supplementation (including vitamin B6) has been shown to alleviate symptoms in patients with diabetic neuropathy (Farvid, Homayouni, Amiri, & Adelmanesh, 2011).

Vitamin B12 plays a critical role in DNA synthesis and regulation, energy production and fatty acid synthesis. Methylcobalamin (physiological equivalent of vitamin B12), by itself or in combination with other drugs, has shown significant neuroprotective effects in disorders, such as diabetic neuropathy (Dongre & Swami, 2013; Shibuya et al., 2014) and subacute herpetic neuralgia (Xu, Lv, Feng, Tang, & Xu, 2013). Studies indicate that methylcobalamin exerts its effects by promoting regeneration of injured nerves, inhibiting ectopic spontaneous discharge and improving nerve conduction velocity (Zhang, Han, Hu, & Xu, 2013). Other arguments to support the relationship between vitamin B12 and CIPN include the fact that vitamin B12 deficiency can develop during chemotherapy and that a history of vitamin B12 deficiency has been identified as an additional risk factor for developing CIPN (Schloss, Colosimo, Airey, & Vitetta, 2015).

Several studies and case reports identified potential benefits of different B vitamins, especially thiamine, pyridoxine, and cyanocobalamin and their derivatives, in the treatment of diabetic peripheral neuropathy in both animal studies and in the clinical setting. A Cochrane review published in 2008 identified 13 randomized and quasi-randomized clinical studies involving B vitamins and diabetic or alcoholic neuropathy that included over 700 participants. The authors concluded that the evidence available is insufficient for determining whether B vitamins can alleviate these types of neuropathies (Ang et al., 2008).

Massive doses of B vitamins, especially vitamin B6 can have neurotoxic effects. Several case reports and case series present the development of severe sensory neuropathy after chronic supplementation of vitamin B6 (daily doses of over 1 g for more than 2 years) that was associated in some cases with motor neuropathy (Friedman, Resnick, & Baer, 1986; Gdynia et al., 2008; Morra et al., 1993; Schaumburg et al., 1983).

Fundamental Studies

B vitamins have been tested in preclinical studies in several settings: on their own (especially vitamin B1 and B12), administered together (vitamin B complex) or in most cases in combination with other analgesic drugs.

Regarding single-vitamin administration, thermal hyperalgesia and neural hyperexcitability were significantly reversed in 10–14 days of vitamin B1 administration (66 mg/kg b.w.) in a rat model of neuropathic pain obtained by chronic DRG compression (Song, Huang, & Song, 2009). Also, an active metabolite of thiamine, thiamine pyrophosphate (20 mg/kg b.w.), was shown to significantly prevent oxidative changes induced by cisplatin administration in rat brain tissue (Turan et al., 2014).

B12 was also tested on its own—both single and repeated intraperitoneal administrations of methylcobalamin significantly alleviated mechanical allodynia in a chronic compression injury animal model. Furthermore, B12 (1.25 and 2.5 mg/kg b.w.) inhibited both neuronal spontaneous activity in A-type sensory neurons and the excitability of medium-sized DRG neurons in neuropathic animals, thus suggesting its potential effect in CIPN (Zhang et al., 2015).

Systemic intraperitoneal administration of a B vitamin complex (B1/B6/B12 at 33/33/0.5 mg/kg, i.p., daily, for 7–14 consecutive days) prevented spinal cord alterations and exerted neuroprotective and antinociceptive effects in a rat model of spinal cord ischemia–reperfusion injury (Yu et al., 2014). Similar results had been previously obtained by Wang et al., who showed that a combination of vitamins B1, B6, and B12 (same doses) is effective in alleviating thermal hyperalgesia in rats with neuropathic pain secondary to spinal ganglia compression or sciatic nerve ligation (Wang, Gan, Rupert, Zeng, & Song, 2005).

Among the drugs concurrently administered with B vitamins in order to assess their efficacy as coanalgesics, positive outcomes were reported from combining them with carbamazepine (Kopruszinski, Reis, & Chichorro, 2012), vitamin E acetate (Morani & Bodhankar, 2010), diclofenac (Granados-Soto et al., 2004), and gabapentin (Reyes-García, Caram-Salas, Medina-Santillán, & Granados-Soto, 2004).

Clinical Studies

The effect of B vitamins was assessed not only in peripheral neuropathy, but also in the prevention and treatment of other neurological (central and peripheral) side effects of chemotherapy. Also, they were mostly assessed in combination with chemotherapy drugs that are not associated with a very high CIPN incidence, such as cyclophosphamide, ifosfamide, and capecitabine.

Thiamine has been reported as being effective in treating ifosfamide-induced encephalopathy. Several case reports and series indicated complete resolution or significant improvement of symptoms in patients that developed encephalopathy and were treated with i.v. thiamin 100 mg every 4 h until symptom improvement (Buesa, García-Teijido, Losa, & Fra, 2003; Imtiaz & Muzaffar, 2010). The prophylactic role of thiamin (300 mg every 12 h p.o. or 100 mg i.v. every 4–6 h) administered during ifosfamide treatment was also reported (Buesa et al., 2003; Hamadani & Awan, 2006). However, not all reports are in agreement—a retrospective chart review published in 2011 assessed the efficacy of thiamine in preventing ifosfamide-induced encephalopathy and concluded that vitamin B1 prophylaxis did not decrease the incidence of this side effect (Richards, Marshall, & McQuary, 2011).

Pyridoxine was assessed in the clinical setting for its ability to prevent vincristine-induced neuropathy (VIPN). Adding 1.5 g of vitamin B6 per day during chemotherapy did not change the incidence of neurotoxic symptoms, indicating that pyridoxine supplementation has no effect in VIPN (Jackson et al., 1986). However, subsequent papers stated that these results are a consequence of the high, neurotoxic pyridoxine dose used. Indeed, several more recent case reports have shown good central and peripheral neurologic outcomes after B6 administration in vincristine-induced neuropathic patients, with vitamin doses ranging from 150 to 300 $mg/m^2/day$ (Bay, Yilmaz, Yilmaz, & Oner, 2006; Ozyurek et al., 2007, 2009). A case series of four pediatric patients with VIPN showed that all patients recovered in 1–2 weeks after the initiation of pyridoxine (150 $mg/m^2/day$) and pyridostigmine treatment (pyridostigmine was used for decreasing gastrointestinal motility associated with vincristine) (Akbayram et al., 2010).

The effect of pyridoxine on cisplatin-induced neuropathy was assessed in only one clinical trial published over 20 years ago, the authors analyzed ovarian carcinoma patients treated with different cisplatin–hexamethylmelamine regimens and found that pyridoxine administration (300 $mg/m^2/day$) significantly reduced neurotoxicity, but seemed to decrease chemotherapy response duration (Wiernik et al., 1992).

Regarding the effect of vitamin B12 in PIPN prevention or treatment, our literature search revealed one case report that presented a breast cancer patient undergoing cyclophosphamide–doxorubicin chemotherapy that developed CIPN during treatment. B12 levels were within normal range at the baseline and were significantly decreased when CIPN occurred. B complex supplementation partly reversed CIPN as assessed by the total neuropathy score (Schloss et al., 2015).

Conclusions

Regarding the efficacy of B vitamins in treating or preventing CIPN, available data is scattered and mostly outdated. Although B vitamins were efficient in animal models, fear of interfering with chemotherapy's efficacy (as was shown in the B6 and cisplatin clinical trial) has significantly hindered subsequent research. Also, it seems that B vitamin supplementation is useful only in the case of decreased plasma levels, and not routinely as prophylaxis—it is well-known that vitamin B deficiency will lead to neuropathy on its own and preexisting B vitamin deficiencies will worsen CIPN (alcoholism is a known risk factor for CIPN). Although B vitamins have shown good results in diabetic neuropathy, CIPN has an entirely different mechanism. Taking into account the very little information available, the American guidelines for CIPN do not discuss B vitamin prophylaxis/treatment in their CIPN guidelines (Hershman et al., 2014).

One promising area of research in this field, however, is the effect of B vitamins as coadjuvants having shown very promising results in several fundamental studies. To our knowledge, there are clinical trials already published which have assessed the combination of a B vitamin complex associated with another analgesic or antiinflammatory drug.

NUTRITIONAL SUPPLEMENTS

Acetyl-L-Carnitine

Theoretical Background—Why it Should Work

Acetyl L-carnitine (ALCAR) is an acetyl ester of carnitine with an essential metabolic role in the oxidation of free fatty acids; because it is a substrate in energy production reactions, it plays an important part in mitochondrial functioning. ALCAR administration promotes peripheral nerve regeneration, restores motor function, and seems to have a direct analgesic role through modulating glutamatergic and cholinergic pathways (Flatters et al., 2006). Also, ALCAR is involved in the acetylation of tubulin (Hershman et al., 2013) and ameliorates mitochondrial dysfunction (Xiao & Bennett, 2008), a feature more and more involved in the pathogenesis of PIPN.

Fundamental Studies

ALCAR was tested in various models of CIPN and all reports indicated it had a neuroprotective effect. Subcutaneous administration of 100 mg/kg b.w. ALCAR protected against paclitaxel-induced, cisplatin-induced, and vincristine-induced peripheral neuropathy in a study by Ghirardi et al., as assessed by mechanical paw withdrawal latencies. The authors also showed that ALCAR is efficient in restoring nerve function in rats with established CIPN (Ghirardi et al., 2005b). The same team assessed the effect of ALCAR on OIPN through both behavioral and neurophysiological tests and reached similar conclusions—ALCAR is effective in both preventing and reversing neuropathy (Ghirardi et al., 2005a). Some years later, it was shown that ALCAR inhibited mechanical allodynia and prevented mitochondrial deficits in rats treated with paclitaxel and oxaliplatin, suggesting that the main mechanism by which ALCAR is neuroprotective involves mitochondrial pathways (Huaien Zheng, Xiao, & Bennett, 2011).

Although the neuroprotective effects of ALCAR have been shown in all these models of CIPN, most of the fundamental studies focused on the relationship between paclitaxel neuropathy and ALCAR. Oral ALCAR supplementation (50 or 100 mg/kg b.w.) was administered in two rodent models to assess its effect on preventing and treating PIPN as assessed by behavioral tests; results indicated a role for ALCAR (both doses) in preventing PIPN, but only a small effect on already-established mechanical allodynia (Flatters et al., 2006). Two years later, members of the same team reported more in-depth assessments of ALCAR's effect on PIPN—100 mg/kg b.w. ALCAR administered concurrently with paclitaxel completely prevented atypical C-fiber mitochondria formation and mechanical allodynia. However, ALCAR treatment did not significantly decrease intraepidermal nerve fiber reduction, Langerhans cell counts nor did it decrease the number of A-fiber atypical mitochondria (Jin, Flatters, Xiao, Mulhern, & Bennett, 2008).

More recently, based on the promising results obtained from other models of CIPN, ALCAR has been tested in BIPN. Supplementation with oral ALCAR (100 mg/mL/kg b.w.) throughout bortezomib therapy and 12 days after led to inhibition of mechanic allodynia and prevented mitochondrial dysfunction as assessed by mitochondrial respiration and ATP production, suggesting ALCAR's neuroprotective effect in this neuropathic model (Zheng, Xiao, & Bennett, 2012).

Clinical Studies

In the clinical setting, ALCAR was assessed both as a prophylactic and as a therapeutic agent. In 2005, the results of two small trials that administered ALCAR as treatment for cisplatin- and paclitaxel-induced neuropathy were published. Maestri et al. (2005) enrolled 26 patients that received ALCAR 1 g i.v. for 10 days and showed that 73% had at least a partial alleviation of symptoms and Bianchi et al. (2005) tested oral ALCAR (1 g twice daily for 8 weeks) in patients with grade 2–3 neuropathy and found that the treatment led to symptomatic relief in 92% of the patients (as assessed by the total neuropathy score) and to significantly improved sensory action potentials when compared to the baseline.

In 2013, the results of a large prospective randomized trial (409 patients) assessing oral ALCAR (3 g/day) supplementation for the prevention of PIPN in women undergoing adjuvant taxane-based breast cancer therapy became available. Twelve weeks after beginning anticancer treatment, there was no statistically significant difference in neuropathy incidence and severity between groups. Even more, after 24 weeks, the group receiving ALCAR had decreased functional status and an increased neuropathy incidence when compared with the placebo group—at this time point, 38% patients in the ALCAR group had more than a 10% decrease in neuropathy score (FACT–NTX score) compared with 28% in the placebo group (Hershman et al., 2013). After the outcome become public, the American Cancer Guidelines declared that using ALCAR as a preventive agent is strongly discouraged and there were no further trials assessing ALCAR as a therapeutic agent in treating PIPN.

Other chemotherapy agents in association with which ALCAR has been investigated include bortezomib—a small clinical trial (19 patients) was designed, based on the promising preclinical results obtained in this type of neuropathy. The results, however, showed that oral ALCAR supplementation (1.5 g twice daily) did not protect against neuropathy induced by the bortezomib and doxorubicin treatment (Callander et al., 2014).

Conclusions

ALCAR was widely investigated in CIPN. It is one of the few nutritional supplements that have been proposed both for prevention and as a treatment for CIPN. The available data suggest ALCAR could be harmful if administered as a preventive agent for CIPN (see the trial performed by Hershman et al.). The role of ALCAR in treating already-established neuropathy remains unclear due to little available of evidence. However, taking into account the clinical results obtained from the prevention study, to further study the potential role of ALCAR in treating CIPN could lead to harmful effects on the patients. In light of the information available, the American guidelines for CIPN are strongly against using ALCAR in CIPN prevention and state that ALCAR's role in CIPN treatment cannot be established at the moment (Hershman et al., 2014).

Omega-3 Fatty Acids

Theoretical Background—Why it Should Work

Omega-3 fatty acids are polyunsaturated fatty acids that are major structural components of the neuronal membrane phospholipids. It has been suggested that increased consumption of Omega-3 fatty acids can protect against cardiovascular diseases and overall morbidity and mortality and can have neuroprotective effects in both central and peripheral models of nerve injury (Ghoreishi et al., 2012). One of the proposed mechanisms for Omega-3 neuroprotection is its antiinflammatory effect—the Omega-6/Omega-3 fatty acid ratio is considered a marker of inflammatory stress and can be decreased by increasing Omega-3 supplementation (Coppey, Davidson, Obrosov, & Yorek, 2015). Omega-3 fatty acids stimulate neuritis growth and modulate voltage-dependent sodium currents (Lauretani et al., 2007), both of which are mechanisms currently involved in the pathogenesis of CIPN. Also, linoleic acid plasma levels, one of the three Omega-3 fatty acids, were shown to correlate with peroneal nerve conduction velocity in an elderly population (Lauretani et al., 2007).

Omega-3 fatty acids have been investigated in diabetic neuropathy, with good outcomes in both preclinical and clinical studies. Menhaden oil, a natural source of Omega-3 fatty acids, was shown to both prevent and treat diabetic neuropathy in diabetic rats (Coppey et al., 2015). In humans, type 2 diabetic patients that received eicosapentaenoic acid (a type of Omega-2 fatty acid) experienced an improvement in their peripheral neuropathy, as well as in other diabetic complications, such as nephropathy and macroangiopathy (Okuda et al., 1996).

Fundamental Studies

In the preclinical setting, resolvin E1, a compound derived from Omega-3 fatty acids has been tested in a model of chronic constriction injury. Intrathecal resolvin administration 3 days prior to sciatic nerve ligation significantly reduced mechanical allodynia in rats. The same group assessed resolvin's effect as a therapeutic agent—rats with established neuropathy showed an alleviation of both mechanical allodynia and heat hyperalgesia after resolvin intrathecal administration (Xu, Berta, & Ji, 2013). Alpha-lipoic acid, an Omega-3 fatty acid, exhibited dose-dependent neuroprotective effects in rats with VIPN with both mechanical and cold allodynia partly reversed after the drug's intraperitoneal administration (Kahng, Kim, Chung, Kim, & Moon, 2015).

Clinical Studies

A case series was reported in 2010, where five patients with different types of established neuropathic pain (varying from cervical radiculopathy to burn injury) were treated with high oral doses of Omega 3 fish oil (2.4–7.2 g/day). Results indicated a significant improvement in function and a decrease in pain intensity as assessed by different patient-reported outcome scales, objective neurological tests, and nerve conduction studies (Ko, Nowacki, Arseneau, Eitel, & Hum, 2010). Two years later, the results of a double-blind RCT that enrolled 69 breast cancer patients about to receive paclitaxel were published. Omega-3 fatty acid supplementation (640 mg 3 times daily during chemotherapy up until 1 month after the end of treatment) was associated with a lower PIPN incidence (30% vs. 59.3%) and with a nonsignificant decrease in PIPN severity when compared with the placebo (Ghoreishi et al., 2012). Another study enrolled 92 lung cancer patients with advanced nonsmall cell lung cancer and each randomly received either eicosapentaenoic acid supplementation (obtained from an oral nutritional supplement) or a placebo during chemotherapy. Results were also in favor of dietary supplementation—the group that received eicosapentaenoic acid had a decreased incidence of neuropathy, fatigue, and loss of appetite, with no difference in overall survival or response rates (Sánchez-Lara et al., 2014).

Subsequently, a National Cancer Institute registered trial was designed and began recruiting in 2013 in order to determine if Omega-3 fatty acids can treat pain in patients with breast or ovarian cancer receiving paclitaxel. Primary data will most likely be available in June 2016 (NCI-Supported Clinical Trials, n.d.).

Conclusions

Omega-3 fatty acid supplementation has so far been reported as effective in PIPN. However, the available clinical data come from a small number of patients from two differently-designed clinical trials. From past experience, several other potential neuroprotective agents have been reported as beneficial in small trials and were shown to be inefficient in larger population samples. The results of the ongoing study should contribute to determining the benefits of Omega-3 fatty acid supplementation in PIPN. In light of the information available, the American guidelines for CIPN state that currently no conclusion can be drawn in the matter of Omega-3 fatty acids and their efficacy in PIPN (Hershman et al., 2014).

Alpha-Lipoic Acid

Theoretical Background—Why it Should Work

Alpha-lipoic acid (ALA) is essential to the cell energy metabolism through its role in the Krebs cycle. It has antioxidant effects by reducing free radical formation and increasing the activity of glutathione peroxidase (Melli et al., 2008). Reports indicate that ALA normalizes endoneural blood flow, improves vascular dysfunction (Gedlicka, Scheithauer, Schüll, & Kornek, 2002), plays a part in calcium homeostasis, and protects mitochondria (Melli et al., 2008).

ALA exerted neuroprotective effects in both fundamental and clinical studies of diabetic neuropathy. A metaanalysis published in 2012 concluded that i.v. ALA (600 mg/day) for 3 weeks is associated with a significant alleviation of neuropathic pain in diabetic patients and that the evidence available is enough to issue a grade A recommendation (Mijnhout, Kollen, Alkhalaf, Kleefstra, & Bilo, 2012). Also, adding ALA (600 mg/day for 60 days) and superoxide dismutase (SOD) treatment to physiotherapy was associated with a better outcome than physiotherapy alone in patients with chronic neck pain (Letizia Mauro, Cataldo, Barbera, & Sanfilippo, 2014). Similar results were obtained in patients with chronic lower back pain—whereas almost 75% of the 98 patients enrolled used analgesics at the beginning of the trial, only 8% still required them after ALA/SOD supplementation (Battisti, Albanese, Guerra, Argnani, & Giordano, 2013).

Fundamental Studies

In vitro, ALA significantly protected against DRG changes induced by both paclitaxel and cisplatin (Melli et al., 2008). Subsequently, ALA was shown to have an inhibitory effect on several cancer cell lines and to enhance paclitaxel's cytotoxic effect on breast cancer cells (Li, Hao, Ren, & Gong, 2015) and fluorouracil's effect on colon cancer cells in vitro (Damnjanovic et al., 2014), suggesting it is not only a neuroprotective agent, but also a potential anticancer adjuvant.

The effect of ALA was assessed in an animal model of cisplatin-induced neuropathy. The authors concluded that ALA supplementation (100 mg/kg/day) during cisplatin treatment reversed electrophysiological changes induced by chemotherapy (Tuncer, Dalkilic, Akif Dunbar, & Keles, 2010). An association between ALA and monosodium glutamate was shown to be effective in a rat model of CisIPN as assessed by behavioral testing, nerve conduction velocity tests and biochemical assessment of oxidative status (Bhadri, Sanji, Madakasira Guggilla, & Razdan, 2013).

ALA was assessed in the treatment of VIPN—a study published as early as 1983 showed that ALA supplementation reduced vincristine toxicity without impacting the drug's efficacy (Berger, Habs, & Schmähl, 1983). A more recent paper assessed ALA's role as a therapeutic agent. In this study, rats were injected with vincristine and assessed for the presence of mechanical allodynia. Those that exhibited neuropathic symptoms were then treated with single-dose ALA (1, 5, or 10 mg/kg b.w.). The authors found that ALA reduced allodynia in a dose-dependent manner in which the duration of the effect was greatest when the single dose administered was the 10 mg dose (Kahng et al., 2015).

Clinical Studies

ALA was first used in the treatment of CIPN. In 2002, the results of a small study were published—15 patients that were diagnosed with at least grade 2 peripheral neuropathy after oxaliplatin chemotherapy received i.v. ALA 600 mg weekly (from 3 to 5 weeks) followed by oral administration (600 mg 3 times daily) for 6 months or until recovery. Eight of the patients responded to ALA treatment as assessed by patient reported outcomes, suggesting a potential therapeutic effect of this supplement (Gedlicka et al., 2002). One year after, the same research department published the results of another small clinical study investigating the effect of ALA (same administration schedule) in patients with established neuropathy secondary to the docetaxel–cisplatin treatment. ALA proved to be effective as a therapeutic agent, reducing the intensity of symptoms in 8 of the 14 enrolled patients (Gedlicka, Kornek, Schmid, & Scheithauer, 2003).

A recent prospective trial enrolled patients about to receive platinum-based chemotherapy and randomized them to receive either ALA 600 mg/3e times daily or a placebo for 24 weeks. The treatment was interrupted 2 days before up until 4 days after delivery of each dose of platinum in order to avoid ALA-cisplatin/oxaliplatin interactions. Although the planned enrollment included over 200 patients, only 72 completed the 24 week schedule mostly due to consent withdrawal. The high rates of attrition were attributed to the large number of pills that participants were supposed to take (6 pills/day) and due to the large duration of the study. The authors found no significant differences in neuropathy as assessed by patient-reported outcomes between the two groups (Guo et al., 2014).

Conclusions

The study by Guo et al., did not reach its primary endpoint and the data available from the 72 patients did not give this study enough power to perform a conclusive statistical analysis. However, it suggests that ALA does not prevent CIPN. All other clinical and most of the preclinical data, however, suggest the supplement's main benefit is in treating already-established neuropathy and not in preventing it. A trial assessing ALA's benefits in chronic platinum neuropathy is needed to determine if this agent is beneficial. Due to the fact that the trial performed by Guo et al., was published in 2014, it was not included in the latest version of the American CIPN guidelines (Hershman et al., 2014).

Glutathione

Theoretical Background—Why it Should Work

Glutathione (GSH) is an important scavenger with an essential role in the body's defense against oxidative damage (Leal et al., 2014). It can circle between its oxidized and reduced forms with the help of NADPH and the ratio between these two GSH forms is a measure of the cell's redox status (Pastore et al., 2001). Furthermore, it has a high affinity for heavy metals, which is why it was hypothesized it may act as a protective agent in platinum-induced neuropathy (Avan et al., 2015). One other argument in favor of the neuroprotective role of GSH came from studies performed in other types of neuropathy—using these supplements yielded favorable outcomes in optic (Ghelli et al., 2008) and diabetic (Ueno et al., 2002) neuropathy.

Fundamental Studies

GSH is among the first agents investigated in CIPN management—a clinical trial from 1990's that investigated GSH's role in preventing cisplatin-induced renal toxicity reported that patients with GSH supplementation seemed to exhibit less neuropathic symptoms. Subsequently, a Dutch team investigated the potential effect of GSH in a rat model of CisIPN and reported positive outcomes as assessed by nerve conduction velocity tests (Hamers et al., 1993). Their results were confirmed by another animal study 1 year later—the authors found that GSH not only improves nerve conduction velocity, but also partly reverses morphological changes induced by cisplatin (Tredici et al., 1994).

Clinical Studies

There are numerous small clinical studies that reported the effects of GSH supplementation in different types of CIPN. GSH was first investigated in cisplatin neuropathy—in 1992 the results of a randomized trial that enrolled 33 relapsed ovarian cancer patients indicated that the GSH-supplementation group had a significantly decreased incidence of neuropathy when compared with the other groups (Bogliun, Marzorati, Cavaletti, & Frattola, 1992). GSH supplementation (2.5 g/week i.v. or 1.5 g/m^2 before administration followed by 600 mg i.m. in days 2–5 after chemotherapy) was associated with positive outcomes in patients treated with weekly cisplatin (Cascinu, Cordella, Del Ferro, Fronzoni, & Catalano, 1995; Colombo et al., 1995), cisplatin every 3 weeks (GSH supplementation 2.5 or 3 g/m^2 before each chemotherapy cycle) (Bogliun et al., 1996; Smyth et al., 1997) or an association of cisplatin–cyclophosphamide (Pirovano et al., 1992). Not all trials were positive—1 trial that enrolled 20 patients treated with cisplatin-etoposide or cisplatin-fluorouracil found that GSH supplementation (5 g GSH every 4 weeks) does not significantly improve the incidence or severity of neuropathy (Schmidinger et al., 2000).

GSH has also been investigated as a prophylactic agent in oxaliplatin neurotoxicity. In 2002, a randomized prospective study that enrolled 52 patients randomly received a placebo or GSH (1.5 g/m^2) before each oxaliplatin administration reported that GSH supplementation maintained normal nerve conduction during chemotherapy and was associated with a decrease in all-grade neurotoxicity incidence (Cascinu et al., 2002). Subsequently, the results of two other studies also identified a benefit for GSH supplementation in terms of neuroprotection. One was performed in an Asian population and assessed both GSH and calcium–magnesium (Ca/Mg) infusions compared with the placebo (Takimoto et al., 2008). The other was conducted by an Italian team and enrolled 27 patients receiving adjuvant chemotherapy that were assessed by means of platinum-DNA adduct formation, platinum pharmacokinetics, and neurotoxicity. The results showed that GSH supplementation significantly reduced the neuropathic side effect without affecting the formation pf platinum-DNA adducts (Milla et al., 2009). Not all published trials were positive—one assessed Ca/Mg versus GSH versus placebo in 93 oxaliplatin-treated patients and found that neither Ca/Mg nor GSH is superior to control in terms of acute and chronic neuropathy (Dong, Xing, Liu, Feng, & Shi, 2010).

In the light of favorable outcomes reported from previous trial, the NCCTG N08CA prospective multicenter study was designed to assess the effect of GSH on CIPN. Patients scheduled to receive chemotherapy with carboplatin and paclitaxel were randomized to receive either GSH 1.5 g/m^2 i.v. or a placebo 15 min before each chemotherapy cycle. Data obtained from 195 enrolled patients with a median follow-up of over 300 days indicated that GSH administration does not protect against acute and chronic CIPN as assessed by patient-reported outcomes and by the common toxicity criteria (Leal et al., 2014).

Conclusions

GSH supplementation had no effect in the trial performed by Leal et al., most likely because the chemotherapy regimen was based on paclitaxel and carboplatin and not oxaliplatin or cisplatin, with which all of the other previous studies had been performed. Evidence demonstrating that GSH has no effect in PIPN is conclusive. However, almost all studies in which GSH was administered for the prevention of OIPN or CisIPN had positive outcomes, even though they were all small studies. We need trials with a design similar to that performed by Leal et al., to assess if GSH can have a neuroprotective effect in these other two types of neuropathies (OIPN and CisIPN).

In light of the information available, the American guidelines for CIPN are moderately against using GSH in neuropathy secondary to carboplatin–paclitaxel treatment, but state that currently no conclusion can be drawn in the matter of GSH and its efficacy in OIPN and CisIPN (Hershman et al., 2014).

Glutamate and Glutamine

Theoretical Background—Why it Should Work

Glutamine is a major tissue component of the skeletal muscle, representing up to 60% of the total free amino acid pool. Although it is the most abundant nonessential amino-acid in the blood, during stress states, such as cancer/chemotherapy/radiotherapy, its consumption exceeds its synthesis and glutamine becomes a conditionally essential amino-acid (Gaurav, Goel, Shukla, & Pandey, 2012). After dietary uptake in the small intestine, glutamine is exported from skeletal muscle and lung in the nervous system (it can cross the blood–brain barrier) and is converted in glutamate (glutamic acid). Glutamate, a precursor of gamma-aminobutyric acid (GABA acid) is a neurotransmitter essential to the central and peripheral nervous system. After the neurons release glutamate in the synapse, astrocytes transport glutamate, and metabolize it once again in glutamine, as part of the glutamine–glutamate cycle (Vahdat et al., 2001).

Assessing glutamate/glutamine in CIPN is supported by several potential mechanisms. On the one hand, the decreased levels of glutamate observed in cancer patients during cancer treatment may be responsible for tissue damage and tissue malfunction (which affects the peripheral nervous system). On the other hand, glutamate is a precursor of GABA and the GABA neurotransmitter system is significantly involved in the pathogenesis of CIPN; it has been hypothesized that high systemic levels of glutamine may down regulate the conversion of glutamine to an excitatory neuropeptide, glutamate (Wang et al., 2007). Last, but not the least, glutamine upregulates NGF mRNA and NGF levels are known to decrease during chemotherapy (Vahdat et al., 2001).

Fundamental Studies

Glutamine has been one of the first dietary supplements investigated in cancer patients. Animal studies assessing the benefit of adding glutamate/glutamine to chemotherapy treatment have been performed as early as the 1980s. A study published in 1996 indicated that oral glutamate supplementation (500 mg/kg/day) during vincristine chemotherapy significantly improved motor and sensory behavioral signs of peripheral neuropathy without interfering with the antineoplastic drug's efficacy (Boyle, Wheeler, & Shenfield, 1996). Three years later, the same team investigated the effect of glutamate on Cisplatin-induced and paclitaxel-induced neuropathy and found that glutamate has neuroprotective effects for both animal models and does not interfere with the two drugs' cytotoxic effect (Boyle, Wheeler, & Shenfield, 1999). More recently, different combinations of monosodium glutamate with either resveratrol, alpha-lipoic acid, or coenzyme Q_{10} were assessed in a rat model of cisplatin-induced neuropathy. Results indicated that all combinations partly reversed behavioral, electrophysiological, and biochemical changes induced by cisplatin. However, the most effective combination was deemed to be the one between glutamate and resveratrol (Bhadri et al., 2013).

Clinical Studies

Glutamic acid supplementation (1.5 g 3 times daily during chemotherapy) was shown to decrease the incidence of chemotherapy dose-modifications in breast cancer patients receiving vincristine in the adjuvant setting (Jackson et al., 1984). Subsequently, the same group designed a prospective trial that included 84 patients assigned to receive vincristine and randomized to glutamic acid supplementation (0.5 g thrice daily during chemotherapy) or control. Results showed that the incidence of moderate paresthesias was almost two times lower in the glutamic acid group (Jackson et al., 1988). As the use of vincristine in adult cancer therapy decreased, clinical trials involving this drug were performed in pediatric patients—a prospective randomized pilot study from 2010 assessed the effect of glutamic acid (1.5 g thrice daily during chemotherapy) in a 54 pediatric patients and found that supplementation with glutamate led to a significant delay to the onset of neurotoxicity (Mokhtar, Shaaban, Elbarbary, & Fayed, 2010). In 2015, the results of a larger prospective trial that included pediatric cancer patients were published. The authors found that glutamic acid supplementation (250 mg/m^2 thrice daily starting before chemotherapy and until 7 days after the last cycle) provided no benefit regarding neuropathy incidence, severity, or onset. There was a trend toward a statistically significant difference in children aged 13 or older that indicated a potential neuroprotective effect of glutamic acid, but the study was not powered to correctly detect that difference (Bradfield, Sandler, Geller, Tamura, & Krischer, 2015).

In a study on stage IV breast cancer patients receiving very large doses of paclitaxel (825 mg/m^2) with G-CSF and stem cell support, oral glutamine supplementation (10 g thrice daily for 4 days after paclitaxel administration) led to fewer neuropathic signs and symptoms when compared with the control although nerve conduction studies revealed no significant differences between the two groups (Vahdat et al., 2001). A subsequent nonrandomized small study performed by members of the same team enrolled similar patients that received high-dose Paclitaxel (825 mg/m^2) and found that glutamine supplementation was associated with a decrease in weakness, numbness, and loss of vibratory perception. The authors also assessed motor and sensory nerve action potentials and found that chemotherapy-induced changes were less important in the glutamine-treated group, but this result was not significant from a statistical point of view (Stubblefield et al., 2005).

After the reported outcome of these two trials, a multicenter prospective RCT was designed. Women with ovarian cancer assigned to receive paclitaxel (175 mg/m^2) and carboplatin (AUC = 6) therapy were randomized to receive oral supplementation with either glutamate (500 mg thrice daily) or placebo starting from the first day of chemotherapy until week three after the 6th cycle. There were 43 patients available for analysis; results indicated that although glutamate supplementation led to a decrease in the severity score for neuropathic symptoms, electro-diagnostic assessment showed no difference in the two groups (Loven et al., 2009).

Glutamine has also been evaluated for preventing neuropathy induced by platinum cytotoxic drugs. Wang et al. (2007) published the results of a pilot study that enrolled 86 colorectal cancer patients that started oxaliplatin-based chemotherapy and randomized them to receive oral glutamine supplementation (15 g twice a day for 7 consecutive days every 2 weeks starting on the day of oxaliplatin infusion) or not. Patients were assessed for neuropathy by means of neurologic examination and in some cases electrophysiological testing at baseline and every two cycles until the 6th cycle. The authors found that glutamine supplementation significantly reduced the incidence and severity of oxaliplatin-induced neuropathy for all grades of neuropathy, but it did not protect against nerve deterioration assessed by electrophysiological testing. Patients in the glutamine-treated group required modifications less often as compared to those in the oxaliplatin-alone group and had similar survival and response rates when compared with the control group (Wang et al., 2007). Another small-randomized prospective study compared i.v. glutamine administration with Ca/Mg supplementation and found that glutamine reduced the severity of symptomatic platinum-induced neuropathy (Huang et al., 2015).

Conclusions

Although glutamate (glutamic acid) has shown neuroprotective effects in different animal models, its efficacy was not clearly demonstrated in clinical trials assessing VIPN. The studies available for adult cancer patients are outdated and involve a small number of patients, whereas those in pediatric cancer patients have had contradictory results. However, since all studies agree that supplementation with glutamate does not interfere with chemotherapy efficacy or with response rates, other clinical trials should be designed to assess its effect.

Regarding the effect of glutamate/glutamine on PIPN, the existing clinical studies enrolled a small number of patients and had significant differences in methodology. While the study performed by Loven et al., used glutamate supplementation, the other two studies administered oral glutamine supplements. Although related, the two amino-acids are not identical in terms of absorption, pharmacokinetics, and distribution. Other potential confounders that might explain the difference between the first two studies and the third include dose and duration of glutamine/glutamate supplementation, other chemotherapy drugs used with paclitaxel, the small number of patients enrolled and different methods performed at different time points for CIPN assessment. In our opinion, the role of glutamate/glutamine in PIPN has not yet been established.

Regarding platinum agents, current available clinical trials, indicate that glutamine is effective in reducing oxaliplatin-induced neuropathy. However, the same issue of insufficient data applies here as well. American guidelines do not currently recommend glutamate/glutamine supplementation due to the low level of evidence available, although they state that the trials performed so far have shown some benefit in some measures of neuropathy (Hershman et al., 2014).

MINERALS AND TRACE ELEMENTS

Ca and Mg Infusions

Theoretical Background—Why it Should Work

Calcium (Ca) homeostasis dysregulations are frequently incriminated in the pathogenesis of CIPN. Although several chemotherapy agents induce Ca alterations, oxaliplatin is best-researched due to its metabolite, oxalate, that specifically chelates both Ca and magnesium (Mg) ions, a fact that significantly appears to contribute to oxaliplatin-induced neuropathy (Weickhardt, Wells, & Messersmith, 2011). Mg ions block the NMDA receptor, which is as well involved in CIPN and other types of chronic pain. In this setting, Ca/Mg infusions were suggested as potential protectors against CIPN—the theoretical background was that the Ca and Mg ions would bind the oxalate and prevent its chelative effect (Weickhardt et al., 2011), influencing the NMDA receptor and increasing extracellular calcium, which in turn would stimulate sodium channel closing, thus decreasing hyperexcitability (Wolf, Barton, Kottschade, Grothey, & Loprinzi, 2008).

Fundamental Studies

In PC12 cells, oxaliplatin and oxalate suppressed neurite outgrowth due to their neurotoxicity, an effect that was attenuated by Ca/Mg addition (Takeshita et al., 2011). In animal models, oxalate was shown to induce significant cold allodynia, a behavioral change that was completely prevented by Ca/Mg administration (Sakurai et al., 2009).

Clinical Studies

The effectiveness of Ca/Mg administration in preventing CIPN has been a continuous subject of debate for over 10 years. Gamelin (2004) retrospectively assessed the efficacy of Ca/Mg administration in preventing acute and chronic neuropathy in colon cancer patients that were treated in the second line with oxaliplatin-based chemotherapy; a part of these patients received 1 g calcium gluconate and 1 g magnesium sulfate before and after oxaliplatin infusion (subsequent clinical trials used similar doses). The results indicated that Ca/Mg infusion was associated with a significant benefit in terms of decreasing the incidence of acute neuropathic symptoms, grade 3 paresthesia and chronic neuropathy (Gamelin, 2004). This conclusion led to the approval of several prospective randomized trials, all of which used the same dose for the Ca/Mg infusion.

The CONcePT trial was designed to evaluate two strategies for decreasing oxaliplatin-induced neuropathy: the impact of intermittent versus continuous oxaliplatin administration and the effect of Ca/Mg infusion. After 174 patients had been included, the trial was prematurely discontinued due to an independent assessment that suggested lower response rates for patients that received Ca/Mg (Hochster, Grothey, & Childs, 2007). A subsequent independent analysis did not confirm this observation (Grothey et al., 2008). Data analysis for the already-enrolled patients indicated a slight nonstatistically significant benefit for the Ca/Mg arm (Hochster et al., 2014). Subsequent studies explained this negative result as a consequence of its early closure and insufficient statistical power.

After the safety concerns raised by the CONcePT trial became public, several other prospective trials with similar designs enrolling at the time were prematurely closed (Chay et al., 2010; Grothey et al., 2011; Ishibashi, Okada, Miyazaki, Sano, & Ishida, 2010). Two of them were performed in Asian populations; analysis of data already available showed no statistically significant difference between the two study arms. The third was the NCCTG N04C7 trial that was supposed to enroll 300 patients, but had only 102 patients included when the safety concerns were issued. Results indicated a significant effect of Ca/Mg on neuropathy—the incidence of grade 2 or higher neurotoxicity was reduced (22% vs. 41% in the placebo group) and the time to first neuropathic symptoms was increased (Grothey et al., 2011). The results of this study were not accepted by all the members of the scientific community, especially because neuropathy assessment was performed by subjective measures and there was no long-term data available (Park et al., 2011).

Other available data at the time included a retrospective analysis of more than 750 patients that reported favorable outcomes from Ca/Mg supplementation in preventing OIPN (Knijn et al., 2011), the preliminary results of the French NEUROXA trial (which also indicated that Ca/Mg supplementation is beneficial) (Gamelin et al., 2008, and the results of two small studies which reported no significant difference between Ca/Mg infusion and placebo (Dong et al., 2010; Han, Khwaounjoo, Kilfoyle, Hill, & McKeage, 2013).

To address these conflicting data, a large placebo-controlled multicenter randomized trial (NCCTG N08CB) was designed. The trial included over 350 colon cancer patients undergoing oxaliplatin-based adjuvant chemotherapy that were randomized to receive either (1) Ca/Mg infusions before and after chemotherapy, (2) Ca/Mg infusion before chemotherapy and placebo after chemotherapy, or (3) placebo before and after chemotherapy. The study failed to identify a benefit for Ca/Mg treatment in terms of acute/chronic neuropathy incidence or intensity of symptoms (Loprinzi et al., 2014).

Conclusions

There have been numerous trials designed to unequivocally determine the benefit of Ca/Mg infusions in preventing OIPN. The NCCTG N08CB trial was well designed and included a large number of patients. Its results are a convincing argument that i.v. Ca/Mg supplementation is not effective in preventing OIPN. In light of these data, the American Society of Clinical Oncology's guidelines are "moderately against" Ca/Mg administration for the prevention of CIPN and conclude that this treatment is associated with little benefit, but also with little harm (Hershman et al., 2014).

Selenium

Theoretical Background—Why it Should Work

Selenium is an essential trace element vital for the CNS and found in over 25 human proteins (selenoproteins) involved in antioxidant and immune defense. Studies show that selenium administration protects against oxidative stress and excessive cytosolic calcium release (Uğuz & Nazıroğlu, 2012), enhances antioxidant status, reduced proapoptotic signaling, stimulates the activity of GSH peroxidase (Santamaría et al., 2005), and protects mitochondria from chronic stress (Wojewoda, Duszyński, Więckowski, & Szczepanowska, 2012). Coadministration of selenium and amyloid β-peptide indicated a significant neuroprotective effect of the trace element in an in vitro model of Alzheimer's disease (Godoi et al., 2013).

Fundamental Studies

Regarding its potential effects in preventing neuropathy, sodium selenite improved nerve conduction velocity in an animal model of diabetic neuropathy (Murat & Hulagu, 2011). Selol, a selenium-based mixture synthesized from sunflower oil was shown to have moderate neuroprotective effects on its own and significantly improve the effects of opioids in a model of VIPN (Bujalska & Gumułka, 2008). A preliminary animal study found that repeated selenium administration partly reverses electrophysiological and histopathological changes induced by cisplatin (Erken et al., 2014).

Clinical Studies

In the clinical setting, the results of a small study on 48 patients with radiation-associated lymphedema that received from 4 to 6 weeks of selenium supplementation indicated that the treatment is well tolerated and beneficial in terms of toxicity (Micke et al., 2003). Another study on 31 ovarian cancer patients indicated that selenium supplementation (200 μg/day) is associated with a significant decrease in different types of chemotherapy side effects—from hair loss to weakness, abdominal pain, and loss of appetite (Sieja & Talerczyk, 2004).

Conclusions

So far, there are no clinical studies powered for assessing the effect of selenium in CIPN. However, taking into account the fact that it has been explored both as a coanalgesic and as a protective agent, further studies would be of use for exploring the benefits of selenium supplementation in different types of cancer pain. In light of the very little information available, the American guidelines for CIPN do not discuss selenium prophylaxis/treatment in their CIPN guidelines (Hershman et al., 2014).

Lithium

Theoretical Background—Why it Should Work

Lithium has been an essential part of treatment in bipolar disorders for the past 50 years. More recently, it has been investigated as a neuroprotective agent in several neurodegenerative disorders, such as Alzheimer's disease, ischemic brain injury, Huntington's and Parkinson's disease (Luo, 2010). Although its mechanism of action is still a matter of controversy, studies indicate it is a specific inhibitor of GSK-3β (Huang et al., 2014), thus stimulating axonal regeneration in peripheral nerves. Also, lithium promotes the activity of some antiapoptotic proteins while inhibiting the activation of proapoptotic signaling (Aminzadeh, Dehpour, Safa, Mirzamohammadi, & Sharifi, 2014) and influences the synthesis and release of several neurotransmitters, such as serotonin, dopamine, and norepinephrine (Bhalla, Garg, & Dhawan, 2010).

Excessive lithium administration has neurotoxic effects—in bipolar patients this can be encountered due to lithium's narrow therapeutic index. Lithium neurotoxicity can be either acute or chronic and induces drowsiness, slurred speech, apathy, confusion, ataxia, tremor, dysarthria, and even dementia (Ivkovic & Stern, 2014).

Fundamental Studies

Lithium was first investigated in VIPN. A study published in 1999 indicated that lithium (12.8 mg/kg b.w. daily throughout chemotherapy) alleviated behavioral changes induced by vincristine in mice as assessed by hot plate and balance tests (Petrini et al., 1999). A more comprehensive study was performed some years later in which not only behavioral, but also histopathological and electrophysiological studies were used. Lithium was shown to reduce all types of vincristine-induced neuropathic changes (Alimoradi et al., 2012).

Oral lithium (300 mg/L) supplementation through drinking water was shown to significantly protect against paclitaxel-induced neuropathy in rats. Lithium partly reversed electrophysiological, histopathological and behavioral changes (as assessed by nerve conduction velocity studies, light microscopy examination of the sciatic nerve, hot plate, and spontaneous exploratory activity) (Pourmohammadi et al., 2012). One other study showed that single-dose lithium administration (12.8 mg/kg b.w.) before each paclitaxel dose prevented peripheral neuropathy and neuronal calcium sensor 1 degradation whilst maintaining adequate neuronal calcium signaling (Mo, Erdelyi, Szigeti-Buck, Benbow, & Ehrlich, 2012). A different dose of lithium (2 mM/kg) administered in rats undergoing paclitaxel treatment had a similar beneficial outcome; the authors demonstrated that lithium exerts its neuroprotective effect through regulating GSK3β signaling, suppression of glial activation, and of proinflammatory cytokines (Gao, Yan, & Weng, 2013).

Clinical Studies

The same team that performed among the first assessments of lithium's efficacy in VIPN also performed the only clinical trial currently published, to our knowledge in which 10 patients undergoing vincristine-based chemotherapy for different types of lymphoproliferative disorders that had developed significant neuropathy received lithium salts (600 mg/day) and subsequently eight patients reported partial alleviation of symptoms, one patient reported complete recovery and one patient had no improvement (Petrini et al., 1999).

Currently, one trial supported by the National Cancer Institute aims to study the effect of lithium on memory in small-cell lung cancer patients receiving prophylactic cranial irradiation (NCI-Supported Clinical Trials, n.d.).

Conclusions

There is an excellent theoretic background supporting lithium's effect in PIPN and VIPN. However, the only clinical trial currently assessing lithium's role in cancer therapy is not powered to detect any benefits of this metal in CIPN. Taking into account the very little information available, the American guidelines for CIPN do not discuss lithium prophylaxis/treatment in their CIPN guidelines (Hershman et al., 2014).

SPECIFIC TYPES OF DIETS

Polyamine-Reduced Diet

Theoretical Background—Why it Should Work

Changes in NMDA-receptors are known to play an essential part in different types of painful neuropathies. In 2011, Mihara et al., demonstrated, that these receptors are also involved in CIPN–NMDA receptor agonists completely reversed OIPN (Mihara et al., 2011). However, in the clinical setting, treatment with NMDA-receptor agonists is limited by side effects. NMDA-receptors are modulated by several endogenous molecules, including polyamines (Berger, Bitar, Waitner, Rebernik, & O'Sullivan, 2006) that have a specific recognition site in the NMDA-receptor complex. Polyamines are biogenic amines that positively modulate the NMDA-receptor system, thus contributing to pain sensitization (Simonnet, Laboureyras, & Sergheraert, 2013). The main sources of polyamines are diet and bacterial metabolism in the gut (Rivat et al., 2008). Based on these data, it was hypothesized that a polyamine-deficient diet (PDD) would protect against OIPN.

Animal Studies

Rivat et al. (2008) tested the effects of a PDD in different types of rat pain models that included a neuropathic pain model (chronic constrictive injury of the sciatic). In rats with established neuropathy, following the PDD progressively decreased pain hypersensitivity and increased the analgesic effect of a small dose of morphine (Rivat et al., 2008). A more recent study assessed the potential prophylactic effects of PDD in an animal model of OIPN. PDD was initiated 7 days prior to single-dose chemotherapy administration. Throughout the experiment, rats on PPD showed no difference in sensibility to mechanical and cold stimuli when compared with the control group (no chemotherapy). Rats that followed a normal diet showed a significant decrease in terms of paw withdrawal thresholds after exposure to cold or mechanical stimuli (Ferrier et al., 2013).

Clinical Trials

In 2013, a randomized clinical trial assessed the effects of 12-day PDD on surgery-related pain. Patients undergoing laminectomy were assigned to total or partial PPD. Results indicated that patients receiving total PPD had decreased pain and an increased quality of life (Estebe et al., 2013). Currently, there is one on-going clinical trial (NEUROXAPOL) that aims to assess the effects of PPD on OIPN in cancer patients that receive the FOLFOX4 chemotherapy protocol. The study should enroll 80 patients. It is a prospective, single-center interventional study that has started in January 2013 and is expected to end in June 2016 (Balayssac et al., 2015).

Conclusions

Modulating pain by dietary interventions has emerged as an attractive possibility in the last years. Promising results have so far been reported from different types of chronic pain that most often have a neuropathic component as well. From a theoretical point of view, modulating the NMDA receptor without notable side effects is a safe and long-lasting therapeutic option for patients in need of chronic treatment. Since the results of the NEUROXAPOL study will probably be available in the last part of 2016 or in early 2017, we will then have more information regarding the feasibility of transferring preclinical data for PDD in clinical studies.

Fasting and Dietary Restriction

Theoretical Background—Why it Should Work

Dietary restriction has been shown to lower the incidence of neurodegeneration, loss of function and even cancer. Prolonged fasting (PF) redistributes energy toward cellular maintenance and repair rather than cell division and down-regulates two important cellular pathways: the glucose-sensing Ras/adenylate cyclase/PKA pathway and the amino acid-sensing Tor/Sch9 (S6K) pathway (Cheng et al., 2014). PF depletes the body of glycogen and then forces it to use fat and ketone bodies. It decreases plasma levels of insulin-like growth factor-1 (IGF-1), an effect that was shown to be protective against chemotherapy toxicity in mice (Cheng et al., 2014). Also, caloric restriction enhances resistance to stress and decreases oxidative damage (Safdie et al., 2009) and protects normal cells only (and not cancer cells) against high chemotherapy doses.

Fundamental Studies

Mice that underwent PF for 48 h before repeated cyclophosphamide administration had a decreased mortality and a shorter hematologic recovery time when compared with mice that had ad libitum access to food (Cheng et al., 2014). Also, 60-h PF led to a better survival in mice receiving high-dose doxorubicin when compared to the control group (89% vs. 16%). Mice that underwent PF also showed no visible signs of toxicity, stress, or pain and there was no influence on chemotherapy's anticancer efficacy (Brandhorst, Wei, Hwang, Morgan, & Longo, 2013).

Clinical Studies

A phase I human study indicated that 72 h fasting before platinum-based chemotherapy was associated with a significantly higher lymphocyte count after two cycles (Cheng et al., 2014). One other study enrolled 10 patients with different types of solid tumors. All patients underwent several cycles of chemotherapy and for some or all of the cycles opted to fast for a variable period anywhere from 48 to 140 h prior to and/or 5–56 h following chemotherapy. Results indicated that most chemotherapy-related toxicities were significantly reduced when fasting prior to chemotherapy (Safdie et al., 2009). Currently, there are four National Cancer Institute-registered trials that assess the benefits of PF or caloric restriction on chemotherapy tolerance and response—one is designed to enroll patients receiving cisplatin-based chemotherapy and randomize them to different short-term starvation schedules before and after each chemotherapy cycle and another is designed for patients receiving taxanes (paclitaxel or docetaxel). These two aforementioned trials will most likely offer information about the incidence of CIPN in the two groups, although they are not specifically powered for this (NCI-Supported Clinical Trials, n.d.).

Conclusions

PF is the result of a novel approach toward CIPN instead of targeting the accumulation of platinum in the nervous system, the idea is to influence the body so that it itself protects the cells. This shift in paradigm is promising and could finally be the key for preventing CIPN in cancer patients.

GLOSSARY

ALA	Alpha-lipoic acid
ALCAR	Acetyl-L-carnitine
BBB	Blood–brain barrier
BIPN	Bortezomib-induced peripheral neuropathy
b.w.	Body weight
Ca	Calcium
CIPN	Chemotherapy-induced peripheral neuropathy
CisIPN	Cisplatin-induced peripheral neuropathy
DRG	Dorsal root ganglia
GABA	Gamma-aminobutyric acid
GSH	Glutathione
IGF-1	Insulin-like growth factor 1
Mg	Magnesium
NADPH	Nicotinamide adenine dinucleotide phosphate
NGF	Nerve growth factor
NMDA	*N*-methyl-D-aspartate
OIPN	Oxaliplatin-induced peripheral neuropathy
PDD	Polyamine-deficient diet
PF	Prolonged fasting
PIPN	Paclitaxel-induced peripheral neuropathy
RCT	Randomized controlled trial
ROS	Reactive oxygen species
TRP	Transient receptor potential
VIPN	Vincristine-induced peripheral neuropathy

References

Afonseca, S. O. de, Cruz, F. M., Cubero, D. de I. G., Lera, A. T., Schindler, F., Okawara, M., … Giglio, A. del. (2013). Vitamin E for prevention of oxaliplatin-induced peripheral neuropathy: a pilot randomized clinical trial. *São Paulo Medical Journal, Revista Paulista de Medicina, 131*(1), 35–38.

Akbayram, S., Akgun, C., Doğan, M., Sayin, R., Caksen, H., & Oner, A. F. (2010). Use of pyridoxine and pyridostigmine in children with vincristine-induced neuropathy. *Indian Journal of Pediatrics, 77*(6), 681–683.

Alessandri-Haber, N., Dina, O. A., Joseph, E. K., Reichling, D. B., & Levine, J. D. (2008). Interaction of transient receptor potential vanilloid 4, integrin, and SRC tyrosine kinase in mechanical hyperalgesia. *The Journal of Neuroscience: The Official Journal of the Society for Neuroscience, 28*(5), 1046–1057.

Alimoradi, H., Pourmohammadi, N., Mehr, S. E., Hassanzadeh, G., Hadian, M. R., Sharifzadeh, M., … Dehpour, A. R. (2012). Effects of lithium on peripheral neuropathy induced by vincristine in rats. *Acta Medica Iranica, 50*(6), 373–379.

Aminzadeh, A., Dehpour, A. R., Safa, M., Mirzamohammadi, S., & Sharifi, A. M. (2014). Investigating the protective effect of lithium against high glucose-induced neurotoxicity in PC12 cells: involvements of ROS, JNK and P38 MAPKs, and apoptotic mitochondria pathway. *Cellular and Molecular Neurobiology, 34*(8), 1143–1150.

Ananth, N., Shetty, B. V., & Vasudevan, D. M. (2003). Vitamin E levels during chemotherapy for ovarian carcinoma. *The National Medical Journal of India, 16*(4), 231–232.

André, N., Braguer, D., Brasseur, G., Gonçalves, A., Lemesle-Meunier, D., Guise, S., … Briand, C. (2000). Paclitaxel induces release of cytochrome c from mitochondria isolated from human neuroblastoma cells'. *Cancer Research, 60*(19), 5349–5353.

Ang, C. D., Alviar, M. J. M., Dans, A. L., Bautista-Velez, G. G. P., Villaruz-Sulit, M. V. C., Tan, J. J., … Roxas, A. A. (2008). Vitamin B for treating peripheral neuropathy. *The Cochrane Database of Systematic Reviews, 16*(3), CD004573.

Areti, A., Yerra, V. G., Naidu, V., & Kumar, A. (2014). Oxidative stress and nerve damage: role in chemotherapy induced peripheral neuropathy. *Redox Biology, 2*, 289–295.

Argyriou, A. A., Chroni, E., Koutras, A., Ellul, J., Papapetropoulos, S., Katsoulas, G., … Kalofonos, H. P. (2005). Vitamin E for prophylaxis against chemotherapy-induced neuropathy: a randomized controlled trial. *Neurology, 64*(1), 26–31.

Argyriou, A. A., Chroni, E., Koutras, A., Iconomou, G., Papapetropoulos, S., Polychronopoulos, P., & Kalofonos, H. P. (2006a). A randomized controlled trial evaluating the efficacy and safety of vitamin E supplementation for protection against cisplatin-induced peripheral neuropathy: final results. *Supportive Care in Cancer: Official Journal of the Multinational Association of Supportive Care in Cancer, 14*(11), 1134–1140.

Argyriou, A. A., Chroni, E., Koutras, A., Iconomou, G., Papapetropoulos, S., Polychronopoulos, P., & Kalofonos, H. P. (2006b). Preventing paclitaxel-induced peripheral neuropathy: a phase II trial of vitamin E supplementation. *Journal of Pain and Symptom Management, 32*(3), 237–244.

Argyriou, A. A., Bruna, J., Marmiroli, P., & Cavaletti, G. (2012). Chemotherapy-induced peripheral neurotoxicity (CIPN): an update. *Critical Reviews in Oncology/hematology, 82*(1), 51–77.

Arrieta, Ó., Hernández-Pedro, N., Fernández-González-Aragón, M. C., Saavedra-Pérez, D., Campos-Parra, A. D., Ríos-Trejo, M. Á., … Sotelo, J. (2011). Retinoic acid reduces chemotherapy-induced neuropathy in an animal model and patients with lung cancer. *Neurology, 77*(10), 987–995.

Avan, A., Postma, T. J., Ceresa, C., Avan, A., Cavaletti, G., Giovannetti, E., & Peters, G. J. (2015). Platinum-induced neurotoxicity and preventive strategies: past, present, and future. *The Oncologist, 20*(4), 411–432.

Balayssac, D., Ferrier, J., Pereira, B., Gillet, B., Pétorin, C., Vein, J., … Pezet, D. (2015). Prevention of oxaliplatin-induced peripheral neuropathy by a polyamine-reduced diet-NEUROXAPOL: protocol of a prospective, randomised, controlled, single-blind and monocentric trial. *BMJ Open, 5*(4), e007479.

Battisti, E., Albanese, A., Guerra, L., Argnani, L., & Giordano, N. (2013). Alpha lipoic acid and superoxide dismutase in the treatment of chronic low back pain. *European Journal of Physical and Rehabilitation Medicine*, *49*(5), 659–664.

Bay, A., Yilmaz, C., Yilmaz, N., & Oner, A. F. (2006). Vincristine induced cranial polyneuropathy. *The Indian Journal of Pediatrics*, *73*(6), 531–533.

Bell, R. F., Borzan, J., Kalso, E., & Simonnet, G. (2012). Food, pain, and drugs: does it matter what pain patients eat? *Pain*, *153*(10), 1993–1996.

Berger, M., Habs, M., & Schmähl, D. (1983). [Effect of thioctic acid (alpha-limpoic acid) on the chemotherapeutic efficacy of cyclophosphamide and vincristine sulfate]. *Arzneimittel-Forschung*, *33*(9), 1286–1288.

Berger, M. L., Bitar, A. Y., Waitner, M. J., Rebernik, P., & O'Sullivan, M. C. (2006). Polyamines and the NMDA receptor: modifying intrinsic activities with aromatic substituents. *Bioorganic and Medicinal Chemistry Letters*, *16*(11), 2837–2841.

Bhadri, N., Sanji, T., Madakasira Guggilla, H., & Razdan, R. (2013). Amelioration of behavioural, biochemical, and neurophysiological deficits by combination of monosodium glutamate with resveratrol/alpha-lipoic acid/coenzyme Q_{10} in rat model of cisplatin-induced peripheral neuropathy. *The Scientific World Journal*, *2013*, 565813.

Bhalla, P., Garg, M. L., & Dhawan, D. K. (2010). Protective role of lithium during aluminium-induced neurotoxicity. *Neurochemistry International*, *56*(2), 256–262.

Bianchi, G., Vitali, G., Caraceni, A., Ravaglia, S., Capri, G., Cundari, S., … Gianni, L. (2005). Symptomatic and neurophysiological responses of paclitaxel- or cisplatin-induced neuropathy to oral acetyl-L-carnitine. *European Journal of Cancer* (*Oxford, England: 1990*), *41*(12), 1746-1750.

Boehmerle, W., Zhang, K., Sivula, M., Heidrich, F. M., Lee, Y., Jordt, S. -E., Ehrlich, B. E. (2007). Chronic exposure to paclitaxel diminishes phosphoinositide signaling by calpain-mediated neuronal calcium sensor-1 degradation. Proceedings of the National Academy of Sciences of the United States of America. 104(26), 11103–11108.

Bogliun, G., Marzorati, L., Cavaletti, G., & Frattola, L. (1992). Evaluation by somatosensory evoked potentials of the neurotoxicity of cisplatin alone or in combination with glutathione. *Italian Journal of Neurological Sciences*, *13*(8), 643–647.

Bogliun, G., Marzorati, L., Marzola, M., Miceli, M. D., Cantu, M. G., & Cavaletti, G. (1996). Neurotoxicity of cisplatin +/− reduced glutathione in the first-line treatment of advanced ovarian cancer. *International Journal of Gynecological Cancer*, *6*(5), 415–419.

Bove, L., Picardo, M., Maresca, V., Jandolo, B., & Pace, A. (2001). A pilot study on the relation between cisplatin neuropathy and vitamin E. *Journal of Experimental and Clinical Cancer Research: CR*, *20*(2), 277–280.

Boyle, F. M., Wheeler, H. R., & Shenfield, G. M. (1996). Glutamate ameliorates experimental vincristine neuropathy. *The Journal of Pharmacology and Experimental Therapeutics*, *279*(1), 410–415.

Boyle, F. M., Wheeler, H. R., & Shenfield, G. M. (1999). Amelioration of Experimental Cisplatin and Paclitaxel Neuropathy with Glutamate. *Journal of Neuro-Oncology*, *41*(2), 107–116.

Bradfield, S. M., Sandler, E., Geller, T., Tamura, R. N., & Krischer, J. P. (2015). Glutamic acid not beneficial for the prevention of vincristine neurotoxicity in children with cancer. *Pediatric Blood and Cancer*, *62*(6), 1004–1010.

Brandhorst, S., Wei, M., Hwang, S., Morgan, T. E., & Longo, V. D. (2013). Short-term calorie and protein restriction provide partial protection from chemotoxicity but do not delay glioma progression. *Experimental Gerontology*, *48*(10), 1120–1128.

Broyl, A., Corthals, S. L., Jongen, J. L., van der Holt, B., Kuiper, R., de Knegt, Y., … Sonneveld, P. (2010). Mechanisms of peripheral neuropathy associated with bortezomib and vincristine in patients with newly diagnosed multiple myeloma: a prospective analysis of data from the HOVON-65/GMMG-HD4 trial. *The Lancet. Oncology*, *11*(11), 1057-65.

Buesa, J. M., García-Teijido, P., Losa, R., & Fra, J. (2003). Treatment of ifosfamide encephalopathy with intravenous thiamin. *Clinical Cancer Research: An Official Journal of the American Association for Cancer Research*, *9*(12), 4636–4637.

Bujalska, M., & Gumułka, S. W. (2008). Effect of selenium compound (selol) on the opioid activity in vincristine induced hyperalgesia. *Neuro Endocrinology Letters*, *29*(4), 552–557.

Callander, N., Markovina, S., Eickhoff, J., Hutson, P., Campbell, T., Hematti, P., … Miyamoto, S. (2014). Acetyl-L-carnitine (ALCAR) for the prevention of chemotherapy-induced peripheral neuropathy in patients with relapsed or refractory multiple myeloma treated with bortezomib, doxorubicin and low-dose dexamethasone: a study from the Wisconsin Oncology Netwo. *Cancer Chemotherapy and Pharmacology*, *74*(4), 875–882.

Carozzi, V. A., Canta, A., & Chiorazzi, A. (2015). Chemotherapy-induced peripheral neuropathy: what do we know about mechanisms? *Neuroscience Letters*, *596*, 90–107.

Cascinu, S., Cordella, L., Del Ferro, E., Fronzoni, M., & Catalano, G. (1995). Neuroprotective effect of reduced glutathione on cisplatin-based chemotherapy in advanced gastric cancer: a randomized double-blind placebo-controlled trial. *Journal of Clinical Oncology: Official Journal of the American Society of Clinical Oncology*, *13*(1), 26–32.

Cascinu, S., Catalano, V., Cordella, L., Labianca, R., Giordani, P., Baldelli, A. M., … Catalano, G. (2002). Neuroprotective effect of reduced glutathione on oxaliplatin-based chemotherapy in advanced colorectal cancer: a randomized, double-blind, placebo-controlled trial. *Journal of Clinical Oncology: Official Journal of the American Society of Clinical Oncology*, *20*(16), 3478–3483.

Cata, J. P., Weng, H. R., Lee, B. N., Reuben, J. M., & Dougherty, P. M. (2006). Clinical and experimental findings in humans and animals with chemotherapy-induced peripheral neuropathy. *Minerva Anestesiologica*, *72*(3), 151–169.

Chawla, J., & Kvarnberg, D. (2014). Hydrosoluble vitamins. *Handbook of Clinical Neurology*, *120*, 891–914.

Chay, W. -Y., Tan, S. -H., Lo, Y. -L., Ong, S. Y. -K., Ng, H. -C., Gao, F., … Choo, S. -P. (2010). Use of calcium and magnesium infusions in prevention of oxaliplatin induced sensory neuropathy. *Asia-Pacific Journal of Clinical Oncology*, *6*(4), 270–277.

Cheng, C. -W., Adams, G. B., Perin, L., Wei, M., Zhou, X., Lam, B. S., … Longo, V. D. (2014). Prolonged fasting reduces IGF-1/PKA to promote hematopoietic-stem-cell-based regeneration and reverse immunosuppression. *Cell Stem Cell*, *14*(6), 810–823.

Chroni, E., Georgiou, S., Monastirli, A., Paschalis, C., & Tsambaos, D. (2001). Effects of short-term oral acitretin therapy on peripheral nerve function: a prospective neurological and neurophysiological study. *Acta Dermato-Venereologica*, *81*(6), 423–425.

Chroni, E., Monastirli, A., Georgiou, S., Pasmatzi, E., Papathanasopoulos, P., & Tsambaos, D. (2014). Sensorimotor polyneuropathy after a 1-month treatment with oral acitretin. *Clinical Neuropharmacology*, *37*(5), 151–153.

Colombo, N., Bini, S., Miceli, D., Bogliun, G., Marzorati, L., Cavaletti, G., … Mangioni, C. (1995). Weekly cisplatin +/− glutathione in relapsed ovarian carcinoma. *International Journal of Gynecological Cancer: Official Journal of the International Gynecological Cancer Society*, *5*(2), 81–86.

Coppey, L. J., Davidson, E. P., Obrosov, A., & Yorek, M. A. (2015). Enriching the diet with menhaden oil improves peripheral neuropathy in streptozotocin-induced type 1 diabetic rats. *Journal of Neurophysiology*, *113*(3), 701–708.

Crawford, L. J., Walker, B., & Irvine, A. E. (2011). Proteasome inhibitors in cancer therapy. *Journal of Cell Communication and Signaling*, *5*(2), 101–110.

Damnjanovic, I., Kocic, G., Najman, S., Stojanovic, S., Stojanovic, D., Veljkovic, A., … Pesic, S. (2014). Chemopreventive potential of alpha lipoic acid in the treatment of colon and cervix cancer cell lines. *Bratislavské Lekárske Listy*, *115*(10), 611–616.

Dong, M., Xing, P., Liu, P., Feng, F., & Shi, Y. (2010). Assessment of the protective effect of calcium-magnesium infusion and glutathione on oxaliplatin-induced neurotoxicity. *Zhonghua Zhong Liu Za Zhi [Chinese Journal of Oncology]*, *32*(3), 208–211.

Dongre, Y. U., & Swami, O. C. (2013). Sustained-release pregabalin with methylcobalamin in neuropathic pain: an Indian real-life experience. *International Journal of General Medicine*, *6*, 413–417.

Erken, H. A., Koç, E. R., Yazıcı, H., Yay, A., Önder, G. Ö., & Sarıcı, S. F. (2014). Selenium partially prevents cisplatin-induced neurotoxicity: a preliminary study. *Neurotoxicology*, *42*, 71–75.

Estebe, J. -P., Degryse, C., Rezzadori, G., Dimache, F., Daccache, D., Le Naoures, A., ... Schoeffer, P. (2013). Effet d'un régime alimentaire carencé en polyamines sur la douleur périopératoire lors d'une chirurgie rachidienne de l'adulte. *Annales Françaises d'Anesthésie et de Réanimation*, *32*, A10.

Ewertz, M., Qvortrup, C., & Eckhoff, L. (2015). Chemotherapy-induced peripheral neuropathy in patients treated with taxanes and platinum derivatives. *Acta Oncologica*, *54*(5), 587–591.

Farvid, M. S., Homayouni, F., Amiri, Z., & Adelmanesh, F. (2011). Improving neuropathy scores in type 2 diabetic patients using micronutrients supplementation. *Diabetes Research and Clinical Practice*, *93*(1), 86–94.

Fehrenbacher, J. C. (2015). Chemotherapy-induced peripheral neuropathy. *Progress in Molecular Biology and Translational Science*, *131*, 471–508.

Ferrier, J., Bayet-Robert, M., Pereira, B., Daulhac, L., Eschalier, A., Pezet, D., ... Balayssac, D. (2013). A polyamine-deficient diet prevents oxaliplatin-induced acute cold and mechanical hypersensitivity in rats. *PloS One*, *8*(10), e77828.

Flatters, S. J. L., & Bennett, G. J. (2006). Studies of peripheral sensory nerves in paclitaxel-induced painful peripheral neuropathy: evidence for mitochondrial dysfunction. *Pain*, *122*(3), 245–257.

Flatters, S. J. L., Xiao, W. -H., & Bennett, G. J. (2006). Acetyl-L-carnitine prevents and reduces paclitaxel-induced painful peripheral neuropathy. *Neuroscience Letters*, *397*(3), 219–223.

Friedman, M. A., Resnick, J. S., & Baer, R. L. (1986). Subepidermal vesicular dermatosis and sensory peripheral neuropathy caused by pyridoxine abuse. *Journal of the American Academy of Dermatology*, *14*(5 Pt 2), 915–917.

Gamelin, L. (2004). Prevention of Oxaliplatin-Related Neurotoxicity by Calcium and Magnesium Infusions: A Retrospective Study of 161 Patients Receiving Oxaliplatin Combined with 5-Fluorouracil and Leucovorin for Advanced Colorectal Cancer. *Clinical Cancer Research*, *10*(12), 4055–4061.

Gamelin, L., Boisdron-Celle, M., Morel, A., Poirier, A. L., Berger, V., Gamelin, E., ... de Gramont, A. (2008). Oxaliplatin-related neurotoxicity: interest of calcium-magnesium infusion and no impact on its efficacy. *Journal of Clinical Oncology: Official Journal of the American Society of Clinical Oncology*, *26*(7), 1188–1189; author reply 1189–1190.

Gao, M., Yan, X., & Weng, H. -R. (2013). Inhibition of glycogen synthase kinase 3β activity with lithium prevents and attenuates paclitaxel-induced neuropathic pain. *Neuroscience*, *254*, 301–311.

Gaurav, K., Goel, R. K., Shukla, M., & Pandey, M. (2012). Glutamine: A novel approach to chemotherapy-induced toxicity. *Indian Journal of Medical and Paediatric Oncology: Official Journal of Indian Society of Medical & Paediatric Oncology*, *33*(1), 13–20.

Gdynia, H. -J., Müller, T., Sperfeld, A. -D., Kühnlein, P., Otto, M., Kassubek, J., & Ludolph, A. C. (2008). Severe sensorimotor neuropathy after intake of highest dosages of vitamin B6. *Neuromuscular Disorders: NMD*, *18*(2), 156–158.

Gedlicka, C., Scheithauer, W., Schüll, B., & Kornek, G. V. (2002). Effective treatment of oxaliplatin-induced cumulative polyneuropathy with alpha-lipoic acid. *Journal of Clinical Oncology: Official Journal of the American Society of Clinical Oncology*, *20*(15), 3359–3361.

Gedlicka, C., Kornek, G. V., Schmid, K., & Scheithauer, W. (2003). Amelioration of docetaxel/cisplatin induced polyneuropathy by alpha-lipoic acid. *Annals of Oncology: Official Journal of the European Society for Medical Oncology/ESMO*, *14*(2), 339–340.

Ghelli, A., Porcelli, A. M., Zanna, C., Martinuzzi, A., Carelli, V., & Rugolo, M. (2008). Protection against oxidant-induced apoptosis by exogenous glutathione in Leber hereditary optic neuropathy cybrids. *Investigative Ophthalmology and Visual Science*, *49*(2), 671–676.

Ghirardi, O., Lo Giudice, P., Pisano, C., Vertechy, M., Bellucci, A., Vesci, L., ... Carminati, P. (2005a). Acetyl-L-carnitine prevents and reverts experimental chronic neurotoxicity induced by oxaliplatin, without altering its antitumor properties. *Anticancer Research*, *25*(4), 2681–2687.

Ghirardi, O., Vertechy, M., Vesci, L., Canta, A., Nicolini, G., Galbiati, S., ... Rigamonti, L. M. (2005b). Chemotherapy-induced allodinia: neuroprotective effect of acetyl-L-carnitine. *In Vivo (Athens, Greece)*, *19*(3), 631–637.

Ghoreishi, Z., Esfahani, A., Djazayeri, A., Djalali, M., Golestan, B., Ayromlou, H., ... Darabi, M. (2012). Omega-3 fatty acids are protective against paclitaxel-induced peripheral neuropathy: a randomized double-blind placebo controlled trial. *BMC Cancer*, *12*, 355.

Godoi, G. L., de Oliveira Porciúncula, L., Schulz, J. F., Kaufmann, F. N., da Rocha, J. B., de Souza, D. O. G., ... de Almeida, H. L. (2013). Selenium compounds prevent amyloid β-peptide neurotoxicity in rat primary hippocampal neurons. *Neurochemical Research*, *38*(11), 2359–2363.

Granados-Soto, V., Sánchez-Ramirez, G., la Torre, M. R., Caram-Salas, N. L., Medina-Santillán, R., & Reyes-García, G. (2004). Effect of diclofenac on the antiallodynic activity of vitamin B12 in a neuropathic pain model in the rat. *Proceedings of the Western Pharmacology Society*, *47*, 92–94.

Greeshma, N., Prasanth, K. G., & Balaji, B. (2015). Tetrahydrocurcumin exerts protective effect on vincristine induced neuropathy: behavioral, biochemical, neurophysiological and histological evidence. *Chemico-Biological Interactions*, *238*, 118–128.

Grothey, A., Hart, L. L., Rowland, K. M., Ansari, R. H., Alberts, S. R., Chowhan, N. M., ... Hochster, H. S. (2008). Intermittent oxaliplatin (oxali) administration and time-to-treatment-failure (TTF) in metastatic colorectal cancer (mCRC): final results of the phase III CONcePT trial. *ASCO Meeting Abstracts*, *26*(Suppl. 15), 4010.

Grothey, A., Nikcevich, D. A., Sloan, J. A., Kugler, J. W., Silberstein, P. T., Dentchev, T., ... Loprinzi, C. L. (2011). Intravenous calcium and magnesium for oxaliplatin-induced sensory neurotoxicity in adjuvant colon cancer: NCCTG N04C7. *Journal of Clinical Oncology*: Official Journal of the American Society of Clinical Oncology, *29*(4), 421–427.

Guo, Y., Jones, D., Palmer, J. L., Forman, A., Dakhil, S. R., Velasco, M. R., ... Fisch, M. J. (2014). Oral alpha-lipoic acid to prevent chemotherapy-induced peripheral neuropathy: a randomized, double-blind, placebo-controlled trial. *Supportive Care in Cancer: Official Journal of the Multinational Association of Supportive Care in Cancer*, *22*(5), 1223–1231.

Hamadani, M., & Awan, F. (2006). Role of thiamine in managing ifosfamide-induced encephalopathy. *Journal of Oncology Pharmacy Practice: Official Publication of the International Society of Oncology Pharmacy Practitioners*, *12*(4), 237–239.

Hamers, F. P., Brakkee, J. H., Cavalletti, E., Tedeschi, M., Marmonti, L., Pezzoni, G., ... Gispen, W. H. (1993). Reduced glutathione protects against cisplatin-induced neurotoxicity in rats. *Cancer Research*, *53*(3), 544–549.

Han, C. H., Khwaounjoo, P., Kilfoyle, D. H., Hill, A., & McKeage, M. J. (2013). Phase I drug-interaction study of effects of calcium and magnesium infusions on oxaliplatin pharmacokinetics and acute neurotoxicity in colorectal cancer patients. *BMC Cancer*, *13*, 495.

Hernández-Pedro, N., Granados-Soto, V., Ordoñez, G., Pineda, B., Rangel-López, E., Salazar-Ramiro, A., … Sotelo, J. (2014). Vitamin A increases nerve growth factor and retinoic acid receptor beta and improves diabetic neuropathy in rats. *Translational Research: The Journal of Laboratory and Clinical Medicine*, *164*(3), 196–201.

Hershman, D. L., Unger, J. M., Crew, K. D., Minasian, L. M., Awad, D., Moinpour, C. M., … Albain, K. S. (2013). Randomized double-blind placebo-controlled trial of acetyl-L-carnitine for the prevention of taxane-induced neuropathy in women undergoing adjuvant breast cancer therapy. *Journal of Clinical Oncology: Official Journal of the American Society of Clinical Oncology*, *31*(20), 2627–2633.

Hershman, D. L., Lacchetti, C., Dworkin, R. H., Lavoie Smith, E. M., Bleeker, J., Cavaletti, G., … Loprinzi, C. L. (2014). Prevention and management of chemotherapy-induced peripheral neuropathy in survivors of adult cancers: American Society of Clinical Oncology clinical practice guideline. *Journal of Clinical Oncology: Official Journal of the American Society of Clinical Oncology*, *32*(18), 1941–1967.

Hochster, H. S., Grothey, A., & Childs, B. H. (2007). Use of calcium and magnesium salts to reduce oxaliplatin-related neurotoxicity. *Journal of Clinical Oncology: Official Journal of the American Society of Clinical Oncology*, *25*(25), 4028–4029.

Hochster, H. S., Grothey, A., Hart, L., Rowland, K., Ansari, R., Alberts, S., … Childs, B. H. (2014). Improved time to treatment failure with an intermittent oxaliplatin strategy: results of CONcePT. *Annals of Oncology: Official Journal of the European Society for Medical Oncology/ESMO*, *25*(6), 1172–1178.

Huang, Y., Qin, J., Chen, M., Chao, X., Chen, Z., Ramassamy, C., … Jin, M. (2014). Lithium prevents acrolein-induced neurotoxicity in HT22 mouse hippocampal cells. *Neurochemical Research*, *39*(4), 677–684.

Huang, J. -S., Wu, C. -L., Fan, C. -W., Chen, W. -H., Yeh, K. -Y., & Chang, P. -H. (2015). Intravenous glutamine appears to reduce the severity of symptomatic platinum-induced neuropathy: a prospective randomized study. *Journal of Chemotherapy*, *27*(4), 235–240.

Imtiaz, S., & Muzaffar, N. (2010). Ifosfamide neurotoxicty in a young female with a remarkable response to thiamine. *JPMA. The Journal of the Pakistan Medical Association*, *60*(10), 867–869.

Ishibashi, K., Okada, N., Miyazaki, T., Sano, M., & Ishida, H. (2010). Effect of calcium and magnesium on neurotoxicity and blood platinum concentrations in patients receiving mFOLFOX6 therapy: a prospective randomized study. *International Journal of Clinical Oncology*, *15*(1), 82–87.

Ivkovic, A., & Stern, T. A. (2014). Lithium-induced neurotoxicity: clinical presentations, pathophysiology, and treatment. *Psychosomatics*, *55*(3), 296–302.

Jackson, D. V, Pope, E. K., Case, L. D., Wells, H. B., White, D. R., Cooper, M. R., … Cruz, J. M. (1984). Improved tolerance of vincristine by glutamic acid. A preliminary report. *Journal of Neuro-Oncology*, *2*(3), 219–222.

Jackson, D. V, Pope, E. K., McMahan, R. A., Cooper, M. R., Atkins, J. N., Callahan, R. D., … Muss, H. B. (1986). Clinical trial of pyridoxine to reduce vincristine neurotoxicity. *Journal of Neuro-Oncology*, *4*(1), 37–41.

Jackson, D. V, Wells, H. B., Atkins, J. N., Zekan, P. J., White, D. R., Richards, F., … Muss, H. B. (1988). Amelioration of vincristine neurotoxicity by glutamic acid. *The American Journal of Medicine*, *84*(6), 1016–1022.

Jain, S. K., & Lim, G. (2001). Pyridoxine and pyridoxamine inhibits superoxide radicals and prevents lipid peroxidation, protein glycosylation, and (Na+ + K +)-ATPase activity reduction in high glucose-treated human erythrocytes. *Free Radical Biology and Medicine*, *30*(3), 232–237.

Jin, H. W., Flatters, S. J. L., Xiao, W. H., Mulhern, H. L., & Bennett, G. J. (2008). Prevention of paclitaxel-evoked painful peripheral neuropathy by acetyl-L-carnitine: effects on axonal mitochondria, sensory nerve fiber terminal arbors, and cutaneous Langerhans cells. *Experimental Neurology*, *210*(1), 229–237.

Kahng, J., Kim, T. K., Chung, E. Y., Kim, Y. S., & Moon, J. Y. (2015). The effect of thioctic acid on allodynia in a rat vincristine-induced neuropathy model. *The Journal of International Medical Research*, *43*(3), 350–355.

Kim, H. K., Kim, J. H., Gao, X., Zhou, J. -L., Lee, I., Chung, K., & Chung, J. M. (2006). Analgesic effect of vitamin E is mediated by reducing central sensitization in neuropathic pain. *Pain*, *122*(1–2), 53–62.

Knijn, N., Tol, J., Koopman, M., Werter, M. J. B. P., Imholz, A. L. T., Valster, F. A. A., … Punt, C. J. A. (2011). The effect of prophylactic calcium and magnesium infusions on the incidence of neurotoxicity and clinical outcome of oxaliplatin-based systemic treatment in advanced colorectal cancer patients. *European Journal of Cancer*, *47*(3), 369–374.

Ko, G. D., Nowacki, N. B., Arseneau, L., Eitel, M., & Hum, A. (2010). Omega-3 fatty acids for neuropathic pain: case series. *The Clinical Journal of Pain*, *26*(2), 168–172.

Kopruszinski, C. M., Reis, R. C., & Chichorro, J. G. (2012). B vitamins relieve neuropathic pain behaviors induced by infraorbital nerve constriction in rats. *Life Sciences*, *91*(23–24), 1187–1195.

Kottschade, L. A., Sloan, J. A., Mazurczak, M. A., Johnson, D. B., Murphy, B. P., Rowland, K. M., … Loprinzi, C. L. (2011). The use of vitamin E for the prevention of chemotherapy-induced peripheral neuropathy: results of a randomized phase III clinical trial. *Supportive Care in Cancer*, *19*(11), 1769–1777.

Lauretani, F., Bandinelli, S., Bartali, B., Benedetta, B., Cherubini, A., Iorio, A. D., … Ferrucci, L. (2007). Omega-6 and Omega-3 fatty acids predict accelerated decline of peripheral nerve function in older persons. *European Journal of Neurology*, *14*(7), 801–808.

Leal, A. D., Qin, R., Atherton, P. J., Haluska, P., Behrens, R. J., Tiber, C. H., … Loprinzi, C. L. (2014). North Central Cancer Treatment Group/Alliance trial N08CA-the use of glutathione for prevention of paclitaxel/carboplatin-induced peripheral neuropathy: a phase 3 randomized, double-blind, placebo-controlled study. *Cancer*, *120*(12), 1890–1897.

Leonetti, C., Biroccio, A., Gabellini, C., Scarsella, M., Maresca, V., Flori, E., … Picardo, M. (2003). Alpha-tocopherol protects against cisplatin-induced toxicity without interfering with antitumor efficacy. *International Journal of Cancer. Journal International Du Cancer*, *104*(2), 243–250.

Letizia Mauro, G., Cataldo, P., Barbera, G., & Sanfilippo, A. (2014). α-Lipoic acid and superoxide dismutase in the management of chronic neck pain: a prospective randomized study. *Drugs in R&D*, *14*(1), 1–7.

Li, B. J., Hao, X. Y., Ren, G. H., & Gong, Y. (2015). Effect of lipoic acid combined with paclitaxel on breast cancer cells. *Genetics and Molecular Research: GMR*, *14*(4), 17934–17940.

Loprinzi, C. L., Qin, R., Dakhil, S. R., Fehrenbacher, L., Flynn, K. A., Atherton, P., … Grothey, A. (2014). Phase III randomized, placebo-controlled, double-blind study of intravenous calcium and magnesium to prevent oxaliplatin-induced sensory neurotoxicity (N08CB/Alliance). *Journal of Clinical Oncology*, *32*(10), 997–1005.

Loven, D., Levavi, H., Sabach, G., Zart, R., Andras, M., Fishman, A., … Gadoth, N. (2009). Long-term glutamate supplementation failed to protect against peripheral neurotoxicity of paclitaxel. *European Journal of Cancer Care*, *18*(1), 78–83.

Luo, J. (2010). Lithium-mediated protection against ethanol neurotoxicity. *Frontiers in Neuroscience*, *4*, 41.

Maestri, A., De Pasquale Ceratti, A., Cundari, S., Zanna, C., Cortesi, E., & Crinò, L. (2005). A pilot study on the effect of acetyl-L-carnitine in paclitaxel- and cisplatin-induced peripheral neuropathy. *Tumori*, *91*(2), 135–138.

McWhinney, S. R., Goldberg, R. M., & McLeod, H. L. (2009). Platinum neurotoxicity pharmacogenetics. *Molecular Cancer Therapeutics*, *8*(1), 10–16.

Melli, G., Taiana, M., Camozzi, F., Triolo, D., Podini, P., Quattrini, A., … Lauria, G. (2008). Alpha-lipoic acid prevents mitochondrial damage and neurotoxicity in experimental chemotherapy neuropathy. *Experimental Neurology*, *214*(2), 276–284.

Micke, O., Bruns, F., Mücke, R., Schäfer, U., Glatzel, M., DeVries, A. F., ... Büntzel, J. (2003). Selenium in the treatment of radiation-associated secondary lymphedema. *International Journal of Radiation Oncology, Biology, Physics*, *56*(1), 40–49.

Mihara, Y., Egashira, N., Sada, H., Kawashiri, T., Ushio, S., Yano, T., ... Oishi, R. (2011). Involvement of spinal NR2B-containing NMDA receptors in oxaliplatin-induced mechanical allodynia in rats. *Molecular Pain*, *7*, 8.

Mijnhout, G. S., Kollen, B. J., Alkhalaf, A., Kleefstra, N., & Bilo, H. J. G. (2012). Alpha lipoic Acid for symptomatic peripheral neuropathy in patients with diabetes: a meta-analysis of randomized controlled trials. *International Journal of Endocrinology*, *2012*, 456279.

Milla, P., Airoldi, M., Weber, G., Drescher, A., Jaehde, U., & Cattel, L. (2009). Administration of reduced glutathione in FOLFOX4 adjuvant treatment for colorectal cancer: effect on oxaliplatin pharmacokinetics, Pt-DNA adduct formation, and neurotoxicity. *Anti-Cancer Drugs*, *20*(5), 396–402.

Mo, M., Erdelyi, I., Szigeti-Buck, K., Benbow, J. H., & Ehrlich, B. E. (2012). Prevention of paclitaxel-induced peripheral neuropathy by lithium pretreatment. *FASEB Journal: Official Publication of the Federation of American Societies for Experimental Biology*, *26*(11), 4696–4709.

Mokhtar, G. M., Shaaban, S. Y., Elbarbary, N. S., & Fayed, W. A. (2010). A trial to assess the efficacy of glutamic acid in prevention of vincristine-induced neurotoxicity in pediatric malignancies: a pilot study. *Journal of Pediatric Hematology/Oncology*, *32*(8), 594–600.

Moon, H. -I., & Park, W. -H. (2010). Four carotenoids from Pittosporum tobira protect primary cultured rat cortical cells from glutamate-induced toxicity. *Phytotherapy Research: PTR*, *24*(4), 625–628.

Morani, A. S., & Bodhankar, S. L. (2010). Early co-administration of vitamin E acetate and methylcobalamin improves thermal hyperalgesia and motor nerve conduction velocity following sciatic nerve crush injury in rats. *Pharmacological Reports: PR*, *62*(2), 405–409.

Morra, M., Philipszoon, H. D., D'Andrea, G., Cananzi, A. R., L'Erario, R., & Milone, F. F. (1993). Sensory and motor neuropathy caused by excessive ingestion of vitamin B6: a case report. *Functional Neurology*, *8*(6), 429–432.

Moudi, M., Go, R., Yien, C. Y. S., & Nazre, M. (2013). Vinca alkaloids. *International Journal of Preventive Medicine*, *4*(11), 1231–1235.

Murat, A., & Hulagu, K. (2011). Effects of selenium on electrophysiological changes associated with diabetic peripheral neuropathy. *Neural Regeneration Research*, *6*(8), 617–622.

NCI-Supported Clinical Trials. (n.d.). Retrieved January 27, 2016. Available from: http://www.cancer.gov/about-cancer/treatment/clinical-trials/search

Okuda, Y., Mizutani, M., Ogawa, M., Sone, H., Asano, M., Asakura, Y., ... Yamashita, K. (1996). Long-term effects of eicosapentaenoic acid on diabetic peripheral neuropathy and serum lipids in patients with type II diabetes mellitus. *Journal of Diabetes and Its Complications*, *10*(5), 280–287.

Ozyurek, H., Turker, H., Akbalik, M., Bayrak, A. O., Ince, H., & Duru, F. (2007). Pyridoxine and pyridostigmine treatment in vincristine-induced neuropathy. *Pediatric Hematology and Oncology*, *24*(6), 447–452.

Ozyurek, H., Turker, H., Akbalik, M., Bayrak, A. O., Ince, H., & Duru, F. 2009. Pyridoxine and pyridostigmine treatment in vincristine-induced neuropathy, Pediatric hematology and oncology (July 9, 2009). Taylor & Francis. Available from: http://www.tandfonline.com/doi/abs/10.1080/08880010701451327?journalCode=ipho20

Pace, A., Savarese, A., Picardo, M., Maresca, V., Pacetti, U., Del Monte, G., ... Bove, L. (2003). Neuroprotective effect of vitamin E supplementation in patients treated with cisplatin chemotherapy. *Journal of Clinical Oncology*, *21*(5), 927–931.

Pace, A., Giannarelli, D., Galiè, E., Savarese, A., Carpano, S., Della Giulia, M., ... Cognetti, F. (2010). Vitamin E neuroprotection for cisplatin neuropathy: a randomized, placebo-controlled trial. *Neurology*, *74*(9), 762–766.

Palencia, G., Hernández-Pedro, N., Saavedra-Perez, D., Peña-Curiel, O., Ortiz-Plata, A., Ordoñez, G., ... Arrieta, O. (2014). Retinoic acid reduces solvent-induced neuropathy and promotes neural regeneration in mice. *Journal of Neuroscience Research*, *92*(8), 1062–1070.

Papa, L., & Rockwell, P. (2008). Persistent mitochondrial dysfunction and oxidative stress hinder neuronal cell recovery from reversible proteasome inhibition. *Apoptosis: An International Journal on Programmed Cell Death*, *13*(4), 588–599.

Park, S. B., Goldstein, D., Lin, C. S. -Y., Krishnan, A. V., Friedlander, M. L., & Kiernan, M. C. (2011). Neuroprotection for oxaliplatin-induced neurotoxicity: what happened to objective assessment? *Journal of Clinical Oncology: Official Journal of the American Society of Clinical Oncology*, *29*(18), e553–e554.

Pastore, A., Piemonte, F., Locatelli, M., Lo Russo, A., Gaeta, L. M., Tozzi, G., & Federici, G. (2001). Determination of blood total, reduced, and oxidized glutathione in pediatric subjects. *Clinical Chemistry*, *47*(8), 1467–1469.

Perry, M. C. (2012). In M. C. Perry (Ed.), *Perry's The Chemotherapy Source Book* ((5th ed.)). Lippincott Williams & Wilkins.

Peters, C. M., Jimenez-Andrade, J. M., Jonas, B. M., Sevcik, M. A., Koewler, N. J., Ghilardi, J. R., ... Mantyh, P. W. (2007). Intravenous paclitaxel administration in the rat induces a peripheral sensory neuropathy characterized by macrophage infiltration and injury to sensory neurons and their supporting cells. *Experimental Neurology*, *203*(1), 42–54.

Petrini, M., Vaglini, F., Cervetti, G., Cavalletti, M., Sartucci, F., Murri, L., & Corsini, G. U. (1999). Is lithium able to reverse neurological damage induced by vinca alkaloids? (Short communication). *Journal of Neural Transmission*, *106*(5–6), 569–575.

Pirovano, C., Balzarini, A., Böhm, S., Oriana, S., Spatti, G. B., & Zunino, F. (1992). Peripheral neurotoxicity following high-dose cisplatin with glutathione: clinical and neurophysiological assessment. *Tumori*, *78*(4), 253–257.

Pourmohammadi, N., Alimoradi, H., Mehr, S. E., Hassanzadeh, G., Hadian, M. R., Sharifzadeh, M., ... Dehpour, A. R. (2012). Lithium attenuates peripheral neuropathy induced by paclitaxel in rats. *Basic and Clinical Pharmacology and Toxicology*, *110*(3), 231–237.

Rajanandh, M. G., Kosey, S., & Prathiksha, G. (2014). Assessment of antioxidant supplementation on the neuropathic pain score and quality of life in diabetic neuropathy patients—a randomized controlled study. *Pharmacological Reports: PR*, *66*(1), 44–48.

Reiner, D. J., Yu, S. -J., Shen, H., He, Y., Bae, E., & Wang, Y. (2014). 9-Cis retinoic acid protects against methamphetamine-induced neurotoxicity in nigrostriatal dopamine neurons. *Neurotoxicity Research*, *25*(3), 248–261.

Reyes-García, G., Caram-Salas, N. L., Medina-Santillán, R., & Granados-Soto, V. (2004). Oral administration of B vitamins increases the antiallodynic effect of gabapentin in the rat. *Proceedings of the Western Pharmacology Society*, *47*, 76–79.

Richards, A., Marshall, H., & McQuary, A. (2011). Evaluation of methylene blue, thiamine, and/or albumin in the prevention of ifosfamide-related neurotoxicity. *Journal of Oncology Pharmacy Practice: Official Publication of the International Society of Oncology Pharmacy Practitioners*, *17*(4), 372–380.

Rivat, C., Richebé, P., Laboureyras, E., Laulin, J. -P., Havouis, R., Noble, F., ... Simonnet, G. (2008). Polyamine deficient diet to relieve pain hypersensitivity. *Pain*, *137*(1), 125–137.

Rivera, E., & Cianfrocca, M. (2015). Overview of neuropathy associated with taxanes for the treatment of metastatic breast cancer. *Cancer Chemotherapy and Pharmacology*, *75*(4), 659–670.

Safdie, F. M., Dorff, T., Quinn, D., Fontana, L., Wei, M., Lee, C., ... Longo, V. D. (2009). Fasting and cancer treatment in humans: a case series report. *Aging*, *1*(12), 988–1007.

Sahin, M., Karauzum, S. B., Perry, G., Smith, M. A., & Aliciguzel, Y. (2005). Retinoic acid isomers protect hippocampal neurons from amyloid-beta induced neurodegeneration. *Neurotoxicity Research*, *7*(3), 243–250.

Sakamoto, K., Hiraiwa, M., Saito, M., Nakahara, T., Sato, Y., Nagao, T., & Ishii, K. (2010). Protective effect of all-trans retinoic acid on NMDA-induced neuronal cell death in rat retina. *European Journal of Pharmacology*, *635*(1–3), 56–61.

Sakurai, M., Egashira, N., Kawashiri, T., Yano, T., Ikesue, H., & Oishi, R. (2009). Oxaliplatin-induced neuropathy in the rat: involvement of oxalate in cold hyperalgesia but not mechanical allodynia. *Pain*, *147*(1–3), 165–174.

Salehi, Z., & Roayaei, M. (2015). Effect of vitamin E on oxaliplatin-induced peripheral neuropathy prevention: a randomized controlled trial. *International Journal of Preventive Medicine*, *6*, 104.

Sánchez-Lara, K., Turcott, J. G., Juárez-Hernández, E., Nuñez-Valencia, C., Villanueva, G., Guevara, P., … Arrieta, O. (2014). Effects of an oral nutritional supplement containing eicosapentaenoic acid on nutritional and clinical outcomes in patients with advanced non-small cell lung cancer: randomised trial. *Clinical Nutrition*, *33*(6), 1017–1023.

Santamaría, A., Vázquez-Román, B., La Cruz, V. P. -D., González-Cortés, C., Trejo-Solís, M. C., Galván-Arzate, S., … Ali, S. F. (2005). Selenium reduces the proapoptotic signaling associated to NF-kappaB pathway and stimulates glutathione peroxidase activity during excitotoxic damage produced by quinolinate in rat corpus striatum. *Synapse*, *58*(4), 258–266.

Schaumburg, H., Kaplan, J., Windebank, A., Vick, N., Rasmus, S., Pleasure, D., & Brown, M. J. (1983). Sensory neuropathy from pyridoxine abuse. A new megavitamin syndrome. *The New England Journal of Medicine*, *309*(8), 445–448.

Schloss, J. M., Colosimo, M., Airey, C., Masci, P. P., Linnane, A. W., & Vitetta, L. (2013). Nutraceuticals and chemotherapy induced peripheral neuropathy (CIPN): a systematic review. *Clinical Nutrition*, *32*(6), 888–893.

Schloss, J. M., Colosimo, M., Airey, C., & Vitetta, L. (2015). Chemotherapy-induced peripheral neuropathy (CIPN) and vitamin B12 deficiency. *Supportive Care in Cancer: Official Journal of the Multinational Association of Supportive Care in Cancer*, *23*(7), 1843–1850.

Schmidinger, M., Budinsky, A. C., Wenzel, C., Piribauer, M., Brix, R., Kautzky, M., … Steger, G. G. (2000). Glutathione in the prevention of cisplatin induced toxicities. A prospectively randomized pilot trial in patients with head and neck cancer and non small cell lung cancer. *Wiener Klinische Wochenschrift*, *112*(14), 617–623.

Scholz, J., & Woolf, C. J. (2007). The neuropathic pain triad: neurons, immune cells and glia. *Nature Neuroscience*, *10*(11), 1361–1368.

Seretny, M., Currie, G. L., Sena, E. S., Ramnarine, S., Grant, R., MacLeod, M. R., … Fallon, M. (2014). Incidence, prevalence, and predictors of chemotherapy-induced peripheral neuropathy: A systematic review and meta-analysis. *Pain*, *155*(12), 2461–2470.

Shibuya, K., Misawa, S., Nasu, S., Sekiguchi, Y., Beppu, M., Iwai, Y., … Kuwabara, S. (2014). Safety and efficacy of intravenous ultra-high dose methylcobalamin treatment for peripheral neuropathy: a phase I/II open label clinical trial. *Internal Medicine*, *53*(17), 1927–1931.

Shinozaki, Y., Sato, Y., Koizumi, S., Ohno, Y., Nagao, T., & Inoue, K. (2007). Retinoic acids acting through retinoid receptors protect hippocampal neurons from oxygen-glucose deprivation-mediated cell death by inhibition of c-jun-N-terminal kinase and p38 mitogen-activated protein kinase. *Neuroscience*, *147*(1), 153–163.

Sieja, K., & Talerczyk, M. (2004). Selenium as an element in the treatment of ovarian cancer in women receiving chemotherapy. *Gynecologic Oncology*, *93*(2), 320–327.

Simonnet, G., Laboureyras, E., & Sergheraert, L. (2013). Polyamine deficient diet: a nutritional therapy for relieving abnormal and chronic pain. *Pharma Nutrition*, *1*(4), 137–140.

Smyth, J. F., Bowman, A., Perren, T., Wilkinson, P., Prescott, R. J., Quinn, K. J., & Tedeschi, M. (1997). Glutathione reduces the toxicity and improves quality of life of women diagnosed with ovarian cancer treated with cisplatin: results of a double-blind, randomised trial. *Annals of Oncology: Official Journal of the European Society for Medical Oncology/ESMO*, *8*(6), 569–573.

Song, X. -S., Huang, Z. -J., & Song, X. -J. (2009). Thiamine suppresses thermal hyperalgesia, inhibits hyperexcitability, and lessens alterations of sodium currents in injured, dorsal root ganglion neurons in rats. *Anesthesiology*, *110*(2), 387–400.

Stubblefield, M. D., Vahdat, L. T., Balmaceda, C. M., Troxel, A. B., Hesdorffer, C. S., & Gooch, C. L. (2005). Glutamine as a neuroprotective agent in high-dose paclitaxel-induced peripheral neuropathy: a clinical and electrophysiologic study. *Clinical Oncology*, *17*(4), 271–276.

Ta, L. E., Bieber, A. J., Carlton, S. M., Loprinzi, C. L., Low, P. A., & Windebank, A. J. (2010). Transient receptor potential vanilloid 1 is essential for cisplatin-induced heat hyperalgesia in mice. *Molecular Pain*, *6*, 15.

Takeshita, M., Banno, Y., Nakamura, M., Otsuka, M., Teramachi, H., Tsuchiya, T., & Itoh, Y. (2011). The pivotal role of intracellular calcium in oxaliplatin-induced inhibition of neurite outgrowth but not cell death in differentiated PC12 cells. *Chemistry Research in Toxicology*, *24*(11), 1845–1852.

Takimoto, N., Sugawara, S., Iida, A., Sakakibara, T., Mori, K., Sugiura, M., … Adachi, M. (2008). Prevention of oxaliplatin-related neurotoxicity by glutathione infusions. *Gan to Kagaku Ryoho. Cancer and Chemotherapy*, *35*(13), 2373–2376.

Tredici, G., Cavaletti, G., Petruccioli, M. G., Fabbrica, D., Tedeschi, M., & Venturino, P. (1994). Low-dose glutathione administration in the prevention of cisplatin-induced peripheral neuropathy in rats. *Neurotoxicology*, *15*(3), 701–704.

Tredici, G., Tredici, S., Fabbrica, D., Minoia, C., & Cavaletti, G. (1998). Experimental cisplatin neuronopathy in rats and the effect of retinoic acid administration. *Journal of Neuro-Oncology*, *36*(1), 31–40.

Tsambaos, D., Sakkis, T., Chroni, E., Koniavitou, K., Monastirli, A., Pasmatzi, E., & Paschalis, C. (2003). Peripheral sensory neuropathy associated with short-term oral acitretin therapy. *Skin Pharmacology and Applied Skin Physiology*, *16*(1), 46–49.

Tuncer, S., Dalkilic, N., Akif Dunbar, M., & Keles, B. (2010). Comparative effects of α lipoic acid and melatonin on cisplatin-induced neurotoxicity. *The International Journal of Neuroscience*, *120*(10), 655–663.

Turan, M. I., Cayir, A., Cetin, N., Suleyman, H., Siltelioglu Turan, I., & Tan, H. (2014). An investigation of the effect of thiamine pyrophosphate on cisplatin-induced oxidative stress and DNA damage in rat brain tissue compared with thiamine: thiamine and thiamine pyrophosphate effects on cisplatin neurotoxicity. *Human and Experimental Toxicology*, *33*(1), 14–21.

Tütüncü, N. B., Bayraktar, M., & Varli, K. (1998). Reversal of defective nerve conduction with vitamin E supplementation in type 2 diabetes: a preliminary study. *Diabetes Care*, *21*(11), 1915–1918.

Ueno, Y., Kizaki, M., Nakagiri, R., Kamiya, T., Sumi, H., & Osawa, T. (2002). Dietary glutathione protects rats from diabetic nephropathy and neuropathy. *Journal of Nutrition*, *132*(5), 897–900.

Uğuz, A. C., & Nazıroğlu, M. (2012). Effects of selenium on calcium signaling and apoptosis in rat dorsal root ganglion neurons induced by oxidative stress. *Neurochemical Research*, *37*(8), 1631–1638.

Vahdat, L., Papadopoulos, K., Lange, D., Leuin, S., Kaufman, E., Donovan, D., … Balmaceda, C. (2001). Reduction of Paclitaxel-induced Peripheral Neuropathy with Glutamine. *Clinical Cancer Research*, *7*(5), 1192–1197.

Wang, Z. -B., Gan, Q., Rupert, R. L., Zeng, Y. -M., & Song, X. -J. (2005). Thiamine, pyridoxine, cyanocobalamin and their combination inhibit thermal, but not mechanical hyperalgesia in rats with primary sensory neuron injury. *Pain*, *114*(1–2), 266–277.

Wang, W. -S., Lin, J. -K., Lin, T. -C., Chen, W. -S., Jiang, J. -K., Wang, H. -S., … Chen, P. -M. (2007). Oral glutamine is effective for preventing oxaliplatin-induced neuropathy in colorectal cancer patients. *The Oncologist*, *12*(3), 312–319.

Weickhardt, A., Wells, K., & Messersmith, W. (2011). Oxaliplatin-induced neuropathy in colorectal cancer. *Journal of Oncology*, *2011*, 201593.

WHO (2003) Diet, nutrition and the prevention of chronic diseases. *World Health Organization Technical Report Series*, *916*, i–viii, 1–149, backcover.
Wiernik, P. H., Yeap, B., Vogl, S. E., Kaplan, B. H., Comis, R. L., Falkson, G., … Horton, J. (1992). Hexamethylmelamine and low or moderate dose cisplatin with or without pyridoxine for treatment of advanced ovarian carcinoma: a study of the Eastern Cooperative Oncology Group. *Cancer Investigation*, *10*(1), 1–9.
Wojewoda, M., Duszyński, J., Więckowski, M., & Szczepanowska, J. (2012). Effect of selenite on basic mitochondrial function in human osteosarcoma cells with chronic mitochondrial stress. *Mitochondrion*, *12*(1), 149–155.
Wolf, S., Barton, D., Kottschade, L., Grothey, A., & Loprinzi, C. (2008). Chemotherapy-induced peripheral neuropathy: prevention and treatment strategies. *European Journal of Cancer*, *44*(11), 1507–1515.
Xiao, W. H., & Bennett, G. J. (2008). Chemotherapy-evoked neuropathic pain: abnormal spontaneous discharge in A-fiber and C-fiber primary afferent neurons and its suppression by acetyl-L-carnitine. *Pain*, *135*(3), 262–270.
Xu, G., Lv, Z. -W., Feng, Y., Tang, W. -Z., & Xu, G. X. (2013a). A single-center randomized controlled trial of local methylcobalamin injection for subacute herpetic neuralgia. *Pain Medicine (Malden, Mass)*, *14*(6), 884–894.
Xu, Z. -Z., Berta, T., & Ji, R. -R. (2013b). Resolvin E1 inhibits neuropathic pain and spinal cord microglial activation following peripheral nerve injury. *Journal of Neuroimmune Pharmacology: The Official Journal of the Society on NeuroImmune Pharmacology*, *8*(1), 37–41.
Yu, C. -Z., Liu, Y. -P., Liu, S., Yan, M., Hu, S. -J., & Song, X. -J. (2014). Systematic administration of B vitamins attenuates neuropathic hyperalgesia and reduces spinal neuron injury following temporary spinal cord ischaemia in rats. *European Journal of Pain*, *18*(1), 76–85.
Zhang, M., Han, W., Hu, S., & Xu, H. (2013). Methylcobalamin: a potential vitamin of pain killer. *Neural Plasticity*, *2013*, 424651.
Zhang, M., Han, W., Zheng, J., Meng, F., Jiao, X., Hu, S., & Xu, H. (2015). Inhibition of hyperpolarization-activated cation current in medium-sized drg neurons contributed to the antiallodynic effect of methylcobalamin in the rat of a chronic compression of the DRG. *Neural Plasticity*, *2015*, 197392.
Zheng, H., Xiao, W. H., & Bennett, G. J. (2011). Functional deficits in peripheral nerve mitochondria in rats with paclitaxel- and oxaliplatin-evoked painful peripheral neuropathy. *Experimental Neurology*, *232*(2), 154–161.
Zheng, H., Xiao, W. H., & Bennett, G. J. (2012). Mitotoxicity and bortezomib-induced chronic painful peripheral neuropathy. *Experimental Neurology*, *238*(2), 225–234.

CHAPTER

3

Migraine: Burden of Disease, Treatment, and Prevention

N.N. Bray, H. Katz

Broward Health Medical Center, Fort Lauderdale, FL, United States

INTRODUCTION

Headaches are a very common complaint seen by primary care physicians and neurologists. Migraines are the second most common primary headache disorder and accounts for 16% of all primary headaches (Bray, Health, & Militello, 2013). Migraine symptoms are usually gradual onset, crescendo pattern with complete resolution, unilateral, and pulsatile with associated symptoms of light (photophobia) and sound intolerance (phonophobia) and nausea (Bray et al., 2013). Migraines can last between 4 and 72 h with a mean duration of 24 h. Migraines can cause severe impairment requiring bed rest and an inability to function (Bray et al., 2013). Approximately 25% of migraine patients have headaches one or more times per week (Lipton, Stewart, Diamond, Diamond, & Reed, 2001) and 62.7% of patients had headaches more than once per month (Lipton et al., 2007). The severe nature of this headache disorder can lead to lower quality of life, decreased work production and thus lower income and social status (Zheng et al., 2015). It is important to understand the implications of this disease process as migraines and its associated symptoms cost approximately $24 billion annually (Evans et al., 2015).

CLINICAL PRESENTATION OF MIGRAINE

Migraines have been divided into migraine with aura (classic or neurologic migraine) and migraine without aura (common migraine) by the International Headache Society, Table 3.1. While only 20% of migraine sufferers experience an aura prior to headache onset, 60–70% of migraine sufferers report a prodrome (Lipton et al., 2001). Prodrome, as opposed to auras, occur up to 24 h before the headache and can consist of a feeling of euphoria, depression, fatigue, hypomania, food cravings, dizziness, cognitive slowing, or asthenia (Bray et al., 2013). Auras occur minutes to hours prior to headache onset and most often consist of visual disturbance (in over 90% or patients), particularly hemianopic field defects and scotomas (blind spots) and scintillations (flickering) that enlarge and spread peripherally (Dodick, 2006). Other aura symptoms can include sensory disorders (pins and needles and/or numbness), speech disorders, and motor weakness (hemiplegic migraine) (IHS, 2013). Other common presenting symptoms include pulsatile pain (85%), photophobia (80%), phonophobia (76%), nausea (73%), and unilateral pain (60%) (Lipton et al., 2001).

In the evaluation of patient presenting with headache it is important to differentiate the patient with migraine from patients with other primary headache syndromes and secondary headaches. It is critical to eliminate secondary headaches from the differential for a patient over the age of 50 who presents for evaluation of a new headache. Other symptoms that suggest a secondary cause of headache include a change in intensity, frequency, or pattern of headache, daily or continuous headache, positional headache, exertional headache, headache upon awakening from sleep, headache refractory to previously effective treatment, jaw pain, history of head trauma, sensory or motor symptoms inconsistent with previous aura, or sudden onset of severe pain (worst headache of life) (Forde, Druarte, & Rosen, 2016). Serious secondary causes of headache include subarachnoid hemorrhage, acute or chronic subdural hematoma, meningitis,

Nutritional Modulators of Pain in the Aging Population. http://dx.doi.org/10.1016/B978-0-12-805186-3.00003-5
Copyright © 2017 Elsevier Inc. All rights reserved.

TABLE 3.1 Diagnostic Criteria for Migraine Disorders (IHS, 2013)

Classification	Diagnosis criteria

Migraine without aura	At least five attacks fulfilling the following criteria:
	• Headache attacks lasting 4–72 h (untreated or unsuccessfully treated)[a]
	• Headache has at least two of the following characteristics:
	  • unilateral location
	  • pulsating quality;
	  • moderate or severe pain intensity
	  • aggravation by or causing avoidance of routine physical activity
	• During headache at least one of the following:
	  • nausea and/or vomiting
	  • photophobia and/or phonophobia
	• Not attributed to another disorder

Migraine with aura typical aura	At least two attacks fulfilling the following criteria:
	• One or more of the following fully reversible aura symptoms:
	  • visual
	  • sensory
	  • speech and/or language
	    - excludes any motor, brainstem, and/or retina symptoms
	• At least two of the following four characteristics:
	  • At least one aura symptom spreads gradually over 5 min and/or two or more symptoms occur in succession.
	  • Each individual aura symptoms lasts 5–60 min.[b]
	  • At least one aura symptoms is unilateral.
	  • The aura is accompanied, or followed within 60 min by headache.
	• Not attributed to another disorder (transient ischemic attack has been excluded)

Migraine with aura brainstem aura	At least two attacks fulfilling the following criteria:
	• One or more of the following fully reversible aura symptoms:
	  • visual
	  • sensory
	  • speech and/or language
	    - Excludes any motor and/or retina symptoms
	• Aura consisting of at least two of the following brainstem symptoms:
	  • dysarthria
	  • vertigo
	  • tinnitus
	  • hypacusis
	  • diplopia
	  • ataxia
	  • diminished level of consciousness
	• At least two of the following:
	  • At least one aura develops gradually over ≥5 min and/or two or more aura symptoms occur in succession.
	  • Each aura symptom lasts ≥5 min–≤60 min.
	  • At least one aura symptoms is unilateral.
	  • The aura is accompanied, or followed within 60 min, by headache.
	• Not attributed to another disorder (transient ischemic attack has been excluded)

Migraine with aura hemiplegic migraine	At least two attacks fulfilling the following criteria:[c]
	• Aura consisting of both of the following:
	  • fully reversible motor weakness
	  • fully reversible visual, sensory, and/or speech/language symptoms
	• At least two of the following:
	  • at least one aura symptom develops gradually over ≥5 min and/or different aura symptoms occur in succession over ≥5 min
	  • each nonmotor symptoms lasts ≥5 min and ≤60 min, and motor symptoms last <72 h
	  • At least one aura symptoms is unilateral
	  • the aura is accompanied, or followed within 60 min, by headache
	• Not attributed to another disorder (transient ischemic attack and stroke has been excluded)

Chronic migraine	• Headache ≥15 days per month for ≥3 months • Occurring in a patient who has at least five attacks of migraine without aura or migraine with aura • Headache ≥8 days per month for ≥3 months: criteria for migraine without aura or migraine with aura are met and/or the headache is treated and relieved by triptan(s) or ergot • Not attributed to another disorder (there is no medication overuse or secondary cause)
Medication-overuse headache	• Headache ≥15 days per month in a patient with a preexisting headache disorder • Regular overuse for > 3 months of one or drugs that can be taken for acute and/or symptomatic treatment of headache • Not attributed to another disorder

[a] *In children <18 years of age, attacks may last 2–72 h.*
[b] *If there are three different aura symptoms, the maximum duration would be 3 × 60 min. Motor aura can last up to 72 h.*
[c] *Familial hemiplegic migraine meets above criteria and patient has at least one first- or second-degree relative has hemiplegic migraine. Termed sporadic hemiplegic migraine if no first- or second-degree relative effected.*

TABLE 3.2 Indication for Neuroimaging in Headache Patients (Scottish Intercollegiate Guidelines Network, 2008)

Nonacute headache	New-onset or acute headache
Abnormal findings on neurologic examination Focal neurologic symptoms (limb weakness, aura <5 min or >60 min) Non focal neurologic findings (Cognitive disturbance)	Sudden onset severe headache (thunderclap headache)
Change in headache frequency, characteristics, or associated symptoms	New onset in patient age >50
Headache that changes with posture	Fever
Headache exacerbated by exertion or valsalva	Neck stiffness
Headache that wakes the patient up from sleep	New onset of headache in patient with a history of human immunodeficiency virus (HIV) infection
Headache that do not meet migraine or other primary headache disorder diagnostic criteria	New onset of headache in patient with a history of cancer
Patient with risk factors for cerebral venous sinus thrombosis	
Jaw claudication or visual disturbance (new)	

encephalitis, intracranial neoplasm, benign intracranial hypertension, giant cell arteritis, acute sever hypertension, carbon monoxide poisoning, acute glaucoma, and carotid dissection. While neuroimaging is not indicated for patients with stable headaches who meet diagnostic criteria for migraines, Table 3.2 provides indications for neuroimaging in patients being evaluated for headache.

PREVALENCE AND DISEASE BURDEN

Migraine is a highly prevalent and largely familiar disorder that often begin in childhood, adolescence, or early adulthood and recur with diminishing frequency during advancing years (Lipton et al., 2007). The World Health Organization estimates migraine headache as the third most common disease in the world (behind dental caries and tension-type headaches) in both males and females (Steiner et al., 2013).

According to the American Migraine Prevalence and Prevention study, 17% of women and 6% of men have migraines. It is more commonly seen in women than men and in whites greater than blacks. The peak incidence of occurrence of migraines is between 30 and 39 years old. People (75%) with migraines have decreased ability to function and 33% require bed rest. Both episodic and chronic migraine headaches are associated with lower quality of life, lower work productivity leading to lower incomes, social status, and worse emotional well-being (Zheng et al., 2015). On the basis of disability, migraine was ranked seventh highest among causes of global disability responsible for 2.9% of all years of life lost to disability (Steiner et al., 2013).

The mean annual cost of care per migraine patient in the United States is $611 (Hu, Markson, Lipton, Stewart, & Berger, 1999). This accounts for $1 billion in direct medical cost and $16 billion in lost productivity each year (Jackson et al., 2015). More recent studies has estimated that the total annual cost of headache therapy for adults (age 18–65) in the European Union is €173 billion, with migraine headaches accounting for €111 billion (Linde et al., 2012). This large economic burden combined with morbidity of disease position migraine headaches as a global public health challenge.

PATHOPHYSIOLOGY OF MIGRAINES

The pathophysiology of migraines is a complex system that involves not only afferent input but modulation by different areas of the brainstem and diencephalic structures and sensitization of the dural vasculature (Bernstein & Burstein, 2012; Akerman, Holland, & Goadsby, 2011). Headaches are caused by activation of the primary afferent fibers that supply mainly meningeal and cerebral blood vessels (Cecil). According to Estemalik & Tepper, 2013, the site of initiation of attacks remains debatable. The two leading theories involve cortical spreading depression (CSD) or a brainstem generator. CSD consists of cortical neuronal activation, followed by a postictal depression of neuronal firing. In contrast to the spreading oligemia of migraine with aura, regional cerebral blood flow imaging has failed to demonstrate changes supporting the theory of CSD in patients with migraine without aura (IHS, 2013). There is literature that supports the concept of glial waves or other cortical events involving the messenger molecules of nitric oxide (NO), 5-hydroxytrptamine (5-HT) and calcitonin gene-related peptide (CGRP) may be involved in migraine without aura (IHS, 2013).

Although the pain associated with migraine was previously contributed to vascular etiologies, the importance of sanitization of pain pathways has been gained increased attention. Meningeal pain mechanisms that

TABLE 3.3 Effect of Dietary Substance on Migraine Headache

Substance	Food	Mechanism of action
Nitrates and nitrites	Preservative used in food coloring, prevention of botulism, and to add a cured or smoked flavor	Release of NO and subsequent vasodilation
Monosodium glutamate	Flavor enhancer widely used in Chinese food, meat tenderizer, and many canned, packaged[a] and prepared foods	Unknown Theories—direct vasoconstrictor effect (high-dose), stimulatory glutamate receptor agonist, or activation of neurotransmission pathway (NO released in endothelial cells leading to vasodilation)
Aspartame	Artificial sweetener (NutraSweet)	Unknown
Tyramine	Aged cheese, cured meats, smoked fish, beer, fermented food, yeast extract	Release of norepinephrine from sympathetic nerve terminals
Phenylethylamine	Cacao	Release of vasoactive amines (serotonin and catecholamine)
Caffeine	Coffee, tea, soda, chocolate Prescription medicationsfioricet, fiorinal, esgic Over-the-counter medication—Excedrin, Anacin	Blockage of inhibitory and excitatory adenosine receptors in the brain and vasculature, resulting in vasoconstriction and release of excitatory neurotransmitters.

[a]Packaged as "hydrolyzed vegetable protein," "autolyzed yeast," "sodium caseinate," "yeast extract," "hydrolyzed oat flour," "texturized protein," or "calcium casinate."
(Sun-Edelstein & Mauskop, 2009)

release inflammatory cytokines, neuroinflammatory peptides, and calcitonin gene related peptide (CGRP), causing cerebral vasodilation start at the trigeminovascular sensory fibers via the trigeminal ganglion to the trigeminal nucleus caudalis in the medullary spinal cord (Estemalik & Tepper, 2013). From the trigeminocervical complex (TCC) these neurons project in the quintothalmic tract and after decussating in the brainstem, synapse on neurons in the thalamus. Important modulation of the trigeminovascular nociceptive input comes from the dorsal raphe nucleus, locus coeruleus, and nucleus raphe magnus (Goadsby, Charbit, Andreou, Akerman, & Holland, 2009). The important role of the trigeminocervial complex in migraine pathophysiology serve as a target for many therapeutic interventions.

TRIGGERS OF MIGRAINES

The brain of patients who suffer from migraines are particularly sensitive to environmental and sensory stimuli. This sensitivity is amplified by females during the menstrual cycle. Migraine triggers are factors that temporarily increase the probability that a migraine headache will develop. Migraines can be triggered or amplified by many things including hunger, dietary, environment, stress, and lack of sleep. The mean number of triggers identified by individual patients with migraine is approximately six (Kelman, 2007). The five most common triggers identified by migraine patients are stress, missing meals or fasting, weather change, under sleeping, and in women, hormonal changes (Kelman, 2007).

Diet

Approximately, one third of migraine sufferers, identify dietary triggers. The mechanism of this trigger is felt to involve chemical sensitivities or pharmacologic effect, but there is some new literature that suggests the possibility of an IgG mediated mechanism (Alpay et al., 2010). Food triggers vary widely between patients. Patients with migraines do not need to avoid all potential triggers but need to work with their providers to identify their individual triggers. Food diaries can be helpful in sorting out which foods are problematic for each patient, however, this is complicated by the fact that food triggers can occur up to 24 h after exposure and exposure does not always equate to the development of a migraine (Sun-Edelstein & Mauskop, 2009).

Common foods implicated include chocolate, aged cheeses, and alcohol. Chemicals found in food that are commonly cited include nitrates and nitrites, monosodium glutamate, aspartame, tyramine, phenythylamine, histamine, phenolic flavonoids, alcohol, and caffeine (Sun-Edelstein & Mauskop, 2009). See Table 3.3 for description of proposed mechanism of action of dietary compounds in headache pathophysiology.

Headaches associated with alcohol can be due either to the acute ingestion or the post ingestion, alcohol hangover headache (AHH). Wine contains tyramine, sulfites, histamine, and phenolic flavonoids all of which have been reported as independent triggers of migraines. AHH commonly occurs after the consumption of a large amount of alcohol; however, it is not always dose-related and occurs more commonly in light or moderate drinkers than in regular heavy drinkers. Dark colored alcoholic

TABLE 3.4 Lifestyle Modifications for Migraine Management (Forde et al., 2016; Becker, 2012)

Lifestyle modifications for migraine management	
Sleep hygiene	Appropriate duration of sleep Regular pattern of sleep
Eat regular meals	Hunger (likely via low blood sugar) can trigger headaches Avoid dehydration
Exercise	Regular exerciseimproves stress and physical fitness
Stress management	Excess stress may trigger migraine attacks Relaxation techniques may reduce headache frequency
Limit caffeine	Caffeine can trigger headache and disrupt sleep Caffeine withdrawal can trigger headaches

beverages, such as red wine, whiskey, and bourbon contain congeners, a natural byproduct of alcohol fermentation, and have a higher association with AHH. There are several theories for the mechanism of AHH that include vasodilation of the intracranial vasculature, disruption of sleep patterns, inflammation due to alteration of cytokine pathways and prostaglandin release, and/or magnesium depletion (Sun-Edelstein & Mauskop, 2009).

Environment

Environmental triggers include changes to weather and climate, glare, bright lights, sounds, and strong odors or perfumes.

Other

Physical exertion, stress, hormonal fluctuations associated with menstruation, irregular sleep patterns, and irregular eating can also trigger migraines.

MIGRAINE THERAPY

Treatment of headaches is divided into abortive therapy aimed at treatment of an acute headache or prophylactic treatment aimed at reducing the frequency and severity of future headaches (Jackson et al., 2015). There are many ways to prevent and treat migraines including pharmacologic agents, supplements, manual, and alternative therapies. Patients play a key role in management of this disease. Use of headache journals can help patients and providers identify lifestyle effects and triggers of migraine headaches. Regardless of treatment modalities utilized, lifestyle modification, and trigger management are critical to the successful management of patients with migraines (Martin, 2010).

Lifestyle Modifications

The goal of patient engagement in the treatment of migraine headaches is to assist patients in developing the needed skills and knowledge to effectively manage their disease. It is important for patients to have proper understanding of the role of acute abortive therapy and prophylactic medications and when to employ each type of therapy. The goal of migraine preventive (prophylactic therapy) is to decrease the frequency and severity of headache attacks by 50% (Bray et al., 2013). Patients should be counseled on the importance of sleep hygiene, a regular exercise program, eating regular meals, limitation of caffeine intake, and the importance of stress management (Forde et al., 2016). Table 3.4 provides an overview of lifestyle modification in the management of migraine headaches.

Acute Abortive Therapy

The goal of acute treatment of migraines is designed to relieve the pain and associated symptoms in a rapid fashion with minimum need for back-up medications (opioids or butalitol). These medications should be easy for self-administration, be cost-effective and have minimum to no side effects. Abortive treatment should be initiated as soon as an aura, prodorome, or pain is noted, ideally within 2 h. The American College of Neurology via the 2000 US Headache Consortium Guidelines recommends NSAIDs as first line abortive treatments for migraines because they are safe, available, tolerable, and have a low side effect profile (Silberstein, 2000). Triptans are recommended as first-line for patients with severe migraine symptoms or patients with a history of migraines refractory to NSAID therapy.

A wide variety of other nonmigraine-specific medications have been used for the management of acute migraines. Antiemetic medications, metoclopramide IV, and prochlorperazine IV/IM/PR, may provide migraine relief in some patients (Grade B) (Silberstein, 2000). There are no randomized, placebo-controlled studies that support the use of butalbital-containing agents in the treatment of acute migraine headaches; caution should be exercised in their use due to concerns over medication-overuse headaches and withdrawal (Silberstein, 2000).

Migraine-Specific Therapy

Migraine-specific medications include triptans and dihydroergotamin (DHE). Triptans, HT1B/1D receptor agonists are also potent 5-HT1F receptor agonists. 5-HT1F activation inhibits trigeminal nucleus fos activation and neuronal firing in response to dural stimulation thus aborting the headache. Triptans are available in oral, nasal sprays and subcutaneous dosing. There is a large body of literature supporting the use of triptans in the management of migraine headaches (Silberstein et al., 2012). This class of medication provides migraine suffers with a quick and effective treatment modality with a minimal side-effect profile (Bray et al., 2013). Physicians should avoid prescribing triptans to patients with uncontrolled hypertension, ischemic heart disease, history of stroke, and during pregnancy. Caution should be exercised in the use of triptan medication in patients with hemiplegic migraine, migraine with prolonged aura, or migrinous infarction. The concomitant use of triptans with other serotonergic medications (monoamine oxidase inhibitors, ergotamine, serotonin reuptake inhibitors) increases the risk of serotonin syndrome. Dihydroergotamine therapy is a potent cranial and peripheral constrictor to counter act the cerebral vasodilation that occurs during migraines (Bray et al., 2013). DHE is available in IV, intramuscular, subcutaneous, and intranasal forms and is effective in patients with moderate to severe migraine and patients who are unable to take oral medications (Freitag & Schloemer, 2014).

In patients requiring the use of acute abortive medications more than two times per week need to be evaluated for the use of prophylactic therapy due to the risk of conversion to medication-overuse headache (Snow, Weiss, Wall, & Mottur-Pilson, 2002).

Prophylactic Therapy

The goal of initiating a pharmacologic agent to prevent lower morbidity suffered by migraine patients is to reduce the severity and frequency of headache by 50%. Other goals of therapy include improve responsiveness to treatment of acute attacks, prevent progression or transformation of episodic migraine to chronic migraine and to reduce the risk of neurologic damage in patients with uncommon migraine conditions (Silberstein, 2000). Despite evidence of decreased morbidity associated with migraines, it is estimated that nearly half of males and a third of females who meet treatment criteria for migraine prophylaxis are not receiving it (Jackson et al., 2015). All migraine management plans should include limiting patient-specific triggers, as well as patient education related to their condition and available treatment options. Patients should be placed on preventive therapy who, have six or more migraine days per month, impairment associated with four or more headache days per month, or sever impairment or need for bed rest three or more headache days per month. Preventive therapy is not indicated in patients with migraine patients with less than 4 days of headache per month and no impairment or less than one headache per month regardless of impairment (Lipton et al., 2007). Other patients who will benefit from prophylaxis therapy include patients with contraindications to or failure of abortive therapy, the use of abortive medication more than twice per week, the presence of uncommon migraine conditions (hemiplegic migraine, migraine with prolonged aura, or migrinous infarction) (Snow et al., 2002).

According to the FDA, pharmacologic agents that prevent migraines include propranalol, timolol, valproate, and topiramate (Estemalik & Tepper, 2013). Beta Blockers, such as propranolol and timolol work by reducing the adrenergic tone and reduces the activity at the level of the adrenergic locus ceruleus. Valproate works by increasing GABA in the brain and thus suppresses neurogenic inflammation. Topiramate blocks calcium and sodium channels and inhibits excitatory glutamatergic receptors and enhances GABA inhibitor activity. Topiramate also inhibits central activation of trigeminal nucleus caudalis and upper spinal cord (Estemalik & Tepper, 2013). Histamine has also been shown to reduce migraines (Estemalik & Tepper, 2013; Holland et al., 2012). The 2012 guidelines did not find sufficient evidence to support the use of daily NSAID or montelukast the prevention of migraine headaches (Estemalik & Tepper, 2013).

Selection of prophylactic treatment should be individualized to the patient based on the individual patient characteristics, comorbidities, medication costs, side effects, and contraindications. A large metaanalysis attempted to compare the efficacy and side effects of prophylactic treatment of migraine headaches in adults using oral pharmacological medications (Jackson et al., 2015). The metaanalysis concluded that there is good evidence supporting the use of propranolol, timolol, valproate, and topiramate. In contrast to the 2012 guidelines from the AAN/AHS that stated Amitriptyline is not an effective medication for migraine prevention, the study concluded that Amitriptyline had the greatest benefit in preventing migraine headaches. They do note that this has not been supported in direct comparison trials (including SSRI, topiramate, and propranolol) (Jackson et al., 2015). Table 3.5 outlines available medications for migraine prophylaxis including the level of evidence supporting their use (Silberstein et al., 2012).

Patient's comorbid medical and psychiatric diagnosis, as well as the medication side effects should be taking into account when choosing a migraine prophylactic medication. Patients should be counseled at the time of initiation of prophylactic medication that the goal is to decrease the frequency and severity of headaches that they suffer by 50% and to improve responsiveness to

TABLE 3.5 Prophylactic Medication for Migraine Management

Medication	Class	Level of evidence[a]	Dose range (mg/day)	Notes
Metoprolol	β-Blockers	A	50–200 (divide dose BID)	Adverse effect: dizziness, fatigue, depression
Propanolol[b]		A	80–240 (divide dose BID)	Avoid in patients with: erectile dysfunction, peripheral vascular disease, Raynaud phenomenon, bradycardia, hypotension
Timolol[b]		A	10–30 (divide dose BID)	Use with caution: asthma, diabetes mellitus, depression, patient age >60, smokers
Atenolol		B	25–150	
Nadolol		B	20–240	
Verapamil	Calcium channel blockers	U	120–240 (divide dose TID)	Tolerance may develop. Minimize by increasing dose or switching to a different calcium channel blocker
Lisinopril	ACE inhibitor	C	10–60	
Candesartan	Angiotensin inhibitor	C	16	
Clonidine	Alpha blocker	C		
Divalproex sodium	Antiepileptic medications	A	250–1500	Common adverse effects: weight gain, hair loss, somnolence, tremor, and teratogenic potential (pregnancy category D)
Sodium valproate[b]		A		
Topiramate[b]		A	25–150	Common side effects: paresthesia, tiredness, GI disturbance, teratogenic potential (pregnancy category D)
Amitriptyline	Tricyclic antidepressants	B	10–150	Side effect: weight gain, sedating, dry mouth, constipation, tachycardia, palpitations, orthostatic hypotension, blurred vision, urinary retention (Pringsheim et al., 2012)
Venlafaxine	SSNRI	B	37.5–150	Consider in patients with panic disorder, generalized anxiety disorder or social anxiety disorder (Banzi et al., 2015)
Frovatriptan	Triptan	A		Short-term prophylaxis of menstrual migraines
Naratriptan	Triptan	B		
Zolmitriptan	Triptan	B		

[a]*Silberstein et al. (2012).*
[b]*FDA approved for the prevention of migraine headaches: Level A, medications with established efficacy (>2 class I trials); Level B, medications are probably effective (1 class I or 2 class II studies); Level C, medications are possible effective (1 class II study); Level U, inadequate or conflicting data to support or refute medication use.*

treatment of acute attacks. To avoid side effects, medications initiated for migraine prevention should be started with a low dose and the dose titrated up slowly every 2–4 weeks. Medications should be given a 2–3 months trial at optimal dose to establish efficacy prior to changing prophylactic medications (Rizzoli, 2014). Patients should be encouraged to keep a headache journal to monitor the frequency and severity of headaches, as well as the need for acute abortive therapy.

The Role of Onabotulinum Toxin a in Migraine Therapy

Onabotulinum toxin type A (Botox) dosed every 12 weeks received FDA approval for the treatment of chronic migraine in October of 2010. Chronic migraine is defined as greater than 15 headache days a month for more than 3 months and at least 8 of these days have migraine features. The proposed mechanism of action includes regulation of pain pathways via inhibition of release of substance P, glutamate, and CGRP. It is theorized that that the inhibition of neuropeptide and neurotransmitter release from the peripheral trigeminal sensory system mitigates the sensitization process (Forde et al., 2016).

The Role of Supplements in Migraine Therapy

The utilization of complementary and alternative medicine (CAM) has increased in the United States. In 2007, it was estimated that Americans spent $34 billion (11.2%) out-of-pocket for CAM treatments (Barnes, Bloom, & Naheen, 2008). The role of supplements in prophylactic migraine management has been widely studied.

Supplements including butterbur, coenzyme Q_{10}, magnesium oxide, riboflavin, and alphalipoic acid, are used to decrease the amount of migraine attacks (Schiapparelli et al., 2010). The quality of the studies used to support their use varies from large randomized double-blind placebo controlled studies to observational cohort studies. Butterbur (*Petasites hybridus*), a perennial waterside plant, decreases the frequency of migraine attacks. People who used Butterbur had improvement of symptoms by >50% over 3–4 months (Holland et al., 2012). Butterbur is thought to act via calcium channel regulation and inhibition of leukotriene synthesis, which are released in migraines inflammation (Estemalik & Tepper, 2013) and also inhibits cycloxygenase 2, which is found in the inflammatory cascade (Orr, 2015). The butterbur plant contains hepatotoxic and carcinogenic compounds, pyrrolizidine alkaloids that are removed in the commercially available preparations, such as Petadolex. Treatment at a dose of either 50 or 75 mg twice daily was well tolerated in clinical trials with only reports of mild gastrointestinal upset (Sun-Edelstein & Mauskop, 2009).

Postmarketing surveillance in Europe of Petadolex has revealed cases of hepatotoxicity and has led to the Swiss Agency for Therapeutic Products and German Federal Institute of Medical Devices has banned its use (Prieto, 2014). Butterbur should be avoided during pregnancy due to concern over it being teratogenic (Loder, 2007).

Magnesium is an essential cation and is important in many physiologic functions in the body. Studies of patients with migraines have demonstrated low magnesium levels during acute attacks (Ramadan, Halvorson, & Vande-Linde, 1989). Possible mechanism of action in migraine pathogenesis may include counteracting vasospasm, inhibiting platelet aggregation, and stabilization of cell membranes.

Magnesium concentration has been demonstrated to influence vascular tone, as well as serotonin receptors, NO synthesis and release, inflammatory mediators, and various other endogenous hormones and neurotransmitters (Bianchi et al., 2004). Low magnesium increases glutamate activity and CSD thus magnesium blocks glutamate activity and thus prevents cortical spreading (Holland et al., 2012).

Study results on role of magnesium in the treatment and prevention of migraine have been mixed. Two double-blind, placebo controlled trials have shown that oral magnesium supplementation is effective in the prevention of headaches (Facchinetti, Snaces, Borella, Genazzani, & Nappi, 1991; Peikart, Wilimzig, & Kohne-Volland, 1996) and a third study was negative (Pfaffenrath et al., 1996). The study by Pfaffenrath had a high discontinuation rate of the oral magnesium salt due to diarrhea. In patients with low ionized magnesium levels, intravenous magnesium has been shown to be effective in acute symptom management (Mauskop et al., 1995).

Feverfew is an herbal preparation, that is, the dread leaves of the weed plant tanacetum pathenium. Parthenolides within the leaves is believed to inhibit serotonin release from platelets and white blood cells and inhibit platelet aggregation. Inhibition of prostaglandin synthesis and phospholipase A may account for the observed anti-inflammatory activity (Sun-Edelstein & Mauskop, 2009). MIG-99 is a more stable feverfew extract has been studied in a total of seven studies. Six studies have demonstrated that feverfew (either alone or in combination with other treatment modalities) had a reduction in number of migraine attacks per month. Most common side effects include gastrointestinal system disorder or respiratory system disorder (Holland et al., 2012).

Riboflavin, vitamin B2, at a dose of 400 mg daily for 3 months has been shown to reduce attacks by 50% in 59% of patients receiving it (Schiapparelli et al., 2010; Holland et al., 2012). Riboflavin, a precursor for flavin mononucleotides, are essential for membrane stability and energy-related cellular functions (Evans & Taylor, 2006). Adverse effects associated with riboflavin supplementation were minor and included diarrhea and polyuria. Riboflavin supplementation is thought to reduce migraines due to augmentation of the activity of mitochondrial complexes and mitochondrial dysfunction plays a role in migraine pathophysiology.

Histamine has been studied in three single-center trials demonstrating a statistically significant reduction in migraine frequency, severity, and duration with subcutaneous injection twice weekly. Adverse effect include, transient itching at the injection site (Holland et al., 2012).

Coenzyme Q_{10} (CoQ_{10}), has been shown to significantly decrease attack frequency, headache days, and days with nausea (Schiapparelli et al., 2010; Holland et al., 2012). CoQ_{10} is an endogenous enzyme cofactor made by all cells in the body. Its primary role is to promote mitochondrial proton–electron translocation (Sun-Edelstein & Mauskop, 2009). Adverse effects reported at low rates in clinical trials included gastrointestinal disturbances and cutaneous allergy (Sun-Edelstein & Mauskop, 2009).

Finally, Alpha lipoic also has proved to cause a significant reduction in attack frequency, headache days, and headache severity (Schiapparelli et al., 2010). Alpha lipoic acid enhances mitochondrial oxygen metabolism and ATP production, similar to riboflavin and CoQ_{10}. While there was a clear trend for reduction in migraine frequency after treatment at 600 mg of alpha lipoic acid daily for 3 months, the only published randomized, placebo-controlled study did not have significant results (Magis et al., 2007).

In 2012, The American Academy of Neurology (ANN) concluded that Petasites (butterbur) is effective for migraine prophylactic based on level A evidence (Holland et al., 2012). However, postmarketing reports have revealed cases of hepatotoxicity. MIIG-99 (feverfew), riboflavin, magnesium, and histamine SC are probably effective for migraine prophylactic based on level B evidence (Holland et al., 2012). Co-Q_{10} and estrogen are possibly effective and may be considered for migraine prevention based on level C evidence (Holland et al., 2012).

The Role of Behavioral Therapy in Migraine Therapy

Medications are not the only options to reduce headaches. Behavioral treatment to include relaxation training, thermal biofeedback with relaxation training, EMG biofeedback, and cognitive behavioral therapy have been shown to reduce migraine frequency and may be considered as treatment options for migraines (Campbell, Penzien, & Wall, 2000). Despite having Grade A recommendation, specific recommendations regarding which of these to use for specific patients cannot be made. The combination of preventive drug therapy with behavioral therapy (relaxation or biofeedback) may achieve additional clinical improvement for migraine relief.

There is limited evidence to support the use of hypnosis, acupuncture, TENS, cervical manipulation, occlusal adjustment, and hyperbaric oxygen as preventive or acute therapy for migraine (Campbell et al., 2000).

Relaxation training to include progressive muscle relaxation, autogenic training, and meditation or passive relaxation were analyzed in a metaanalysis that revealed a 32% improvement in headache frequency (Campbell et al., 2000). Thermal biofeedback training showed an average of 37% improvement in headache activity. Studies evaluating combination of relaxation training and thermal biofeedback found a mean average improvement of 33% in headache activity (Campbell et al., 2000).

The Role of Alternative Therapies in Migraine Therapy

Alternative therapies including acupuncture and osteopathic manipulation have been shown to lead to fewer headaches. Acupuncture has been shown to have higher response rates and fewer headaches and was associated with better outcomes than prophylactic medicine (Da Silva, 2015; Zheng et al., 2015; Schiapparelli et al., 2010). Acupuncture is one of the main treatment modalities of traditional Chinese medicine and is one of the most commonly used complementary therapies. A 2001 Cochrane review on idiopathic headache judged acupuncture effective in a preventive therapy for migraine headaches, however, effectiveness in treatment for acute headache was unable to be determined due to methodological errors in the included studies (Melchart et al., 2001). Subsequent to that publication, several large and strictly controlled trials have occurred and an updated Cochrane review was published in 2009 that included 22 randomized controlled trails. The 2009 Cochrane review looked at the efficacy of acupuncture in migraine prophylaxis with one of three controlled interventions: acupuncture versus no prophylactic treatment or routine care only; acupuncture versus "sham" (placebo) acupuncture; acupuncture versus pharmacological prophylaxis. Based on this review, the authors concluded that "acupuncture should be considered as a treatment option for migraine patients needing prophylactic treatment due to frequent or insufficiently controlled migraine attacks, particularly in patients refusing prophylactic drug treatment or experiencing adverse effect from such treatments" (Linde et al., 2009).

Multiple small studies have evaluated the role of Osteopathic manipulative therapy (OMT) and spinal manipulative therapy (SMT) in the treatment and prevention of migraines. The study results are mixed (Bray et al., 2013). A randomized controlled trial of 42 female patient with migraines demonstrated patient in the OMT treatment group decreases pain intensity, reduces number of migraines and improved health related quality of life (Voigt et al., 2001). Additional studies have demonstrated that OMT therapy resulted in a reduction in cost of care per patient and when SMT was combined with amitriptyline a reduction in headache index (Schabert & Crow, 2009; Keays, Neher, Safranek, & Webb, 2008).

The Role of Diet in Migraine Therapy

Finally, diet plays a significant role in migraines and thus adjusting ones diet can be used to prevent and treat migraines. Given the inflammatory processes underlying migraines both metabolic abnormalities and food allergies are implicated in migraines (Evans & Taylor, 2006). The Elimination diet has proven to be affective. The elimination diet rids a person from eating any foods that have IgG antibodies to food antigens since IgG antibodies against food antigens correlate with inflammation(Orr, 2015; Alpay et al., 2010). Decreased sodium intake has also been effective at preventing migraines. Orr et al., shows that a low sodium diet leads to a decrease in headache in the last 7 days of the low sodium diet. Less proinflammatory Omega 6 fatty acids and more antiinflammatory Omega 3 fatty acids should be use to prevent headaches (Evans & Taylor, 2006). High Omega 3 and low Omega 6 fatty acids had a greater impact on headaches than just low Omega 6 fatty acids alone (Orr, 2015). Low fat diets also play a role in reducing migraines as it decreases prostaglandin synthesis, decreases headache frequency and intensity. As previously reviewed avoidance of food triggers is also important including monosodium glutamate, chocolate, aspartame, and alcohol intake.

CONCLUSIONS

Migraine headache is a complicated disorder with a high burden of disease and morbidity for patients who experience this disorder. The approach to care for these patients should be multifaceted with attention to both prevention via avoidance of triggers, lifestyle modifications to minimize suffering, management of acute headaches, as well as prevention of headaches. There are a wide number of medications, herbal preparations, behavioral, and manual medicine techniques that are supported to decrease the pain and frequency of episodes in patients who suffer from migraine headaches. The approach to these patients should be individualized based on patient-preference and comorbidities with a goal to minimize suffering and maximize function. With continued research into the pathophysiology of disease, the efficacy of different treatment modalities and the partnership between healthcare providers and patients, migraines will continue to become a manageable chronic medical condition.

References

Akerman, S., Holland, P. R., & Goadsby, P. J. (2011). Diencephalic and brainstem mechanisms in migraine. *Nature Reveiws Neuroscience, 12*(10), 570–584.

Alpay, K., Ertaş, M., Orhan, E. K., Üstay, D. K., Lieners, C., & Baykan, B. (2010). Diet restriction in migraine, based on IgG against foods: a clinical double-blind, randomised, cross-over trial. *Cephalalgia, 30*(7), 829–837.

Banzi, R., Cusi, C., Randazzo, C., Sterzi, R., Tedesco, D., & Moja, L. (2015). Selective serotonin reuptake inhibitors (SSRIs) and serotonin-norepinephrine reuptake inhibitors (SNRIs) for the prevention of migraine in adults. *Cochrane Database System Review, 4*.

Barnes, P. M., Bloom, B., & Nahin, R. L. (2008). Complementary and alternative medicine use among adults and children: United States, 2007. *National Health Statistical Report, 12*, 1–23.

Becker, W. J. (2012). Headache triggers, lifestyle factors, and behavioural therapies in migraine – appendix I. *Canadian Journal of Neurological Science, 39*(S2), S48–53.

Bernstein, C., & Burstein, R. (2012). Sensitization of the trigeminovascular pathway: perspective and implications to migraine pathophysiology. *Journal of Clinical Neurology (Seoul, Korea), 8*(2), 89–99.

Bianchi, A., Salomone, S., Caraci, F., Pizza, V., Bernardini, R., & D'Amato, C. C. (2004). Role of magnesium, coenzyme Q_{10}, riboflavin, and vitamin B12 in migraine prophylaxis. *Vitamins and Hormones, 69*, 297–312.

Bray, N., Heath, A., & Militello, J. (2013). Miraine: Burden of disease, treatment, and prevention. *Osteopathic Family Physician, 5*, 116–122.

Campbell, J. K., Penzien, D. B., Wall, E M. (2000). Evidence based guidelines for migraine headaches: Behavioral and physical treatments. US Headache Consortium. Available from: www.aan.com/public/practiceguidelines/headache

Da Silva, A. N. (2015). Acupuncture for migraine prevention. *Headache, 55*(3.), 470–473.

Dodick, D. W. (2006). Chronic daily headache. *New England Journal Medicine, 354*, 158–165.

Estemalik, E., & Tepper, S. (2013). Preventive treatment in migraine and the new US guidelines. *Neuropsychiatric Disease and Treatment, 9*, 709–720.

Evans, R. W., & Taylor, F. R. (2006). Expert opinion: "Natural" or alternative medications for migraine prevention. *Headache, 46*, 1012–1018.

Evans, E. W., Lipton, R. B., Peterlin, B. L., Raynor, H. A., Thomas, J. G., O'Leary, K. C., Pavlovic, J., Wing, R. R., & Bond, D. S. (2015). Dietary intake patterns and diet quality in a nationally representative sample of women with and without severe headache or migraine. *Headache, 55*(4), 550–561.

Facchinetti, F., Sances, G., Borella, P., Genazzani, A. R., & Nappi, G. (1991). Magnesium prophylaxis of menstrual migraine: effects of intracellular magnesium. *Headache, 31*, 298–301.

Forde, G., Durarte, R. A., & Rosen, N. (2016). Managing chronic headache disorders. *Medical Clinics of North America, 100*(1), 117–141.

Freitag, F. G., & Schloemer, F. (2014). Medical management of adult headache. *Otolaryngology Clinic North America, 47*, 221–237.

Goadsby, P. J., Charbit, A. R., Andreou, A. P., Akerman, S., & Holland, P. R. (2009). Neurobiology of migraine. *Neuroscience, 161*(2), 327–341.

Headache Classification Committee of the International Headache Society (IHS) (2013). The international classification of headache disorders, 3rd ed. (beta version). *Cephalgia, 33*(9), 629–808.

Holland, S., Silberstein, S. D., Freitag, F., Dodick, D. W., Argoff, C., & Ashman, E. (2012). Evidence-Based Guideline update: NSAIDs and other complementary treatments for episodic migraine prevention in adults. *Neurology, 78*, 1346–1353.

Hu, X. H., Markson, L. E., Lipton, R. B., Stewart, W. F., & Berger, M. L. (1999). Burden of migraine in the United States: disability and economic costs. *Archives of Internal Medicine, 159*, 813–818.

Jackson, J. L., Cogbill, E., Santana-Davila, R., Eldredge, C., Collier, W., et al. (2015). A comparative effectiveness meta-analysis of drugs for the prophylaxis of migraine headache. *PLoS One, 10*(7), e0130733.

Keays, A. C., Neher, J. O., Safranek, S., & Webb, C. W. (2008). Clinical inquiries. Is osteopathic manipulation effective for headaches? *Journal of Family Practice, 57*(3), 190–191.

Kelman, L. (2007). The triggers of precipitants of the acute migraine attack. *Cephalalgia, 27*(5), 394–402.

Linde, K., Allais, G., Brinkhaus, B., Manheimer, E., Vickers, A., & White, A. R. (2009). Acupuncture for migraine prophylaxis. *Cochrane Database Systems Review*,(1), .

Linde, M., Gustavsson, A., Stovner, L. J., Steiner, T. J., Barre, J., Katsarave, Z., Lainez, J. M., Lampl, C., Lanteri-Minet, M., Rastenvte, D., Ruiz de la Torre, E., Tassorelli, C., & Andree, C. (2012). The cost of headache disorders in Europe: the Eurolight project. *European Journal of Neurology, 19*(5), 703–711.

Lipton, R. B., Stewart, W. F., Diamond, S., Diamond, M. L., & Reed, M. (2001). Prevalence and burden of migraine in the United States: data from the American Migraine Study II. *Headache, 41*, 646–657.

Lipton, R. B., Bigal, M. E., Diamond, M., Freitag, F., Reed, M. L., & Stewart, W. F. AMPP Advisory Group. (2007). Migraine prevalence, disease burden, and the need for preventive therapy. *Neurology, 68*, 343–349.

Loder, E. (2007). Migraine in pregnancy. *Seminar of Neurology, 27*, 425–433.

Magis, D., Ambrosini, A., Sandor, P., Jacquy, J., Laloux, P., & Schoenen, I. (2007). A randomized double-blind placebo-controlled trial of thiocitic acid in migraine prophylaxis. *Headache, 47*, 52–57.

Martin, P. R. (2010). Behavioral management of migraine headache tirggers: learning to cope with triggers. *Current Pain Headache Reports, 14*, 221–227.

Mauskop, A., Altura, B. T., Cracco, R. Q., & Altura, B. M. (1995). Intravenous magnesium sulfate relieves migraine attacks in patients with low serum ionized magnesium levels; a pilot study. *Clinical Science, 89*, 633–636.

Melchart, D., Linde, K., Fisher, P., Berman, B., White, A., Vickers, A., & Allais, G. (2001). Acupuncture for idiopathic headache. *Cochrane Database Systems Review*,(1), .

Orr, S. L. (2015). Diet and nutraceutical interventions for headache management: a review of the evidence. *Cephalalgia*, 1–22. doi:10.1177/0333102415590239.

Peikart, A., Wilimzig, C., & Kohne-Volland, R. (1996). Prophylaxis of migraine with oral magnesium: results from a prospective, multicenter, placebo-controlled and double-blind randomized study. *Cephalalgia*, *16*, 257–263.

Pfaffenrath, V., Wessely, P., Meyer, C., Isler, H. R., Evers, S., Grotemeyer, K. H., Taneri, Z., Soyka, D., Gobel, H., & Fischer, M. (1996). Magnesium in the prophylaxis of migraine-a double-blind placebo-controlled study. *Cephalagia*, *16*, 436–440.

Prieto, J. M. (2014). Update on the efficacy and safety of Petadolex, a butterbur extract for migraine prophylaxis. *Bots Targets Thererapy*, *4*, 1–9.

Pringsheim, T., Davenport, W., Mackie, G., Worthington, I., Aubé, M., Christie, S. N., Gladstone, J., & Becker, W. J. Canadian Headache Society Prophylactic Guidelines Development Group. (2012). Canadian Headache Society guideline for migraine prophylaxis. *Canadian Journal of Neurological Science*, *39*(Suppl. 2), S1–S59.

Ramadan, N. M., Halvorson, H., & Vande-Linde, A. (1989). Low brain magnesium in migraine. *Headache*, *29*, 590–593.

Rizzoli, P. (2014). Preventive pharmacotherapy in migraine. *Headache*, *54*(2), 364–369.

Schabert, E., & Crow, W. T. (2009). Impact of osteopathic manipulative treatment on cost of care for patients with migraine headache: a retrospective review of patient records. *Journal of American Osteopathic Association*, *109*(8), 403–407.

Schiapparelli, P., Allais, G., Gabellari, I. C., Rolando, S., Terzi, M. G., & Benedetto, C. (2010). Non-pharmacological approach to migraine prophylaxis: part II. *Neurologic Science*, *31*(Suppl. 1), S137–S139.

Scottish Intercollegiate Guidelines Network (2008). Diagnosis and management of headache in adults. A national clinical guideline (Vol. 81). Edinburgh, ON.p. 107. Available from: www.sign.ac.uk

Silberstein, S. D. (2000). Practice parameter: evidence-based guidelines for migraine headache (an evidence-based review): report of the Quality Standards Subcommittee of the American Academy of Neurology. *Neurology*, *55*, 754–762.

Silberstein, S. D., Holland, S., Freitag, F., Dodick, D. W., Aroff, C., & Ashman, E. (2012). Evidence-based guideline update: pharmacologic treatment for episodic migraine prevention in adults: Report of the Quality Standards Subcommittee of the American Academy of Neurology and the American Headache Society. *Neurology*, *78*, 1337–1345.

Snow, V., Weiss, K., Wall, E., & Mottur-Pilson, C. (2002). Pharmacologic management of acute attacks of migraine and prevention of migraine headache. *Annals of Internal Medicine*, *137*, 840–849.

Steiner, T. J., Stovner, L. J., & Birbeck, G. L. (2013). Migraine: the seventh disabler. *The Journal of Headache and Pain*, *14*(1), 1.

Sun-Edelstein, C., & Mauskop, A. (2009). Foods and supplements in the management of migraine headaches. *Clinical Journal of Pain*, *25*(5), 446–452.

Voigt, K., Liebnitzky, J., Burmeister, U., Sihvonen-Riemenschneider, H., Beck, M., Voigt, R., & Bergmann, A. (2001). Efficacy of osteopathic manipulative treatment of female patients with migraine: results of a randomized controlled trial. *Journal of Alternate and Complementary Medicine*, *17*(3), 225–230.

Zheng, H., Chen, M., Huang, D., Li, J., Chen, Q., & Fang, J. (2015). Interventions for migraine prophylaxis: protocol of an umbrella systematic review and network meta-analysis. *BMJ Open*, *5*(5).

CHAPTER

4

Myelinodegeneration and Its Influence on Pain: Aging, Diets, and Genetic Dysregulation

J. Chen*,**,†, S.-M. Guan‡

*Institute for Biomedical Sciences of Pain, Tangdu Hospital, The Fourth Military Medical University, Xi'an, People's Republic of China; **Key Laboratory of Brain Stress and Behavior, PLA, Xi'an, People's Republic of China; †Beijing Institute for Brain Disorders, Beijing, People's Republic of China; ‡School of Stomatology, The Fourth Military Medical University, Xi'an, People's Republic of China

INTRODUCTION

In the *World Report on Ageing and Health* published in 2015, the World Health Organization (WHO) proclaimed that it is a transition for the first time in history that most people can expect to live into their 60s and beyond (World Health Organization, 2015). In a systematic analysis for the Global Burden of Disease (GBD) study 2013, it was revealed that globally, life expectancy at birth rose by 6.2 years (from 65.3 to 71.5 years) between 1990 and 2013, healthy life expectancy (HALE) at birth rose by 5.4 years (from 56.9 to 62.3 years) (Global Burden of Disease 2013 DALYs and HALE Collaborators, 2015).

However, through up-to-date analysis of global data for years lived with disability (YLDs) for 301 diseases and injuries from 188 countries between 1990–2013, it was estimated that YLDs rose by 42.3% from 537.6 million to 764.8 million due to aging and population growth (Global Burden of Disease Study 2013 Collaborators, 2015). The transition from communicable diseases to specific noncommunicable diseases accounts for the age-related causal relationship between diseases and increase in YLDs and disability adjusted life years (DALYs) (Global Burden of Disease 2013 DALYs and HALE Collaborators, 2015). The leading causes of YLDs are mostly associated with chronic pain problems, such as low back pain, neck pain, migraine, other musculoskeletal disorders, and osteoarthritis that rank among the top 13 illnesses. These are followed by common pain comorbidities, such as major depression, diabetes, anxiety, falls, bipolar disorder, medication overuse headache, Alzheimer's disease (AD), alcohol use disorders and epilepsy that rank among the top 25 causes of YLDs. The data of GBD study 2013 suggest that people are living longer, but with more diseases and increased disability (multimorbidities) driven mainly by increase in pain, musculoskeletal, mental, neurological disorders, substance use, diabetes, and frailty (Dansie, Turk, Martin, Van Domelen, & Patel, 2014; Forbes et al., 2016; Mansfield, Sim, Jordan, & Jordan, 2016; Patel, Dansie, & Turk, 2013a; Patel, Guralnik, Dansie, & Turk, 2013b; Patel et al., 2014, 2016; Wade et al., 2016). These comorbid states and pain reciprocally interact and greatly limit functional ability and daily physical activity in older people (Dansie et al., 2014; Patel et al., 2013a,b, 2014, 2016). For example, the results of the 2011 National Health and Aging Trends Study revealed that the overall prevalence of bothersome pain in the United States of America was 52.9%, affecting 18.7 million older adults (Patel et al., 2013b). It is astonishing to find that 74.9% of older adults have multiple sites of pain that limit the physical activity and influence functional ability (Patel et al., 2013b, 2014). Among the 7,601 individuals aged 65 and older representing 35.3 million Medicare beneficiaries, 53.0% reported to have bothersome pain, and among them 19.5% had recurrent falls and 18.0% had fear of falling, respectively (Patel et al., 2014). The prevalence of impaired balance and coordination in these older people increased with

Nutritional Modulators of Pain in the Aging Population. http://dx.doi.org/10.1016/B978-0-12-805186-3.00004-7
Copyright © 2017 Elsevier Inc. All rights reserved.

increasing sites of pain and limitation of physical activity, namely 11.6% with one site of pain, 17.7% with two sites, 25.0% with three sites, and 41.4% with four or more sites (Patel et al., 2014).

Biologically, aging is defined as a gradual, lifelong accumulation of molecular and cellular damage that results in a progressive, generalized impairment in many body functions, an increased vulnerability to environmental challenges and a growing risk of disease and death that is accompanied by a broad range of psychosocial changes (World Health Organization, 2015). Thus, maintaining healthy aging is a great challenge worldwide. Based on the WHO report, healthy aging is defined as "the process of developing and maintaining the functional ability that enables well-being in older age" (World Health Organization, 2015). Functional ability includes (1) the intrinsic capacity comprising of all the physical and mental capacities of an individual; (2) the relevant environments comprising of all the factors in the extrinsic world that form the context of an individual's life, including the built environment (home, communities, and the broader society) and people's relationships, attitudes, and values, health and social policies, the systems that support them, and the services that they implement characteristics; and (3) the interactions between the individual and these characteristics. Thus, exposures to various negative environmental influences across the life course can no doubt change the individual's health status.

In another systematic analysis for the GBD Study 2013, data of 79 behavioral, environmental, and occupational, and metabolic risks or clusters of risks collected from 188 countries during 1990–2013 were evaluated for DALYs (Global Burden of Disease 2013 Risk Factors Collaborators, 2015). In that study, it was concluded that behavioral, environmental, and occupational, and metabolic risks can explain half of global mortality and more than one-third of global DALYs (Global Burden of Disease 2013 Risk Factors Collaborators, 2015). It has also been revealed that dietary risks account for 11.3 million deaths and 241.4 million DALYs and high-salt food associated high systolic blood pressure accounts for 10.4 million deaths and 208.1 million DALYs, suggesting that diet is one of the major risk factors to healthy aging. High energy and high sodium foods and low intake of fruit, whole grains, vegetables, nuts, and seeds are the most important contributors to the increased YLDs although diet patterns and components vary substantially by region and country over the world (Bishwajit, 2015; Global Burden of Disease 2013 Risk Factors Collaborators, 2015). These data suggest that there is a close relationship between diet and YLDs and pain, especially in older persons.

The distinct psychophysical properties of pain in elderly people are characterized as follows: (1) increase in pain threshold to a variety of sensory stimulus modalities (heat, cold, mechanical, electrical); (2) decrease in pain tolerance; (3) decrease in sensory discrimination accuracy; (4) bluntness in acute pain, but predisposition and vulnerability to chronic pain; (5) multisites of pain; (6) multimorbidities (metabolic syndrome, diabetes, stroke, cardiovascular diseases, and musculoskeletal diseases, etc.); (7) decline in other functional abilities, such as hearing loss, visual loss, motor disorders, cognitive decline, and coping ability; (8) comorbidity with emotional disorders (e.g., depression) (Gibson & Weiner, 2005; Harkins, Price, Bush, & Small, 1994; World Health Organization, 2015). These properties of pain in the elderly are likely to be associated with age-related neurodegeneration in both the peripheral (PNS) and the central nervous system (CNS). However, the link between the above properties of pain in elderly people and the biological basis of age-related neurodegeneration has been largely neglected and underestimated. Over the past several decades most of the animal studies on neurobiology of aging have been targeted on single genes and molecules that are likely to be involved in certain neurodegenerative diseases (such as AD and Parkinson's disease), the overall lifespan changes in the nervous system have been less studied (López-Otín, Blasco, Partridge, Serrano, & Kroemer, 2013; Masoro & Austad, 2011). Due to limitations of the use of transgenetic (knock-in or knock-out) techniques in studying the lifespan changes of the whole nervous system in mammals, *Caenorhabditis elegans*, *Drosophila melanogaster*, zebrafish, and mammalian senescent cells were widely used as surrogates in the study of neurobiology of aging and neurodegenerative diseases. What happened in these surrogates may be quite different from what would happen in the elderly people who are exposed to different behavioral, environmental, and metabolic risk factors during their 6–8 decades of lifespan (Global Burden of Disease 2013 Risk Factors Collaborators, 2015; Masoro & Austad, 2011; World Health Organization, 2015). Thus, life-long observations of changes in the mammals' nervous system are of critical importance in unraveling the mechanisms of age-related changes in functional ability and diseases, especially pain, and its comorbidities.

Thus, in this chapter, first we would like to review advances in emerging studies of the age-related changes in the nervous system of normal elderly people (*Homo sapiens*) that highly support presence of a close relationship between widespread white matter changes (WMCs), also referred to as Binswanger's disease, leukoaraiosis (leukoaraiosis), leukoencephalopathy, periventricular (or white matter) hyperintensity, cerebral small vessel disease, and white matter lesions (WML), and decline of various functional abilities in older aged people (Baezner et al., 2008; Baloh, Ying, & Jacobson, 2003; Bhadelia et al., 2009; Black, Gao, & Bilbao, 2009; Blahak et al., 2009; Burton et al., 2004; de Laat et al., 2010; Della Nave et al., 2007; Kertesz et al., 1988; Kirkpatrick & Hayman, 1987; Murray et al., 2010; Prins et al., 2005; Sullivan, Pary, Telang, Rifai, & Zubenko, 1990; Tang, Nyengaard, Pakkenberg, & Gundersen, 1997). The WMCs or myelin breakdown have also been found to be correlated with early onset of AD (Bartzokis, 2011; Bartzokis et al., 2010, 2012; Haroutunian et al., 2014; Lu et al., 2014) and Parkinson's disease (PD) (Bohnen & Albin, 2011). Second, discoveries of age-related WMCs in nonhuman primates (mainly rhesus monkey or *Macaca mulatta*) and their relationship with decline of cognitive functions would be described (Peters, 2002, 2009; Peters & Kemper, 2012). Third, discoveries of lifespan changes in myelin structures and functions since birth (postnatal day, PND 1) to very old (more than 26 months after birth or >PND 728) in rats (*Rattus norvegicus*) would be introduced and then the risk factors of myelinodegeneration including aging, diets, and genetic dysregulation would also be described based on the published and unpublished data collected from rats (Xie et al., 2013a; Xie, Zhang, Fu, & Chen, 2013b; Xie et al., 2014a; Xie, Liang, Fu, Zhang, & Chen, 2014b). Finally, a working hypothesis on the molecular and cellular mechanisms of myelinodegeneration was proposed.

AGE-RELATED WHITE MATTER CHANGES IN THE NERVOUS SYSTEM AND THEIR RELATIONSHIPS WITH DECLINE OF VARIOUS FUNCTIONAL ABILITIES IN NORMAL ELDERLY PEOPLE

The phenomenon of WMCs in healthy elderly people was first noticed in clinic by W.G. Bradley and coworkers with the use of high spatial resolution magnetic resonance imaging (MRI) in 1984. The age-related WMCs were then confirmed by many observations detected on T_2-weighted MRI and diffusion tensor imaging (DTI). The age-related WMCs are featured structurally by patchy WML in 20–30% of neurologically healthy elderly subjects (52–72 years old, $n = 15$) (Kirkpatrick & Hayman, 1987) or by periventricular and subcortical hyperintensities appeared as periventricular rim (74%) and caps (17%) around the frontal and occipital poles of the lateral ventricles in healthy volunteer control group (50–78 years old, $n = 58$) (Kertesz et al., 1988). Unidentified bright objects in subcortical, cortical, and periventricular structures of the brain were also found in 8.6% of healthy aged people (Kertesz et al., 1988). The age-related MRI periventricular and subcortical hyperintensities were not likely to be vascular origin but highly correlated with age, hypertension, cardiac disease, and diabetes (Sullivan et al., 1990).

Anatomically, the brain is generally composed of gray matter (GM) and white matter (WM). GM is made up of aggregated neuronal cell bodies (or called nuclear groups) and neuropil comprised of dendrites, axon hillock, some passing-by myelinated fibers, buttons, synapses, and glial cells (astrocyes, oligodendrocytes, and microglial cells). WM is mainly composed of fat-rich myelinated fiber bundles or tracts in the subcortical commissural structures and long-projection fiber tracts originated from the spinal cord or the brain stem to the cerebral cortex. Each individual myelinated fiber contains myelin sheath that wraps up each axon at internodal (node of Ranvier) segment with compact myelin lamellae along the whole length of nerve fibers (Armati & Mathey, 2010; Dyck, Thomas, & Lambert, 1975; Kettenmann & Ransom, 1995; Lazzarini, 2004). In the CNS, neuroglial oligodendrocytes (OD) are myelinating cells (Figs. 4.1 and 4.3). Each OD wraps up at least 50 axonal fibers (1:50) and forms compact myelin lamellae of myelin sheath. In the PNS, myelinating cells are referred to as Schwann cells (SC) (Fig. 4.2). There is another type of Schwann cells (SC2) that have no myelinating function and surround a bundle of unmyelinated C fibers (diameter: 0.2–1.5 μm) by a layer of process (Fig. 2B, Xie et al., 2013a). Unlike OD, myelinating SC (SC1) only wraps up one axonal fiber (1:1) and forms similar compact myelin lamellae (Fig. 4.2A). Generally, in the adult WM almost all axonal fibers are surrounded by myelin sheath (Fig. 4.1B), however, in the PNS only large diameter (6–20 μm) and small diameter (1.6–5 μm) nerve fibers are surrounded by myelin sheath (Fig.2B, Xie et al., 2013a). For example, in the somatosensory system, the pseudounipolar primary sensory neurons of the dorsal root ganglia (DRG) can be divided into three classes according to the anatomical and electrophysiological properties of the peripheral branches they innervate: large myelinated Aβ fibers, small myelinated Aδ fibers, and unmyelinated C fibers (Chen et al., 2013). The integrity of myelin sheath is very important in maintaining the neuronal information exchange in the nervous system because of its properties of interaxonal insulation and fast saltatory conduction, propagation of action potentials along the myelinated axons from one node of Ranvier to the next node, increasing conduction velocity of action potentials. The integrity of myelin sheath is also essential for development, maturity, and survival of axon fibers in the nervous system and for neural regeneration in the PNS. Thus, the immature development of myelin sheath due to genetic mutation of various myelin protein coding genes or demyelination (such as multiple sclerosis, MS) due to autoimmune reaction would result in severe clinical problems that are intractable and resistant to most of the clinical treatments (Armati & Mathey, 2010; Dyck et al., 1975; Kettenmann & Ransom, 1995; Lazzarini, 2004).

Using a stereological method, Tang and coworkers examined age-related WMCs in autopsied normal human brains (average age 74 vs. 38, $n = 5$ for each group) and found that there was a distinct loss of the total volume of WM (15%) and the total volume of the myelinated fibers

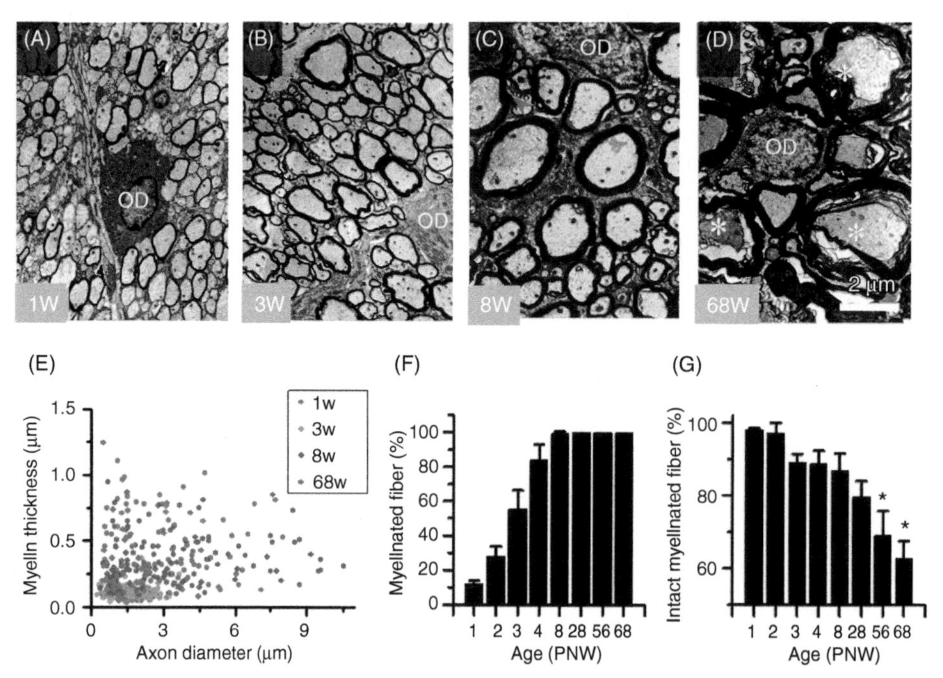

FIG. 4.1 **Age-related changes in myelin structure of the spinal dorsal column in rats from 1 to 68 weeks old.** (A–D) Ultrastructural micrographs showing age-related changes in myelin sheath. (E) A scatter graph showing correlation between the size of axon diameter and the thickness of myelin sheath. (F) Age-related percent changes in myelinated fibers. (G) Age-related percent changes in intact myelinated fibers. OD, Oligodendrocyte; asterisks in D indicate three typical axons with degeneration; *$p < 0.05$ in G; scale bars = 2 μm for A–D.

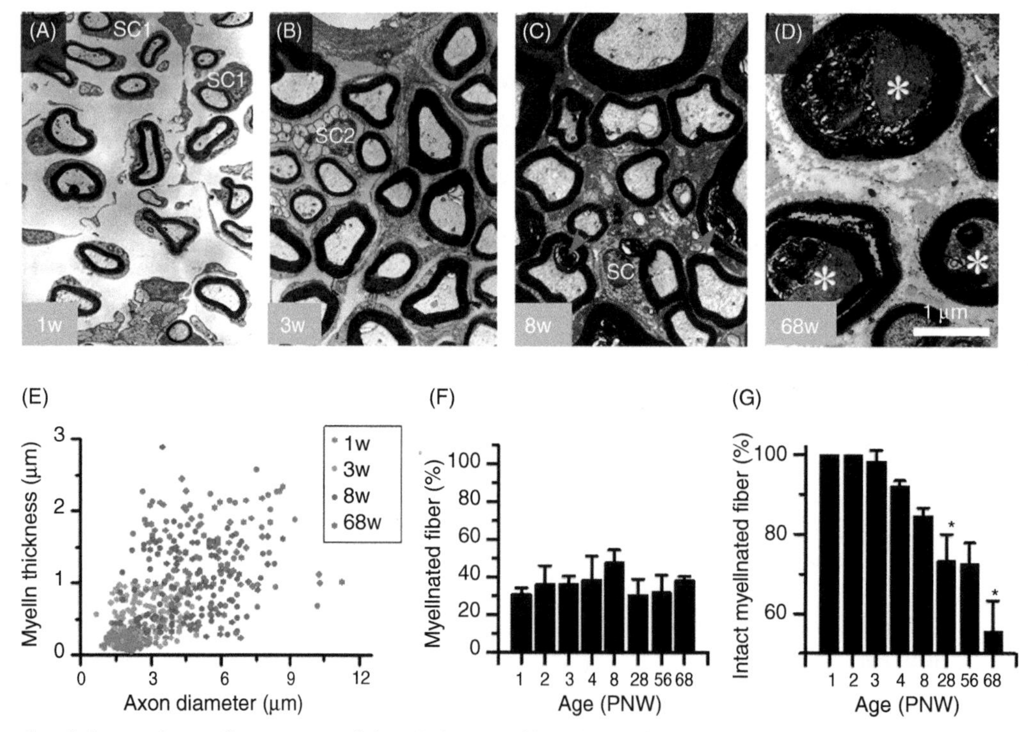

FIG. 4.2 **Age-related changes in myelin structure of the sciatic nerve fibers in rats from 1 to 68 weeks old.** (A–D) Ultrastructural micrographs showing age-related changes in myelin sheath. (E) A scatter graph showing correlation between the size of axon diameter and the thickness of myelin sheath. (F) Age-related percent changes in myelinated fibers. (G) Age-related percent changes in intact myelinated fibers. Arrow in C indicates intraaxonal myelin-like inclusion. Asterisks in D indicate three typical axons with degeneration; Schwann cell (SC), SC1 myelinating type, SC2, nonmyelinating type surrounded by many unmyelinated C fibers; *, $p < 0.05$ in G; scale bars = 1 μm for A–D.

(17%) in the old group relative to the young group (Tang et al., 1997). Moreover, the total length of the myelinated fibers of the WM in the elderly group was significantly decreased by 27% (Tang et al., 1997). Consistency of the MRI and the brain histological results implicates existence of dramatic WMLs with age.

In the past decade, studies have been focused on the correlations between the age-related WMLs and age-related decline in various functional abilities in the elderly aged people. Accumulating evidence showed a great association and correlation between WMLs and functional disabilities that include gait and balance dysfunction (Baezner et al., 2008; Baloh et al., 2003; Bhadelia et al., 2009; de Laat et al., 2010; Murray et al., 2010), falls (Blahak et al., 2009), decline in information processing speed and executive function (Prins et al., 2005), and impairment of attention, memory, and global cognitive performance (Della Nave et al., 2007; Prins et al., 2005), in normal old people. In a longitudinal study, Baloh and coworkers measured visual acuity, vestibulo-ocular response, pure-tone hearing thresholds, vibration sense, deep tendon reflexes, and gait/balance performance in 59 normal older subjects with averaged age of 78.5 on entry (Baloh et al., 2003). During the 8–10 years of observation, there was a significant age-related decrease in vestibulo-ocular response and increase in pure-tone hearing thresholds, decrease in vibration sense and deep tendon reflexes in the feet, and decrease in total Tinetti score of gait and balance (Baloh et al., 2003). The WM hyperintensities were highly correlated with gait and balance dysfunction. In another cross-sectional analysis sponsored by the Leukoaraiosis and Disability Study of 11 European centers, deficiencies in gait and balance performance were demonstrated to be correlated with the severity of age-related WMLs (Baezner et al., 2008). The age-related gait dysfunction was significantly associated with WMLs in the genu of the corpus callosum detected by DTI (Bhadelia et al., 2009; de Laat et al., 2010). Based upon the accumulating evidence from cohort and clinical neuroimaging studies and pathological examinations, it can be concluded that in "normal" older aged people there are widespread myelin damages in the whole nervous system that are highly correlated with various functional disabilities involving the visual, auditory, somatosensory, somatomotoric, and even memory, and cognitive functions.

LIFESPAN TRAJECTORY OF MYELIN INTEGRITY AND MYELIN BREAKDOWN MODEL OF AD AND NEUROPSYCHIATRIC DISORDERS

Age-related damage or breakdown of myelin structures has been proposed to be the initial risk factor of AD (Bartzokis, 2011; Bartzokis et al., 2010, 2012; Haroutunian et al., 2014; Lu et al., 2014), PD (Bohnen & Albin, 2011), and even impairment of memory, attention and global cognitive performance in older stroke patients (Black et al., 2009; Burton et al., 2004). Bartzokis and colleagues proposed a myelin-breakdown model for the development of AD and other psychiatric disorders, saying that "the interplay between the continuous developmental processes of myelination and degenerative processes acting on several prominent vulnerabilities of oligodendrocytes and the myelin they sustain. These vulnerabilities make oligodendrocytes and their myelin the "weakest link" that will succumb to a variety of suboptimal genetic variants and environmental insults" (Bartzokis, 2011). Bartzokis's myelin-breakdown model was mostly based upon a quadratic like (inverted "U") curve of lifespan trajectories of human brain myelination that are supported by the MRI data and postmortem myelin staining data from frontal and temporal lobes of normal individuals (see Fig. 1 of both Bartzokis, 2011 and Haroutunian et al., 2014). It was shown that the human brain reaches maturity in middle age when myelin content reaches its peak at approximately 25% of brain volume according to both neuroimaging and histological staining data (Bartzokis, 2011; Haroutunian et al., 2014). In general at about 45 years old, age-related myelin breakdown begins that might be associated with increase in age-related functional disabilities described previously (Bartzokis, 2011; Bartzokis et al., 2010, 2012; Haroutunian et al., 2014; Lu et al., 2014). Moreover, the unique properties of ODs and myelin production are as follows: (1) brain cholesterol, the major constituent of myelin, is synthesized almost exclusively de novo by neuroglial cells that would be sensitive to lipid metabolism; (2) ODs have the highest iron content of all brain cell types that is required by cholesterol and lipid synthesizing enzymes; (3) the production and maintenance of the myelin sheaths that is up to 600 times the surface area of OD soma membrane and 100 times the weight of the soma makes the energy consumption of myelinating cells two- to threefold higher than nonmyelinating cells in the brain; (4) ODs are more vulnerable to genetic and interior or exterior environmental changes due to life-long myelination, demyelination, and remyelination; (5) myelin is vulnerable to age and metabolism dysfunctions (Bartzokis, 2011; Haroutunian et al., 2014; Xie et al., 2013a). Thus, it is believed that the production, maintenance, and repair of the human brain's pervasive myelin sheaths would underlie human unique vulnerability to highly prevalent neuropsychiatric disorders ranging from schizophrenia to degenerative disorders, such as AD (Bartzokis, 2011; Haroutunian et al., 2014). Yet, the proposed human age-related myelin breakdown model requires proof from animal studies.

AGE-RELATED DEGENERATIVE CHANGES IN MYELIN AND NERVE FIBERS IN MONKEY CNS

Age-related alterations in myelin structures in the CNS of animals had long been neglected or underestimated until the late 1990s. There had been at least two major impediments that delayed the progress in discovery of age-related myelin damage and its relationship with functional disabilities and diseases. One was the century predominance of Cajal's neuronal doctrine in the field of neuroscience by which only neurons and synapses were thought to be the central players of brain functions and diseases. The other was technical limitation. As aforementioned, the WMLs had not been widely noticed until the uses of MRI and even DTI in detection of both GM and WM in human brains. High quality postmortem brain slice staining of myelin was not possible due to rapid lipid degradation after death. It was also very difficult to well preserve myelin-containing brain structures, because artifact-like alterations in myelin structures were produced due to fixative-induced shrinkage of the nerve fibers and poor sample preparation (Peters, 2002). Due to discoveries of age-related myelin changes in human brains and technical advances in sample preparation and observations, age-related alterations in myelin structures in animal CNS can be intensively conducted.

The effects of normal aging on the CNS myelin sheath and axonal fibers have been carefully studied in rhesus monkeys by Peters and coworkers with elegant pioneering TEM observations (see reviews Peters, 2002, 2009; Peters & Kemper, 2012). The observations have been mainly concentrated on cerebral cortices including visual cortex, striate cortex, and frontal cortex, and nerve trunks and fiber tracts in WM, such as the optic nerve, the optic radiation, the anterior commissure, and the corpus callosum, in an attempt to establish the relationships between the myelin changes and the development of age-related cognitive disorders. Through repeated examinations of young-, middle-, and old-aged rhesus monkeys' brain, Peters and coworkers confirmed that there are age-related degenerative changes in myelin sheath and nerve fibers due to advancement in the aging process. The use of rhesus monkeys as subjects has great advantages in the study of normal aging effects: (1) they have a lifespan of only 35 years, one third of human lifespan (75–90 years) that makes the study possible for one single scientist; (2) they develop cognitive decline similar to humans but rarely have AD-like pathology in the aged brain that is appropriate to observations of normal aging effects; (3) the methods used for assessment of cognitive functions between humans and monkeys are comparable; (4) the procedures for sample preparations are well-established and the brain tissues can be well preserved for the purpose of further ultrastructural observations (Peters, 2002, 2009; Peters & Kemper, 2012).

From long term studies of normal aging effects on myelin in rhesus monkeys, distinct histological characteristics of age-related myelinodegeneration can be summarized based on descriptions by Peters and his coworkers (Peters, 2002, 2009; Peters & Kemper, 2012): (1) age-related myelinodegeneration is a global effect in both WM and GM although the associative fibers in the cortex (GM) are relatively better preserved than in the subcortical structures, such as commissural fibers; (2) age-related myelinodegeneration under TEM are distinct from the shearing defect caused by fixation artifacts and identifiable in structural appearance, displaying as split myelin sheaths, myelin balloons, redundant myelin, and sheath with electron dense cytoplasm; (3) age-related myelinodegeneration is often accompanied by loss of myelinated nerve fibers due to axonopathy; (4) age-related myelinodegeneration is accompanied by swelling of OD processes, increased numbers of ODs and increased numbers of dense inclusions in the OD perikarya; (5) age-related myelinodegeneration is also accompanied by continuous remyelination; (6) age-related myelinodegeneration is accompanied by activation of microglial cells that are involved in the processes of phagocytosis. The previous age-related myelinopathology and secondary myelinopathological responses of ODs and microglial cells are consistent with the age-related WMLs in the human brain and highly support their possible roles in development of age-related cognitive dysfunctions and other functional disabilities.

In search of brain structures that are related to both myelinopathology and cognitive decline with age, many studies have been carried out (see Tables 1–3 of Peters & Kemper, 2012). Overall, total brain weight, total cortical thickness, and total volumes of the prefrontal cortex, the hippocampus, and the calcarine cortex were not found to be significantly changed with age. Moreover, numbers of neurons in the primary somatomotoric cortex, the hippocampus, the entorhinal cortex, visual cortex, prefrontal area 46, and occipital area 17 were not significantly lost with age. However, frequency of altered myelin sheaths and loss of nerve fibers, axonal buttons, dendritic spines, and synapses in the prefrontal area 46 were increased significantly with age. The loss of commissural nerve fibers could be 26–30% in the fornix, the splenium of corpus callosum, and the anterior commissure. About 30–60% loss of synapses could also be seen for both asymmetrical type and symmetrical type across layer 1 to layers 2/3 in the area 46 of the prefrontal cortex. These structural changes were highly correlated with both age and cognitive deficit. Brodmann's area 46 is a subregion of the dorsolateral prefrontal cortex. Area 46 has complex connections with somatosensory, visual, visuomotor, motor, and limbic systems and plays a key role in cognition (Peters & Kemper, 2012). The age-related myelinodegeneration and myelinopathological changes have also been demonstrated to be involved in changes in electrophysiological properties of neuronal excitability and synaptic transmission in monkeys. For example, the layer 3 pyramidal neurons of area 46 in older monkeys fired more frequently than young ones (Peters & Kemper, 2012). As for the synaptic transmission and modulation, brain slice patch-clamp recordings were carried out in area 46, it was found that the frequency of spontaneous excitatory postsynaptic currents (sEPSCs) in layer three neurons were significantly reduced with age, while the frequency of GABA-mediated spontaneous inhibitory postsynaptic currents (sIPSCs) were significantly increased with age (Peters & Kemper, 2012). The decrease in frequency of sEPSCs is probably caused by loss of excitatory synaptic inputs from other brain regions due to loss of nerve fibers (deafferentation), while the increase in frequency of sIPSCs is probably caused by disinhibition of GABA release due to loss of presynaptic input, and this imbalance between excitatory and inhibitory systems would lead to cognitive dysfunction.

Unfortunately, so far the relationship between age-related myelinodegeneration and pain has not been studied in either monkeys or humans. The limitation of these studies on monkey's myelin is that only ultrastructural data from TEM observations have been provided, the underlying molecular/cellular and genetic mechanisms of age-related myelinodegeneration remain largely unknown. Thus, studies on the underlying mechanisms of age-related myelinodegeneration and its relationship with functional disabilities with age are required.

LIFESPAN CHANGES IN MYELIN STRUCTURES OF RAT NERVOUS SYSTEM

Age-related changes in myelin sheath and myelinated axon fibers in the peripheral somatosensory and motor systems have long been noticed in both humans and animals that are referred to as neuropathy or polyneuropathies according to the number of nerve fibers involved in the defects (Dyck et al., 1975; Lazzarini, 2004). Age-related functional changes of myelinated fibers in the PNS have also been widely reported in terms of decrease in nerve conduction velocity and other functional disabilities (Dyck et al., 1975; Lazzarini, 2004; Thomas, King, & Sharma, 1980). However, the fine structural characteristics of age-related myelinodegeneration have been well studied only in rats. For instance, in the tibial and plantar nerves of Wistar rats with ages of 2, 4, 6, 9, 12, 15, 18, 21, and 24 months, the occurrence of abnormalities were mainly identified in large myelinated nerve fibers (Sharma, Bajada, & Thomas, 1980). The results showed a distinct increase in fiber diameter with age followed by slight axonal degeneration after 15–18 months of age and severe (approximately 30%) axonal degeneration and impaired conduction velocity after 24 months of age (Sharma et al., 1980). Under TEM, segmental demyelination (also referred to as myelinopathy) and axonal degeneration (also referred to as axonopathy) were found to be prominent in the tibial and plantar nerves of rats with 18–24 months of age (Thomas et al., 1980). Afterward, the age-related myelinopathy and axonopathy have been widely discovered in rats (Bergman & Ulfhake, 2002; Johansson, Stenström, & Hildebrand, 1996; Knox, Kokmen, & Dyck, 1989; Krinke et al., 1988; for reviews see Dyck et al., 1975; Lazzarini, 2004). Similar age-related myelinopathy and axonopathy were also found in mice (Ceballos, Cuadras, Verdú, & Navarro, 1999; Shen, Zhang, Gao, Gu, & Ding, 2011) and cats (Adinolfi, Yamuy, Morales, & Chase, 1991). Importantly, myelinopathy or myelinodegeneration discovered in animals might be the initial pathological processes of painful diabetic and prediabetic neuropathy and polyneuropathies in humans (American Diabetes Association, 2010; Dyck et al., 1975; Lazzarini, 2004; Papanas, Vinik, & Ziegler, 2011; Sumner, Sheth, Griffin, Cornblath, & Polydefkis, 2003; Tabak, Herder, Rathmann, Brunner, & Kivimaki, 2012; Tesfaye et al., 2010; Tracy & Dyck, 2008; Xie et al., 2013a). Unlike the pathological changes in the experimental models of MS, which shows acute disappearance of myelin sheath at internodal segment (demyelination) in nature (Lazzarini, 2004), the pathological changes of age-related myelinopathy or myelinodegeneration under TEM was featured with widespread myelin breakdown and axonopathy. Like what happened in the CNS of rhesus monkeys, the age-related myelinodegeneration in rodents is also characterized by distinct myelin abnormalities, such as myelin balloon (bubbling), myelin invagination (infolding), and exvagination (outfolding), outward slippage (giant and swollen axons with a ultrathin myelin sheath), inward slippage (disproportionate thick myelin sheath with atrophic axons), loss of circularity, focal split myelin lamellae and myelin breakdown, intramyelin dense inclusions and intraaxonal dense inclusions, and intraaxonal accumulation of glycogen bodies (Adinolfi et al., 1991; Bergman & Ulfhake, 2002; Ceballos et al., 1999; Knox et al., 1989; Krinke et al., 1988; Thomas et al., 1980; Verdú, Ceballos, Vilches, & Navarro, 2000; for reviews see Dyck et al., 1975; Lazzarini, 2004). Moreover, age-related myelinopathy in the PNS is also accompanied by increased extracellular interstitial tissue space (loss of matrix substances), macrophagocytosis, neogenesis of SCs, and remyelination that are thought to be essential for protection of axons from myelinopathy-associated axonal degeneration as demonstrated in both the CNS and PNS (Irvine & Blakemore, 2008; Lasiene, Matsui, Sawa, Wong, & Horner, 2009; Verdú et al., 2000; for reviews see Armati & Mathey, 2010; Lazzarini, 2004).

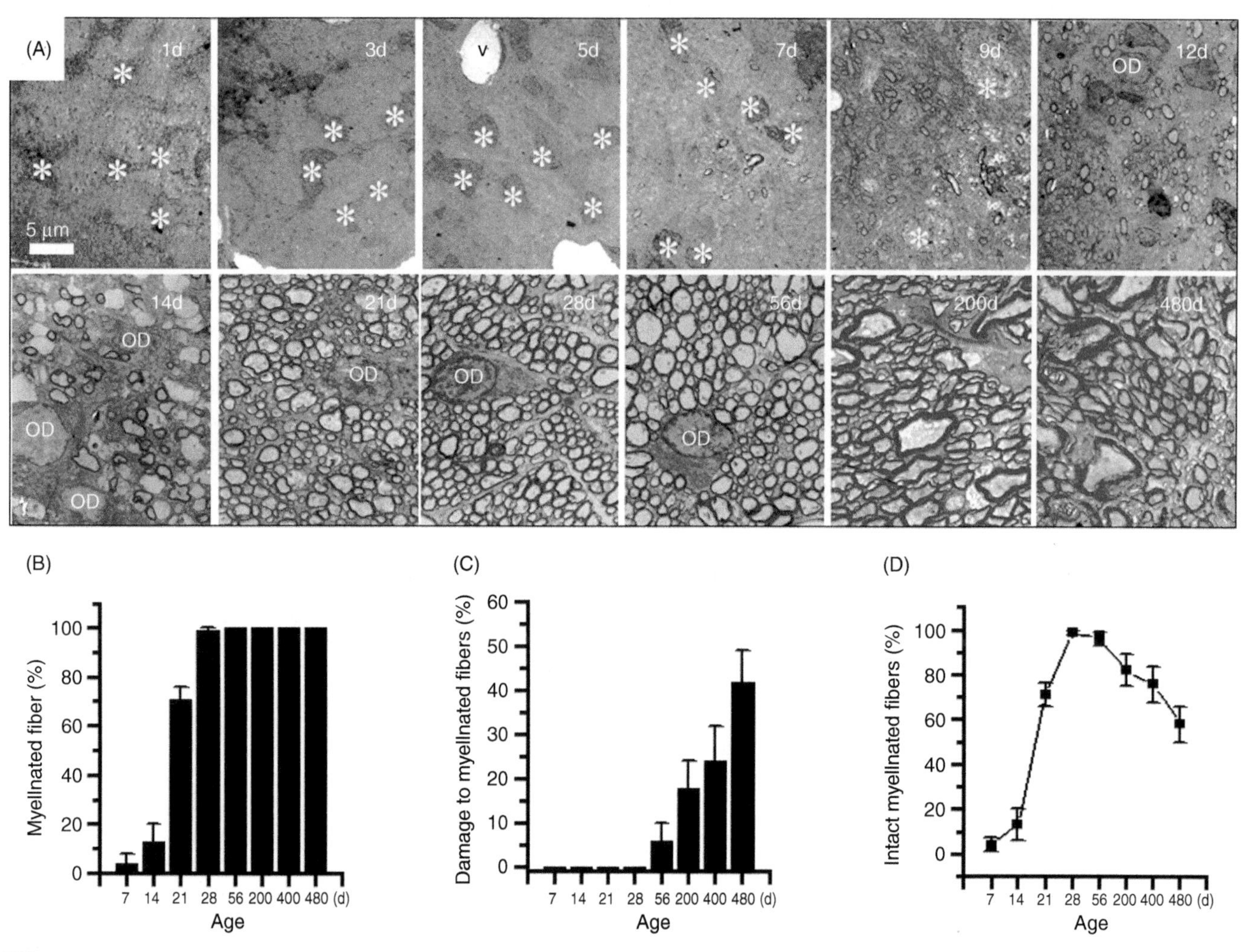

FIG. 4.3 **Postnatal development, maturity and aging of the optic nerve fibers in rats from 1 to 480 days old**. (A) Ultrastructural micrographs showing age-related changes in myelin sheaths. (B) Age-related percent changes in myelinated fibers. (C) Age-related percent damage to myelinated fibers. (D) Age-related percent changes in intact myelinated fibers. Asterisks indicate OD progenitor cells; oligodendrocyte (OD); scale bars = 5 μm for A-1d to −480d.

It is implicated that the pathology of age-related myelinodegeneration in both the PNS and the CNS across different species ranging from rodents to cats, from nonhuman primates to humans is very much similar and might share common underlying mechanisms.

In order to get insights into the underlying mechanisms of age-related changes in myelin structures, lifespan observations of global myelin trajectories in terms of development, maturity, and aging in both the CNS and PNS have been made in rats with ages from birth to older fed in the SPF laboratory animal facility at Institute for Biomedical Sciences of Pain, Tangdu Hospital, Fourth Military Medical University (see Xie et al., 2013b, 2014a,b). The natural lifespan of rats studied ranged from 370 to 844 days after birth (580 days for 50% survival rate, $n = 130$) (unpublished data recorded from April 2008–December 2015).

The onset of myelinated fibers was generally determined by region, distance, and feature of different classes of nerve fibers. The onset was defined as the time when myelination began to appear and only several very thinly myelinated fibers can be identified per mesh under TEM in our studies [Fig. 4.3A(7d)]. In the CNS, nerve fibers are classified into long-projection fibers, commissural fibers and associative fibers. Long-projection fibers and commissural fibers form the whole WM in the CNS, while associative fibers are intracortical fibers that connect different part of cortices. Generally, both the central (spinal dorsal column) and peripheral (sciatic nerve) axonal fibers of the DRG neurons in the somatosensory system were the first ones to be myelinated before birth (Figs. 4.1 and 4.2), followed by onset of long-projecting fibers including the optic nerve (Fig. 4.3), the corticospinal tract and the middle cerebellar peduncles at postnatal day 7 (PND7). The corpus calosum and the anterior commissure were much later than the above regions and began to myelinate by PND21 (unpublished data).

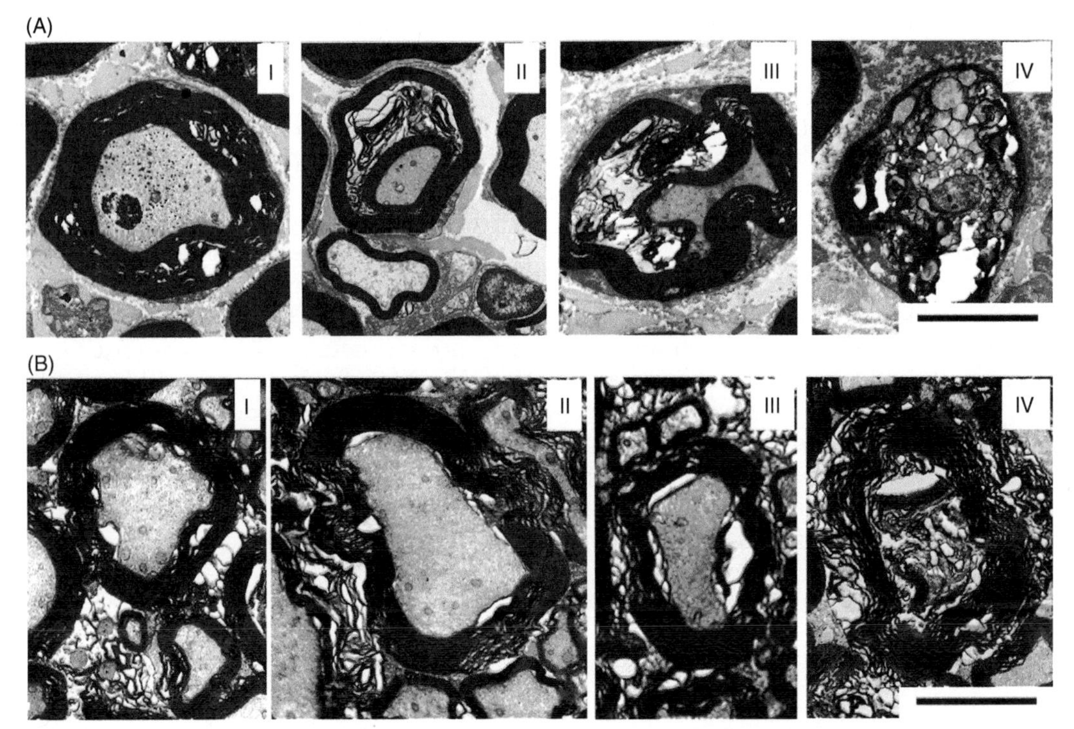

FIG. 4.4 **Pathological grade classification of myelinodegeneration.** (A) The sciatic nerves. (B) The spinal dorsal column. Dysintegrity and deformity of myelin sheath, infolding, and outfolding of myelin sheath, focal, or widespread split myelin lamellae, and intramyelin balloon and inclusions can be seen in both PNS and CNS. Scale bar = 5 μm for A and 2 μm for B. *From Xie, F., Fu, H., Hou, J. F., Jiao, K., Costigan, M., & Chen, J. (2013a). High energy diets-induced metabolic and prediabetic painful polyneuropathy in rats.* PLoS One, 8, *e57427.(supplemental Fig. 4.1) with permission according to CC BY license of open access journals.*

The maturity of myelination was defined as the time when integrity of all myelin sheaths reached best [Figs. 4.1C, 4.2C, and 4.3A(28 and 56d)]. The size of fibers and the thickness of myelin sheaths cannot be used as parameters of growth indices because they are increased with age (Figs. 1E and 2E, see Xie et al., 2014b). Nor G-ratio can be used due to the same reason (see Xie et al., 2013a, 2014b).

According to the ultrastructural characteristics of myelinopathology described previously, slight and statistically nonsignificant myelinopathic or myelinodegenerative changes were first identified just soon after maturity of myelin structures, showing as loss of myelin integrity (dysintegrity) including one or two of the following pathological changes, such as deformity, loss of circularity, focal myelin defect, intramyelin inclusions, and slight increased electron density [Fig. 4.1C, 4.2C, and 4.3(200d)]. However, significant and severe myelin dysintegrity that is referred to as myelinopathy or myelinodegeneration could only be identified at quarter-life for the peripheral sensory and motor nerves, at half-life for the central long-projection fibers and at three quarters of life for the commissural fibers based upon lifespan observations across the whole nervous system in rats (Figs. 1–3 and unpublished data). The myelinopathology under TEM in aged rats was impressive and distinct on first sight and it included collectively: (1) overall increased electron density indicating degenerative-like changes; (2) widespread split myelin lamellae and myelin breakdown; (3) intramyelin or intraaxonal balloon(s); (4) intraaxonal myelin-like or unidentified inclusions; (5) axonal degeneration and loss (for details see Figs. 4.1D, 4.2D, 4.3 (480d) and Fig. 4.4). Moreover, in the PNS, degeneration of unmyelinated C fibers were also seen in advanced aged rats (unpublished data), while small myelinated fibers remain less changed with age (Fig. 4.2C). These lifespan changes in myelin in rat CNS (Fig. 4.3D) are largely consistent with the quadratic like (inverted "U") curve of lifespan trajectories of human brain myelination (Fig. 1 of both Bartzokis, 2011 and Haroutunian et al., 2014). The lifespan observations of cortical associative fibers in rats are not available and remain to be provided in future.

GRADE-BASED CLASSIFICATION OF MYELINOPATHOLOGY

Because traditional measurement of myelinated fibers, such as thickness of myelin, size of axon, and G-ratio cannot be used as indices due to lifespan changes, grade classification of the damaged fibers was adopted in our previous studies (Xie et al., 2013a, 2014a, 2014b). They were classified into three or four grades according to the intensity and extensity of destruction of myelin sheaths and axons for both the PNS (Fig. 4.4A) and the CNS (Fig. 4.4B). The pathologically-classified grade I (pI) is a slight pathological change including myelin sheath deformity, myelin lamina rarefaction, focal demyelination, or vacuolization with the axon being less affected; pII, pI plus more than one half damage of myelin sheath; pIII, moderate pathological changes including myelin lamina reticulation, focal demyelination, vacuolization, and axonal changes including increased electron density and intraaxonal myelin-like inclusions, lipofuscin deposition, glycogen granules, dense microfilament, and microtubule; pIV, the most severe pathological changes including dramatic myelin damage or disruption that are accompanied by axonal degeneration and loss including widespread split myelin lamellae and myelin breakdown, intramyelin or intraaxonal balloon(s). Using this grade classification of myelinopathology, qualitative, and quantitative analysis of myelinopathy and myelinodegeneration can be made (Fig. 4.4).

DIETS AS RISK FACTORS OF MYELINOPATHY AND MYELINODEGENERATION

It has been well accepted that peripheral neuropathy, with clinical manifestations of pain, sensory, autonomic, and even motor dysfunctions, is a major common complication of both diabetes and prediabetes (American Diabetes Association, 2010; Papanas et al., 2011; Tabak et al., 2012; Tesfaye et al., 2010; Xie et al., 2013a). Most of the painful peripheral neuropathy involves damage of both myelinated and unmyelinated fibers in the peripheral sensory fibers (American Diabetes Association, 2010; Papanas et al., 2011; Tabak et al., 2012; Tesfaye et al., 2010; Xie et al., 2013a). To establish the role of the metabolic state in the pathogenesis of polyneuropathy and myelinodegeneration, an age- and sex-matched, longitudinal study in rats fed with high-fat and high-sucrose diet (HFSD), or high-fat, high-sucrose and high-salt diet (HFSSD) relative to conventional diet (CD) was performed (Xie et al., 2013a). The composition of the CD, HFSD, and HFSSD and the mass or energy proportion of carbohydrate, protein, and fat in the three groups are described in detail (see supplemental Tables 1 and 2 of Xie et al., 2013a). Body weight, foodstuff consumption, and systolic blood pressure of each rat were measured. Blood was collected for biochemical measurements and analysis of fasting plasma glucose (FPG), insulin, free fatty acids (FFA), homeostasis model assessment-insulin resistance index (HOMA-IR), thermal and mechanical sensitivity and motor coordination were measured in parallel during post diet day (PDD) 1–120. Finally, large and small myelinated fibers, as well as unmyelinated fibers in the sciatic nerves and ascending fibers in the spinal dorsal column were quantitatively assessed under TEM. As a result, early metabolic syndrome (hyperinsulinemia, dyslipidemia, and hypertension) and prediabetic conditions (impaired fasting glucose) could be induced by both high-energy and high-sodium diets in rats which later developed painful polyneuropathy that was characterized by myelinopathy and myelinodegeneration, such as myelin breakdown and loss of large myelinated fibers in both peripheral and central branches of primary afferent DRG neurons [Figs. 4.5 and 4.6, from Xie et al., 2013a (Figs. 6 and 8, pp7–8)]. Similar to what seen in aged rats described previously, small myelinated fibers were far less damaged [Fig. 4.5, from Xie et al., 2013a (Fig. 6, pp7)]. Unmyelinated C fibers were slightly affected, particularly in rats fed with HFSSD (also see Fig. 5 of Xie et al., 2013a).

ASSOCIATION OF MYELINODEGENERATION WITH PAIN

Both age-related and high-energy/high-sodium diet-related myelinodegeneration can produce great impact upon pain perception and nociceptive responses.

In a previous observation in rats, the paw withdrawal response threshold and latency to both mechanical and thermal nociceptive stimuli were all increased with age (Ge, Chen, Li, & Chen, 2002). Compared with rats of 2 and 12 months old, only rats of 26 months old showed significant elevation of pain mechanical threshold and thermal latency when about 50% of large myelinated Aβ fibers and 20% of unmyelinated C fibers were severely damaged (Unpublished data). Upon receiving subcutaneous injection of bee venom, a model of acute inflammatory pain (Chen & Lariviere, 2010), rats with advanced age showed 30 min delay in peak response of spontaneous paw flinches relative to those of young and middle ages (Unpublished data). This result was in consistency with our previous reports showing a similar time delay in spike responses of spinal dorsal horn wide-dynamic-range neurons (Zheng, Chen, & Arendt-Nielsen, 2004a; Zheng, Feng, & Jian, Chen, 2004b). Moreover, neurogenic inflammatory responses, such as paw edema mediated partially by unmyelinated C-fibers (Chen et al., 2013) was also impaired in rats of advanced age (Unpublished data). In contrast to heightened pain threshold and lowered pain response, it was interesting to observe that the duration of mechanical hyperalgesia or allodynia, but not thermal hyperalgesia, was much more prolonged in aged rats, suggesting transit facilitation from acute to chronic conditions by aging. Herein, age-related myelinodegeneration might be a predisposing factor to chronicity of pain. Collectively, these published and unpublished observations highly support a

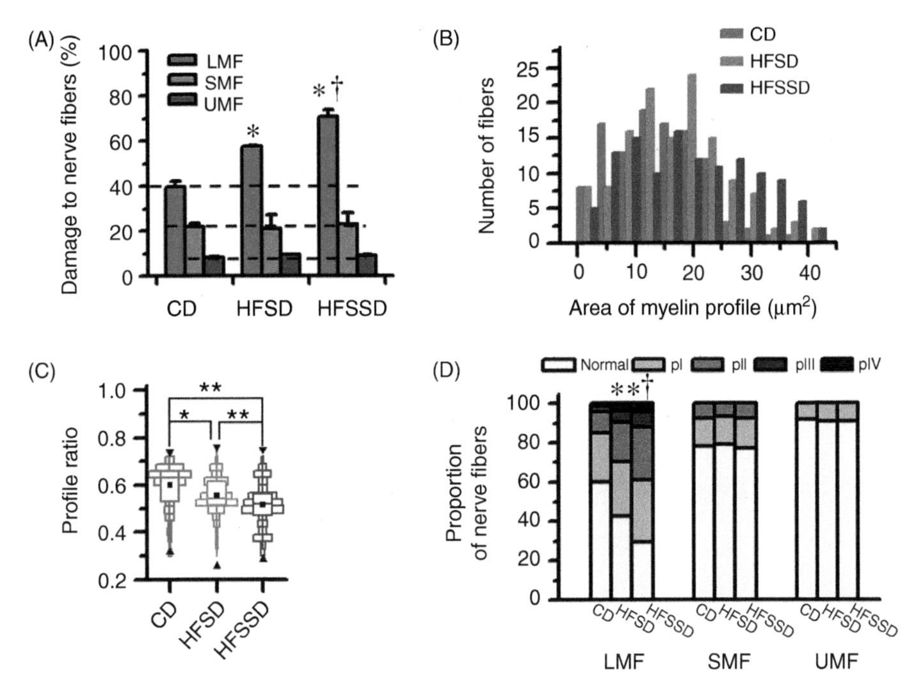

FIG. 4.5 Quantitative analysis of structural changes in large myelinated fiber (LMF), small myelinated fiber (SMF), and unmyelinated fiber (UMF) in the sciatic nerves of rats fed conventional diet (CD), high-fat/high-sucrose diet (HFSD) and high-fat/high-sucrose/high salt diet (HFSSD), respectively. (A) Percent damage to LMF, SMF, and UMF. (B) Distributional histograms of profile areas of myelinated fibers. (C) Boxplots show changes in profile ratios (changes in myelin profile) obtained by dividing area of axon profiles with area of fiber profiles of the myelinated fibers. (D) Proportion of nerve fibers with different pathologically-classified grades (grades pI–pIV). Horizontal lines in A indicate level of percentage damage to nerve fibers in CD. Upper reverse black triangles, lower upright black triangles, horizontal lines across each box and black squares in each box represent maximum, minimum, median, and mean of profile ratios in C. * and †, $p < 0.05$, **, $p < 0.01$. Error bars in A: ± SEM. *From Xie, F., Fu, H., Hou, J. F., Jiao, K., Costigan, M., & Chen, J. (2013a). High energy diets-induced metabolic and prediabetic painful polyneuropathy in rats.* PLoS One, 8, *e57427. (Fig. 6, pp.7) with permission according to CC BY license of open access journals.*

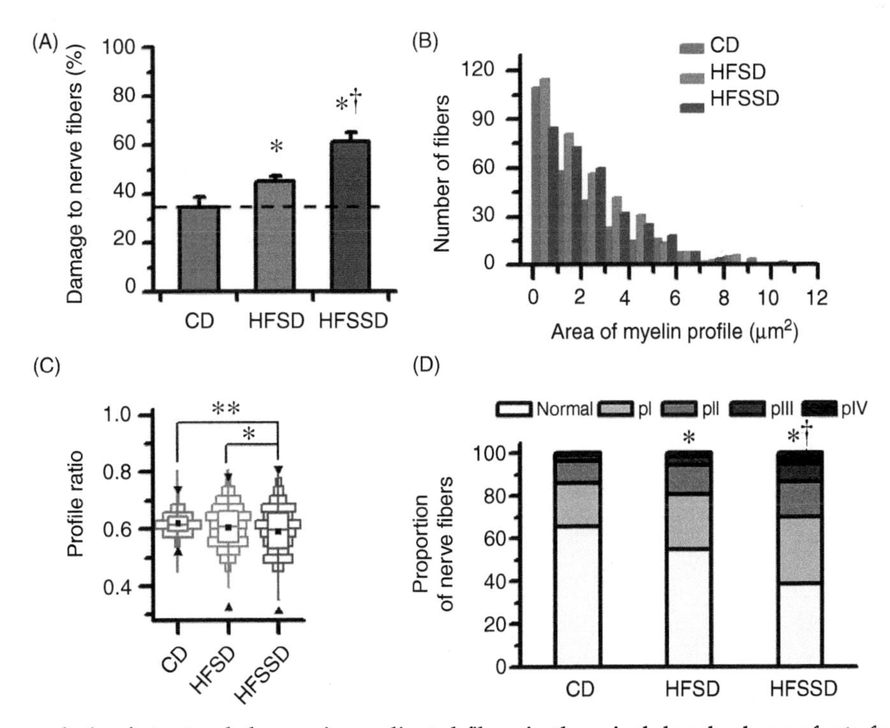

FIG. 4.6 **Quantitative analysis of structural changes in myelinated fibers in the spinal dorsal column of rats fed with CD, HFSD, and HFSSD, respectively.** For annotations of A–D seen Fig. 5. * and †, $p < 0.05$, **, $p < 0.01$. Error bars in A: ± SEM. *From Xie, F., Fu, H., Hou, J. F., Jiao, K., Costigan, M., & Chen, J. (2013a). High energy diets-induced metabolic and prediabetic painful polyneuropathy in rats.* PLoS One, 8, *e57427. (Fig. 8, pp.8) with permission according to CC BY license of open access journals.*

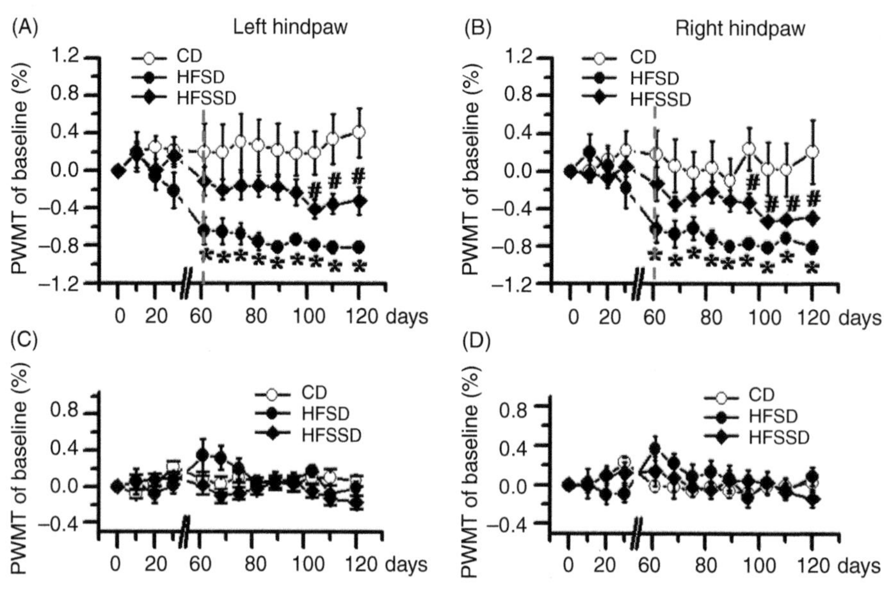

FIG. 4.7 **Time courses of the effects of CD, HFSD, and HFSSD on the somatic sensory functions measured in conscious rats.** Changes in mechanical pain sensitivity (A–B) and thermal pain sensitivity (C–D) of bilateral hind paws were shown ($n = 5–6$ animals). Paw withdrawal mechanical threshold (PWMT); paw withdrawal thermal latency (PWTL). * $p < 0.05$, HFSD versus CD; # $p < 0.05$, HFSSD versus CD. Vertical dashed lines in A and B indicate initial significant changes in PWMT caused by the diets. Error bars: ± SEM. *From Xie, F., Fu, H., Hou, J. F., Jiao, K., Costigan, M., & Chen, J. (2013a). High energy diets-induced metabolic and prediabetic painful polyneuropathy in rats.* PLoS One, 8, e57427. *(Fig. 3, pp.5) with permission according to CC BY license of open access journals.*

tight relationship between age-related changes in nociceptive responses (pain perception) and age-related myelinodegeneration. The heightened pain threshold, delayed pain response and prolonged duration of chronic pain have been frequently seen in elderly people (Gibson & Weiner, 2005; Harkins et al., 1994), suggesting that the rat model of the effects of aging on pain would be valid and useful in studying the underlying mechanisms of pain in elderly human.

Hereinabove, nutrients or diets have been shown to pose a risk to myelinodegeneration in adult rats of young and middle ages (Xie et al., 2013a). Could high-energy diets-induced myelinodegeneration be in close association with the development of chronic pain? Also in the age- and sex-matched longitudinal study in rats fed with HFSD or HFSSD, mechanical, but not thermal, hyperalgesia could be identified since PDD60 that lasted without recovery until the termination of observation on PDD120. Because insulin-resistance and prediabetic condition occurred 35 days (since PDD25) earlier than the occurrence of mechanical hyperalgesia (PDD60) [Fig. 4.7, from Xie et al. (2013a), (Fig. 3, p. 5)], it did not support direct involvement of hyperinsulinemia and dyslipidemia in the production of mechanical hyperalgesia. Thus, high-energy diets-induced myelinodegeneration was proposed to play a critical role in development of mechanical hyperalgesia (Xie et al., 2013a). In fact, in clinic and subclinic, neuropathy is a common condition of prediabetes (Papanas et al., 2011). Prediabetics are referred to as an intermediate group of individuals who have impaired fasting glucose or impaired glucose tolerance, but with their blood glucose concentrations being lower than the diabetic threshold (Tabak et al., 2012). In clinic, nerve and blood vessel structures have been studied in patients with diabetic painful neuropathy and it was concluded that large fiber demyelination, axonal degeneration, and loss, epineurial arterioles obliteration and epineurial inflammation are frequently observed in this syndrome (Tracy & Dyck, 2008). The spectrum of neuropathy in prediabetic condition with identified impaired glucose tolerance has also been studied and damage was shown to various types of peripheral nerve fibers, accounting for 42.3% small sensory fiber neuropathy, 15.3% large sensory fiber neuropathy, and 42.3% sensorimotor neuropathy (Sumner et al., 2003). As most diabetics and prediabetics are more than 50 years old, age and diet may both serve as risk factors to development of complex myelinodegeneration, and consequently more fibers would be damaged in both the PNS and CNS, leading to multiple sites of pain and multiple comorbidities, such as motor deficit, learning, and cognitive disorders. In aged rats with severe myelinodegeneration, performances of rota-rod treadmill test, hole-exploring open field test and Morris water maze test were all evaluated and it was shown that besides development of mechanical pain hypersensitivity, all the performances significantly declined (Unpublished data). Moreover, because myelin is mainly (>70%) made up of lipids that depend upon lipid synthesis and metabolism, it is more vulnerable to high-energy diets, which may lead to insulin resistance and dysregulation of lipid metabolism (Kettenmann & Ransom, 1995).

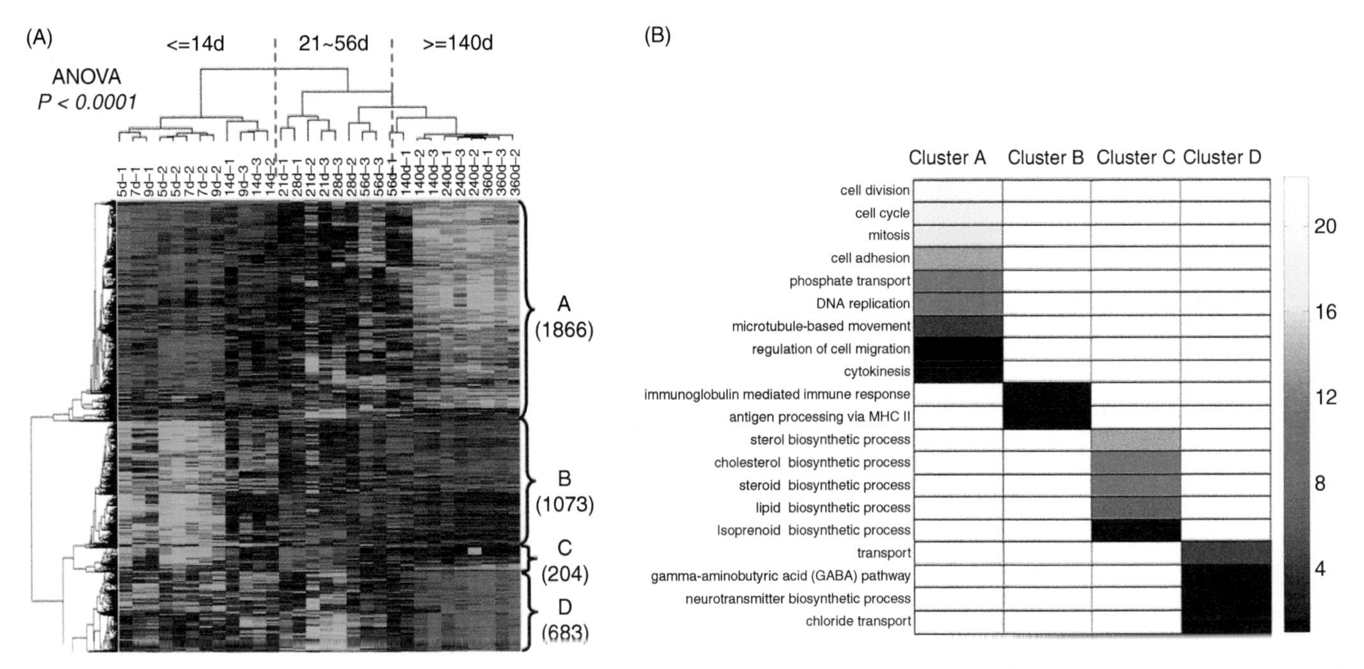

FIG. 4.8 **Age-related changes in functionally-identified gene profiling in the optic nerves of rats with 5, 7, 9, 14, 21, 28, 56, 140, 240, and 360 days old.** (A) Four hierarchical clusters (A–D) were obtained from cluster analysis of 3826 transcripts showing statistical significance of age-related difference in expressions ($p < 0.0001$). Each row represents the expression level for one gene during development. Each column is time point. (B) Biological functions of cluster A–D annotated according to gene ontology analysis using GO database version 2.2.11. Enriched functions of gene at each cluster are listed in the left table, with color representing the significance level (scaled by the negative log of corrected P-value). *From Xie, F., Fu, H., Hou, J. F., Jiao, K., Costigan, M., & Chen, J. (2013a). High energy diets-induced metabolic and prediabetic painful polyneuropathy in rats.* PLoS One, 8, *e57427. (Figs. 3 and 4, p.220) with permission from Spandidos Publications.*

GENETIC AND MOLECULAR BASIS OF AGE-RELATED MYELINODEGENERATION

Why are myelin structures so vulnerable to age and diets? To answer this question, genetic and molecular basis of myelin vulnerability should be studied. Based on our lifespan observations of myelin trajectories described previously, we selected 10 time points (PND5, 7, 9, 14, 21, 28, 56, 140, 240, 360) that covered the whole lifespan changes of myelin structures from birth to old age in terms of development, maturity, and degeneration (Xie et al., 2014a). We selected the optic nerves as tissue samples because: (1) the onset of myelination begins from PND7 that allows us to identify gene profile changes from nonmyelination stage (PND5) to the initial stage of myelination (PND7, 9, 14, and 21), and then to the mature stage (PND28, 56), and finally to the initial and advanced degeneration stages (PND140, 240, 360) (Fig. 4.3); (2) the optic nerves belong to the CNS but are isolated from the brain, which render them appropriate for studying myelinated axon fibers of retinal gangalion cells without involving neuronal cell bodies; (3) the samples are predominant with axons and neuroglial cells (OD and astrocytes) and microglial cells; (4) functional measurements of nerve conduction velocity and visual evoked potentials are easily handled without any invasive injury, largely excluding injury-induced changes in genetic expressions; (5) age-related changes in gene expression profiling can be compared with age-related changes in myelin structures in the corresponding time points, which are more advantageous over previous reports that only examined gene expression profiling (Lee, Weindruch, & Prolla, 2000; Verdier et al., 2012).

Using high-through one-way ANOVA analysis, in all age points a total of 3826 genes were identified that showed differences in expression ($P < 0.0001$). Hierarchical clustering analysis was used on those differentially expressed genes to investigate the categorized characteristics of lifespan changes in gene expressions [Fig. 4.8A, from Xie et al., 2014a (Fig. 3, pp. 220)]. Based upon life changes in gene expression profiling, the rat myelin lifespan could be divided into three stages: (1) myelin developing period from PND5 to PND14; (2) maturing period of myelin sheath from PND21 to PND56; (3) degenerative period of myelin due to aging process started from PND140. Clustering analysis also divided the differentially expressed genes into four subsets according to their expression tendency: (1) Cluster A including 1866 transcripts which expressed at high level only in early developing period; (2) Cluster B including 1073 transcripts which had low expression in developing period but maintained high level of expression since maturing period; (3) Cluster C with 204 transcripts which were expressed low in developing period, greatly upregulated in maturing period, but dropped to very low level again in degenerative period; (4) Cluster D with 683 transcripts which were upregulated only in degenerative period [Fig. 4.8A, from Xie et al., 2014a (Fig. 3, pp. 220)]. Through web-based functional enrichment analysis along with GO annotation of the main functions of the genes in each cluster subset, we got to understand that [Fig. 4.8B, from Xie et al., 2014a (Fig. 4, pp. 220)]: (1) genes in cluster A are mainly involved in functions of cellular differentiation and proliferation, such as the biological processes of cell division, cell cycle, mitosis, DNA replication, and so on; (2) genes in cluster B are mainly involved in immune response and the antigen presenting processes; (3) genes in cluster C are mainly involved in lipid biosynthesis and metabolisms; (4) genes in cluster D are mainly involved in transmitter biosynthetic process and transportation, particularly GABA and its chloride channel receptor transport.

The age-related changes in gene expression profiling of the optic nerves are unique and well represent genes required for myelinating cell differentiation and proliferation, OD growth and myelination, and processes of myelinodegeneration and microglial cell activation and macrophagocytosis. At the developing period after birth, OD progenitor cells are aggregated (see asterisks in Fig. 4.3A-1d, -3d, -5d, and -7d) and differentiated into myelinating cells which begin to myelinate by wrapping the axons nearby (see myelinating OD in Fig. 4.3-12d and Fig. 4.3-14d). Thus, the genes in cluster A are significantly upregulated from PND5 to PND14 followed by dramatic decline after maturity. While at the maturing stage during PND21-56, myelination reaches peak when large amount of lipid synthesis are dramatically required for formation of thick and compact lamellae of myelin sheath due to increases in axonal size and length with age. Thus the genes in cluster C remain upregulated during the maturing period but are downregulated at the developing and degenerative periods. Surprisingly, at both the maturing and the degenerative period of myelin, the genes in cluster B remain upregulated without any signs of decline until PND360 and are further increased in level with age. This suggests that myelin damage or myelin changes may start very early in life. At the maturing and degenerative periods, microglia-mediated immune responses, such as phagocytosis (Brown & Neher, 2014; Prinz & Priller, 2014), are probably actively involved and play very important roles for redundant myelin truncation and for injured myelin repair. Meanwhile, life-long remyelination would also occur due to demyelination or myelinodegeneration (Irvine & Blakemore, 2008; Kerezoudi & Thomas, 1999). However, remyelination and peripheral axonal fiber regeneration could be greatly affected by age (Irvine & Blakemore, 2008; Kerezoudi & Thomas, 1999; Verdú et al., 2000). In another previous report (Xie et al., 2013b), using immunocytochemical and Western blot techniques, age-related downregulation of myelin basic protein (MBP) and myelin oligodendrocyte glycoprotein (MOG) was found to be negatively correlated with upregulation of immunoreactive products of glial fibrillary acidic protein (GFAP) and ionized calcium-binding adaptor molecule 1 (Iba1), biomarkers of activation of astrocytic and microglial cells, respectively [Fig. 4.9 modified from Xie et al., 2013b (Fig. 4, pp. 1024; Fig. 7, p. 1026)]. Fig. 4.10 is an example of photomicrographs showing different intensities of MOG-like immunoreactivities on coronal sections across neural axis of the whole CNS from forebrain to the lumbar spinal cord of 2 months old and 18 months old rats [from Xie et al., 2013b (Fig. 1, p. 1023)]. The MOG-like immunoreactivities were very strong in the whole CNS of 2 months old rats, while global loss of MOG in the whole CNS was detected in 18 months old aged rats (Xie et al., 2013b). This age-related difference in immunohistochemical staining results may explain why many previous efforts failed in immunostaining of myelin proteins using immunocytochemistry (Kettenmann & Ransom, 1995). Myelin contains about 40% water and 60% dry mass substances. About 70–85% dry mass is lipids and 15–30% is proteins (Kettenmann & Ransom, 1995). There are many myelin proteins serving as "glue" to adhere inner surfaces of cytoplasm membrane of an OD processes and outer surfaces of adjacent OD cytoplasm membrane processes of compact myelin lamellae. In the CNS, under TEM the inner surfaces of cytoplasm membrane of OD processes form the major dense lines (MDLs) along which MBP (30%), proteolipid protein (PLP, 50%) and 2′,3′-cyclic nucleotide 3′- phosphodiesterase (4%) are major myelin proteins (Armati & Mathey, 2010; Kettenmann & Ransom, 1995; Lazzarini, 2004). While the outer surfaces of adjacent OD cytoplasm membrane processes form the intraperiod lines (IPLs) along which PLP (50%), and MOG (0.05%) are major myelin proteins (Armati & Mathey, 2010; Kettenmann & Ransom, 1995; Lazzarini, 2004). At the very beginning of myelination, an OD extends its processes to interact with a segment of axons to form OD membrane-axolemma or inner tongue process that requires myelin-associated glycoprotein (1%). In the PNS, protein zero (P0), MBP and peripheral myelin protein 22 serve as major myelin proteins to stabilize compact myelin sheath (Kettenmann & Ransom, 1995; Lazzarini, 2004). Thus, age-related decrease in various myelin proteins would no doubt result in lamellae split from both the MDLs and IPLs (Xie et al., 2014b), leading to widespread myelin breakdown, intramyelin balloon(s), intramyelin inclusions, and other myelinodegenerative changes. In our unpublished work, it was found that the myelinodegenerative changes may lead to release of various alarmins, such as high mobility group box-1 protein (HMGB1) from injured myelin structures or other resources (Chan et al., 2012). The release of HMGB1

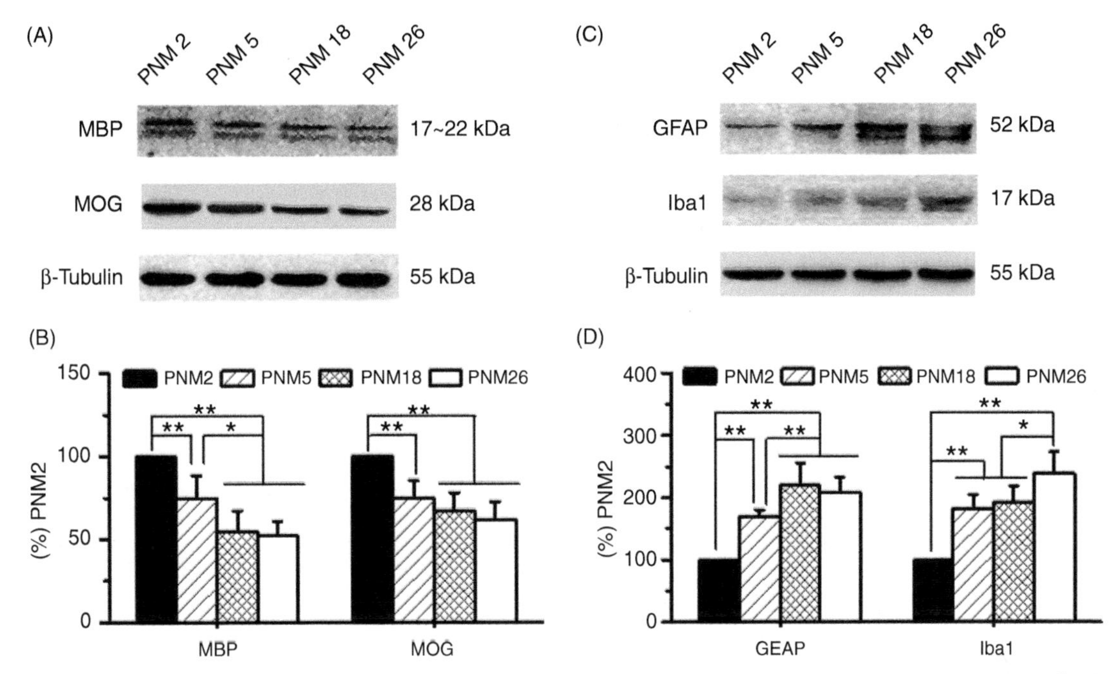

FIG. 4.9 **Age-related negative correlation between myelin protein decline and activation of microglial and astrocytic cells in rat CNS.** (A) Age-related changes in expression of myelin basic protein (MBP) and myelin oligodendrocyte glycoprotein (MOG) in rats with ages of 2, 5, 18, 26 months old (PNM2, 5, 18, and 26, whole brain tissue homogenate excluding the cerebellum: $n = 4$ per time point). (B) Averaged level of age-related percent changes in expressions of MBP and MOG. * $p < 0.05$; ** $p < 0.01$; error bars: ± SEM. (C) Age-related expression of glial fibrillary acidic protein (GFAP), an astrocyte biomarker, and ionized calcium-binding adaptor molecule 1 (Iba1), a microglial biomarker, in rats. (D) Averaged level of age-related percent changes in expressions of GFAP and Iba1. * $p < 0.05$; ** $p < 0.01$; Error bars: ± SEM. *From Xie, F., Zhang, J. C., Fu, H., & Chen, J. (2013b). Age-related decline of myelin proteins is highly correlated with activation of astrocytes and microglia in the rat CNS.* International Journal of Molecular Medicine, *32, 1021–1028. (Fig. 4, p.1024 and Fig. 7, p.1026) with permission from Spandidos Publications.*

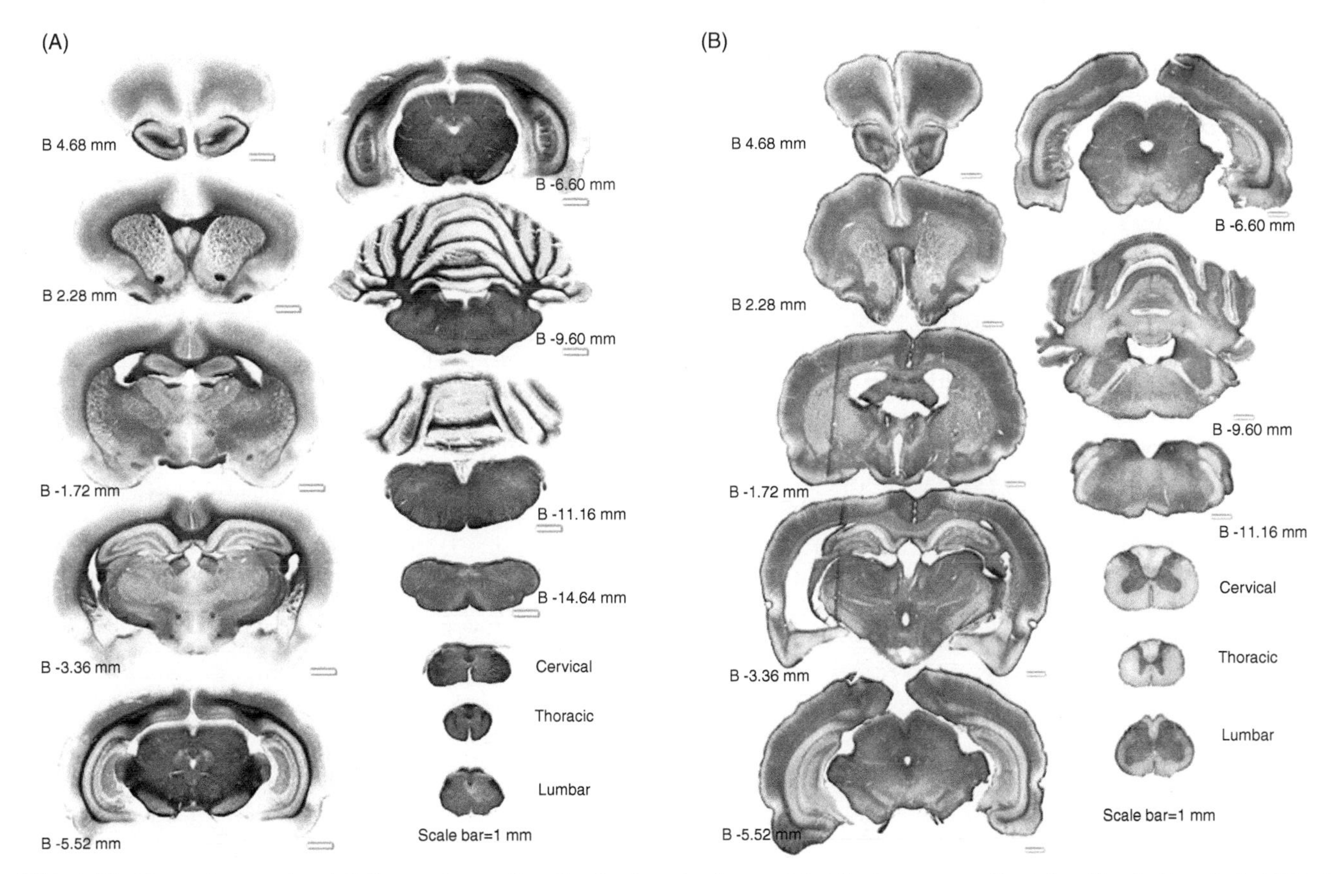

FIG. 4.10 **Dramatic age-related difference in myelin oligodendrocyte glycoprotein-like immunoreactive intensities in the whole CNS of rats between 2 and 18 months old.** *From Xie, F., Zhang, J. C., Fu, H., & Chen, J. (2013b). Age-related decline of myelin proteins is highly correlated with activation of astrocytes and microglia in the rat CNS.* International Journal of Molecular Medicine, *32, 1021–1028. (Fig. 1, pp.1023) with permission from Spandidos Publications.*

might serve as one of alarmins to activate microglial cells and further act on their toll-like receptors (TLRs) and/or receptors of advanced glycation end product (RAGEs) to promote production of proinflammatory mediators, such as tumor necrosis factor α (TNFα), cytokines, chemokines, and so on through regulation of nuclear transcriptional factor kappa B (NF-κB) cascade. The exposure of the axons to the extracellular inflammatory environment due to myelin breakdown would probably cause proinflammatory programmed cell death (pyroptosis) and necroptosis (Cookson & Brennan, 2001; Fink & Cookson, 2005), resulting in consequent axonal degeneration and loss. Since it was suggested more recently that aging may involve several hallmarks, such as genomic instability, telomere attrition, epigenetic alterations, loss of proteostasis, deregulated nutrient sensing, mitochondrial dysfunction, and oxidants over burden, cellular senescence, inhibition of autophagy, stem cell exhaustion, and intercellular communication (López-Otín et al., 2013; Masoro & Austad 2011), more complex mechanisms may be involved in age and diets-related myelinodegeneration.

As for why age- and diet-related myelinodegeneration can cause mechanical pain hypersensitivity or facilitate pain transit from acute to chronic state, little is known for the answers. However, widespread activation of microglial cells in the spinal dorsal horn caused by myelin damage and axonal loss at the adjacent dorsal column may be involved in central sensitization of dorsal horn pain-signaling neurons by actions of cytokines and chemokines (Chen et al., 2013). Meanwhile, sensitization of primary sensory cells at the DRG might also be involved in the processes due to Nav1.8 upregulation through SDF1-CXCR4 signaling-mediated satellite glial cell-neuronal interactions (Yang et al., 2015, 2016).

Myelinoscience is just an emerging field that requires more attentions. Unraveling the molecular and cellular mechanisms of myelinodegeneration would be one of the most important directions for brain health in aged people. Any advances in understanding of the molecular and cellular mechanisms of myelinodegeneration may shed new light on discovery of new therapeutic targets and delay the processes of age-related functional disabilities and keep aging healthy. Moreover, since high-energy diets facilitate myelinodegenerative changes even in young and middle aged animals, it would be helpful to change one's life-styles as early as possible so as to protect myelin structures from damage.

References

Adinolfi, A. M., Yamuy, J., Morales, F. R., & Chase, M. H. (1991). Segmental demyelination in peripheral nerves of old cats. *Neurobiology of Aging, 12*, 175–179.

American Diabetes Association. (2010). Diagnosis and classification of diabetes mellitus. *Diabetes Care, 33*(Suppl. 1), S62–S69.

Armati, P. J., & Mathey, E. K. (2010). *The biology of oligodendrocytes.* Cambridge: Cambridge University Press.

Baezner, H., Blahak, C., Poggesi, A., Pantoni, L., Inzitari, D., Chabriat, H., Erkinjuntti, T., Fazekas, F., Ferro, J. M., Langhorne, P., O'Brien, J., Scheltens, P., Visser, M. C., Wahlund, L. O., Waldemar, G., Wallin, A., & Hennerici, M. G. LADIS Study Group. (2008). Association of gait and balance disorders with age-related white matter changes: the LADIS study. *Neurology, 70*, 935–942.

Baloh, R. W., Ying, S. H., & Jacobson, K. M. (2003). A longitudinal study of gait and balance dysfunction in normal older people. *Archives of Neurology, 60*, 835–839.

Bartzokis, G. (2011). Alzheimer's disease as homeostatic responses to age-related myelin breakdown. *Neurobiology of Aging, 32*, 1341–1371.

Bartzokis, G., Lu, P. H., Heydari, P., Couvrette, A., Lee, G. J., Kalashyan, G., Freeman, F., Grinstead, J. W., Villablanca, P., Finn, J. P., Mintz, J., Alger, J. R., & Altshuler, L. L. (2012). Multimodal magnetic resonance imaging assessment of white matter aging trajectories over the lifespan of healthy individuals. *Biological Psychiatry, 72*, 1026–1034.

Bartzokis, G., Lu, P. H., Tingus, K., Mendez, M. F., Richard, A., Peters, D. G., Oluwadara, B., Barrall, K. A., Finn, J. P., Villablanca, P., Thompson, P. M., & Mintz, J. (2010). Lifespan trajectory of myelin integrity and maximum motor speed. *Neurobiology of Aging, 31*, 1554–1562.

Bergman, E., & Ulfhake, B. (2002). Evidence for loss of myelinated input to the spinal cord in senescent rats. *Neurobiology of Aging, 23*, 271–286.

Bhadelia, R. A., Price, L. L., Tedesco, K. L., Scott, T., Qiu, W. Q., Patz, S., Folstein, M., Rosenberg, I., Caplan, L. R., & Bergethon, P. (2009). Diffusion tensor imaging, white matter lesions, the corpus callosum, and gait in the elderly. *Stroke, 40*, 3816–3820.

Bishwajit, G. (2015). Nutrition transition in South Asia: the emergence of non-communicable chronic diseases. Version 2. F1000, Res, *4*, 8.

Black, S., Gao, F., & Bilbao, J. (2009). Understanding white matter disease: imaging-pathological correlations in vascular cognitive impairment. *Stroke, 40*(Suppl. 3), S48–S52.

Blahak, C., Baezner, H., Pantoni, L., Poggesi, A., Chabriat, H., Erkinjuntti, T., Fazekas, F., Ferro, J. M., Langhorne, P., O'Brien, J., Visser, M. C., Wahlund, L. O., Waldemar, G., Wallin, A., Inzitari, D., & Hennerici, M. G. LADIS Study Group. (2009). Deep frontal and periventricular age related white matter changes but not basal ganglia and infratentorial hyperintensities are associated with falls: cross sectional results from the LADIS study. *J Neurol Neurosurg Psychiatry, 80*, 608–613.

Bohnen, N. I., & Albin, R. L. (2011). White matter lesions in Parkinson disease. *Nature Review Neurology, 7*, 229–236.

Brown, G. C., & Neher, J. J. (2014). Microglial phagocytosis of live neurons. *Nature Reviews Neuroscience, 15*, 209–216.

Burton, E. J., Kenny, R. A., O'Brien, J., Stephens, S., Bradbury, M., Rowan, E., Kalaria, R., Firbank, M., Wesnes, K., & Ballard, C. (2004). White matter hyperintensities are associated with impairment of memory, attention, and global cognitive performance in older stroke patients. *Stroke, 35*, 1270–1275.

Ceballos, D., Cuadras, J., Verdú, E., & Navarro, X. (1999). Morphometric and ultrastructural changes with ageing in mouse peripheral nerve. *Journal of Anatomy, 195*(Pt4), 563–576.

Chan, J. K., Roth, J., Oppenheim, J. J., Tracey, K. J., Vogl, T., Feldmann, M., Horwood, N., & Nanchahal, J. (2012). Alarmins: awaiting a clinical response. *Journal of Clinical Investigation, 122*, 2711–2719.

Chen, J., Han, J. S., Zhao, Z. Q., Wei, F., Hsieh, J. C., Bao, L., Chen, A. C. N., Dai, Y., Fan, B. F., Gu, J. G., Hao, S. L., Hu, S. J., Ji, Y. H., Li, Y. J., Li, Y. Q., Lin, Q., Liu, X. G., Liu, Y. Q., Lu, Y., Luo, F., Ma, C., Qui, Y. H., Rao, Z. R., Shi, L., Shyu, B. C., Song, X. J., Tang, J. S., Tao, Y. X., Wan, Y., Wang, J. S., Wang, K. W., Wang, Y., Xu, G. Y., Xu, T. L., You, H. J., Yu, L. C., Yu, S. Y., Zhang, D. Y., Zhang, D. R., Zhang, J. M., Zhang, X., Zhang, Y. Q., & Zhuo, M. (2013). Pain. In D.

W. Pfaff (Ed.), *Neuroscience in the 21st Century: From Basic to Clinical* (pp. 965–1023). New York: Springer.

Chen, J., & Lariviere, W. R. (2010). The nociceptive and anti-nociceptive effects of bee venom injection and therapy: a double-edged sword. *Progress in Neurobiology, 92*, 151–183.

Cookson, B. T., & Brennan, M. A. (2001). Pro-inflammatory programmed cell death. *Trends in Microbiology, 9*, 113–114.

Dansie, E. J., Turk, D. C., Martin, K. R., Van Domelen, D. R., & Patel, K. V. (2014). Association of chronic widespread pain with objectively measured physical activity in adults: findings from the National Health and Nutrition Examination survey. *Journal of Pain, 15*, 507–515.

de Laat, K. F., Tuladhar, A. M., van Norden, A. G., Norris, D. G., Zwiers, M. P., & de Leeuw, F. E. (2010). Loss of white matter integrity is associated with gait disorders in cerebral small vessel disease. *Brain, 134*, 73–83.

Della Nave, R., Foresti, S., Pratesi, A., Ginestroni, A., Inzitari, M., Salvadori, E., Giannelli, M., Diciotti, S., Inzitari, D., & Mascalchi, M. (2007). Whole-brain histogram and voxel-based analyses of diffusion tensor imaging in patients with leukoaraiosis: correlation with motor and cognitive impairment. *AJNR American Journal of Neuroradiology, 28*, 1313–1319.

Dyck, P. J., Thomas, P. K., & Lambert, E. H. (1975). *Peripheral neuropathy*. Philadelphia: W.B. Saunders Company.

Fink, S. L., & Cookson, B. T. (2005). Apoptosis, pyroptosis, and necrosis: mechanistic description of dead and dying eukaryotic cells. *Infection and Immunity, 73*, 1907–1916.

Forbes, H. J., Thomas, S. L., Smeeth, L., Clayton, T., Farmer, R., Bhaskaran, K., & Langan, S. M. (2016). A systematic review and meta-analysis of risk factors for postherpetic neuralgia. *Pain, 157*, 30–54.

Ge, W., Chen, J., Li, Y., & Chen, H. S. (2002). Pain-related behavioral response of elderly rats to peripheral different chemical tissue injury. *Journal of Fourth Military Medical University, 23*, 433–436.

Gibson, S. J., & Weiner, D. K. (2005). *Pain in older persons*. Seattle: IASP Press.

Global Burden of Disease 2013 DALYs and HALE Collaborators. (2015). Global, regional, and national disability-adjusted life years (DALYs) for 306 diseases and injuries and healthy life expectancy (HALE) for 188 countries, 1990–2013: quantifying the epidemiological transition. *Lancet, 386*, 2145–2191.

Global Burden of Disease 2013 Risk Factors Collaborators. (2015). Global, regional, and national comparative risk assessment of 79 behavioural, environmental and occupational, and metabolic risks or clusters of risks in 188 countries, 1990–2013: a systematic analysis for the Global Burden of Disease Study 2013. *Lancet, 386*, 2287–2323.

Global Burden of Disease Study 2013 Collaborators. (2015). Global, regional, and national incidence, prevalence, and years lived with disability for 301 acute and chronic diseases and injuries in 188 countries, 1990–2013: a systematic analysis for the Global Burden of Disease Study 2013. *Lancet, 386*, 743–800.

Harkins, S. W., Price, D. D., Bush, F. M., & Small, R. E. (1994). Geriatric pain. In P. D. Wall, & R. Melzack (Eds.), *Textbook of pain*, (3rd ed., pp. 769–784). Edinburgh: Churchill Linvingstone.

Haroutunian, V., Katsel, P., Roussos, P., Davis, K. L., Altshuler, L. L., & Bartzokis, G. (2014). Myelination, oligodendrocytes, and serious mental illness. *Glia, 62*, 1856–1877.

Irvine, K. A., & Blakemore, W. F. (2008). Remyelination protects axons from demyelination-associated axon degeneration. *Brain, 131*(Pt 6), 1464–1477.

Johansson, C. S., Stenström, M., & Hildebrand, C. (1996). Target influence on aging of myelinated sensory nerve fibres. *Neurobiology of Aging, 17*, 61–66.

Kerezoudi, E., & Thomas, P. K. (1999). Influence of age on regeneration in the peripheral nervous system. *Gerontology, 45*, 301–306.

Kertesz, A., Black, S. E., Tokar, G., Benke, T., Carr, T., & Nicholson, L. (1988). Periventricular and subcortical hyperintensities on magnetic resonance imaging. Rims, caps, and unidentified bright objects. *Archives of Neurology, 45*, 404–408.

Kettenmann, H., & Ransom, B. R. (1995). *Neuroglia*. New York: Oxford University Press.

Kirkpatrick, J. B., & Hayman, L. A. (1987). White-matter lesions in MR imaging of clinically healthy brains of elderly subjects: possible pathologic basis. *Radiology, 162*, 509–511.

Knox, C. A., Kokmen, E., & Dyck, P. J. (1989). Morphometric alteration of rat myelinated fibers with aging. *Journal of Neuropathology and Experimental Neurology, 48*, 119–139.

Krinke, G., Froehlich, E., Herrmann, M., Schnider, K., Da Silva, F., Suter, J., & Traber, K. (1988). Adjustment of the myelin sheath to axonal atrophy in the rat spinal root by the formation of infolded myelin loops. *Acta Anatomica (Basel), 131*, 182–187.

Lasiene, J., Matsui, A., Sawa, Y., Wong, F., & Horner, P. J. (2009). Age-related myelin dynamics revealed by increased oligodendrogenesis and short internodes. *Aging Cell, 8*, 201–213.

Lazzarini, R. A. (2004). *Myelin biology and disorders*. Amsterdam: Elsevier Academic Press.

Lee, C. K., Weindruch, R., & Prolla, T. A. (2000). Gene-expression profile of the ageing brain in mice. *Nature Genetics, 25*, 294–297.

López-Otín, C., Blasco, M. A., Partridge, L., Serrano, M., & Kroemer, G. (2013). The hallmarks of aging. *Cell, 153*, 1194–1217.

Lu, P. H., Lee, G. J., Shapira, J., Jimenez, E., Mather, M. J., Thompson, P. M., Bartzokis, G., & Mendez, M. F. (2014). Regional differences in white matter breakdown between frontotemporal dementia and early-onset Alzheimer's disease. *Journal of Alzheimers Disease, 39*, 261–269.

Mansfield, K. E., Sim, J., Jordan, J. L., & Jordan, K. P. (2016). A systematic review and meta-analysis of the prevalence of chronic widespread pain in the general population. *Pain, 157*, 55–64.

Masoro, E. J., & Austad, S. N. (2011). *Handbook of the neurobiology of aging*. Amsterdam: Elsevier.

Murray, M. E., Senjem, M. L., Petersen, R. C., Hollman, J. H., Preboske, G. M., Weigand, S. D., Knopman, D. S., Ferman, T. J., Dickson, D. W., & Jack, C. R., Jr. (2010). Functional impact of white matter hyperintensities in cognitively normal elderly subjects. *Archives of Neurology, 67*, 1379–1385.

Papanas, N., Vinik, A. I., & Ziegler, D. (2011). Neuropathy in prediabetes: does the clock start ticking early? *Nature Reviews Endocrinology, 7*, 682–690.

Patel, K. V., Cochrane, B. B., Turk, D. C., Bastian, L. A., Haskell, S. G., Woods, N. F., Zaslavsky, O., Wallace, R. B., & Kerns, R. D. (2016). Association of pain with physical function, depressive symptoms, fatigue, and sleep quality among veteran and non-veteran postmenopausal women. *Gerontologist, 56*(Suppl. 1), S91–S101.

Patel, K. V., Dansie, E. J., & Turk, D. C. (2013a). Impact of chronic musculoskeletal pain on objectively measured daily physical activity: a review of current findings. *Pain Management, 3*, 467–474.

Patel, K. V., Guralnik, J. M., Dansie, E. J., & Turk, D. C. (2013b). Prevalence and impact of pain among older adults in the United States: findings from the 2011 National Health and Aging Trends Study. *Pain, 154*, 2649–2657.

Patel, K. V., Phelan, E. A., Leveille, S. G., Lamb, S. E., Missikpode, C., Wallace, R. B., Guralnik, J. M., & Turk, D. C. (2014). High prevalence of falls, fear of falling, and impaired balance in older adults with pain in the United States: findings from the 2011 National Health and Aging Trends Study. *Journal of American Geriatrics Society, 62*, 1844–1852.

Peters, A. (2002). The effects of normal aging on myelin and nerve fibers: a review. *Journal of Neurocytology, 31*, 581–593.

Peters, A. (2009). The effects of normal aging on myelinated nerve fibers in monkey central nervous system. *Frontiers in Neuroanatomy, 3*, 11.

Peters, A., & Kemper, T. (2012). A review of the structural alterations in the cerebral hemispheres of the aging rhesus monkey. *Neurobiology of Aging*, *33*, 2357–2372.

Prins, N. D., van Dijk, E. J., den Heijer, T., Vermeer, S. E., Jolles, J., Koudstaal, P. J., Hofman, A., & Breteler, M. M. (2005). Cerebral small-vessel disease and decline in information processing speed, executive function and memory. *Brain*, *128*(Pt9), 2034–2041.

Prinz, M., & Priller, J. (2014). Microglia and brain macrophages in the molecular age: from origin to neuropsychiatric disease. *Nature Reviews Neuroscience*, *15*, 300–312.

Sharma, A. K., Bajada, S., & Thomas, P. K. (1980). Age changes in the tibial and plantar nerves of the rat. *Journal of Anatomy*, *130*(Pt 2), 417–428.

Shen, D., Zhang, Q., Gao, X., Gu, X., & Ding, F. (2011). Age-related changes in myelin morphology, electrophysiological property and myelin-associated protein expression of mouse sciatic nerves. *Neuroscience Letters*, *502*, 162–167.

Sullivan, P., Pary, R., Telang, F., Rifai, A. H., & Zubenko, G. S. (1990). Risk factors for white matter changes detected by magnetic resonance imaging in the elderly. *Stroke*, *21*, 1424–1428.

Sumner, C. J., Sheth, S., Griffin, J. W., Cornblath, D. R., & Polydefkis, M. (2003). The spectrum of neuropathy in diabetes and impaired glucose tolerance. *Neurology*, *60*, 108–111.

Tabak, A. G., Herder, C., Rathmann, W., Brunner, E. J., & Kivimaki, M. (2012). Prediabetes: a high-risk state for diabetes development. *Lancet*, *379*, 2279–2290.

Tang, Y., Nyengaard, J. R., Pakkenberg, B., & Gundersen, H. J. (1997). Age-induced white matter changes in the human brain: a stereological investigation. *Neurobiology of Aging*, *18*, 609–615.

Tesfaye, S., Boulton, A. J., Dyck, P. J., Freeman, R., Horowitz, M., Kempler, P., Lauria, G., Malik, R. A., Spallone, V., Vinik, A., Bernardi, L., & Valensi, P. Toronto Diabetic Neuropathy Expert Group. (2010). Diabetic neuropathies: update on definitions, diagnostic criteria, estimation of severity, and treatments. *Diabetes Care*, *33*, 2285–2293.

Thomas, P. K., King, R. H., & Sharma, A. K. (1980). Changes with age in the peripheral nerves of the rat. An ultrastructural study. *Acta Neuropathology*, *52*, 1–6.

Tracy, J. A., & Dyck, P. J. (2008). The spectrum of diabetic neuropathies. *Physical Medicine and Rehabilitation Clinics North America*, *19*, 1–26.

Verdier, V., Csárdi, G., de Preux-Charles, A. S., Médard, J. J., Smit, A. B., Verheijen, M. H., Bergmann, S., & Chrast, R. (2012). Aging of myelinating glial cells predominantly affects lipid metabolism and immune response pathways. *Glia*, *60*, 751–760.

Verdú, E., Ceballos, D., Vilches, J. J., & Navarro, X. (2000). Influence of aging on peripheral nerve function and regeneration. *Journal of Peripheral Nervous System*, *5*, 191–208.

Wade, K. F., Lee, D. M., McBeth, J., Ravindrarajah, R., Gielen, E., Pye, S. R., Vanderschueren, D., Pendleton, N., Finn, J. D., Bartfai, G., Casanueva, F. F., Forti, G., Giwercman, A., Huhtaniemi, I. T., Kula, K., Punab, M., Wu, F. C., & O'Neill, T. W. (2016). Chronic widespread pain is associated with worsening frailty in European men. *Age Ageing*, *45*, 268–274.

World Health Organization (2015). *World report on ageing and health*. Geneva: WHO Press. Available from: http://apps.who.int/iris/bitstream/10665/186463/1/9789240694811_eng.pdf.

Xie, F., Fu, H., Hou, J. F., Jiao, K., Costigan, M., & Chen, J. (2013a). High energy diets-induced metabolic and prediabetic painful polyneuropathy in rats. *PLoS One*, *8*, e57427.

Xie, F., Fu, H., Zhang, J. C., Chen, X. F., Wang, X. L., & Chen, J. (2014a). Gene profiling in the dynamic regulation of the lifespan of the myelin sheath structure in the optic nerve of rats. *Molecular Medicine Reports*, *10*, 217–222.

Xie, F., Liang, P., Fu, H., Zhang, J. C., & Chen, J. (2014b). Effects of normal aging on myelin sheath ultrastructures in the somatic sensorimotor system of rats. *Molecular Medicine Reports*, *10*, 459–466.

Xie, F., Zhang, J. C., Fu, H., & Chen, J. (2013b). Age-related decline of myelin proteins is highly correlated with activation of astrocytes and microglia in the rat CNS. *International Journal of Molecular Medicine*, *32*, 1021–1028.

Yang, F., Sun, W., Yang, Y., Wang, Y., Li, C. L., Fu, H., Wang, X. L., Yang, F., He, T., & Chen, J. (2015). SDF1-CXCR4 signaling contributes to persistent pain and hypersensitivity via regulating excitability of primary nociceptive neurons: involvement of ERK-dependent Nav1.8 up-regulation. *Journal of Neuroinflammation*, *12*, 219.

Yang, F., Sun, W., Luo, W. J., Yang, Y., Yang, F., Wang, X. L., & Chen, J. (2016). SDF1-CXCR4 signalling contributes to the transition from acute to chronic pain. *Molecular Neurobiology*.

Zheng, J. H., Chen, J., & Arendt-Nielsen, L. (2004a). Complexity of tissue injury-induced nociceptive discharge of dorsal horn wide dynamic range neurons in the rat, correlation with effects of systemic morphine. *Brain Research*, *1001*, 143–149.

Zheng, J. H., Feng, W., Jian, Z., & Chen, J. (2004b). Age-related change in deterministic behaviors of nociceptive firing of rat dorsal horn neurons. *Acta Physiologica Sinica*, *56*, 178–182.

SECTION B

HERBS AND EXTRACTS IN PAIN MANAGEMENT

CHAPTER

5

Getting to the Root of Chronic Inflammation: Ginger's Antiinflammatory Properties

P. Inserra, A. Brooks***

*John Tyler Community College, Chester, VA, United States; **Virginia Polytechnic Institute and State University, Blacksburg, VA, United States

INTRODUCTION

Zingiber officinale, most commonly known as ginger, is a plant that belongs to the family Zingiberaceae. This plant is native to India, but is cultivated in many countries within Asia, Africa, Australia, and Latin America (Mashhadi et al., 2013). The root of the ginger plant, also referred to as a rhizome, is a horizontal underground stem, which grows continuously into lateral shoots (Khodaie & Sadeghpoor, 2015). Perennial in nature, ginger root, grows year after year on its own. This quality allows ginger root to be a hardy and more readily produced plant.

Ginger is rich in phytochemicals which can be extracted as an oil, dried, and also ground into a powder form. Gingerol and shogaol, two of the bioactive molecules found in ginger, have shown antioxidant activity, among other benefits, in various contexts (Mashhadi et al., 2013). The phenol [6]-gingerol, and a dehydrated analog, [6]-shogaol, is the primary bioactive compounds derived from ginger.

Benefits of ginger's phytochemical properties have given it timeless popularity. Its varying uses include, but are not limited to, administration as a medicinal remedy, as a nutritional supplement, as an aromatherapy agent, as a seasoning in cuisines, and as a flavoring in beverages, such as tea.

Traditionally, ginger has been used for a variety of conditions, many of which are similar to its present-day uses including, treatment of colds, digestive maladies, and fevers (White, 2007). The most popular present day use for ginger is as a treatment for nausea and vomiting associated with pregnancy and motion sickness.

Ginger rhizome can be consumed in several forms. It can be found in the form of a capsule containing the dried and ground root, as an oil, that can be applied for topical treatment, and as a dried and ground spice which can be added to food or drink.

Although ginger is categorized as a food additive by the US Food and Drug Administration, the field of complementary and alternative medicine considers ginger to be an evidence-based treatment for several medical disorders and symptoms. Recent interest in the possibility that the ginger rhizome, does in fact, hold the key to medicinal benefits and powerful treatments for chronic diseases and disorders, such as arthritis, type 2 diabetes mellitus (DM), dysmenorrhea, cancer, and respiratory conditions, among others, has led to several clinical trials in order to test its rate of efficacy.

When the efficacy of *Z. officinale* as a treatment for inflammation and pain was evaluated, several in vitro and animal experiments found ginger extract to be more potent than the antiinflammatory compounds found in aspirin (Chrubasik, Pittler, & Roufogalis, 2005).

ARTHRITIS

Arthritis is a group of debilitating conditions including osteoarthritis and rheumatoid arthritis, which result in damage to the articular cartilage associated with joints. The etiology of osteoarthritis is due to excessive

Nutritional Modulators of Pain in the Aging Population. http://dx.doi.org/10.1016/B978-0-12-805186-3.00005-9
Copyright © 2017 Elsevier Inc. All rights reserved.

wear and tear on the joints and is therefore associated with older age and obesity. Osteoarthritis is the most common form of arthritis and is a major debilitating degenerative disease affecting the elderly. It leads to joint swelling, stiffness, and deformation, inflammation, pain, and impaired function and activity. It has been estimated to affect 30.8 million Americans (Cisternas et al., 2016) and nearly half of all Americans 85 years of age or older (Murphy et al., 2008). Rheumatoid arthritis is an autoimmune disease resulting in destruction in the articular cartilage affecting 1.5 million people in the United States (Myasoedova, Crowson, Kremers, Therneau, & Gabriel, 2010) and 1 in 250 children (Sacks, Helmick, Luo, Ilowite, & Bowyer, 2007). Both conditions benefit from antiinflammatory treatment. Traditionally NSAIDS (nonsteroidal antiinflammatory) have been used, however use of these drugs are associated with a high incidence of peptic ulcers presumably due to inhibition of cyclooxygenase-1 (COX-1) (Steen, 2001). Although newer therapies selectively target COX-2, they too have been associated with adverse gastrointestinal effects (Cheung et al., 2010). Recent investigations have therefore focused on the potential of natural antiinflammatory substances, like ginger, as effective therapies to minimize these adverse effects.

In a study by Drozdov, Kim, Tkachenko, and Varvanina (2012) 43 patients with osteoarthritis of the knee and hip were randomized into two groups and given either 340 mg ginger EV.EXT 35 *Z. officinale* extract or 100 mg diclofenac daily for 4 weeks, with both groups also receiving 1000 mg glucosamine daily. The study group consisting of 35 women and 8 men. Results of this study indicated that the ginger combination therapy administered to the study participants was equally effective as the diclofenac NSAID treatment administered. Patients in the diclofenac group experienced increased dyspepsia symptoms, such as esophageal reflux, with one patient forming a duodenal ulcer which required administration to be discontinued. Ginger combination therapy was concluded to be safer in the treatment of osteoarthritis, as it did not affect the stomach mucosa or worsen dyspepsia in the patients who received it.

In a study by Villalvilla et al. (2013), the researchers sought to discover if ginger derivatives held the ability to control innate immune responses, particularly if ginger derivatives held antiinflammatory and anticatabolic properties. [6]-shogaol, a derivative obtained from ginger powder, was utilized in the study in order to determine whether or not this compound exhibited benefits to bone and cartilage in the body. A mixture of proinflammatory chemicals were added to both cultured fetal bovine and human cartilage. [6]-Shogaol effectively blocked the TLR4-mediated innate immune response, thereby slowing chondrocyte degradation. This data suggests that diets supplemented with ginger may play a role in the reduction of osteoarthritis symptoms caused by continuous inflammation and chondrocyte degradation.

DIABETES MELLITUS

DM is a group of diseases characterized by hyperglycemia. Type 2 DM is the most common form in the United States. It is a progressive disorder first associated with insulin resistance and typically seen in overweight and obese individuals. The incidence of Type 2 DM is on the rise and parallels the incidence of obesity. Historically this disease was only seen in adults, but as overweight and obesity rates rise in children and adolescents, it is now observed at alarming rates in younger populations. Type 2 DM has been estimated to account for up to 95% of all adult diabetes cases in the United States and more than 20,000 cases in individuals younger than 20 years of age (Centers for Disease Control and Prevention, 2014).

Complications of Type 2 DM contribute to a large portion of the disease's morbidity and mortality, while also significantly impacting quality of life. Comorbidities include atherosclerosis, renal disease, stroke, metabolic syndrome, and other inflammatory diseases. Recently, chronic-low grade inflammation has been shown to be associated with Type 2 DM. It is therefore not surprising that antiinflammatory dietary components, such as ginger, may play a role in preventing or managing inflammatory diseases like Type 2 DM.

In a study by Mahluji et al. (2013), the effects of *Z. officinale* were studied in relation to their abilities to affect proinflammatory cytokines and acute phase proteins, which cause low-grade inflammation. The study consisted of 64 Type 2 DM patients randomly assigned to receive 2 ginger tablets per day for 2 months or placebo 2 times per day for 2 months. Patients participating in insulin therapy were not included in the study. Baseline measurements of serum concentrations of proinflammatory cytokines, such as IL-6 and acute phase proteins were obtained. These measurements were also obtained at the end of the study period. The researchers found reduced measures of inflammation in the group receiving ginger supplementation. This data suggests that ginger is a viable treatment option to decrease inflammation related to type 2 DM.

In a double-blind study conducted by Khandouzi et al. (2015), the effects of ginger on fasting blood sugar, hemoglobin A1c, and Apo A-1 were evaluated. Fifty participants with type 2 DM received either 1 g capsules of dried ginger or placebo. Study participants were given a 24-h diet recall questionnaire, anthropometric data, such as height and weight was collected, and blood values were assessed for the markers being evaluated at baseline and at the end of the 12 week study period. Participants receiving ginger had decreased fasting blood sugar, hemoglobin A1c, Apo B, and Apo A-1. These findings indicate that ginger can contribute to the treatment of high blood glucose levels and hemoglobin A1c levels in those with type 2 DM.

A double blind placebo controlled study conducted by Arablou et al. (2014), assessed the effects ginger on lipid profile and glycemic status in the 70 diabetic participants. Participants received either 1600 mg of ginger per day or placebo for 12 weeks. Levels of lipids, c-reactive proteins, and serum sugars were measured both before and after the provided interventions, with results showing a decrease in fasting plasma glucose, hemoglobin A1c, and insulin in participants receiving ginger. These results are consistent with other studies and further demonstrate the effectiveness of ginger in diabetes management.

A 3 month double blind placebo controlled trial conducted by Shidfar et al. (2015), examined the effects of 3 g ginger powder as a treatment for diabetes and found significant improvements in the glycemic levels after ginger supplementation. Clinically relevant decreases in blood glucose of 19.4 mg/dL were observed, while participants receiving placebo saw a slight increase of 1.6 mg/dL.

In a study by Imani et al. (2015), the effects of 1000 mg of ginger per day for a 10 week period were tested on 36 peritoneal dialysis patients. The purpose of this study was to determine if the prescribed dosage of daily ginger would have an effect on serum glucose levels and inflammation markers. Subjects were randomly selected to receive 1000 mg ginger or placebo for 10 weeks. The researchers found that serum fasting glucose was reduced by 2 mmol/L with ginger supplementation, indicating that small reductions in glycemic markers can be seen in nondiabetic patients. This data suggests that ginger could confer a preventative role in diabetes, although future research is needed to test this hypothesis.

DYSMENORRHEA

Primary dysmenorrhea is a medical condition characterized by pain and cramping in the lower back and abdomen associated with menstruation. It typically begins 24–48 h before menstruation and can last for several days. Symptoms vary amongst women, but range from mild to severe and can contribute to fatigue, decreased productivity and work absenteeism, and are experienced by over 80% of women of reproductive age (Grandi & Cagnacci, 2012). Although the etiology of dysmenorrhea is not completely understood, it is hypothesized to involve inflammatory mediators, such as prostaglandins released from endometrial cells as they are sloughed off during menstruation. Inflammatory mediators stimulate uterine contraction and nerve endings, resulting in pain and inflammation. This is further demonstrated by several studies which have shown that NSAIDS are an effective treatment to manage symptoms in women with dysmenorrhea by inhibiting COX-2 and subsequent prostaglandin secretion (Daniels, Torri, & Desjardins, 2005; Edwards, Moore, & McQuay, 2004). Recently, several clinical trials have been conducted to test the efficacy of ginger supplementation on improving dysmenorrhea.

In a study conducted by Halder (2012), the efficacy of oral ginger intake on symptoms of dysmenorrhea were compared to the practice of progressive muscle relaxation. Progressive muscle relaxation consists of consciously squeezing muscle groups until tense and then releasing the tension while actively reflecting on the feeling of the practice being performed.

The 75 nursing students recruited for this study were divided into three groups. Two experimental groups received either oral ginger supplementation or employed progressive muscle relaxation techniques. Ginger supplementation was provided in the form of 1 g of powder dissolved in warm water after a meal. The control group received no intervention or treatment for menstrual related pain and discomfort. Halder (2012), determined that both progressive muscle relaxation and oral ginger intake were successful in reducing the symptoms of dysmenorrhea, but that oral ginger supplementation was more effective, in that it reduced a larger variety of symptoms. Ginger powder was able to decrease symptoms, such as cramping in the lower abdomen, nausea, and diarrhea, offering a novel method for managing symptoms associated with dysmenorrhea.

In a study conducted by Shirvani, Motahari-Tabari, and Alipour, (2014) the effects of ginger on pain relief in primary dysmenorrhea were evaluated in comparison to treatment with mefenamic acid. With NSAIDs being employed as a primary treatment method for symptoms of dysmenorrhea, such as cramping and lower back pain, the researchers in this study sought to determine if ginger was a viable treatment option with fewer potential side effects. One hundred and 22 female students who experienced severe primary dysmenorrhea in at least 50% of their menstrual cycles participated. Pain intensity also was required to be rated at least 40 mm based on a 100 mm visual analog scale. The study participants were randomly placed into two treatment groups. Participants in the mefenamic acid group receiving capsules in the amount of 250 mg every 8 h. Those in the ginger group received capsules in the amount of 250 mg every 6 h. These capsules were given from the onset of menstruation and until pain relief endured for two menstrual cycles. Participants were asked to rate the intensity of their pain through the use of a visual analog scale. Upon completion of the clinical trial at the end of two complete menstrual cycles, it was determined that pain intensity was reduced in both groups of participants. Those participants receiving mefenamic acid capsules and those receiving ginger capsules both reported that there was a decrease in the severity of dysmenorrhea, duration of pain, volume of menstrual bleeding, and length of menstrual cycle. The researchers concluded that ginger is equally effective in the treatment of dysmenorrhea to that of mefenamic acid, with the benefit of having no known adverse side effects.

Jenabi (2013), studied the effectiveness of ginger as a pain reliever for symptoms of primary dysmenorrhea in contrast to that of no provided treatment. The clinical trial was conducted with 70 female students as participants. The average age of participant was approximately 21 years with the average age of menarch being 13.66 years. Participants were randomly divided into two groups, one receiving a 500 mg ginger capsule and the other group receiving a placebo. The intervention or placebo were administered in rounds of 3 capsules daily during the first menstrual cycle for 3 days, for a total of 1500 mg administered per day. At the beginning of the study, participants were asked to rate a variety of primary dysmenorrhea symptoms through the use of a five-point Likert scale. Post-intervention, the participants were asked to complete the same evaluation using the same five-point Likert scale. Findings from this study indicated that those receiving ginger reported that their symptoms were better (40%) or much better (42.6%). Research outcomes indicated that ginger can be considered as an effective treatment for pain management in primary dysmenorrhea, with a decreased incidence of side effects when compared to current use of anti-inflammatory drugs among those experiencing primary dysmenorrhea symptoms.

In a study conducted by Rahnama, Montazeri, Huseini, Kianbakht, and Naseri (2012), ginger was tested against a placebo in order to determine the effectiveness of ginger root in reducing symptoms associated with dysmenorrhea in a double-blind trial. The researchers selected 118 female students with an average age of 21, experiencing moderate or severe primary dysmenorrhea. They were assigned to two groups composed of 59 students. The study was conducted using two different cycles with differing protocols. During the first cycle of the study, one group of 59 students received 500 mg capsules of ginger root powder 3 times per day, while the second group of 59 students received 500 mg of encapsulated placebo 3 times per day. Treatments were administered 2 days prior to the onset of the menstrual cycles of the participants and treatment continued throughout the first 3 days of the menstrual cycle. During the second cycle of the study, ginger and placebo treatments were given for only the first 3 days of the menstrual cycle. Throughout the study, both before administration of treatment and after administration of treatment, the severity of pain as a result of dysmenorrhea was evaluated using a visual analog scale and a verbal multidimensional system for scoring. Participants were also asked to keep a written log of any adverse side effects experienced throughout the study. At the conclusion of the study, results suggested that ginger might be an effective therapy for the relief of pain associated with primary dysmenorrhea. This was found to be true when the ginger was administered at the onset or during the 3 days prior to the menstrual cycle.

CANCER

Colon cancer is the second leading cause of cancer in the United States. In 2012, 134,784 people were diagnosed and 51,516 people died from colorectal cancer. Although mortality rates have been declining, black men and women have disproportionately higher risk of both incidence and mortality. Screening through colonoscopy has been effective in early diagnosis and removal of precancerous polyps. Unfortunately, due to the invasiveness of this procedure, public health campaigns have not been successful in eliminating this disease. Risk for colorectal cancer has been shown to be increased by dietary factors and lack of exercise, as well as genetic predisposition. It has also been hypothesized that development of colorectal cancer is related to inflammation (Coussens & Werb, 2002). A large prospective study has demonstrated higher levels of inflammatory markers in individuals who subsequently developed the disease (Erlinger, 2004) and numerous studies have shown the effectiveness of NSAIDS in the prevention of this disease (Rostom, 2007). An alternative approach to preventing colon cancer could be the use of antiinflammatory agents, either pharmacological in nature or natural compounds, such as ginger. Several clinical trials have been conducted and are evaluated in the proceeding section.

In a study conducted by Jiang et al. (2013), the effects of oral supplementation with ginger root on elevated inflammatory markers present in those at normal risk and those at high risk for colorectal cancer. The researchers aimed to determine whether or not ginger's reported antiinflammatory activities were able to decrease the potential for colorectal cancer. This study was comprised of 50 total participants, with 30 at a normal risk for the development of colorectal cancer and 20 at increased risk for the cancer. The participants were assigned at random to either the placebo group or the ginger supplementation group. Those in the ginger group were administered a 2.0 g/day ginger tablet for 28 days. At baseline and at the conclusion of the study, the researchers obtained colon biopsies from all 50 participants obtained via flexible sigmoidoscopy techniques. Ginger consumption was found to decrease COX-1 protein levels in the colon by 23.8% in those at an increased risk for the cancer. In the placebo group, 18.9% of participants had a decrease in COX-1 protein levels. Normal risk participants had no changes in COX-1 levels. Although individuals with normal risk for colorectal cancer did not benefit from ginger, ginger supplementation does confer benefits to individuals at high risk for colorectal cancer. Although additional research is needed in a larger population with a longer period of intervention, ginger supplementation may have a beneficial role in the prevention of colon cancer in high risk groups.

In a study conducted by Zick et al. (2014), the effects of ginger root extract on eicosanoids in colonic mucosa was investigated. Due to previous studies exhibiting that oral supplementation with ginger root was able to effectively lower COX-1 protein levels in those at increased risk for colorectal cancer, the researchers in this study wished to determine if inhibition of COX-1 would alter the production of proinflammatory eicosanoids in the colon.

The 20 participants in this study were assigned to either a ginger or placebo group at random. The ginger group received 2.0 g/day of ginger root in the form of oral capsules for 28 days. Flexible sigmoidoscopy was used to obtained colon biopsies in all participants at both the beginning of the study and at the conclusion of the study.

Findings from this study indicated that there was a lack of ability for ginger to decrease the eicosanoid levels in individuals with increased risk for colorectal cancer. Ginger was concluded to be both tolerable and safe by all participants in the study. The researchers of this study concluded that further investigation should be pursued with more of a focus on other markers for colorectal cancer risk among populations with increased risk for this type of cancer.

A rare type of breast cancer occurring in approximately 1% of cases is an inflammatory form of breast cancer. Similar to colon cancer, the inflammatory nature of this disease could benefit from antiinflammatory agents, such as ginger. In a study conducted by Karimi and Roshan (2013), the researchers sought to discover whether interventions, such as ginger supplementation, with or without water-based exercise, would cause a change in biomarkers related to inflammation and oxidative stress in women diagnosed with breast cancer. Women selected for this study were not only diagnosed with breast cancer, but qualified as obese according to measured BMI. The combination of both obesity and existing cancer allowed for study participants who were likely experiencing large quantities of inflammation.

Forty women with an average age of approximately 48 years volunteered to participate in the study. The ginger supplement groups received 4 capsules of ginger containing 750 mg each daily for a total of 6 weeks. The exercise protocol, for those enrolled in a group with water-based exercise with or without ginger supplementation, consisted of a program with progressive intensity and time in a pool, at a frequency of 4 times per week for 6 weeks. Fasting blood samples were collected from the participants. These samples were collected pre- and postintervention. After 6 weeks of supplementation with ginger, adiponectin levels increased by 6.31% in comparison to the baseline measurement. The control group, those who were sedentary and did not receive ginger supplementation, had no change in stress-related biomarkers. Water-based exercise interventions caused a 17.22% increase in serum adiponectin levels. Findings from this study suggested that a combination of oral ginger supplementation and water-based exercise have an effect on increasing antioxidants in the body and decreasing inflammatory markers. This suggests that an increase in physical activity and use of ginger as a natural treatment may be considered as a viable treatment option for inflammation in obese women with breast cancer.

RESPIRATORY

Respiratory diseases, such as acute respiratory distress syndrome (ARDS) and chronic obstructive pulmonary disease (COPD), although two distinct diseases, share similar features of inflammation of the airways. ARDS can be a life threatening condition. Injury, infection, and other exposures lead to inflammation and fluid buildup in the alveolar air sacs, thus impeding gas exchange and leading to low blood oxygen levels. Lack of or low levels of oxygen in the blood impairs organ function throughout the body with the brain, kidneys, and heart being most susceptible. Individuals with ARDS often require mechanical ventilation which can further exacerbate the inflammatory response (Uhlig, Ranieri, & Slutsky, 2004).

COPD actually refers to a group of diseases, including emphysema, chronic bronchitis, and asthma, all of which impair ventilation. COPD often is a result of inflammation of the small airways which prevents air from reaching the alveoli and the subsequent gas exchange from taking place (Hogg et al., 2004). The hallmark of both of these serious respiratory diseases is inflammation and decreased gas exchange in the alveoli, although the inflammation arises from distinct areas of the respiratory system. Due to the inflammatory nature of these diseases, treatment regimens typically focus on decreasing inflammatory mediators; corticosteroids. However, corticosteroids have not been shown to be effective, and resistance to corticosteroid treatment has been observed (Meduri & Yates, 2004). Natural antiinflammatory agents have been the target of recent investigations. Here we review the antiinflammatory effects of ginger on respiratory diseases.

In a study by Brockwell et al. (2014), the authors aimed to test a newly patented formulation- AKL1, comprised of standardized extracts of *Picrorhiza kurroa, Ginko biloba, and Z. officinale* as an adjuvant therapy for patients with COPD experiencing chronic cough despite medical management. These compounds have been shown to have antiinflammatory properties. The randomized double-blind placebo-controlled parallel-group trial tested the safety and efficacy of the formulation and the authors hypothesized that AKL1 would improve cough-related quality of life as assessed using the LCQ and St. George's Respiratory Questionnaire (SGRQ). Seventy-eight patients were screened and participated in the run-in period of the study to determine eligibility in the experimental period and 33 eligible participants were then randomly assigned to receive either placebo or AKL1 in addition to their current medications. LCQ scores were determined at baseline, week 4, and week 8. Statistically significant improvements were seen in the treatment group in respect to cough-related quality of life as measured through the LCQ and SGRQ however, 13 out of 20 and 9 out of 13 subjects in the treatments versus placebo groups had data for all time points and were included in the analysis. Although these results are promising and consistent with pilot data (unpublished), more research is needed to assess the effects of ALK1 as an add-on therapy in larger populations, and controlling for the type of relevant medication participants are receiving.

Another trial was conducted to evaluate the effect of ginger on inflammatory factors in the respiratory profile of patients with ARDS. Thirty-two ARDS patients were randomized to receive ginger or placebo. Ginger supplementation was found to significantly lower inflammatory cytokines; IL-1, IL-6, and TNF-α. Improvements in oxygenation were also observed with ginger supplementation. This data shows promise for the use in ginger in enteral diets and formulations for patients with ARDS, potentially improving gas exchange, decreasing the duration of mechanical ventilation and ICU stays.

CONCLUSIONS

Ginger has been used as a natural botanical remedy for a variety of diseases throughout history. We are only now coming to understand the scientific mechanism by which ginger acts. The recent and abundant clinical trials reviewed here demonstrate compelling evidence for ginger's antiinflammatory properties and potential use as a treatment for a variety of inflammatory diseases that plague industrialized nations. All 16 trials reviewed in this chapter demonstrated powerful antiinflammatory properties. Future research needs to focus on determining the optimal dose, route of administration, and form of ginger supplementation required to induce its antiinflammatory properties. Although each of the clinical trials reviewed here demonstrated a decrease in inflammation with supplemented ginger, dosing ranged from 250 mg to 3 g and was given in a variety of formulations. Additionally, the duration of supplementation varied from 3 days to 3 months. Once the optimal dosing, length of supplementation, and formulation is determined, future studies, and clinical protocols can be developed, as ginger offers a safe, effective, and natural way to control chronic inflammation and pain for the treatment and prevention of a variety of chronic diseases. Ginger supplementation could then be tested as part of an overall natural antiinflammatory diet or supplement and include other well-known compounds, such as eicosapentaenoic acid (EPA), docosahexaenoic acid (DHA), and turmeric, as synergistic effects of these compounds offer promise to be as, or more, effective than NSAIDS or corticosteroid treatments.

References

Arablou, T., Aryaeian, N., Valizadeh, M., Sharifi, F., Hosseini, A., & Djalali, M. (2014). The effect of ginger consumption on glycemic status, lipid profile and some inflammatory markers in patients with type 2 diabetes mellitus. *International Journal of Food Sciences and Nutrition, 65*(4), 515–520.

Brockwell, C., Ampikaipakan, S., Sexton, D., Price, D., Freeman, D., Ali, M., & Wilson, A. M. (2014). Adjunctive treatment with oral AKL1, a botanical nutraceutical, in chronic obstructive pulmonary disease. *International Journal of Chronic Obstructive Pulmonary Disease COPD*, 715–721. doi: 10.2147/copd.s54276.

Centers for Disease Control and Prevention. (2014). *National diabetes statistics report: estimates of diabetes and its burden in the United States, 2014*. Atlanta, GA: U.S. Department of Health and Human Services, Centers for Disease Control and Prevention.

Cheung, R., Cheng, T., Dong, Y., Lin, H., Lai, K., Lau, C., & Parsons, B. (2010). Incidence of gastroduodenal ulcers during treatment with celecoxib or diclofenac: Pooled results from three 12-week trials in Chinese patients with osteoarthritis or rheumatoid arthritis. *International Journal of Rheumatic Diseases, 13*(2), 151–157.

Chrubasik, S., Pittler, M., & Roufogalis, B. (2005). *Zingiberis rhizoma*: a comprehensive review on the ginger effect and efficacy profiles. *Phytomedicine, 12*(9), 684–701.

Cisternas, M. G., Murphy, L., Sacks, J. J., Solomon, D. H., Pasta, D. J., & Helmick, C. G. (2016). Alternative methods for defining osteoarthritis and the impact on estimating prevalence in a US population-based survey. *Arthritis Care and Research, 68*(5), 574–580.

Coussens, L. M., & Werb, Z. (2002). Inflammation and cancer. *Nature, 420*(6917), 860–867.

Daniels, S. E., Torri, S., & Desjardins, P. J. (2005). Valdecoxib for treatment of primary dysmenorrhea. *Journal of General Internal Medicine, 20*(1), 62–67.

Drozdov, V. N., Kim, V. A., Tkachenko, E. V., & Varvanina, G. G. (2012). Influence of a specific ginger combination on gastropathy conditions in patients with osteoarthritis of the knee or hip. *The Journal of Alternative and Complementary Medicine, 18*(6), 583–588.

Edwards, J. E., Moore, R. A., & McQuay, H. J. (2004). Rofecoxib for dysmenorrhea: meta- analysis using individual patient data. *BMC Womens' Health, 4*(1), 5.

Erlinger, T. P. (2004). C-reactive protein and the risk of incident colorectal cancer. *Jama, 291*(5), 585.

Grandi, G., F., X., C., P., V., & Cagnacci, A. (2012). Prevalence of menstrual pain in young women: What is dysmenorrhea? *JPR Journal of Pain Research*, 169–174. doi:10.2147/jpr.s30602.

Halder, A. (2012). Effect of progressive muscle relaxation versus intake of ginger powder on dysmenorrhea amongst the nursing students in Pune. *The Nursing journal of India, 103*(4), 152–156.

Hogg, J. C., Chu, F., Utokaparch, S., Woods, R., Elliott, W. M., Buzatu, L., Cherniack, R. M., Sciurba, F. C., Coxson, H. O., & Pare, P. D. (2004). The nature of small-airway obstruction in chronic obstructive pulmonary disease. *New England Journal of Medicine, 351*(13), 1367–11367.

Imani, H., Tabibi, H., Najafi, I., Atabak, S., Hedayati, M., & Rahmani, L. (2015). Effects of ginger on serum glucose, advanced glycation end products, and inflammation in peritoneal dialysis patients. *Nutrition, 31*(5), 703–707.

Jenabi, E. (2013). The effect of ginger for relieving of primary dysmenorrhoea. *JMPA: The Journal of the Pakistan Medical Association, 63*(1), 8–10.

Jiang, Y., Turgeon, D. K., Wright, B. D., Sidahmed, E., Ruffin, M. T., Brenner, D. E., & Zick, S. M. (2013). Effect of ginger root on cyclooxygenase-1 and 15-hydroxyprostaglandin dehydrogenase expression in colonic mucosa of humans at normal and increased risk for colorectal cancer. *European Journal of Cancer Prevention, 22*(5), 455–460.

Karimi, N., & Roshan, V. D. (2013). Change in adiponectin and oxidative stress after modifiable lifestyle interventions in breast cancer cases. *Asian Pacific journal of cancer prevention: APJCP, 14*(5), 2845–2850.

Khandouzi, N., Shidfar, F., Rajab, A., Rahideh, T., Hosseini, P., & Mir Taheri, M. (2015). The effects of ginger on fasting blood sugar, hemoglobin a1c, apolipoprotein B, apolipoprotein a-I and malondialdehyde in type 2 diabetic patients. *Iranian Journal of Pharmaceutical Research: IJPR, 14*(1), 131–140.

Khodaie, L., & Sadeghpoor, O. (2015). Ginger from ancient times to the new outlook. *Jundishapur Journal of Natural Pharmaceutical Products, 10*(1), .

Mashhadi, N. S., Ghiasvand, R., Askari, G., Hariri, M., Darvishi, L., & Mofid, M. R. (2013). Anti-oxidative and anti-inflammatory effects of ginger in health and physical activity: review of current evidence. *International Journal of Preventative Medicine, 4*(Suppl. 1), S36–S42.

Meduri, G. U., & Yates, C. R. (2004). Systemic inflammation-associated glucocorticoid resistance and outcome of ARDS. *Annals of the New York Academy of Sciences, 1024*(1), 24–53.

Mahluji, S., Ostadrahimi, A., Mobasseri, M., Ebrahimzade, A. V., & Payahoo, L. (2013). Anti-inflammatory effects of zingiber officinale in type 2 diabetic patients. *Advanced Pharmaceutical Bulletin, 3*(2), 273–276.

Murphy, L., Schwartz, T. A., Helmick, C. G., Renner, J. B., Tudor, G., Koch, G., & Jordan, J. M. (2008). Lifetime risk of symptomatic knee osteoarthritis. *Arthritis Rheum Arthritis & Rheumatism, 59*(9), 1207–1213.

Myasoedova, E., Crowson, C. S., Kremers, H. M., Therneau, T. M., & Gabriel, S. E. (2010). Is the incidence of rheumatoid arthritis rising?: Results from Olmsted County, Minnesota, 1955-2007. *Arthritis and Rheumatism, 62*(6), 1576–1582.

Rahnama, P., Montazeri, A., Huseini, H. F., Kianbakht, S., & Naseri, M. (2012). Effect of *Zingiber officinale* R. rhizomes (ginger) on pain relief in primary dysmenorrhea: a placebo randomized trial. *BMC Complementary and Alternative Medicine, 12*(1), 92.

Rostom, A. (2007). Nonsteroidal anti-inflammatory drugs and cyclooxygenase-2 inhibitors for primary prevention of colorectal cancer: a systematic review prepared for the U.S. Preventive Services Task Force. *Annals of Internal Medicine, 146*(5), 376.

Sacks, J. J., Helmick, C. G., Luo, Y., Ilowite, N. T., & Bowyer, S. (2007). Prevalence of and annual ambulatory health care visits for pediatric arthritis and other rheumatologic conditions in the United States in 2001–2004. *Arthritis Rheum Arthritis and Rheumatism, 57*(8), 1439–1445.

Shidfar, F., Rajab, A., Rahideh, T., Khandouzi, N., Hosseini, S., & Shidfar, S. (2015). The effect of ginger (*Zingiber officinale*) on glycemic markers in patients with type 2 diabetes. *Journal of Complementary and Integrative Medicine, 12*(2.), .

Shirvani, M. A., Motahari-Tabari, N., & Alipour, A. (2014). The effect of mefenamic acid and ginger on pain relief in primary dysmenorrhea: a randomized clinical trial. *Arch Gynecol Obstet Archives of Gynecology and Obstetrics, 291*(6), 1277–1281.

Steen, K. S. (2001). Incidence of clinically manifest ulcers and their complications in patients with rheumatoid arthritis. *Annals of the Rheumatic Diseases, 60*(5), 443–447.

Uhlig, S., Ranieri, M., & Slutsky, A. S. (2004). Biotrauma Hypothesis of Ventilator-induced Lung Injury. *American Journal of Respiratory and Critical Care Medicine, 169*(2), 314–316.

Villalvilla, A., Silva, J. A., Largo, R., Gualillo, O., Vieira, P. C., Herrero-Beaumont, G., & Gómez, R. (2013). 6-Shogaol inhibits chondrocytes' innate immune responses and cathepsin-K activity. *Molecular Nutrition and Food Research, 58*(2), 256–266.

White, B. (2007). Ginger: an overview. *American Family Physician, 75*(11), 1689–1691.

Zick, S. M., Turgeon, D. K., Ren, J., Ruffin, M. T., Wright, B. D., Sen, A., & Brenner, D. E. (2014). Pilot clinical study of the effects of ginger root extract on eicosanoids in colonic mucosa of subjects at increased risk for colorectal cancer. *Molecular Carcinogenesis, 54*(9), 908–915.

CHAPTER

6

Illegal Adulterations of (Traditional) Herbal Medicines and Dietary Supplements for the Treatment of Pain

E. Deconinck

Division of food, medicines and consumer safety, Section Medicinal Products, Scientific Institute of Public Health (WIV-ISP), Brussels, Belgium

INTRODUCTION

For thousands of years, herbs and plants have played an important role in traditional medicines and herbal derived medicines. The most well-known medicines based on herbs and plants, besides other products, are the traditional Chinese and Indian (Ayurvedic) medicine. Although in different countries, such as Japan (Kampo medicines), the Middle East and South Asia (Unani medicine), and in different countries on the African and the Latin American continent local herbal based medicines can be found (Félix-Silva, Giordani, da Silva-Jr, Zucolotto, & Fernandes-Pedrosa Mde, 2014; Kofi-Tsekpo, 2004; Miraldi, Ferri, & Mostanghimi, 2001; Mosihuzzaman & Choudhary, 2008; Tshibangu et al., 2004).

The interest in plants and herbs, as sources for treatment was and is in fact worldwide. It should not be forgotten that many of the allopathic medicines used today find their origin in herbal products from which new chemical identities were isolated and later synthesized. Some examples are acetyl salicylic acid, digoxin, morphine, paclitaxel, atropine, and vinblastine (Fujii, Fujii, & Yamazaki, 1983; Datta & Srivastava, 1997; Miller, Jolles, & Rapoport, 1973; Phillipson & Handa, 1976; Strobel, Stierle, & Hess, 1994).

Although the original allopathic medicines now serve as reference, over the last decade the interest in traditional medicines and herbal alternatives is increasing, especially in the industrialized world. This is due to a general trend of returning to traditional and natural products, exhaustively promoted in marketing campaigns. These campaigns influence the public opinion about the choice of treatment they use, especially when it concerns complaints that can be treated by self-medication, using over the counter available products. Furthermore, the concerns about the adverse effects of chemical drugs and questioning of the allopathic medicines have stimulated the popularity of herbal medicines (World Health Organization, 2000a).

The fast growing industry of traditional medicines and herbal products increased the concern about the quality and safety of these products. That is why the World Health Organization (WHO) and other regulatory bodies have begun programs in order to set quality parameters and guidelines to conduct quality control (European Medicine Evaluation Agency, 2010a, 2010b; World Health Organization, 1991, 2000a, 2000b, 2005). Quality control of natural products is extremely important since the effectiveness of these products depends on the concentration of certain active components they contain. However, these concentrations of active ingredients are influenced by numerous factors, such as the climate, cultivation conditions, harvest time, drying, storage, and so on. As a result of these influences the concentrations may vary and therefore affect the quality of the product (Bashir & Abu-Goukh, 2003; Chena, Li, Chen, Guo, & Cai, 2010; Cianchino, Acosta, Ortega, Martinez, & Gomez, 2008; European Medicine Evaluation Agency, 2006; Liang, Qu, Luo, & Wang, 2006; Lopez-Feria, Cardenas, Garcia-Mesa, & Valcarcel, 2008; Nathani, Nair, & Kakkar, 2006; Shin, Liu, Nock, Holliday, & Watkins, 2007; Simeoni & Lebot, 2002; Tan et al., 2008;

Nutritional Modulators of Pain in the Aging Population. http://dx.doi.org/10.1016/B978-0-12-805186-3.00006-0
Copyright © 2017 Elsevier Inc. All rights reserved.

Whitton, Lau, Salisbury, Whitehouse, & Evans, 2003). This may cause ineffectiveness on one hand and possible toxicity on the other, both causing a potential risk for public health.

Nowadays the quality control and assurance of herbal products and traditional medicines is based on published monographs, defining the quality parameters to which the considered product should comply. These types of monographs are published by the WHO (Declaration of Alma-Ata, 1978; World Health Organization, 1999, 2003, 2007), The European Medicine Agency (Committee on Herbal Products, 2010) and are part of the European Pharmacopoeia (2010) (Council of Europe 2010) and some national pharmacopoeias, like those of Germany, France, India, and China.

The quality issue of herbs and plants used as traditional medicines or dietary supplements is another increasingly occurring problem, which poses serious threats for public health. It concerns the availability and the distribution of counterfeit medicines and adulterated dietary supplements, which represents a global problem that has increased rapidly in the past decades, mainly due to the development of the internet. Dietary supplements and traditional medicines are now freely available through internet or in some specialty shops. Caution is heavily advised, especially when the products are sold by internet sites not disclosing their identity or through other illegal suppliers. Different research projects clearly showed that three problems are occurring with these products that could endanger consumers' health: (a) the product does not contain the correct herbs or plants. Here different situations are possible: (1) the product contains some dried common plants in order to create a cheap counterfeited product. (2) Confounding took place. Therapeutic properties are often found for one specific plant species, while other related species have less or no therapeutic activity or have other, possibly toxic effects. (b) The herbal product is adulterated with synthetic drugs. These are not labeled on the package and are often present in wrong dosages. The problem here is that the consumer/patient thinks he is taking a natural and safe product, but in fact is taking a medicine. In this case adverse or toxic effects are not immediately related to the dietary supplement, neither by the patient nor by the medical staff. These products can interfere with medical treatments. (c) The product contains some regulated or toxic plants, since these products are not controlled by a regulatory body nor produced following quality norms (Deconinck, Custers, & De Beer, 2015a).

This chapter deals with these three types of illegal practices with a special focus on herbal treatments and dietary supplements sold for the treatment of pain. Different reported cases of incidents with this type of products will be discussed, as well as analytical solutions for distinction and detection of these illegal preparations.

COUNTERFEITING AND CONFOUNDING OF HERBAL TREATMENTS

As mentioned before the activity of an herbal medication is based on the concentration of some active ingredients present in the crude plant material. These concentrations can vary according to different factors such as climate, cultivation conditions, harvest time, drying, storage, extraction procedure, and so on. The large variability in active ingredients may put the patient's health and safety at risk (Bashir & Abu-Goukh, 2003; Chena et al., 2010; Cianchino et al., 2008; Liang et al., 2006; Lopez-Feria et al., 2008; Naithani et al., 2006; Shin et al., 2007; Simeoni & Lebot, 2002; Tan et al., 2008; Whitton et al., 2003).

In order to produce herbal medicines, the plant should be grown, harvested and processed following standard procedures in order to ensure a minimal concentration of the active ingredients and so a minimal activity. This is why quality control of the crude materials is of extreme importance. Therefore many monographs on the quality control of bulk herbal materials were published during the past decades. These monographs can be found in the European Pharmacopoeia (2010) (Council of Europe, 2010), the United States Pharmacopoeia (2010) (United States Pharmacopoeial Convention, 2010) and the Pharmacopoeia of the People's Republic of China (2010) (Chinese Pharmacopoeia Commission, 2010). The identifications are often based on microscopic and macroscopic analysis of the product combined with the use of biomarkers.

These botanical, macroscopic and microscopic identification/authentication methods are very useful for crude plant material, however when dealing with herbal based dietary supplements the situation is completely different, since the crude material is often powdered, mixed with other powders of synthetic and/or herbal origin and compressed to a tablet or filled into a capsule. The identification strategies of the monographs mentioned above does not apply anymore, since macroscopic and microscopic evaluation is no longer possible and the detection of biomarkers can be disturbed (Deconinck, De Leersnijder, Custer, Courselle, & De Beer, 2013a).

The identification of the correct plants in dietary supplements and more generally the quality control of these products is extremely important, especially when dealing with products coming from the Internet market or other nonregulated sources. Products coming from regulated sources are produced following the "good manufacturing procedures" (GMP) guidelines and include a thorough identification of the bulk materials before processing. This cannot be expected from producers selling their products through Internet sites without disclosing their physical address or through other not trustworthy distributors.

Considering that the products are 100% herbal in origin two possible problems might occur. The first is called counterfeiting. The product is sold as a traditional/herbal medicine, but in fact contains only some common cheap plants and therefore contains no active ingredients, or the herbal product is diluted with bulk material, reducing the concentration of the active components and so the efficacy of the product (Applequist & Miller, 2013; Pferschy-Wenzig & Bauer, 2015; Zhang, Wider, Shang, Li, & Ernst, 2012). Examples of such counterfeited/diluted products can be found for ginseng products and Chinese star anise fruit. The Asian ginseng is often diluted with other types of ginseng species, for example, American ginseng. This is problematic since both plants have different saponin profiles and have contradictory effects on the vascular system and blood glucose levels (Pferschy-Wenzig & Bauer, 2015). Chinese star anise fruit has been repeatedly adulterated with Japanese star anise fruit. The latter however contains the neurotoxic sesquiterpene delactone anisatin, a potent noncompetitive GABA (Pferschy-Wenzig & Bauer, 2015; Samuels, Finkelstein, Singer, & Oberbaum, 2008). These adulterations resulted in numerous cases of adverse neurological reactions, such as nausea, hallucinations, and epileptic seizures, especially in infants since star anise tea is often used for infant colic (Pferschy-Wenzig & Bauer, 2015).

The second is called confounding. Here, the product only contains herbs, however, they are the incorrect ones. Often these producers buy their bulk materials as cheap as possible and do not verify identity or quality of it. In this way, the active plants can be confounded with others of the same species or even totally different plants. This can lead to inactivity of the product, unexpected side effects or toxic effects (Deconinck et al., 2015a). Misidentification or confounding happens either at the site of plant collection or at the stage of the processed/dried herbal material, for example due to mistakes on the part of the importer or retailer as consequence of incorrect labeling or similar appearance (Pferschy-Wenzig & Bauer, 2015; Zhang et al., 2012). Confounding is often due to problems with the nomenclature of the plants, since not only the scientific Latin names are used but also pharmacopoeial and local names. For example, in different regions of China a particular trivial name can refer to different plants or drugs containing completely different, possibly toxic compounds (Pferschy-Wenzig & Bauer, 2015; Rivera et al., 2014; Zhang et al., 2012). An example of confounding was discovered in Belgium where it resulted in more than hundred cases of kidney intoxication. The root of *Stephania tetranda* that is mainly harvested in northern China and officially named in the Chinese Pharmacopoeia as "*Hangfangji*", is locally called "*Fangji*". This name is also used in Southern China for the root of *Aristolochia fanghi,* generally referred to as "*Guangfanji*". The latter plant contains some nephrotoxic and carcinogenic aristocholic acid derivatives and was included in a preparation used for weight loss instead of *Stephania tetranda,* resulting in nephrotoxicity (Pferschy-Wenzig & Bauer, 2015; Vanherweghem et al., 1993).

Another potential problem is the presence of toxic or regulated plants in traditional medicines or dietary supplements. This however, is largely a legal problem, since some plants may be legal in one country but illegal or regulated in another. When such products are imported, the distributors are not always aware that these products contain plants that are not allowed in the countries they distribute. An example of this is *Pausinystalia yohimbe,* a plant that is used in herbal treatment for potency problems. This plant is allowed in several countries, but for example forbidden in dietary supplements in Belgium (Koninklijk besluit, 1997) and several other European countries.

CHEMICAL ADULTERATIONS OF HERBAL TREATMENTS

Next to counterfeiting and confounding of herbal and traditional medicines, the chemical adulteration of traditional medicines and dietary supplements is an increasing trend and represents, an even more important threat to public health. Dietary supplements and traditional medicines are freely available through internet and some specialized shops and are marketed to be composed of 100% herbal and natural ingredients and to be 100% safe. Despite this, several investigations revealed the presence of pharmaceutical ingredients as adulterants in these products. When purchasing counterfeit medicines over the internet, the patient can be held partially responsible for the health risk he is willing to take, but this is not the case with these adulterated products. The patient is convinced he is taking harmless supplements and therefore adverse effects are not immediately related to the dietary supplement, neither by the patient nor by the medical staff.

Essentially four different groups of adulterated dietary supplements and traditional medicines can be distinguished: weight loss, potency enhancement, muscle building, and the treatment of pain. This chapter will focus on the latter group. The group of analgesic medicines, found as adulterants, is constituted of a heterogeneous group of molecules that can be pharmaceutically divided into three categories: the analgesics, the narcotic analgesics, and the nonsteroidal inflammatory drugs (NSAIDs) (Deconinck, Kamugisha, Van Campenhout, Courselle, & De Beer, 2015b). Next to the analgesics also the pharmaceutical class of the benzodiazepines can be found as adulterants present in traditional medicines and dietary supplements for the treatment of pain (Choi et al., 2015).

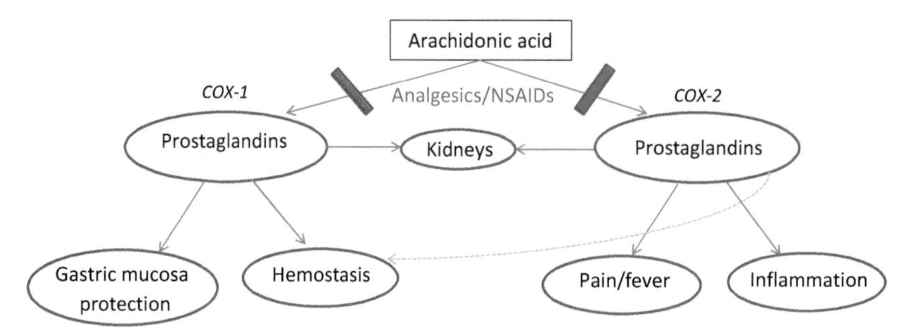

FIGURE 6.1 **Simplified schematic overview of the working mechanism of analgesics and NSAIDs.**

An example of an adulterated traditional medicine was described by Johansson, Fransson, Rundolf, Huynh, & Arvidsson, 2014). They found a dietary supplement claiming to contain the Indian spice turmeric with curcumine I, II, en III as main components. Though liver damage was reported and linked to the product. Analysis showed that the product contained nimesulide, an NSAID of the COX-2 inhibitor type that was not marketed in many countries due to hepatotoxicity. Deconinck et al. (2015b) analyzed five products claiming to be of 100% herbal and natural origin. In the five samples, respectively ibuprofen, paracetamol and caffeine, aceclofenac, diclofenac, and indomethacine were detected. Bogusz, Hassan, Al-Enazi, Ibrahim, & Al-Tufail (2006) found phenylbutazone en dipyrone in a sample of herbal powder "Jamu Ragel" originating from Indonesia and commercialized for the treatment of pain and rheumatism. Kim et al. (2014) screened 214 food and dietary supplements coming from the South Korean market and found that 53 samples were adulterated with analgesics. Ibuprofen, an NSAID, was the most found compound followed by diclofenac, naproxen, piroxicam, paracetamol, and indomethacin. Doménech-Carbó et al. (2013) found lorazepam, a popular benzodiazepine, in three commercial available herbal medicines in Brazil. Also de Carvalho et al. (2010) found benzodiazepines in 4 of 12 phytotherapeutic formulations, bought on a local market in Brazil. These examples show that the adulteration of traditional herbal medicines and herbal-based dietary supplements is a real problem. The more these few examples only show the tip of the iceberg, since the majority of the official laboratories dealing with this problem, do not make their findings public.

Pharmacology of Most Encountered Chemical Adulterants for the Treatment of Pain

The Analgesics

The two most found adulterants in dietary supplements for the treatment of pain belonging to this category are paracetamol (acetaminophen) and acetyl salicylic acid.

The mechanism by which paracetamol induces its analgesic effect remains unclear. It is believed that the primary mechanism of action is the inhibition of the cyclooxygenases (COX), with a predominant effect on COX-2. Inhibition of the cyclooxygenases prevents the metabolism of arachidonic acid to prostaglandin H2, which is further converted to proinflammatory compounds. In the central nervous system this inhibition reduces the concentration of prostaglandin E2, from where the pyretic effect, and activates the descending inhibitory serotonergic pathways resulting in analgesia (Anderson, 2008; Jahr & Lee, 2010; e-compendium, 2015).

A similar mechanism of action can be found for acetyl salicylic acid. It directly and irreversibly inhibits the activity of both COX-1 and COX-2, interfering with the formation of prostaglandins and thromboxanes from arachidonic acid. Where the inhibition of COX-2 results in the analgesic and antipyretic effect, the inhibition of COX-1 results in a suppression of the prostaglandins involved in physiological processes like the protection of the stomach mucosa. This explains the most important side effect of acetyl salicylic acid, that is, gastro intestinal complaints with in severe cases gastrointestinal ulcus and ulcus bleeding (e-compendium, 2015; Vane & Botting, 2003). A schematic representation of the interference with the COX enzymes is given in Fig. 6.1. Another problem that can occur with acetyl salicylic acid as adulterant is that the quality of the bulk product is low and contains high amounts of salicylic acid, a deterioration product of acetyl salicylic acid. Salicylic acid is mainly topically used as a keratoliticum and is not suited for oral administration due to severe toxic effects.

Both molecules are often combined with caffeine, which has a synergetic effect when used in doses of at least 30 mg per dosage unit. This is probably also the reason why caffeine is often found in dietary supplements for the treatment of pain.

The Narcotic Analgesics

Narcotic analgesics are molecules that are based on the natural occurring alkaloids present in the *Papaver somniferum*. Narcotic analgesics, with morphine as typical example, bind to the opioid receptors present in both the

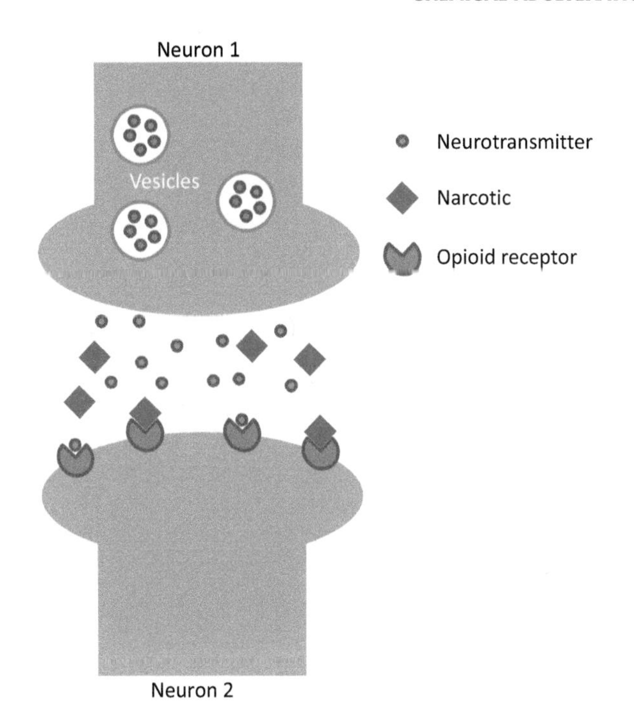

FIGURE 6.2 **Schematic representation of the working mechanism of narcotics.**

central as the peripheral nervous system and block them for the interaction with neurotransmitters (Fig. 6.2). Three types of opioid receptors exist: the mu, the kappa, and the delta receptors. Binding to the three receptors will lead to the analgesic effects, but also to some severe side effects like sedation, euphoria, respiratory depression, constipation, and physical dependence. The different narcotic analgesics may differ in the proportion to which they bind to the different opioid receptors, but may also have some supplementary modes of action (Pasternak, 1993). For example tramadol, a narcotic analgesic marketed to threat moderate to severe acute and chronic pain, binds to the mu-receptors but also acts as a serotonine and norepinephrine reuptake inhibitor (WHO Expert Committee on Drug Dependence, 2014). It also has to be said that the complete working mechanism for most of the narcotic analgesics is not yet known. Examples of narcotic analgesic besides morphine are buprenorphine, fentanyl, and tramadol. Codeine is not used as narcotic analgesic, but is often combined with paracetamol for its synergetic effect (e-compendium, 2015).

Nonsteroidal Inflammatory Drugs (NSAIDs)

In general, it can be said that the different NSAIDs variably interact with the COX enzymes and inhibit the COX-1 and COX-2 enzymes in different moieties (Fig. 6.1). Although exceptions the inhibition fall within three categories (Dannhardt & Kiefer, 2001; Smith et al., 2000):

- rapid competitive and reversible binding to COX-1 and COX-2
- rapid, lower-affinity reversible binding followed by time-dependent, higher-affinity, slowly reversible binding of COX-1 and COX-2
- rapid reversible binding followed by covalent modification of COX-1 and COX-2

Ibuprofen and piroxicam are examples of the first category. Ibuprofen competitively inhibits the prostaglandin synthesis through the arachidonic pathways and dissociate rapidly from the COX-binding sites. The inhibition of COX-2 by ibuprofen is believed to be the working mechanism for its effect in mediating inflammation, pain, fever, and swelling. Though its antipyretic effects may also be due to its action on the hypothalamus resulting in increased peripheral blood flow, vasodilation, and subsequent heat dissipation. The inhibition of COX-1 is thought to be the cause of side effects like gastro-intestinal ulceration (Selinsky, Gupta, Sharkey, & Loll, 2001). Piroxicam, like ibuprofen exerts its antiinflammatory effect through the inhibition of the COX enzymes, but essentially blocks the COX-1 enzyme. Piroxicam also inhibits the migration of leukocytes into sites of inflammation and prevents the formation of thromboxane A2, an aggregating agent, by the platelets (http://www.drugbank.ca/drugs/DB00554 accessed December 8th, 2015).

Typical examples of the second category are diclofenac and indomethacin. The antiinflammatory effect of diclofenac is believed to be due to both the inhibition of the leukocyt migration as the inhibition of the COX-enzymes, where COX-1 and COX-2 are inhibited with relative equipotency (Gan, 2010, http://www.drugbank.ca/drugs/DB00586 accessed December 8th, 2015). For indomethacin the time dependent tight binding could be demonstrated through in vitro experiments. Indomethacin is more selective for COX-1, than for COX-2, which accounts for its increased adverse gastric effects compared to other NSAIDs. Next to the inhibition of the prostaglandin synthesis and the inflammatory reactions, it also suppress the phospholipase A2 activity, the enzyme responsible for releasing arachidonic acid from phospholipids and therefore reinforce the effect of the COX inhibition (Summ & Evers, 2013).

Although acetyl salicylic acid is not always categorized as an NSAID, it is the type example of the third category.

Benzodiazepines

Benzodiazepines are a class of psychoactive drugs that are used for their hypnotic, sedative, and anxiolytic effects. For these indications they are very popular since they are as efficient as the other hypnotic drugs, but are less toxic in case of overdose. In the treatment of pain, especially in case of severe back pain, they are sometimes used for their muscle relaxing effects. No significant clinical difference exists between the different benzodiazepines concerning their hypnotic, sedative, anxiolytic, and muscle relaxing properties. It is only a matter of dosage and pharmacokinetic differences. Though pharmacokinetic properties as the half-life and the occurrence of certain metabolites can influence the duration of the effects. These differences form the basis for the division of the benzodiazepines in short, middle long, and long working molecules (Gecommentarieerd geneesmiddelen repertorium, 2015). Examples of short working benzodiazepines are triazolam and midazolam, of middle long working alprazolam, bromazepam, lorazepam, and lormetazepam and of longworking are clobazan, clonazepam, and diazepam (Gecommentarieerd geneesmiddelen repertorium, 2015).

Benzodiazepines can be used for the treatment of anxiety, insomnia, agitation, seizures, muscle spasms, alcohol withdrawal, and as premedication for medical or dental procedures. Even if these drugs are considered safe and effective for short-term use, they have contraindications like Myastenia Gravis, severe respiratory insufficiency, sleep apnea, and severe liver insufficiency. Due to these contraindications, the illegal presence of benzodiazepines in dietary supplements or traditional medicines can be very dangerous for people suffering from these symptoms. The more the use of benzodiazepines, especially with long term use can cause some side effects like excessive sedation, drowsiness, memory, and concentration disorders, confusion, residual effects (hangover), and paradoxal effects (mainly with children and elder) like increased drowsiness, fear, and even agitation and aggression. The use of benzodiazepines gives rise to tolerance and psychical dependence after 1–2 weeks (Gecommentarieerd geneesmiddelen repertorium, 2015).

Benzodiazepines act as positive allosteric modulators of the Gamma Amino Butyric Acid (GABA)-A receptor, which is a ligand-gated chloride-selective ion channel. GABA is the most common neurotransmitter in the central nervous system and can be found in high concentration in both the cortex as the limbic system. It has an inhibitory effect and reduces the excitability of the neurons, resulting in a calming effect on the brain. Three types of GABA receptors (A, B, and C) exist, but the benzodiazepines interact with the GABA-A receptor. This receptor consists of 5 glycoprotein subunits, two α-, two β-, and 1 γ-subunit. The benzodiazepine-binding site is located in a specific pocket at the intersection of the α- and the γ- subunit. The binding of benzodiazepines induces a conformational change of the GABA-A receptor, inducing a conformational change of the receptor's chloride channel that hyperpolarizes the cell and account for the GABA inhibitory effect throughout the central nervous system (Fox et al., 2011; Griffin, Kaye, Bueno, & Kaye, 2013; Kelly et al., 2002). A schematic on the working mechanism of benzodiazepines is given in Fig. 6.3.

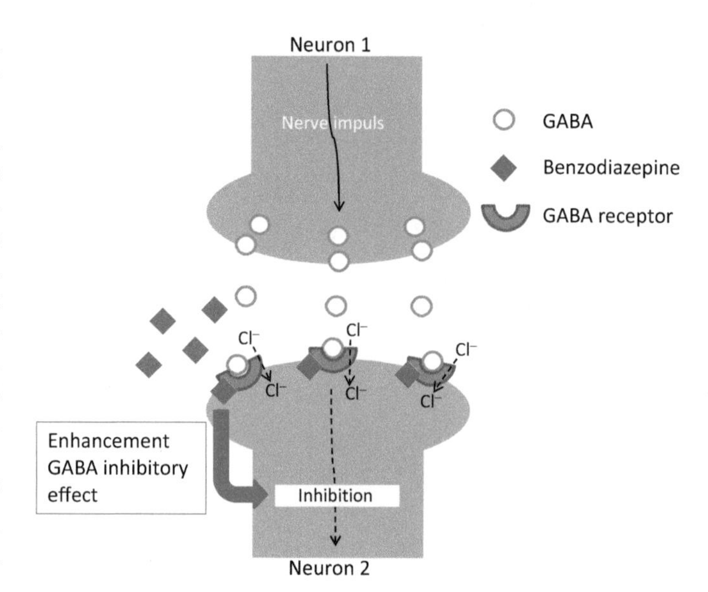

FIGURE 6.3 **Schematic representation of the working mechanism of benzodiazepines.**

Analytical Challenges and Solutions

Several analytical approaches, for the detection of adulteration of traditional medicines and dietary supplements are available. These approaches can be generally classified under the spectroscopic methods and the separation/chromatographic methods.

For chemical adulteration, spectroscopic approaches are often preferred, because they are fast, need minimal, or even no sample preparation and often are nondestructive. The infrared spectroscopic techniques, that is, Fourier-transformed infrared spectroscopy (FT-IR) (Custers et al., 2015; Deconinck et al., 2014; Venhuis et al., 2011), near infrared spectroscopy (NIR) (da Silva Fernandes, da Costa, Valderrama, Março, & de Lima, 2012) and Raman spectroscopy already proved their usefulness in the detection of chemical adulterants. FT-IR was for example used for the detection of sibutramine, by far the most encountered adulterant in dietary supplements for weight loss (Deconinck et al., 2014). The study clearly showed that adulterated and nonadulterated dietary supplement could be discriminated based on their overall infrared spectrum and this in a nondestructive way. In general it can be concluded that methods like FT-IR, NIR, and Raman spectroscopy can be used for a first screening of suspected products for chemical adulterations and this especially at customs or inspection sites, since these instruments are available in portable format and are generally nondestructive (Deconinck et al., 2014; Custers et al., 2015). This allows limitation of the number of nonadulterated, legal products blocked at customs and to focus the work of control laboratories on really suspected products. The problem with these kinds of primary screening methods is that they are based on chemometrics for detection and discrimination and that at the moment each adulterant or group of adulterants has its own combination of chemometric data treatment and so no general multi component screening can be performed (Deconinck et al., 2014; Custers et al., 2015). Nuclear magnetic resonance (NMR) spectroscopy is also used in the field of chemically adulterated herbal products, though it is often used in combination with FT-IR and mass spectrometry in order to elucidate the structure of unknown compounds, often designer molecules, present in the products. Especially for the analysis of herbal products for potency and weight loss, this is an issue (Deconinck, Sacré, Courselle, & De Beer, 2013b). To our knowledge no designer molecules of medicines used for pain treatment were already detected in adulterated traditional medicines or dietary supplements.

The biggest advantage of spectroscopic techniques, especially the infrared methods, is that no or minimal sample preparation is necessary, though this is also their biggest disadvantage. Infrared spectroscopy is a whole sample approach, this means that the recorded spectrum is obtained for the tablet, capsule content, liquid, and so on, as a whole and that it reflects the total composition. This means that matrix components can interfere with the detection of adulterants and that adulterants, which are not targeted by the analysis will not be detected and unknowns cannot be identified. Therefore, laboratories charged with the analysis of suspected traditional medicines or dietary supplements consider chromatographic methods as standard. Chromatographic methods or more in general separation methods allow to separate a product or mixture in its different constituents and to detect them separately. This has the advantage that chemical adulterants can be detected without or with less interference of the matrix, in our case often a herbal based matrix, and a subsequent quantification of the adulterants is possible. In general, liquid chromatography (LC) is used for the screening and analysis of suspected traditional medicines and dietary supplements, but also thin layer chromatographic and gas chromatographic methods are available (Deconinck et al., 2013b). Thin layer chromatography has the advantage of being low cost, especially important in countries that do not have a lot of investment capacity, but also have less sensitivity and specificity. Gas chromatography is more used for the detection of volatile components, such as residual solvents (Deconinck, Canfyn, Sacré, Courselle, & De Beer, 2013c), but is less suited for the detection of adulterants, since the latter would need some volatility, which is not always the case. The two most important detection techniques often hyphenated with liquid chromatography for adulterant detection are ultraviolet spectroscopy (UV) and mass spectrometry (MS). Mass spectrometry is the preferred detection method in this type of analysis, since it allows unambiguous identification of adulterants based on exact mass, in case of high resolution MS, and/or fragmentation patterns, in case of low resolution MS and also allows structure elucidation in case of unknown compounds like designer molecules. Examples of LC–MS screening methods that are able to detect analgesics, NSAIDs, and benzodiazepines as adulterants are described by Bogusz et al. (2006), de Carvalho et al. (2011) and Guo et al. (2015). Although LC–MS is considered as the golden standard, several laboratories do not have access to expensive mass spectrometric technology. An alternative is the use of LC with UV detection. Here the adulterants can be detected and identified based on chromatographic retention time and, if a diode array detector (DAD) is used, based on the UV spectrum. A DAD can be considered as a multiwavelength UV detector. LC–UV or LC–DAD belongs to the standard equipment of laboratories for pharmaceutical quality control. Examples of screening methods, based on LC–UV or DAD, for the detection of analgesics, NSAIDs and benzodiazepines are described by Almeida and Ribeiro (1999); Almeida, Ribeiro, and Polese (2000); Mikami, Goto, Ohno, Oka, and Kanamori (2005); Liu, Woo, and Koh (2001); Deconinck et al. (2015b).

In order to check the presence/absence of certain plants in dietary supplements the chromatographic fingerprint approach often used in pharmacognosy for the identification of crude plant material can be applied. A chromatographic fingerprint is a characteristic profile reflecting the complex chemical composition of a sample, obtained using a chromatographic technique. Chromatographic fingerprints are the most informative type of fingerprints in plant analysis, since by spreading the information contained in the sample over time, one can reveal the individual compounds and their underlying information (Deconinck et al., 2013a, 2015a; Tistaert, Dejaegher, & Vander Heyden, 2011). This is also, why chromatographic fingerprints are probably the best choice for the detection of certain plants in mixtures of herbal and/or synthetic powders. In literature (Deconinck et al., 2013a, 2015a) a general strategy to perform such an identification based on chromatographic fingerprints is described. In short the procedure can be summarized as follows: using a standard sample of crude material or a standard extract of the plant of interest choose the most appropriate extraction solvent and develop a chromatographic method in such a way that an as specific as possible chromatogram for the plant is obtained. Once the characteristic chromatographic profile is obtained, the samples to be tested are extracted with the same extraction solvent and analyzed using the developed chromatographic method for the standard. The chromatographic profiles for samples are now compared to the one of the standard product. This can be done based on a common correlation of the profiles or some

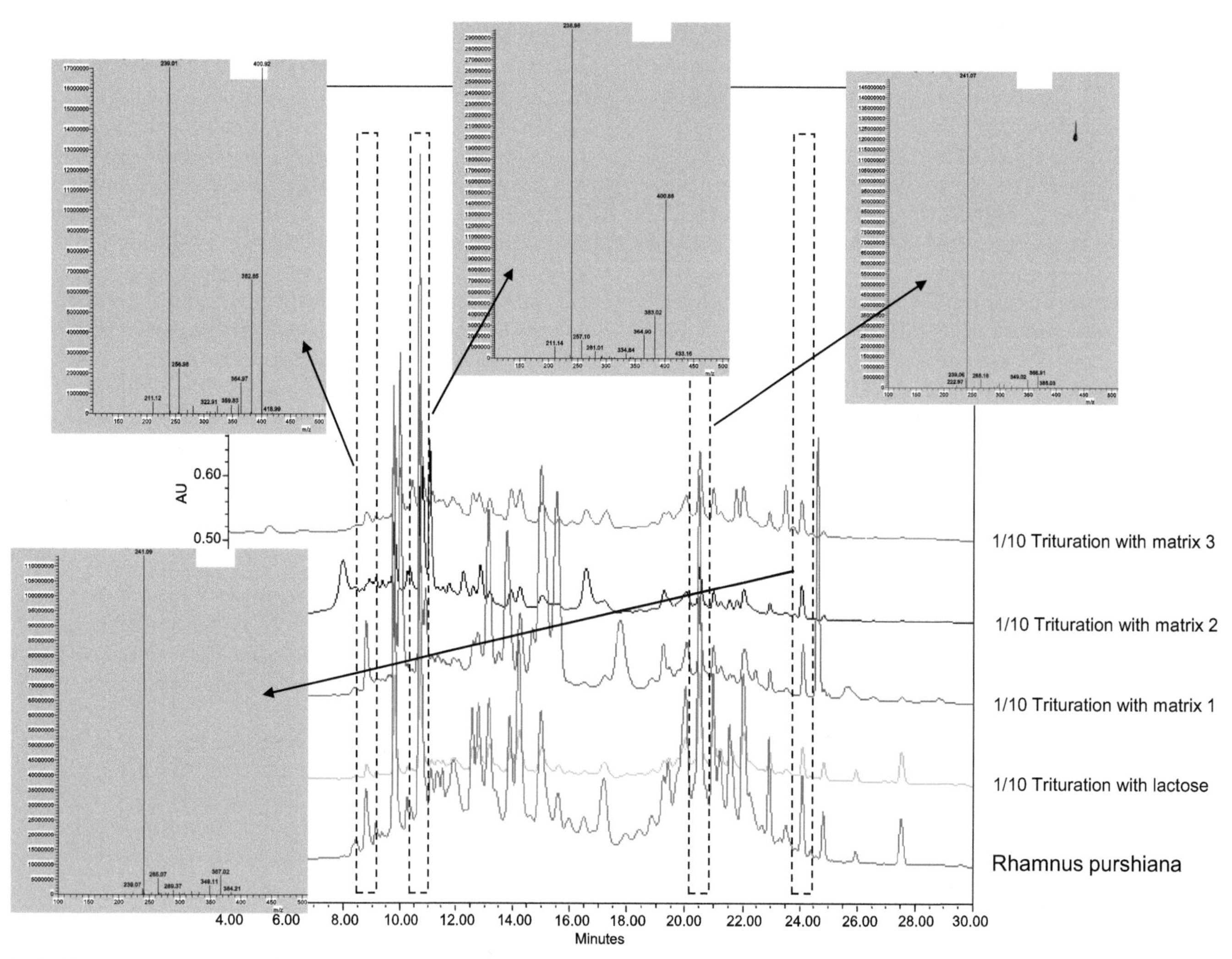

FIGURE 6.4 **Chromatographic fingerprints for *Rhamnus purshiana* and its triturations.**

more advanced chemometrc techniques and will result in a probability of presence of the considered herbal product in the sample. Afterwards a mass spectrometric analysis of the most characteristic peaks, corresponding between standard and sample(s) can be performed in order to confirm that they are identical (Deconinck et al., 2013a, 2015a). As example Fig. 6.4 shows the chromatographic fingerprints for *Rhamnus purshiana* and its trituration in lactose and three herbal matrices together with the mass spectra of the most characteristic peaks.

Although laborious and the fact that for each herbal compound a different method and analysis should be performed, this is for the moment the only way to detect regulated and/or toxic plants in fraudulent dietary supplements and herbal medicines. Based on these analysis people can be warned for certain products, websites can be closed and distributors can be brought to justice. This to contribute to consumers safety and protection of public health.

CONCLUSIONS

In general, it can be concluded that, next to counterfeiting of medicines, the market of traditional medicines and dietary supplements is affected by pharmaceutical crime. While confounding of herbal raw material can be accidental or due to a lack of quality norms and systems with the manufacturer, counterfeiting of herbal products and adulteration of traditional medicines and dietary supplements is considered a crime. The idea is to make as much money as fast as possible. Counterfeiting is clear since cheap herbal material is sold as a traditional product, containing herbal medicines. Adulteration, especially with medicines, is probably a strategy to sell more products. Due to the medicines present, the products are effective and consumers are persuaded to use them for a longer period of time or even to promote the products. Since the medicines added, are cheap bulk products, probably not produced under Good

Manufacturing Procedures (GMP), this strategy will lead to maximal profit.

Authorities worldwide are aware of this problem and are conducting campaigns both on the national as the international level. National agencies are conducting regular controls of the traditional products and the dietary supplements on their market and control laboratories are becoming more efficient in the detection of adulterations. On the European level, the Official Medicines Control laboratories (OMCL) network is constantly monitoring the situation throughout Europe, exchanging information, methodologies and technology throughout the network.

Most of the reported pharmaceutical crime cases, concerning traditional medicines, and dietary supplements, are dealing with products sold for erectile dysfunction, potency enhancements, and weight loss. Though illegal products sold for the treatment of chronic pain or rheumatoid arthritis are encountered. Therefore, people are advised to buy their products from recognized distribution centers, since these are controlled by the regulatory authorities and especially avoid internet websites who do not disclose their identity or physical address.

References

Almeida, A. E., & Ribeiro, M. L. (1999). High-performance liquid chromatographic determination of amfepramone hydrochloride, mazindol, and diazepam in tablets. *Journal of Liquid Chromatography & Related Technologies*, *22*, 1759–1769.

Almeida, A. E., Ribeiro, M. L., & Polese, L. (2000). Determination of amfepramone hydrochloride, femproporex, and diazepam in so-called "natural" capsules used in the treatment of obesity. *Journal of Liquid Chromatography & Related Technologies*, *23*, 1109–1118.

Anderson, B. J. (2008). Paracetamol (acetaminophen): mechanisms of action. *Pediatric Anesthesia*, *18*, 915–921.

Applequist, W. L., & Miller, J. S. (2013). Selection and authentication of botanical materials for the development of analytical methods. *Analytical and Bioanalytical Chemistry*, *405*, 4419–4428.

Bashir, H. A., & Abu-Goukh, A. B. A. (2003). Compositional changes during guava fruit ripening. *Food Chemistry*, *80*, 557–563.

Bogusz, M. J., Hassan, H., Al-Enazi, E., Ibrahim, Z., & Al-Tufail, M. (2006). Application of LC-ESI-MS-MS for detection of synthetic adulterants in herbal remedies. *Journal of Pharmaceutical and Biomedical Analysis*, *41*, 554–564.

Chena, H., Li, X., Chen, J., Guo, S., & Cai, B. (2010). Simultaneous determination of eleven bioactive compounds in *Saururus chinensis* from different harvesting seasons by HPLC-DAD. *Journal of Pharmaceutical and Biomedical Analysis*, *51*, 1142–1146.

Choi, J. Y., Heo, S., Yoo, G. J., Park, S. K., Yoon, C. Y., & Baek, S. Y. (2015). Development and validation of an LC–MS/MS method for the simultaneous analysis of 28 specific narcotic adulterants used in dietary supplements. *Food Additives & Contaminants. Part A, Chemistry, Analysis, Control, Exposure & Risk Assessment*, *32*, 1029–1039.

Cianchino, V., Acosta, G., Ortega, C., Martinez, L. D., & Gomez, M. R. (2008). Analysis of potential adulteration in herbal medicines and dietary supplements for the weight control by capillary electrophoresis. *Food Chemistry*, *108*, 1075–1081.

Committee on Herbal Medicinal Products (HMPC) (2010). *Overview of assessment work—Priority list*. London, UK: European Medicine Evaluation Agency.

Custers, D., Cauwenbergh, T., Bothy, J. L., Courselle, P., De Beer, J. O., Apers, S., & Deconinck, E. (2015). ATR-IR spectroscopy and chemometrics: interesting tools to discriminate and characterize counterfeit medicines? *Journal of Pharmaceutical and Biomedical Analysis*, *112*(2015), 181–189.

Dannhardt, G., & Kiefer, W. (2001). COX inhibitors—current status and future prospects. *European Journal of Medicinal Chemistry*, *36*, 109–126.

da Silva Fernandes, R., da Costa, F. S., Valderrama, P., Março, P. H., & de Lima, K. M. (2012). Non-destructive detection of adulterated tablets of glibenclamide using NIR and solid-phase fluorescence spectroscopy and chemometric methods. *Journal of Pharmaceutical and Biomedical Analysis*, *66*, 85–90.

Datta, A., & Srivastava, P. S. (1997). Variation in vinblastine production by *Catharanthus roseus* during in vivo and in vitro differentiation. *Phytochemistry*, *46*, 135–137.

de Carvalho, L. M., Correia, D., Garcia, S. C., de Bairros, A. V., do Nascimento, P. C., & Bohrer, D. (2010). A new method for the simultaneous determination of 1,4-benzodiazepines and amfepramone as adulterants in phytotherapeutic formulations by voltammetry. *Forensic Science International*, *202*, 75–81.

de Carvalho, L. M., Martini, M., Moreira, A. P., de Lima, A. P., Correia, D., Falcão, T., Garcia, S. C., de Bairros, A. V., do Nascimento, P. C., & Bohrer, D. (2011). Presence of synthetic pharmaceuticals as adulterants in slimming phytotherapeutic formulations and their analytical determination. *Forensic Science International*, *204*, 6–12.

Declaration of Alma-Ata (1978). International Conference on Primary Health Care, Alma-Ata, USSR. Available from: http://www.who.int/hpr/NPH/docs/declarationalmaata.pdf

Deconinck, E., De Leersnijder, C., Custers, D., Courselle, P., & De Beer, J. O. (2013a). A strategy for the identification of plants in illegal pharmaceutical preparations and food supplements using chromatographic fingerprints. *Analytical and Bioanalytical Chemistry*, *405*, 2341–2352.

Deconinck, E., Sacré, P. -Y., Courselle, P., & De Beer, J. O. (2013b). Chromatography in the detection and characterization of illegal pharmaceutical preparations. *Journal of Chromatographic Science*, *51*, 791–806.

Deconinck, E., Canfyn, M., Sacré, P. -Y., Courselle, P., & De Beer, J. O. (2013c). Evaluation of the residual solvent content of counterfeit tablets and capsules. *Journal of Pharmaceutical and Biomedical Analysis*, *81-82*, 80–88.

Deconinck, E., Cauwenbergh, T., Bothy, J. L., Custers, D., Courselle, P., & De Beer, J. O. (2014). Detection of sibutramine in adulterated dietary supplements using Attenuated Total Reflectance-Infrared spectroscopy. *Journal of Pharmaceutical and Biomedical Analysis*, *100*, 279–283.

Deconinck, E., Custers, D., & De Beer, J. O. (2015a). Identification of (antioxidative) plants in herbal pharmaceutical preparations and dietary supplements. *Methods in Molecular Biology*, *1208*, 181–199.

Deconinck, E., Kamugisha, A., Van Campenhout, P., Courselle, P., & De Beer, J. O. (2015b). Development of a Stationary Phase Optimised Selectivity Liquid Chromatography based screening method for adulterations of food supplements for the treatment of pain. *Talanta*, *138*, 240–246.

Doménech-Carbó, A., Martini, M., de Carvalho, L. M., Viana, C., Doménech-Carbó, M. T., & Silva, M. (2013). Standard additions-dilution method for absolute quantification in voltammetry of microparticles. Application for determining psychoactive 1,4-benzodiazepine and antidepressants drugs as adulterants in phytotherapeutic formulations. *Journal of Pharmaceutical and Biomedical Analysis*, *80*, 159–163.

e-compendium (2015). Algemene vereniging van de geneesmiddelen industrie. Available from: www.e-compendium.be

European Medicine Evaluation Agency (2006) Guideline on the environmental risk assessment of medicinal products for human use, London, UK. Available from: http://www.ema.europa.eu/docs/enGB/documentlibrary/Scientificguideline/2009/10/WC500003978.pdf

European Medicine Evaluation Agency. (2010a). Inventory of herbal substances for assessment–Alphabetical order, London, UK. Available from: http://www.ema.europa.eu/docs/enGB/documentlibrary/Other/2009/12/WC500017723.pdf

European Medicine Evaluation Agency. (2010b). Guideline on declaration of herbal substances and herbal preparations in herbal medicinal products/traditional herbal medicinal products, London, UK. Available from: http://www.ema.europa.eu/docs/enGB/documentlibrary/Scientificguideline/2009/09/WC500003283.pdf

European Pharmacopoeia 7.0. (2010). Council of Europe. Strasbourg, France.

Félix-Silva, J., Giordani, R. B., da Silva-Jr, A. A., Zucolotto, S. M., & Fernandes-Pedrosa Mde, F. (2014). *Jatropha gossypiifolia* L. (Euphorbiaceae): A review of traditional uses, phytochemistry, pharmacology, and toxicology of this medicinal plant. *Evidence-Based Complementary and Alternative Medicine*.

Fox, C., Liu, H., Kaye, A. D., Manchikanti, L., Trescot, A. M., Christo, P. J., & Falco, F. J. R. (2011). *Clinical Aspects of Pain Medicine and Interventional Pain Management: A Comprehensive Review*. Paducah, KY: ASIP Publishing, Chapter: Antianxiety agents.

Fujii, Y., Fujii, H., & Yamazaki, M. (1983). Separation and determination of cardiac glycosides in *Digitalis purpurea* leaves by micro high-performance liquid chromatography. *Journal of Chromatography, 258*, 147–153.

Gan, T. J. (2010). Diclofenac: an update on its mechanism of action and safety profile. *Current Medical Research and Opinion, 26*, 1715–1731.

Gecommentarieerd geneesmiddelen repertorium 2015, Belgische Centrum voor Farmacotherapeutische informatie, Brussels, Belgium.

Griffin, C. E., Kaye, A. M., Bueno, F. R., & Kaye, A. D. (2013). Benzodiazepine pharmacology and central nervous system-mediated effects. *Ochsner. Journal, 13*, 214–223.

Guo, B., Wang, M., Liu, Y., Zhou, J., Dai, H., Huang, Z., Shen, L., Zhang, Q., & Chen, B. (2015). Wide-scope screening of illegal adulterants in dietary and herbal supplements via rapid polarity-switching and multistage accurate mass confirmation using an LC-IT/TOF hybrid instrument. *The Journal of Agricultural and Food Chemistry, 63*, 6954–6967.

Jahr, J. S., & Lee, V. K. (2010). Intravenous acetaminophen. *Anesthesiology Clinics, 28*, 619–645.

Johansson, M., Fransson, D., Rundlöf, T., Huynh, N. H., & Arvidsson, T. (2014). A general analytical platform and strategy in search for illegal drugs. *Journal of Pharmaceutical and Biomedical Analysis, 100*, 215–229.

Kelly, M. D., Smith, A., Banks, G., Wingrove, P., Whiting, P. W., Atack, J., Seabrook, G. R., & Maubach, K. A. (2002). Role of the histidine residue at position 105 in the human alpha 5 containing GABA(A) receptor on the affinity and efficacy of benzodiazepine site ligands. *British Journal of Pharmacology, 135*, 248–256.

Kim, H. J., Lee, J. H., Park, H. J., Kim, J. Y., Cho, S., & Kim, W. S. (2014). Determination of non-opioid analgesics in adulterated food and dietary supplements by LC-MS/MS. *Food additives & contaminants. Part A, Chemistry, analysis, control, exposure & risk assessment, 31*, 973–978.

Kofi-Tsekpo, M. (2004). Institutionalization of African traditional medicine in health care systems in Africa. *African Jornal of Health Sciences, 11*(1–2), i–i10.

Koninklijk besluit van 29 Augustus. (1997). Betreffende de fabricage van en de handel in voedingsmiddelen die uit planten of uit plantenbereidingen samengesteld zijn of deze bevatten. Available from: http://health.belgium.be/eportal/foodsafety/foodstuffs/foodsupplements/841608_NL?ie2Term=public?&fodnlang=nl#Planten

Liang, Q., Qu, J., Luo, G., & Wang, Y. (2006). Rapid and reliable determination of illegal adulterant in herbal medicines and dietary supplements by LC/MS/MS. *Journal of Pharmaceutical and Biomedical Analysis, 40*, 305–311.

Liu, S. -Y., Woo, S. -O., & Koh, H. -L. (2001). HPLC and GC–MS screening of Chinese proprietary medicine for undeclared therapeutic substances. *Journal of Pharmaceutical and Biomedical Analysis, 24*, 983–992.

Lopez-Feria, S., Cardenas, S., Garcıa-Mesa, J. A., & Valcarcel, M. (2008). Classification of extra virgin olive oils according to the protected designation of origin, olive variety and geographical origin. *Talanta, 75*, 937–943.

Mikami, E., Goto, T., Ohno, T., Oka, H., & Kanamori, H. (2005). Simultaneous analysis of seven benzodiazepines in dietary supplements as adulterants using high performance liquid chromatography and its application to an identification system for diazepam. *Journal of Health Sciences, 51*, 278–283.

Miller, R. J., Jolles, C., & Rapoport, H. (1973). Morphine metabolism and normorphine in *Papaver somniferum*. *Phytochemistry, 12*, 597–603.

Miraldi, E., Ferri, S., & Mostaghimi, V. (2001). Botanical drugs and preparations in the traditional medicine of West Azerbaijan (Iran). *Journal of Ethnopharmacology, 75*, 77–87.

Mosihuzzaman, M., & Choudhary, M. I. (2008). Protocols on safety, efficacy, standardization, and documentation of herbal medicine (IUPAC technical report). *Pure and Applied Chemistry, 80*, 2195–2230.

Naithani, V., Nair, S., & Kakkar, P. (2006). Decline in antioxidant capacity of Indian herbal teas during storage and its relation to phenolic content. *Food Research International, 39*, 176–181.

Pasternak, G. W. (1993). Pharmacological mechanisms of opioid analgesics. *Clinical Neuropharmacology, 16*, 1–18.

Pferschy-Wenzig, E. M., & Bauer, R. (2015). The relevance of pharmacognosy in pharmacological research on herbal medicinal products. *Epilepsy Behaviour, 52*, 344–362.

Pharmacopoeia of the People's Republic of China–English edition (2010). Chinese Pharmacopoeia Commission, People's Medical Publishing House, Beijing, China.

Phillipson, J. D., & Handa, S. S. (1976). Hyoscyamine N-oxide in *Atropa belladonna*. *Phytochemistry, 15*, 605–608.

Rivera, D., Allkin, R., Obón, C., Alcaraz, F., Verpoorte, R., & Heinrich, M. (2014). What is in a name? The need for accurate scientific nomenclature for plants. *Journal of Ethnopharmacology, 152*, 393–402.

Samuels, N., Finkelstein, Y., Singer, S. R., & Oberbaum, M. (2008). Herbal medicine and epilepsy: proconvulsive effects and interactions with antiepileptic drugs. *Epilepsia, 49*, 373–380.

Selinsky, B. S., Gupta, K., Sharkey, C. T., & Loll, P. J. (2001). Structural analysis of NSAID binding by prostaglandin H_2 synthase: time-dependent and time independent inhibitors elicit identical enzyme conformations. *Biochemistry, 40*, 5172–5180.

Shin, Y., Liu, R. H., Nock, J. F., Holliday, D., & Watkins, C. B. (2007). Temperature and relative humidity effects on quality, total ascorbic acid, phenolics and flavonoid concentrations, and antioxidant activity of strawberry. *Postharvest Biology and Technology, 45*, 349–357.

Simeoni, P., & Lebot, V. (2002). Identification of factors determining kavalactone content and chemotype in Kava (*Piper methysticum* Forst. f.). *Biochemical* Systematics and *Ecology, 30*, 413–424.

Smith, W. L., De Witt, D. L., & Garavito, R. M. (2000). COXs: structural, cellular and molecular biology. *Annual Review of Biochemistry, 69*, 145–182.

Strobel, G., Stierle, A., & Hess, W. M. (1994). The stimulation of taxol production in *Taxus brevifolia* by various growth retardants. *Plant Science, 101*, 115–124.

Summ, O., & Evers, S. (2013). Mechanism of action of indomethacin in indomethacin-responsive headaches. *Current Pain and Headache Reports, 17*, 327.

Tan, X., Li, Q., Chen, X., Wang, Z., Shi, Z., Bi, K., & Jia, Y. (2008). Simultaneous determination of 13 bioactive compounds in Herba Artemisiae Scopariae (Yin Chen) from different harvest seasons by

HPLC–DAD. *Journal of Pharmaceutical and Biomedical Analysis, 47,* 847–853.

Tistaert, C., Dejaegher, B., & Vander Heyden, Y. (2011). Chromatographic separation techniques and data handling methods for herbal fingerprints: a review. *Analytica Chimica Acta, 690,* 148–161.

Tshibangu, K. C., Worku, Z. B., de Jongh, M. A., van Wyk, A. E., Mokwena, S. O., & Peranovic, V. (2004). Assessment of effectiveness of traditional herbal medicine in managing HIV/AIDS patients in South Africa. *East African Medical Journal, 81,* 499–504.

United States Pharmacopoeia 35. (2010). United States Pharmacopoeial Convention, Inc., Rockville, MD.

Vane, J. R., & Botting, R. M. (2003). The mechanism of action of aspirin. *Thrombosis Research, 110,* 255–258.

Vanherweghem, J. L., Depierreux, M., Tielemans, C., Abramowicz, D., Dratwa, M., Jadoul, M., Richard, C., Vandervelde, D., Verbeelen, D., & Vanhaelen-Fastre, R. (1993). Rapidly progressive interstitial renal fibrosis in young women: association with slimming regimen including Chinese herbs. *Lancet, 341,* 387–391.

Venhuis, B. J., Zomer, G., Hamzink, M., Meiring, H. D., Aubin, Y., & de Kaste, D. (2011). The identification of a nitrosated prodrug of the PDE-5 inhibitor aildenafil in a dietary supplement: a Viagra with a pop. *Journal of Pharmaceutical and Biomedical Analysis, 54,* 735–741.

Whitton, P. A., Lau, A., Salisbury, A., Whitehouse, J., & Evans, C. S. (2003). Kava lactones and the kava-kava controversy. *Phytochemistry, 64,* 673–679.

WHO Expert Committee on Drug Dependence (2014): Tramadol, Update Review Report. Available from: http://www.who.int/medicines/areas/quality_safety/6_1_Update.pdf

World Health Organization (1991) Guidelines for the assessment of herbal medicines, Geneva, Switzerland. Available from: http://whqlibdoc.who.int/HQ/1991/WHOTRM91.4.pdf

World Health Organization (1999) WHO monographs on selected medicinal plants (Volume I), Geneva, Switzerland. Available from: http://whqlibdoc.ho.int/publications/1999/9241545178.pdf

World Health Organization (2000a) General Guidelines for Methodologies on Research and Evaluation of Traditional Medicine, Geneva, Switzerland. Available from: http://whqlibdoc.who.int/hq/2000/WHOEDMTRM2000.1.pdf

World Health Organization (2000b) General Guidelines for Methodologies on Research and Evaluation of Traditional Medicine, Geneva, Switzerland. Available from: http://whqlibdoc.who.int/hq/2000/WHOEDMTRM2000.1.pdf

World Health Organization (2003) WHO monographs on selected medicinal plants (Volume II), Geneva, Switzerland. Available from: http://whqlibdoc.who.int/publications/2002/9241545372.pdf

World Health Organization (2005) National policy on traditional medicine and regulation of herbal medicines, Geneva, Switzerland. Available from: http://whqlibdoc.who.int/publications/2005/9241593237.pdf

World Health Organization (2007). WHO monographs on selected medicinal plants (Volume III), Geneva, Switzerland. Available from: http://apps.who.int/medicinedocs/index/assoc/s14213e/s14213e.pdf

Zhang, J., Wider, B., Shang, H., Li, X., & Ernst, E. (2012). Quality of herbal medicines: challenges and solutions. *Complementary Therapies Medicine, 20,* 100–106.

CHAPTER

7

Diabetic Neuropathy Modulation by Zinc and/or Polyphenol Administration

L. Bădescu, M. Ciocoiu**, C. Bădescu*[†]*, M. Bădescu***

*Department of Cell and Molecular Biology, St. Spiridon Hospital, University of Medicine and Pharmacy "Grigore T. Popa", Iasi, Romania; **Department of Pathophysiology, St. Spiridon Hospital, University of Medicine and Pharmacy "Grigore T. Popa", Iasi, Romania; [†]Internal Medicine Clinic, St. Spiridon Hospital, University of Medicine and Pharmacy "Grigore T. Popa", Iasi, Romania

INTRODUCTION

Diabetes mellitus (DM) is a much-feared disease of our century, a metabolic disorder accompanied by many biochemical alterations. It is a chronic condition that involves the state of nutrition of the whole body and the progress of which upsets the intermediate metabolism process of all food substances: carbohydrates, lipids, proteins (American Diabetes Association, 2008). At the same time, according to the WHO data, there are 10,000 new cases of insulin-dependent DM among children in Europe each year. 600,000 cases of diabetes have been diagnosed in Romania, only 400,000 of whom actually receive treatment. It is thought that there are other 400,000 people suffering from diabetes, who have not been diagnosed yet. Diabetic neuropathy is the most common complication of DM, as it affects about 65% of the diabetics and is due to the chronic persistence of hyperglycemia (Bantle et al., 2008; Boulton et al., 2008).

It is the most common form of neuropathy in the developed countries of the world, accounts for more hospitalizations than all the other diabetic complications combined, and is responsible for 50–75% of nontraumatic amputations (Cameron & Cotter, 1994). It may be silent and go undetected while exercising its ravages. It is a heterogeneous disorder that encompasses a wide range of abnormalities affecting proximal and distal peripheral sensory and motor nerves, as well as the autonomic nervous systems (Freeman, 2005). The major morbidity associated with somatic neuropathy is foot ulceration, the precursor of gangrene and limb loss. It is now recognized that a major effect of diabetes is on the small unmyelinated or thinly myelinated C and A delta nerve fibers that subserve autonomic function and thermal and pain perception (Low, Benrud-Larson, Sletten, & Tonette, 2004; Malik, Maser, Sosenko, & Ziegler, 2005).

Rationale for the Research

In the light of the considerations above, our research aims at emphasizing the potentially beneficial effect of zinc and of a particular polyphenol extract on the neurological complications due to the progress of DM. The purpose of this research is to prove the importance of electrodiagnosis in the early detection of asymptomatic diabetic polyneuropathy, to decide whether neuropathy may be improved by Zn or polyphenol administration and to assess its prevalence in patients diagnosed with type II diabetes. Peripheral neuropathy is the most frequent disorder of the peripheral nervous system. Diabetic neuropathy prevalence is thought to vary between very wide limits, that is, 10–90% (Gooch & Podwall, 2004). The EURODIAB study had 35% of the subject that were diagnosed with neuropathy. Over 80% of the diabetic neuropathy patients suffered from a symmetrical form of the disorder. Sensory neuropathy was the most common and it turned into mixed sensory-motor neuropathy in patients with long-lasting progressing diabetes and metabolic imbalance.

According to numerous prestigious studies (Diabetes Control and Complication Trial, United Kingdom Prospective Diabetes Study-UKPDS), glucose level control improvement is the best way to prevent and ameliorate diabetic neuropathy, since hyperglycemia triggers all the

Nutritional Modulators of Pain in the Aging Population. http://dx.doi.org/10.1016/B978-0-12-805186-3.00007-2
Copyright © 2017 Elsevier Inc. All rights reserved.

other mechanisms. We achieved (in prior trials on animals and in the current study) significant glucose level decreases by the administration of soluble zinc salts and polyphenols for variable periods of time (Gorson & Ropper, 2006).

We used polyphenols extracted from *Ginkgo biloba* (GB) leaves. Polyphenols make up one of the main classes of secondary plant metabolites with aromatic structure (phytohormones). Ginko is an extremely powerful antioxidant. Due to the flavonoids it contains, it exerts a protective action on cell membranes and maintains their integrity. Ginko also has a vasodilator effect, as it stimulates the endothelial factor and prostacyclin synthesis. Its pharmacological action is mainly due to glucosides, flavonoids, and ginkgolides. The effect of the *G. biloba* leaf extract, with a standardized content of 24% flavonoid glycosides and 6% terpenoids, was the object of over forty double-blind experiments designed to treat cerebral circulatory failure (Cohen-Boulakia, 2000). The *G. biloba* extract has been proven to largely improve the following symptoms in case of cerebral circulatory failure and diminished cerebral capacities: short-term memory deficiencies, headaches, tinnitus, and depression. It seems that the *G. biloba* extract improves cerebral blood flow and thus leads to a more efficient use of glucose and oxygen. It improves old age-related symptoms and prevents their occurrence (Delia Loggia et al., 1996). In addition, it prevents the occurrence of strokes by diminishing blood viscosity. We administered 2 tablets/day (i.e., 500 mg $\times$ 2 of extract) for 6 months.

The second antioxidant that we used was zinc, a much studied microelement involved in many pathological conditions. Zinc is a trace element, a naturally occurring element found in the soil. In food it occurs in insignificant amounts. Therefore, the necessary zinc intake must have a different source than food. In children, zinc deficiency may lead to growth retardation and to abnormal genitalia development (in boys). In adults, zinc deficiency may cause hair loss, increased nail fragility, trophic skin disorders, or asthenia. Zinc is essential for protein and insulin synthesis. Metabolically speaking, zinc stimulates all the insulin-influenced ways (Al-Maroof & Al-Sharbatti, 2006). Nevertheless, its action mechanism seems to be insulin-independent. Here are a series of arguments supporting this assumption:

- The lipogenesis stimulation capacity of insulin is not significantly reduced by endogenous zinc chelation;
- Unlike insulin, zinc does not inhibit lipolysis;
- The stimulating effect of zinc on glucose incorporation in lipids supplements the effect of certain saturating insulin concentrations;
- Zn does not stimulate autophosphorylation or the kinase activity of the insulin receptor in rat adipocytes;
- Insulin resistance is not accompanied by Zn resistance.

Therefore, insulin seems to act differently than Zinc since the first stages of the signaling cascade (Arquilla, Packer, Tarmas, & Myamoto, 1998).

As dietary supplement, a daily Zinc intake amounting to 15 mg is recommended. In athletes, the daily intake may be as high as 50 mg. A greater zinc intake is recommended to alcoholic and diabetics. We chose the per os administration of 50 mg of amino acid-chelated zinc per day for 6 months (the chelated form ensures perfect absorption and assimilation).

Study Design and Participants

This was a study with a sample composed of patients attending the diabetes outpatient service of the hospital of the Medical University of Iasi (Romania) aged between 51 and 73 years, with an average age of 63 years, having a diagnostic of type 2 diabetes, controlled with diet, or with oral antidiabetics, but not with insulin. Inclusion criteria were (1) type 2 DM; (2) the duration of diabetes beetween 5 and 15 years. Only patients who freely gave informed consent were included in the study.

The study group included 184 patients diagnosed with DM, 96 women and 88 men. *112 patients, 52 women, and 60 men*, were diagnosed with diabetic neuropathy and included in the study.

Only 132 of the 184 patients that had undergone clinical, paraclinical, and biological exams were included in the study and were distributed in 3 study groups, which were relatively homogeneous from the viewpoint of the patients' age, sex, and length of diabetes:

- all of them were administered only oral antidiabetic drugs;
- aged between 40 and 70 years;
- length of diabetes exceeding 4 years.

In addition to the antidiabetic drugs prescribed by the diabetes center, the first group, which included *56 patients* (30 men and 26 women), were also administered a *Zn* supplement (*Unizinc 50 mg*) for a period of 6 months.

The second group, which included other *56 patients* (30 men and 26 women), were also administered an additional therapy consisting of *polyphenols extracted from G. Biloba* for a period of 6 months.

The last group, which included *20 diabetic patients* (10 men and 10 women), were the controls (they were only given the classical antidiabetic therapy).

The following data were evaluated in all the patients: gender (man or women), age, duration of diabetes, anthropometric parameters (height, weight, body mass index BMI); serum cholesterol, HDL-cholesterol fraction, triglycerides; blood pressure and heart rate in standard examination conditions. An electroneurography was subsequently conducted (Dworkin et al., 2003).

Electromyography and motor and sensory nerve conduction velocity changes are disorders due to diabetic neuropathy. When polyneuropathy progresses, the disorders follow a certain path, as they first involve sensory excitability, then motor excitability, fiber conductivity, and EMG path changes, and they finally trigger subjective and objective clinical symptoms (Arezzo & Zotova, 2002).

A Reporter ESAOTE computerized system was used for electrophysiological examinations devoted to surface electromyography and stimulus detection techniques.

In the three groups we aimed at detecting possible diabetic neuropathy cases and different related variables or potential risk factors. The number of patients suffered from diabetic neuropathy is 60.9%.

The association between diabetic neuropathy and potential variables reveals the following aspects (Table 7.1):

- The length of the diabetic condition was significantly higher in patients with diabetic neuropathy ($p < 0.005$).
- The HbA_{1c} level (%) is considerably higher in the group with diabetic neuropathy ($p < 0.001$), when HbA_{1c} is >7%, the predictive value is 93%.
- Hypertension is significantly associated with diabetic neuropathy ($p < 0.001$), the predictive value being 50%.

TABLE 7.1 Prevalence of Diabetic Neuropathy in Patients Diagnosed with Diabetes Mellitus. Association between Diabetic Neuropathy and Potential Variables

	Diabetic neuropathy		
Variables	**Present 112 patients**	**Absent 72 patients**	**Statistical significance**
Length of diabetes mellitus			
Mean	5.0	3.5	$p < 0.005$
Limits	2.0–10.0	0.5–12.5	
Type of treatment [*n* (%)]			
Insulin	18 (10.0)	6 (3.3)	$p < 0.001$
Oral antidiabetic drugs	28 (15.6)	98 (53.3)	
Diet	10 (5.6)	32 (17.8)	
HbA_{1c} [*n* (%)]			
HbA_{1c} (%)	8.49	7.08	$p < 0.001$
>7%	43 (23.9)	69 (38.3)	
<7%	3 (1.7)	67 (37.2)	
Hypertension (*n* (%))	32 (17.8)	56 (31.1)	$p < 0.001$

LABORATORY EVALUATION

Serum Glucose

Metabolic parameters, such as: serum glucose, total cholesterol, LDL, HDL, triglycerides (enzymatic colorimetric method), glycated hemoglobin, and renal function indicators like: creatinine, creatinine clearance.

The individual glucose values of diabetic patients who were also administered additional Zn therapy are not dependent on the age of the patients ($r = -0.09$) and are not correlated with the length of the condition either ($r = -0.17$) (Fig. 7.1).

One may notice, though, a direct correlation between the individual glucose values at the beginning of the experiment and the same values read after 6 months of additional zinc therapy ($r = 0.69$), which reveals that the high initial glucose values were still high after 6 months of additional zinc therapy, although they did not exceed 200 mg/dl. Statistically speaking, the study confirmed that the mean glucose values of female patients who were administered a zinc supplement for 6 months were significantly lower than those of the women under classical therapy (t Student = 2.67; GL = 18; $p < 0.05$).

When we compared the two sexes in the three study groups, we noticed no significant differences between the mean glucose values either in the group under classical antidiabetic therapy, or in the group taking zinc supplements. Differences occurred between the patients taking zinc supplements and their control counterparts: male $p < 0.01$; female $p < 0.05$.

The individual glucose values of diabetic patients taking polyphenol supplements were directly correlated with the patients' age ($r = 0.37$) and length of the condition ($r = 0.40$) (Fig. 7.2).

We also noted a direct correlation between the individual glucose values at the beginning of the experiment and the same values read after 6 months of polyphenol supplement administration ($r = 0.74$), which reveals that the high initial glucose values were still high after 6 months of polyphenol therapy, although they did not exceed 200 mg/dL.

The individual glucose values of diabetic women under polyphenol therapy had a lower variability than the same values of diabetic women under classical antidiabetic therapy (16.52 vs. 22.69). There is a 23% (F-test = 0.23) likelihood that the two sets of glucose values were not significantly different, which supports the assumption that in women the glucose values read after polyphenol administration for 6 months may differ up to 77% from the glucose levels of female patients taking only classical antidiabetic drugs (King, 2004; Ahmed & Thornalley, 2007).

From a statistical point of view, we concluded that the mean glucose values of female patients who had

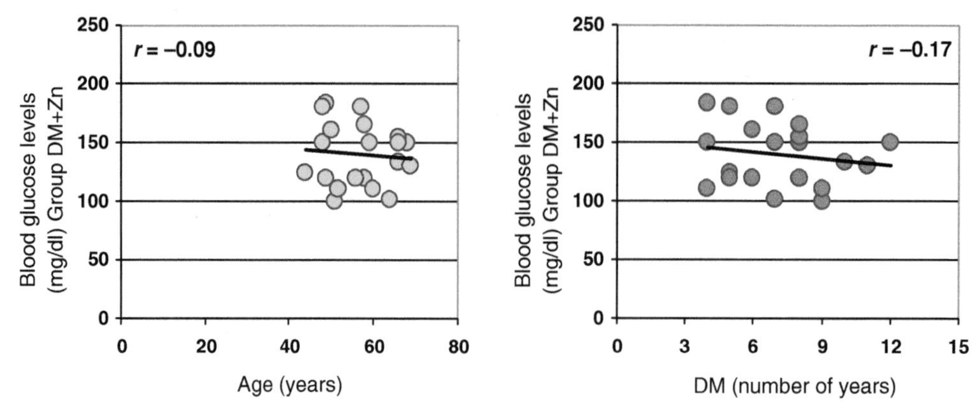

FIGURE 7.1 **Correlation of individual glucose values with age and length of DM in diabetic patients treated with Zn.**

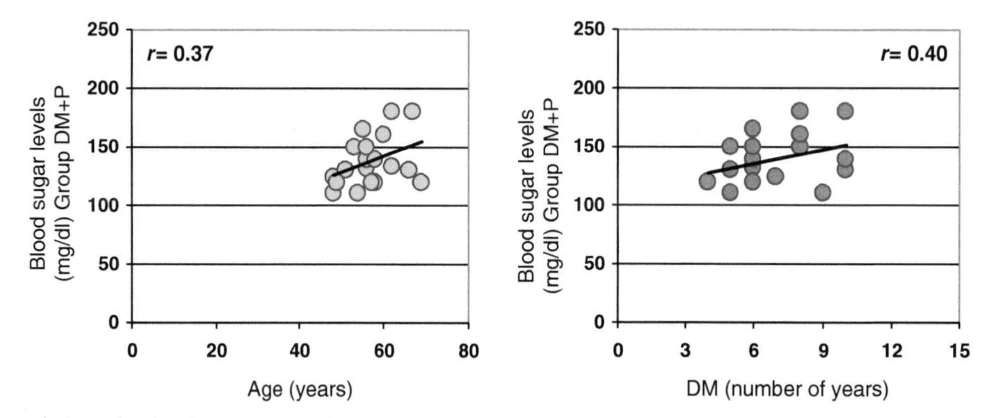

FIGURE 7.2 **Correlation of individual glucose values with age and length of DM in diabetic patients treated with polyphenols.**

been under polyphenol therapy for 6 months were not significantly different from the mean glucose values of female patients taking only classical antidiabetic drugs (t Student = 1.06; GL = 18; $p > 0.05$).

A comparative breakdown of the study groups revealed that the mean glucose values of the two sexes were significantly different in the study group under classical antidiabetic therapy, whereas the polyphenol therapy led to differences between the male patients receiving supplements and their control counterparts $p < 0.002$.

In conclusion, the 6-month follow-up of the glucose levels of diabetic patients enabled us to reach the following findings:

- zinc supplements administered in addition to the regular antidiabetic therapy decreased the mean glucose values by 23.6% in men and by 22% in women;
- poylphenol supplements administered in addition to the regular antidiabetic therapy decreased the mean glucose values by 18.9% in men and by 9.1% in women.

Note that zinc supplements led to a more substantial decrease of the patients' glucose values than polyphenol supplements, both in the male and in the female patients, yet this decrease was not statistically significant, as the mean glucose values of the two sexes after 6 months of additional zinc or polyphenol therapy (Scalbert & Williamson, 2000; Maret, 2002; Al-Maroof & Al-Sharbatti, 2006) were approximately the same.

Glycosylated Hemoglobin

The individual glycosylated hemoglobin [Hb A_1C(%)] values of diabetic patients who also received Zn supplements were independent of their age ($r = 0.09$) and they were not significantly correlated with the length of the condition either ($r = 0.20$).

We noted a direct correlation between the individual glycosylated hemoglobin values at the beginning of the experiment and the same values measured after 6 months of Zinc supplement therapy ($r = 0.77$); 77% of the patients with high initial glycosylated hemoglobin values still had high values after 6 months of Zinc therapy.

From a statistical point of view, the mean Hb A_1C(%) values of female patients who had taken zinc supplements for 6 months were found to be significantly lower than those of female patients under classical antidiabetic therapy (t Student = 4.90; GL = 18; $p < 0.001$) (Fig. 7.3).

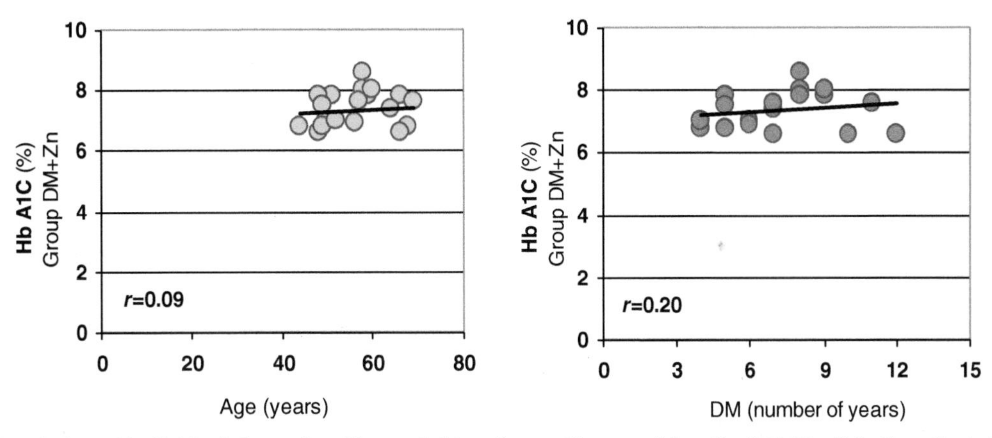

FIGURE 7.3 **Correlation of individual glycosylated hemoglobin values with age and length of DM in diabetic patients taking zinc.**

In the male sex, the individual glycosylated hemoglobin values read between the two moments of the study are equally homogeneous (CV% 8.34 vs. 8.31). There is a 60% ($F = 0.60$) likelihood that the glucose values of the two groups under survey were not different; nevertheless, the mean values showed a considerably significant statistical difference after 6 months of zinc supplement therapy (t Student = 4.78; GL = 18; $p < 0.001$).

When we compared the two sexes in the three study groups, we noticed no significant differences between the mean glycosylated hemoglobin values either in the group under classical antidiabetic therapy, or in the group taking zinc supplements. Differences occurred between the patients taking zinc supplements and their control counterparts, both in the male sex and in the female sex ($p < 0.001$).

The individual glycosylated hemoglobin values of diabetic patients taking additional polyphenol supplements were very weakly indirectly correlated with the age of the patients ($r = -0.11$) and the length of the condition ($r = -0.19$) (Fig. 7.4).

We noted, however, a direct correlation between the individual glycosylated hemoglobin values at the beginning of the experiment and the same values measured after 6 months of polyphenol supplement therapy ($r = 0.79$); 79% of the patients with high initial glycosylated hemoglobin values still had high values after 6 months of poylphenol therapy.

From a statistical point of view, the mean glycosylated hemoglobin values of female patients who had taken polyphenol supplements for 6 months were found to be significantly different than those of female patients under classical antidiabetic therapy (t Student= 3.46; GL = 18; $p < 0.003$).

In conclusion, the 6-month follow-up of the glycosylated hemoglobin levels of diabetic patients enabled us to reach the following findings:

- Zinc supplements administered in addition to the regular antidiabetic therapy decreased the mean glycosylated hemoglobin values by 16.4% in men and by 16.6% in women;

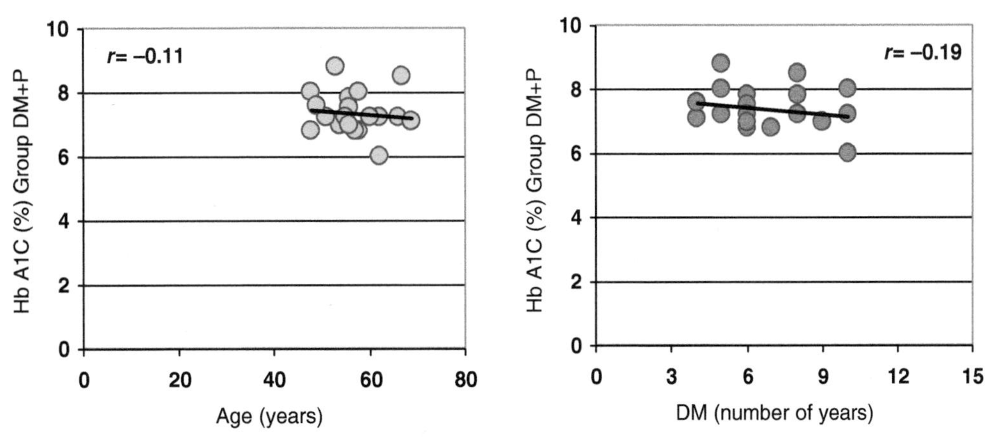

FIGURE 7.4 **Correlation of individual glycosylated hemoglobin values with age and length of diabetes mellitus in diabetic patients taking polyphenols.**

- poylphenol supplements administered in addition to the regular antidiabetic therapy decreased the mean glycosylated hemoglobin values by 12.9% in men and by 13.9% in women.

Note that Zinc supplements led to a more substantial decrease of the patients' glycosylated hemoglobin values in both sexes, as compared to the group that was also administered polyphenol supplements (Raz, Karsai, & Katz, 1989; Ishii & Lupien, 1995; Landrault et al., 2003).

This value reduction does not show significant statistical differences depending on the patients' sex, as the mean glycosylated hemoglobin values after 6 months of zinc or polyphenol supplement administration were approximately the same (Fuhrman, Volkova, Suraski, & Aviram, 2001; Yilmaz & Toledo, 2004).

STIMULUS DETECTION ELECTRODIAGNOSIS

We detected abnormal electrophysiological values in 82 patients of the 112 suffering from type II DM. There were no abnormal values detected in the control group. 64 of the 82 patients with abnormal values were diagnosed with sensory neuropathy and 18 with sensory-motor neuropathy.

The stimulus detection parameters of patients with diabetic neuropathy were also determined after Zn supplement administration (*Unizinc 50 mg-Zn*) for 6 months and after polyphenol supplement administration (*G. Biloba-GB*) also for 6 months.

The stimulus detection examination was conducted in the motor fibers of the median, ulnar, common peroneal and tibial nerves, as well as in the sensory fibers of the median, ulnar, and sural nerves (Gooch & Podwall, 2004; Freeman, 2005).

The following electrophysiological indices were studied for each motor nerve: motor distal latency (MDL), in milliseconds, compound motor action potential (CMAP), measured in mV at proximal and distal stimulation, motor nerve conduction velocity (mNCV) measured in m/s).

The following parameters were measured on sensory nerve examination: sensory latency, sensory nerve action potential (SNAP) expressed in microV, sensory nerve conduction velocity (sNCV) expressed in m/s (Tables 7.2–7.7).

sNCV improved significantly when we administered Unizinc and *G. biloba* supplements. We found that sensory transmission is best recovered after zinc administration, which confirms once again zinc involvement in neuronal physiology regardless of the patients' sex (Figs. 7.5–7.10) (Tables 7.8–7.10).

CMAPp and CMAPd, which had decreased significantly (0.0001 and 0.0004) in diabetic patients

TABLE 7.2 Results of the Stimulus Detection Examination of the *Cubital* Nerve, in Men, at the Beginning of the Study

Cubital nerve	DM group	Control group	*p*
SNAP	8.23 ± 6.5	15.08 ± 6.4	0.0001
sNCV (m/s)	44.8 ± 16.6	58.66 ± 8.2	0.0001
CMAPp	4.6 ± 4.2	6.84 ± 4.4	0.007
CMAPd	5.22 ± 0.8	7.18 ± 0.6	0.005
mNCV (m/s)	49.80 ± 6.6	60.8 ± 8.8	0.0004
MDL (m/s)	4.38 ± 1.2	3.46 ± 0.4	0.04

TABLE 7.3 Results of the Stimulus Detection Examination of the *Cubital* Nerve, in Men, after Zn Administration

Cubital nerve	DM group	Control group	*p*
SNAP	8.82 ± 4.5	15.08 ± 6.4	0.0001
sNCV (m/s)	48.6 ± 14.4	58.66 ± 8.2	0.005
CMAPp	4.5 ± 4.2	6.84 ± 4.4	0.007
CMAPd	5.12 ± 0.7	7.18 ± 0.6	0.005
mNCV (m/s)	54.80 ± 6.6	60.8 ± 8.8	0.0004
MDL (m/s)	4.26 ± 1.4	346 ± 0.4	0.04

TABLE 7.4 Results of the Stimulus Detection Examination of the *Cubital* Nerve, in Men, After G. *biloba* Administration

Cubital nerve	DM group	Control group	*p*
SNAP	8.82 ± 4.5	15.08 ± 6.4	0.0001
sNCV (m/s)	46.8 ± 12.4	58.66 ± 8.2	0.005
CMAPp	4.5 ± 4.2	6.84 ± 4.4	0.007
CMAPd	5.12 ± 0.7	7.18 ± 0.6	0.005
mNCV (m/s)	52.80 ± 4.2	60.8 ± 8.8	0.0004
MDL (m/s)	4.26 ± 1.4	3.46 ± 0.4	0.04

TABLE 7.5 Results of the Stimulus Detection Examination of the *Cubital* Nerve, in Women, at the Beginning of the Study

Cubital nerve	DM group	Control group	*p*
SNAP	10.82 ± 8.6	16.84 ± 3.4	0.001
sNCV (m/s)	40.8 ± 16.6	56.42 ± 8.2	0.001
CMAPp	4.4 ± 1.8	6.60 ± 1.4	0.02
CMAPd	4.8 ± 0.8	6.64 ± 0.6	0.03
mNCV (m/s)	48.28 ± 6.6	56.4 ± 6.2	0.04
MDL (m/s)	2.62 ± 0.68	2.54 ±0.4	0.06

TABLE 7.6 Results of the Stimulus Detection Examination of the *Cubital* Nerve, in Women, After Zn Administration

Cubital nerve	DM group	Control group	*p*
SNAP	10.82 ± 8.6	16.84 ± 3.4	0.001
sNCV (m/s)	48.2 ± 12.8	56.42 ± 8.2	0.005
CMAPp	4.4 ± 1.8	6.60 ± 1.4	0.02
CMAPd	4.8 ± 0.8	6.64 ± 0.6	0.03
mNCV (m/s)	52.66 ± 4.6	56.4 ± 6.2	0.04
MDL (m/s)	2.62 ± 0.68	2.54 ± 0.4	0.06

TABLE 7.7 Results of the Stimulus Detection Examination of the *Cubital* Nerve, in Women, After *G. biloba* Administration

Cubital nerve	DM group	Control group	*p*
SNAP	10.82 ± 8.6	16.84 ± 3.4	0.001
sNCV (m/s)	43.9 ± 12.8	56.42 ± 8.2	0.005
CMAPp	4.4 ± 1.8	6.60 ± 1.4	0.02
CMAPd	4.8 ± 0.8	6.64 ± 0.6	0.03
mNCV (m/s)	50.62 ± 4.6	56.4 ± 6.2	0.04
MDL (m/s)	2.62 ± 0.68	2.54 ± 0.4	0.06

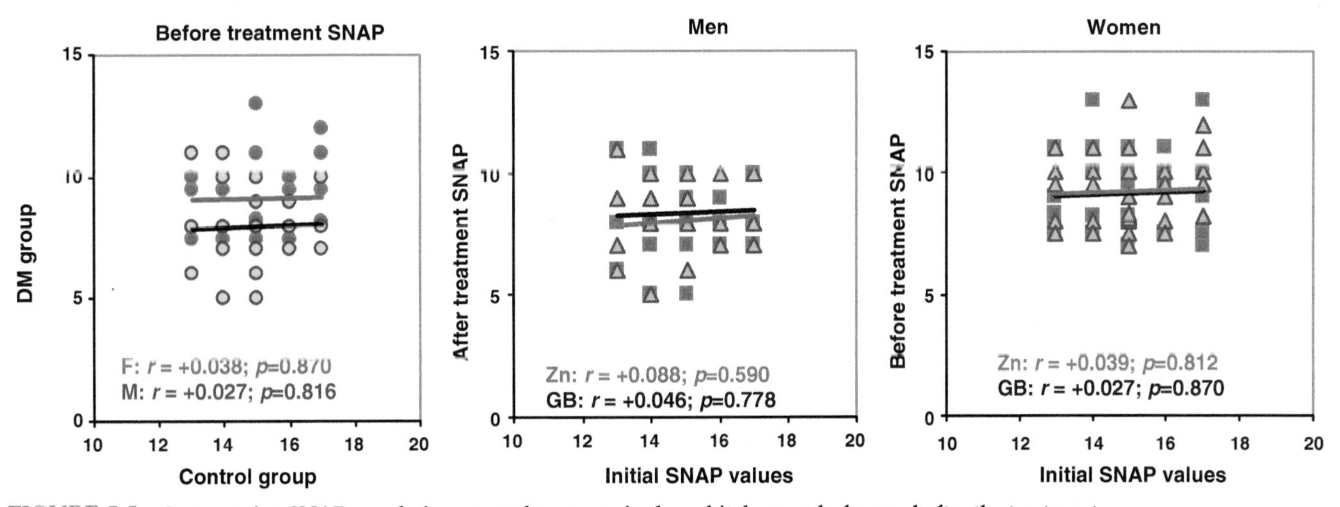

FIGURE 7.5 **Comparative SNAP correlation on study groups, in the cubital nerve, before and after the treatment.**

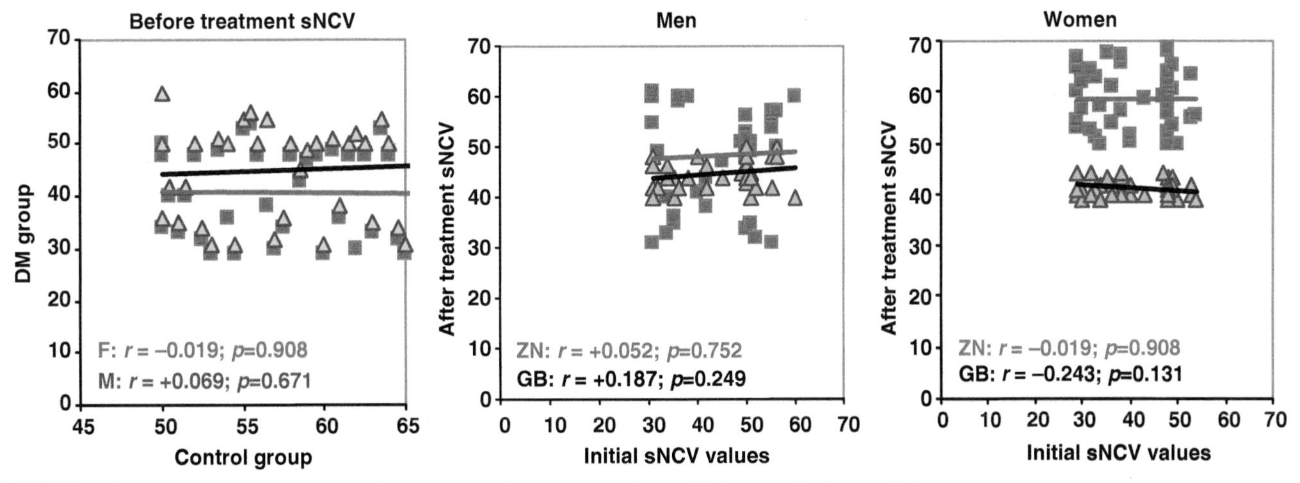

FIGURE 7.6 **Comparative sNCV correlation on study groups, in the cubital nerve, before and after treatment.**

as compared to their control counterparts, were not significantly influenced by zinc administration. However, surprisingly enough, the values were significantly improved in both sexes (more so in the female sex) by polyphenol administration. Zinc or polyphenol administration had no significant effect on the mNCV in the tibial nerve. This proves that both the degree of neuronal involvement and the extent of neuronal involvement are uneven (Said et al., 2003; Watson, Moulin, Watt-Watson, Gordon, & Eisenhoffer, 2003; Gorson & Ropper, 2006) (Figs. 7.11–7.14) (Tables 7.11–7.13).

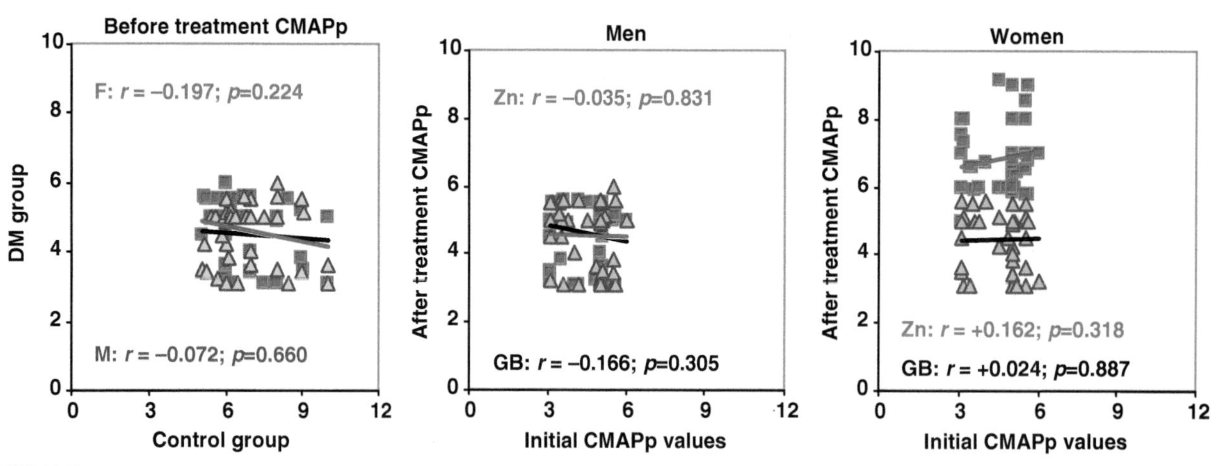

FIGURE 7.7 Comparative CMAPp correlation on study groups, in the cubital nerve, before and after the treatment.

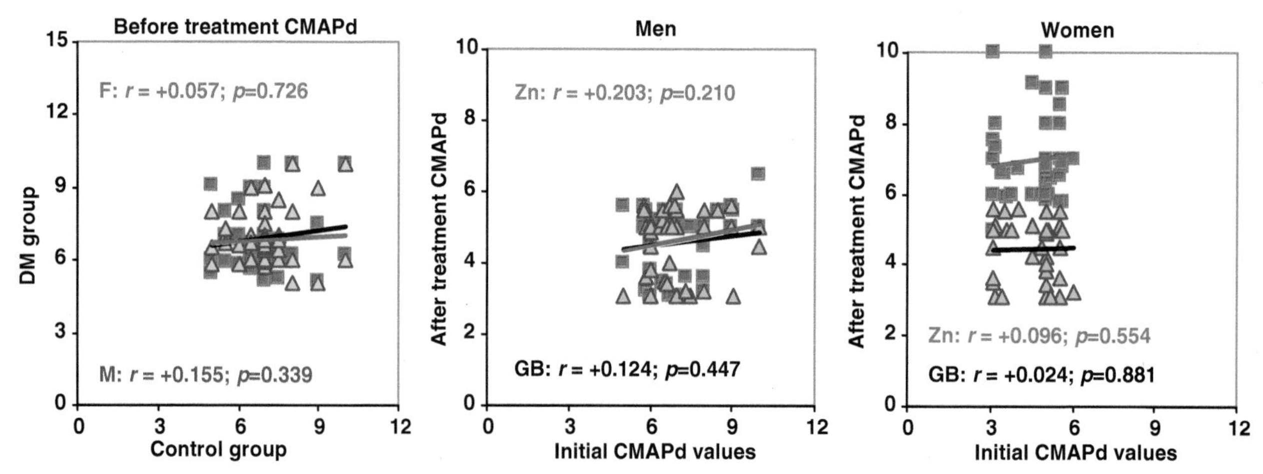

FIGURE 7.8 Comparative CMAPd correlation on study groups, in the cubital nerve, before and after the treatment .

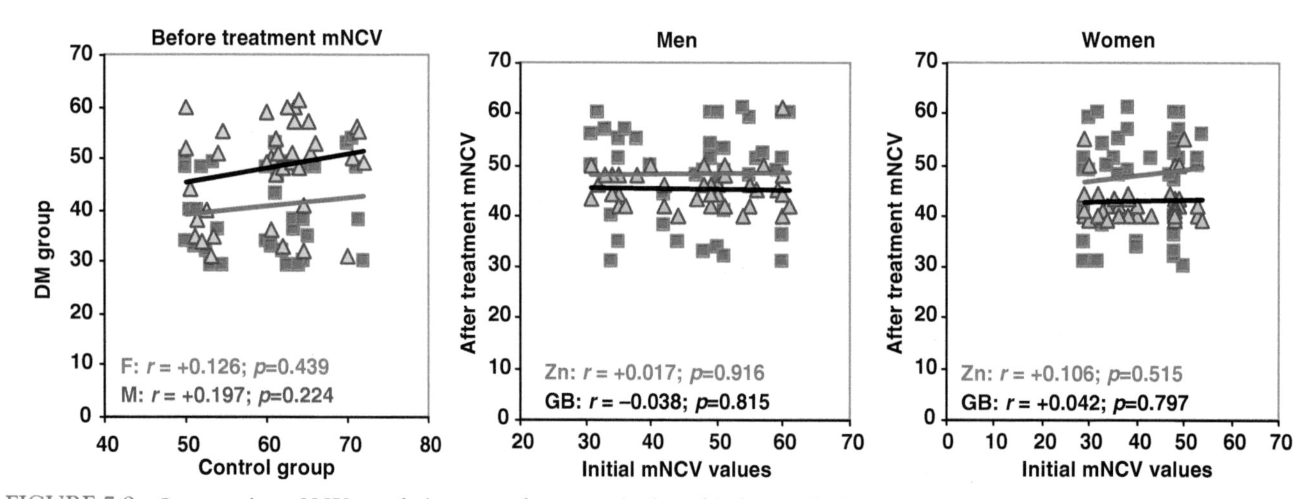

FIGURE 7.9 Comparative mNCV correlation on study groups, in the cubital nerve, before and after the treatment.

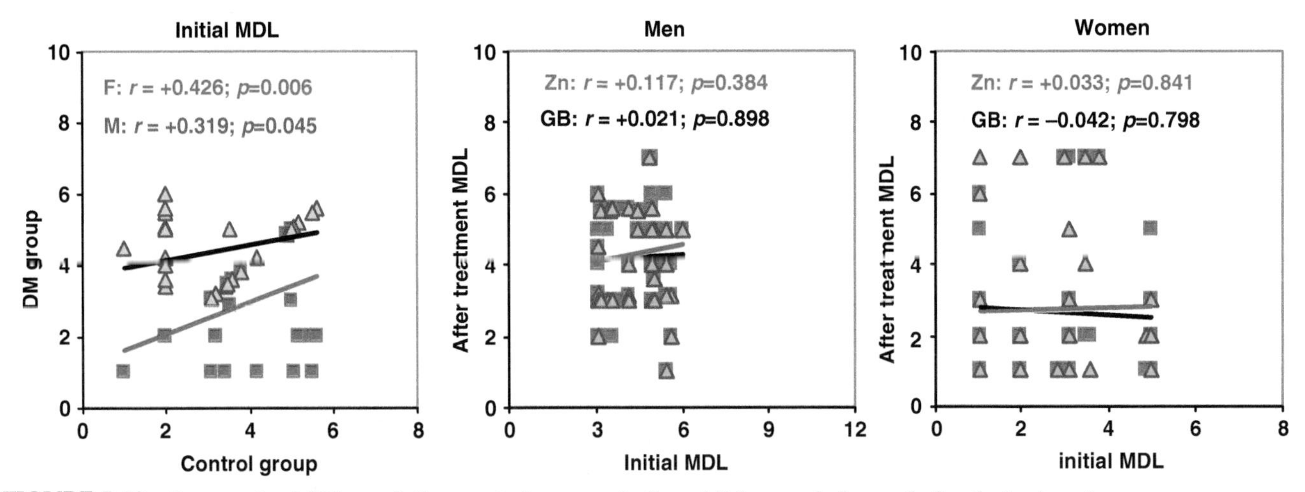

FIGURE 7.10 **Comparative MDL correlation on study groups, in the cubital nerve, before and after the treatment.**

TABLE 7.8 Results of the Stimulus Detection Examination of the *Tibial* Nerve, in Men, at the Beginning of the Study

Tibial nerve	DM group	Control group	*p*
CMAPp	3.2 ± 0.6	7.33 ± 0.8	0.0001
CMAPd	3.82 ± 0.6	8.12 ± 0.8	0.0004
mNCV	42.2 ± 8.24	52.4 ± 4.22	0.0003
MDL	7.6 ± 2.32	4.2 ± 0.42	0.004

TABLE 7.9 Results of the Stimulus Detection Examination of the *Tibial* Nerve, in Men, After Zn Administration

Tibial nerve	DM group	Control group	*p*
CMAPp	5.8 ± 0.4	7.33 ± 0.8	0.0004
CMAPd	6.02 ± 0.4	8.12 ± 0.8	0.007
mNCV	46.4 ± 6.22	52.4 ± 4.22	0.0008
MDL	6.8 ± 4.42	4.2 ± 0.42	0.007

TABLE 7.10 Results of the Stimulus Detection Examination of the *Tibial* Nerve, in Men, After *G. biloba* Administration

Tibial nerve	DM group	Control group	*p*
CMAPp	5.4 ± 0.2	7.33 ± 0.8	0.0004
CMAPd	5.82 ± 1.2	8.12 ± 0.8	0.007
mNCV	47.4 ± 8.24	52.4 ± 4.22	0.0003
MDL	5.8 ± 6.32	4.2 ± 0.42	0.006

The sensory nerves were the most impaired; as concerns the sensitive NCV in the median and ulnar nerves, the differences between the control and the study groups were statistically significant ($p = 0.04$ and $p = 0.02$, respectively).

Diabetic nerve trunks are extremely sensitive to focal neuropathies, which occur in a small number of cases (Martin et al., 2006; Sorensen, Molyneaux, & Yue, 2006). Focal neuropathies are due to repetitive compression, as is the case with the inclination on the ulnar nerve

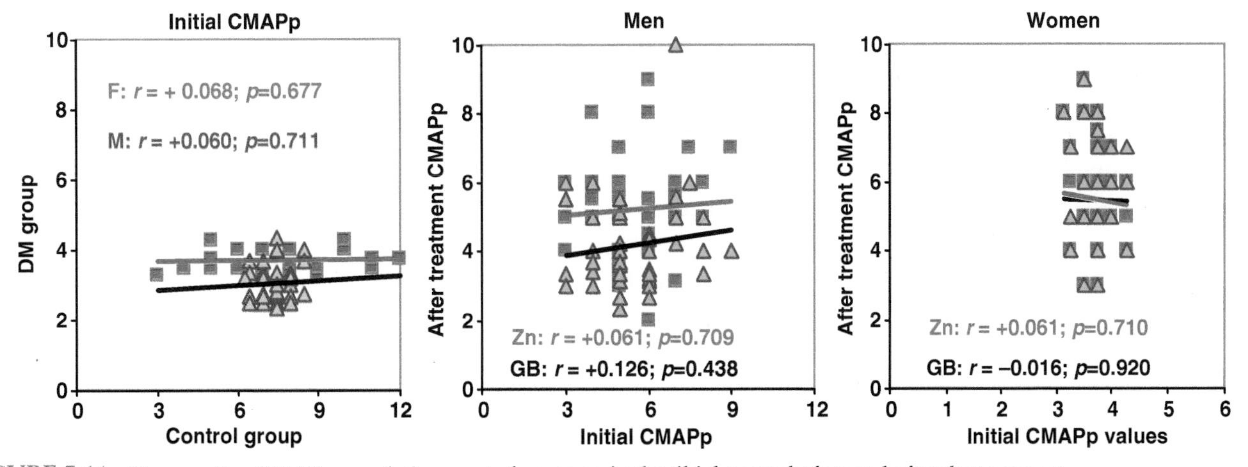

FIGURE 7.11 **Comparative CMAPp correlation on study groups, in the tibial nerve, before and after the treatment.**

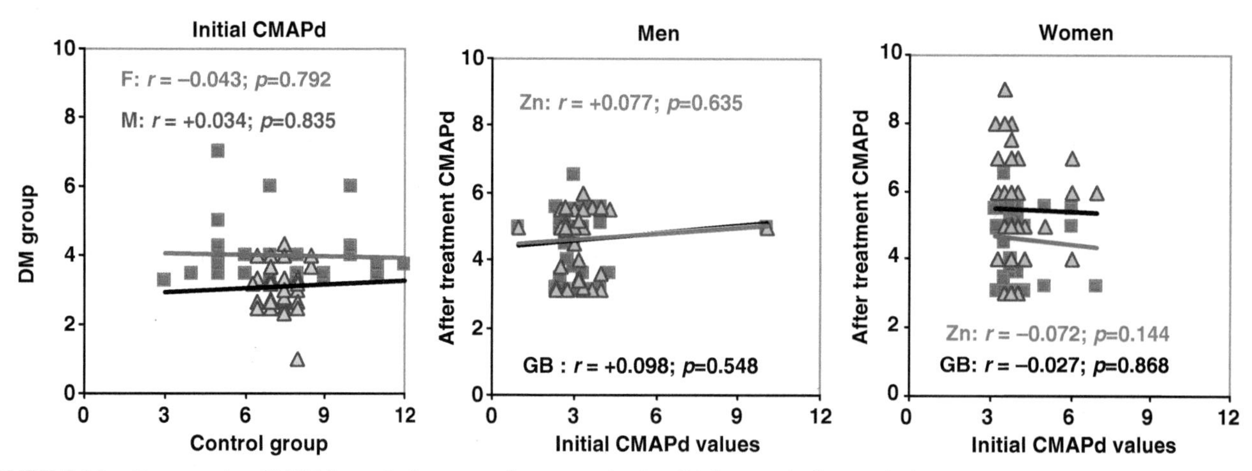

FIGURE 7.12 Comparative CMAPd correlation on study groups, in the tibial nerve, before and after the treatment.

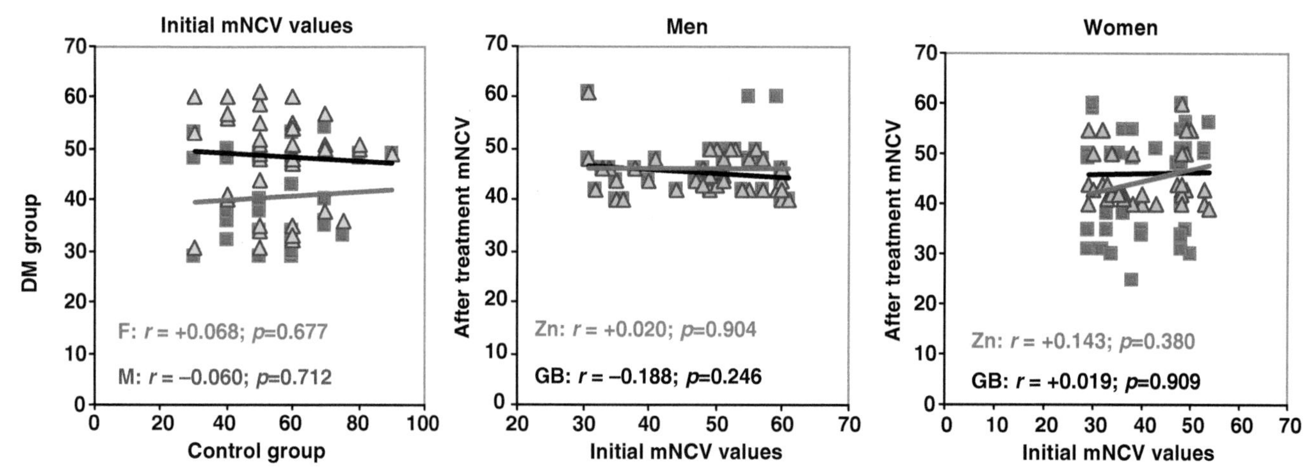

FIGURE 7.13 Comparative mNCV correlation on study groups, in the tibial nerve, before and after the treatment.

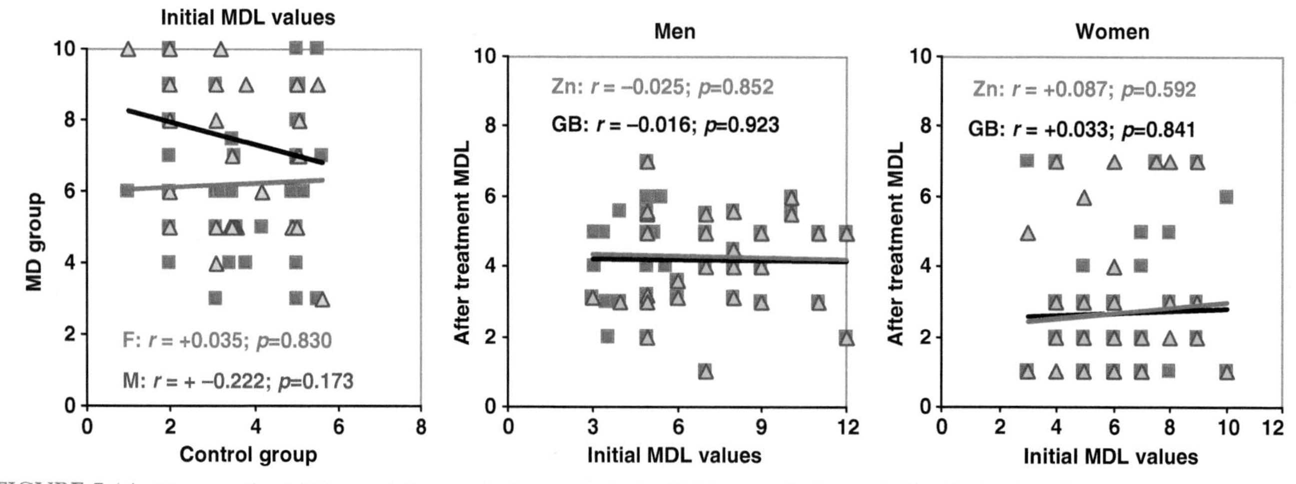

FIGURE 7.14 Comparative MDL correlation on study groups, in the tibial nerve, before and after the treatment.

TABLE 7.11 Results of the Stimulus Detection Examination of the *Tibial* Nerve, in Women, at the Beginning of the Study

Tibial nerve	DM group	Control group	*p*
CMAPp	3.62 ± 0.4	6.83 ± 0.6	0.005
CMAPd	4.12 ± 0.2	7.12 ± 0.8	0.006
mNCV	44.8 ± 4.84	50.4 ± 4.22	0.0001
MDL	6.4 ± 3.32	5.6 ± 0.32	0.004

TABLE 7.12 Results of the Stimulus Detection Examination of the *Tibial* Nerve, in Women, After Zn Administration

Tibial nerve	DM group	Control group	*p*
CMAPp	5.52 ± 0.4	6.83 ± 0.6	0.006
CMAPd	6.02 ± 0.2	7.12 ± 0.8	0.008
mNCV	46.6 ± 4.84	50.4 ± 4.22	0.005
MDL	5.9 ± 3.32	5.6 ± 0.32	0.009

TABLE 7.13 Results of the Stimulus Detection Examination of the *Tibial* Nerve, in Women, After *G. biloba* Administration

Tibial nerve	DM group	Control group	*p*
CMAPp	4.82 ± 0.8	6.83 ± 0.6	0.006
CMAPd	5.12 ± 0.2	7.12 ± 0.8	0.007
mNCV	45.9 ± 4.84	50.4 ± 4.22	0.007
MDL	6.8 ± 3.32	5.6 ± 0.32	0.008

in its groove and with the pressure of the peroneal nerve on the neck of the fibula. The closing may occur inside the carpal tunnel with the median nerve, causing the occurrence of a carpal tunnel syndrome. Its precise physiopathology is unknown (Sluka & Walsh, 2003; Willis, 2004). There is circumstantial evidence suggesting that ischemia combined with mechanical sensitivity may be responsible. Clinical microvascular ischemia symptoms include acute or subacute palsy onset in older patients suffering from cardiovascular diseases. The pathological evidence is limited and includes the occurrence of microinfarcts, multifocal pathology and fibrinoid alteration. There are three sets of findings that occur constantly when chronic diabetic neuropathy is concerned: first, the solidification of the basal vertebral arch blade; second, endothelial cell and smooth muscle proliferation (Herrmann, Griffin, & Hauer, 1999; Lenninger, Edward, Lipshaw, & Feldman, 2006) accompanied by capillary caliber variability and capillary closing; third, the nerve fiber loss tends to be multifocal rather than diffuse. It is very likely that microvascular ischemia combined with connective tissue changes and myelin alterations could predispose the nerve trunk to compression lesions. The nerve conduction velocity values were significantly improved in patients taking Zn and they even tended to become normal in patients with recently diagnosed DM (Llewelyn et al., 1991; Malik et al., 2005).

The conduction velocity (both sNCV and mNCV) improved significantly by the administration of Unizinc and *G. biloba* supplements. Sensory transmission is best recovered after zinc administration, which confirms once again zinc involvement in neuronal physiology regardless of the patients' sex.

The nerve conduction velocity values of diabetic patients taking polyphenols were improved, though insignificantly. It is well known that proanthocyanidins inhibit and reduce excessive free oxygen radical formation in conditions of oxidative stress (as is the case with DM). They also ameliorate tissue hypoxia, which causes certain mental and somatic disorders that may occur due to the diabetic condition. In this case, hypoxia causes the accumulation of reduced substrates (flavins, coenzymes, etc.) generated by the autoxidation of free radicals (Low et al., 2004; Said, 2007). Proanthocyanidins inhibit these free radicals since they are able to cross the hemato-encephalic barrier (Alcaraz & Hoult, 1999; Palma & Taylor, 1999).

In his studies on experimental animal models, (Palma & Taylor, 1999) analyzed the neuro-protective effect of red grape polyphenols. He administered a 2-month diet with polyphenol extract dissolved in ethanol 5% to rats subjected to conditions of oxidative stress. He drew the following conclusions: flavonoids have a neuro-protective effect as they inhibit ROS generation, regulate calcium homeostasis and prevent intracellular glutathione depletion. They have a protective LDL antioxidant effect and inhibit platelet aggregation. Resveratrol has an antioxidant effect and protects the neuronal membrane. It has a platelet aggregation prevention and antioxidant LDL effect, as well as an antiinflammatory effect, and it inhibits cytokine-induced NO production. Quercetin inhibits A_2 phospholipase activity. Catechins have an antioxidant and antiinflammatory effect, and reduce NO synthesis by protecting the nuclear factor (NF-cB). This effect was also noted on macrophage cultures in oxidative stress conditions.

The serum cholesterol of type II DM patients was 231.6 ± 82.7 SD, a value which, was significantly higher ($F = 7.03$, $p = 0.0114$, 95% CI) than the one determined in the control group (166.6 ± 24.6 SD).

The triglycerides value (171.9 ± 77.5 SD) was significantly higher ($F = 5.18$, $p = 0.028$, 95%CI) than in the control group (119 ± 31.9 SD).

The HDL cholesterol values showed no significant differences between the two groups (42.16 ± 3.2 SD-control group, 42.46 ± 4.6 SD-study group, $p = 0.839$).

LDL carries 2/3 of the circulating cholesterol. The increase of the LDL-cholesterol (LDL-C) level in the plasma is one of the main atherogenic risk factors. Blood LDL reaches the vascular intima where, due to the high peroxide concentration, turns into oxidized LDL, which is rapidly bound by the macrophages the receptors of which are not influenced by the LDL cholesterol content. Considerable tissue destruction, including diabetic neuropathy, may occur in pathological conditions, when oxidative stress is present (as is the case with DM) and lipid peroxidation is stimulated, which is a self-propagating reaction.

DISCUSSIONS

Diabetic polyneuropathy detection and staging may be achieved by electrodiagnosis methods (nerve conduction, amplitudes) and by quantitative sensitivity testing. Seven long-term prospective studies were published, which analyzed the effect of enhanced DM therapy on chronic complication prevention and progress. These studies showed that in type II DM patients enhanced antidiabetic therapy slowed down but did not fully prevent diabetic polyneuropathy. Enhanced antidiabetic therapy either had no effect, or slowed down polyneuropathy progress only partially. It is well known that the oxidative stress induced by active oxygen species play an important role in the etiology of neurodegenerative diseases. The plant polyphenols added to a neuronal cell culture subjected to oxidative stress under the action of linoleic acid hydrogen peroxide causes a significant increase of the cell survival rate following the antiradical action of these active principles (Scalbert & Williamson, 2000; Wang, Wang, Fan, Wu, & Ren, 2007).

The active biological properties of flavonoids are closely related to their antioxidant power. In general, their antiradical activity is associated with:

- direct free radical removal; due to their low reduction potential, flavonoids are thermodynamically capable of reducing highly oxidized free radicals, such as superoxide, peroxyl, alkoxyl, or hydroxyl radicals (Yilmaz & Toledo, 2004);
- chelatization of transition metals involved in free radical production;
- inhibition of enzymatic systems involved in free radical generation (for instance, xanthine oxidase) (Takeda, Suzuki, Okada, & Oku, 2000; Karachalias, Babei-Jadidi, & Kupich, 2005).

On the other hand, zinc is the cofactor that over 300 enzymes belonging to the six big enzyme classes need to function. It is common knowledge that in DM the metabolic activity is fully impaired and that the pancreas of diabetic patients only contains 50% of the amount of Zn found in the pancreas of nondiabetic people. The Zn supplement added to the diabetics' diet reduces hyperlipaemia by enhancing lipid catabolism, restores the ability of the pancreas to increase insulin production and diminishes oxidative stress (Raz et al., 1989; Maret, 2002). Therefore, the patient's body must maintain an adequate intracellular zinc concentration in order to ensure cell growth even when its extracellular levels are low. To enhance intracellular zinc concentration cells have developed effective systems that allow them to accumulate Zn when there is not enough zinc. These systems use transport proteins in order to carry zinc through the lipid double layer of the membrane down to plasma level. Once inside the cells, some of the zinc is carried in the intracellular organites, where it serves as cofactor for certain zinc-dependent enzymes and for certain processes occurring in these compartments. For instance, mitochondrial isoenzyme, alcohol dehydrogenase, is a zinc-dependent enzyme. When it occurs in excessive amounts, zinc may also be stored in certain intracellular compartments and used later, when a zinc deficiency occurs. Therefore, Zn supplements are a must in any diabetic patient's diet.

The beneficial effect of zinc and polyphenols may also be due to the antiinflammatory effect of these two agents. Several studies showed that the antiinflammatory activity of certain flavonoids are due to their inhibiting action on certain enzymes involved in arachidonic acid metabolism, such as phospholipase A2, cyclooxygenase (COX) and lipoxygenase (LOX). The in vivo testing of certain *G. biloba* plant extracts has recently shown the suppressing action of the active principles present in this plant, in comparison with the expression of inducible enzymes like COX and nitric oxide synthase. The increase in the activity of these enzymatic systems leads to a prostaglandin and nitric oxide production increase. The high values of the latter trigger the inflammatory process. When using a 1–5 μM/mL serum concentration, ginkgetin, the active principle occurring in the *G. biloba* leaves, causes a approximate 65% reduction of the prostaglandin production in case of skin inflammation induced to laboratory animals (Landrault et al., 2003).

CONCLUSIONS

1. We detected abnormal electrophysiological values in 82 patients of the 112 suffering from type II DM. There were no abnormal values detected in the control group. 64 of the 82 patients with abnormal values were diagnosed with sensory neuropathy and 18 with sensory-motor neuropathy.
2. The glucose values of diabetic patients taking zinc/polyphenol supplements were found to decrease insignificantly.

3. Zinc supplements administered to diabetic patients caused substantial glycosylated hemoglobin value decreases in both sexes, as compared to the group that were administered polyphenol supplements.
4. The analysis of the results of the electrophysiological examination conducted at the beginning of the experiment revealed the fact that the parameters measured for both sensory and motor nerves had significantly lower statistical values in diabetic patients (in both sexes) than in control patients.
5. The extension of the latency period, as well as the change in amplitude, may be an early sign of peripheral polyneuropathy.
6. The sensory nerves were the most impaired; as far as the sensory NCV in the median and ulnar nerves, the differences between the control group and the study group are statistically significant ($p = 0.04$ and $p = 0.02$, respectively). Focal neuropathies are due to repetitive compression, as is the case with the inclination on the ulnar nerve in its groove and with the pressure of the peroneal nerve on the neck of the fibula. The closing may occur inside the carpal tunnel with the median nerve, thus causing the occurrence of a carpal tunnel syndrome.
7. The motor NCV values of the median, ulnar, peroneal, and tibial nerves did not show significant differences between the two groups, whereas the test significance values is lower than 0.05. The comparative sex-dependent NCV analysis did not reveal significant differences between the male and female sexes ($p > 0.05$, 95% CI).
8. The nerve conduction velocity values of diabetic patients taking zinc/polyphenol supplements improved, although not significantly (possibly due to the shortness of the therapy, which only lasted 6 months).

References

Ahmed, N., & Thornalley, P. J. (2007). Advanced glycation endproducts: what is their relevance to diabetic complications? *Diabetes Obesity Metabolism, 9*(3), 233–245.

Alcaraz, M. J., & Hoult, J. R. (1999). Actions of flavonoids and the novel anti-inflammatory flavone, hypolaetin-8-glucoside, on prostaglandin biosynthesis and inactivation. *Biochemical Pharmacology, 34*, 2477–2482.

Al-Maroof, R. A., & Al-Sharbatti, S. S. (2006). Serum zinc levels in diabetic patients and effect of zinc supplementation on glycemic control of type 2 diabetics. *Saudi Medical Journal, 27*(3), 344–350.

American Diabetes Association. (2008). Standards of medical care in diabetes. *Diabetes Care, 31*(Suppl. 1), S12–S54.

Arezzo, J. C., & Zotova, E. (2002). Electrophysiologic measures of diabetic neuropathy: mechanism and meaning. *International Review of Neurobiology, 50*, 229–255.

Arquilla, E., Packer, S., Tarmas, W., & Myamoto, S. (1998). The effect of zinc on insulin metabolism. *Endocrinology, 103*, 1440–2144.

Bantle, J. P., Wylie-Rosett, J., Albright, A. L., Apovian, C. M., Clark, N. G., Franz, M. J., Hoogwerf, B. J., Lichtenstein, A. H., Mayer-Davis, E., Mooradian, A. D., & Wheeler, M. L. (2008). Nutrition recommendations and interventions for diabetes: a position statement of the American Diabetes Association. *Diabetes Care, 31*(Suppl. 1), S61–S78.

Boulton, A. J., Vinik, A. I., Arezzo, J. C., Bril, V., Feldman, E. L., Freeman, R., Malik, R. A., Maser, R. E., Sosenko, J. M., & Ziegler, D. (2008). Diabetic neuropathies. A statement by the American Diabetes Association. *Diabetes Care, 31*(Suppl. 1), S61–S78.

Cameron, N. E., & Cotter, M. A. (1994). The relationship of vascular changes to metabolic factors in diabetes mellitus and their role in the development of peripheral nerve complications. *Diabetes Metabolism Reviews, 10*, 189–224.

Cohen-Boulakia, F. (2000). In vivo sequential study of skeletal muscle capillary permeability in diabetic rats: effect of anthocyanosides. *Metabolism, 49*(7), 880–885.

Delia Loggia, R., Sosa, S., Tubaro, A., Morazzoni, P., Bombardelli, E., & Griffmi, A. (1996). Anti-inflammatory activity of some *Ginkgo biloba* constituents and of their phospholipid-complexes. *Fitoterapia, 67*, 257–263.

Dworkin, R. H., Backonja, M., Rowbotham, M. C., Allen, R. R., Argoff, C. R., Bennett, G. J., Bushnell, M. C., Farrar, J. T., Galer, B. S., Haythornthwaite, J. A., Hewitt, D. J., Loeser, J. D., Max, M. B., Saltarelli, M., Schmader, K. E., Stein, C., Thompson, D., Turk, D. C., Wallace, M. S., Watkins, L. R., & Weinstein, S. M. (2003). Advances in neuropathic pain: diagnosis, mechanisms and treatment recommendations. *Archives of Neurology, 60*(11), 1524–1534.

Freeman, R. (2005). Autonomic peripheral neuropathy. *Lancet, 365*(9466), 1259–1270.

Fuhrman, B., Volkova, N., Suraski, A., & Aviram, M. (2001). White wine with red wine-like properties: increase extraction of grape skin polyphenols improves the antioxidant capacity of the derived white wine. *Journal of Agricultural and Food Chemistry, 49*, 3164–3168.

Gooch, C., & Podwall, D. (2004). The diabetic neuropathies. *Neurologist, 10*(6), 311–322.

Gorson, K. C., & Ropper, A. H. (2006). Additional causes for distal sensory polyneuropathy in diabetic patients. *Journal of Neurology, Neurosurgery, and Psychiatry, 77*, 354–358.

Herrmann, D. N., Griffin, J. W., & Hauer, P. (1999). Intraepidermal nerve fiber density, sural nerve morphometry and electrodiagnosis in peripheral neuropathies. *Neurology, 53*, 1634–1640.

Ishii, D. N., & Lupien, S. B. (1995). Insulin-like growth factors protect against diabetic neuropathy: effects on sensory nerve regeneration in rats. *Journal of Neuroscience Researches, 40*, 138–144.

Karachalias, N., Babaei-Jadidi, R., & Kupich, C. (2005). Highdose thiamine therapy counters dyslipidemia and advanced glycation of plasma protein in streptozotocin-induced diabetic rats. *Annallas of the New York Academy of Sciences, 1043*, 777–783.

King, R. H. (2004). The role of glycation in the pathogenesis of diabetic polyneuropathy. *Molecular Pathology, 54*, 400–408.

Landrault, N., Poucheret, P., Azay, J., Krosniak, M., Gasc, F., Jenin, C., Cros, G., & Teissedre, P. L. (2003). Effect of the polyphenols-enriched chardonnay white wine in diabetic rats. *Journal of Agricultural and Food Chemistry, 51*(1), 311–318.

Leinninger, G. M., Edwards, J. L., Lipshaw, M. J., & Feldman, E. L. (2006). Mechanisms of disease: mitochondria as new therapeutic targets in diabetic neuropathy. *Nature Clinical Practice Neurology, 2*, 620–628.

Llewelyn, J. G., Gilbey, S. G., Thomas, P. K., King, R. H., Muddle, J. R., & Watkins, P. J. (1991). Sural nerve morphometry in diabetic autonomic and painful sensory neuropathy. *Brain, 114*, 867–892.

Low, P. A., Benrud-Larson, L. M., Sletten, D. M., & Tonette, L. (2004). Autonomic symptoms and diabetic neuropathy. A population-based study. *Diabetes Care, 27*, 2942–2947.

Malik, R. A., Tesfaye, S., Newrick, P. G., Walker, D., Rajbhandari, S. M., Siddique, I., Sharma, A. K., Boulton, A. J. M., King, R. H. M., Thomas, P. K., & Ward, J. D. (2005). Sural nerve pathology in diabetic patients with minimal but progressive neuropathy. *Diabetologia, 48*, 578–585.

Maret, W. (2002). The function of zinc metallothionein: a link between cellular zinc and redox state. *Journal of Nutrition, 130*, 1455S–1458S.

Martin, C. L., Albers, J., Herman, H. W., Cleary, P., Waberski, B., Greene, D. A., Stevens, M. J., & Feldman, E. L. (2006). Neuropathy among the Diabetes Control and Complications Trial Cohort 8 years after trial completion. *Diabetes Care, 29*, 340–344.

Palma, M., & Taylor, L. R. (1999). Extraction of polyphenolic compounds from grape seeds with near critical carbon dioxide. *Journal of Chromatography A, 849*, 117–124.

Raz, I., Karsai, D., & Katz, M. (1989). The influence of zinc supplementation on glucose homeostasis in NIDDM. *Diabetes Research, 11*(2), 73–79.

Said, G., Lacroix, C., Lozeron, P., Ropert, A., Planté, V., & Adams, D. (2003). Inflammatory vasculopathy in multifocal diabetic neuropathy. *Brain, 126*, 376–385.

Said, G. (2007). Diabetic neuropathya—review. *Nature Clinical Practice Neurology, 3*, 331–340.

Scalbert, A., & Williamson, G. (2000). Dietary intake and bioavailability of polyphenols. *Journal of Nutrition, 30*, 2073–2085.

Sluka, K. A., & Walsh, D. (2003). Transcutaneous electrical nerve stimulation: basic science mechanisms and clinical effectiveness. *Journal of Pain, 4*, 109–121.

Sorensen, L., Molyneaux, L., & Yue, D. K. (2006). The relationship among pain, sensory loss, and small nerve fibers in diabetes. *Diabetes Care, 29*, 883–887.

Takeda, A., Suzuki, M., Okada, S., & Oku, N. (2000). Influence of histidine on zinc transport into rat brain. *Biological Trace Element Research*(32), 31–38.

Wang, X., Wang, B., Fan, Z., Wu, S., & Ren, J. (2007). Thiamine deficiency induces endoplasmic reticulum stress in neurons. *Neuroscience, 144*(3), 1.045-1.056.

Watson, C. P., Moulin, D., Watt-Watson, J., Gordon, A., & Eisenhoffer, J. (2003). Controlled-release oxycodone relieves neuropathic pain: a randomized controlled trial in painful diabetic neuropathy. *Pain, 105*, 71–78.

Willis, W. D. (2004). Role of neurotransmitters in sensitization of pain responses. *Annal of the New York Academy of Sciences, 933*, 175–184.

Yilmaz, Y., & Toledo, R. (2004). Major flavonoids in grape seeds and skins: antioxidant capacity of catechin, epicatechin and gallic acid. *Journal of Agricultural and Food Chemistry, 52*, 255–260.

CHAPTER

8

Natural Remedies for Treatment of Cancer Pain

M.S. Garud*, M.J. Oza*,**, A.B. Gaikwad†, Y.A. Kulkarni*

*Shobhaben Pratapbhai Patel School of Pharmacy & Technology Management, SVKM's NMIMS, Mumbai, Maharashtra, India; **SVKM's Dr. Bhanuben Nanavati College of Pharmacy, Mumbai, Maharashtra, India; †Department of Pharmacy, Birla Institute of Technology and Science, Pilani Campus, Pilani, Rajasthan, India

INTRODUCTION

The International Association for the Study of Pain (IASP) defines pain as "an unpleasant sensory and emotional experience associated with actual or potential tissue damage, or described in terms of such damage." This definition is derived from the definition given by Harold Merskey in 1964.

Cancer is one of the life threatening diseases in the global population. It has multiple physical symptoms among which the pain is one of the most critical indication related with cancer. Intensity of cancer pain increases with advancement in stage of cancer. A systematic review on prevalence of cancer related pain reported that more than one third patients suffer from moderate to severe pain (van den Beuken-van Everdingen et al., 2007). According to reports of meta-analysis, 64% of patients with metastatic disease suffer from cancer pain, while this percentage is between 59% and 33% for patients receiving antineoplastic therapy and who had received curative cancer treatment respectively (van den Beuken-van et al., 2009; Lee et al., 2015).

To guide cancer pain management worldwide, in 1986 the World Health Organization (WHO) developed a three step analgesic ladder for treatment of cancer pain Fig. 8.1 (Ventafridda & Stjernsward, 1996).

A 10 year prospective study was carried out by Zech, Diefenbach, Radbruch, and Lehmann (1995) for validation of the WHO analgesic ladder which showed that more than 70% of cancer patients attained good pain relief using WHO recommendations. Now it's more than 25 years after development of this ladder and still cancer pain is a major issue having prevalence of as high as 60–80% in advanced cancer patients.

Pain caused by cancer has different reasons or root causes. In many cases the pain is the outcome of underlying cancers (85%), in 17% cases it is secondary to antineoplastic therapies and 9% is related with comorbidities unrelated to cancer (Grond, Zech, Diefenbach, Radbruch, & Lehmann, 1996). Fig. 8.2 summarizes different causes of cancer pain. Among various causes, patients with bone metastases reports severe pain than compared with soft tissue metastases (Ahles et al., 1984; Brescia, Portenoy, Ryan, Krasnoff, & Gray, 1992). Although there is direct relation between prevalence of pain and stage of cancer, severe pain can occur in all cancer stages (Greenwald, Bonica, & Bergner, 1987). Higher prevalence of pain is observed with the patients having cancer of the pancreas, bone, brain, lymphoma, lung, head, and neck (Breivik et al., 2009).

Cancer pain can be categorized under different types, which includes nociceptive pain and neuropathic pain (Fig. 8.3).

Nociceptive pain is caused due to an acute or persistent injury to somatic or visceral tissues. Accordingly it is subclassified as somatic nociceptive pain and visceral nociceptive pain. Somatic nociceptive pain involves injury to bones, joints, or muscles and is described as aching, stabbing, or throbbing. While visceral nociceptive pain results from injury to viscera. If it involves a hollow viscus (like bowel obstruction) and is poorly localized, it is characterized as cramping or gnawing.

Nutritional Modulators of Pain in the Aging Population. http://dx.doi.org/10.1016/B978-0-12-805186-3.00008-4
Copyright © 2017 Elsevier Inc. All rights reserved.

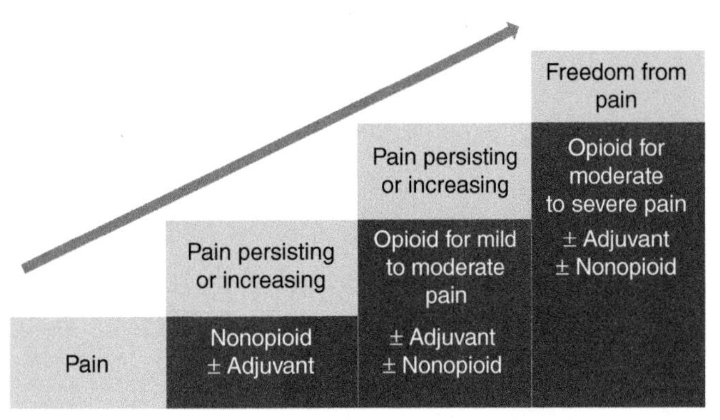

FIGURE 8.1 **Ladder for treatment of cancer pain.** *Source: Adapted from Ventafridda, V., & Stjernsward, J. (1996). Pain control and the World Health Organization analgesic ladder.* JAMA, *275(11), 835–836.*

If it is originating from other visceral structures (like organ capsules, myocardium), it is described as aching, stabbing, sharp and so on (Davis, 2012).

Neuropathic pain is diverse in nature and includes injury to the peripheral and or central nervous system. It is generally related with referred pain which is perceived in a location that is not the source of the pain, allodynia which is a pain caused due to nonpainful stimulus, hyperpathia which is an inflated pain response to nociceptive stimuli. It is also correlated with dysesthesia, which can be perceived as unpleasant, abnormal sensation in an area of neurologic deficit (Woolsey & Martin, 2003).

According to the nature of pain, cancer pain can be categorized as acute pain and chronic pain. Acute pains are generally iatrogenic in nature, that is, they occur generally due to procedures or antineoplastic therapies, as well as they may also be disease related complications. Procedures, include lumbar puncture, biopsy, stent placements, and so on. Antineoplastic therapies include, chemotherapy, hormonal treatments, immunotherapy, radiation therapy, and so on. Related complications include, hemorrhage into a tumor, pathologic fracture, obstruction or perforation of hollow viscus, and so on.

Another type of pain is chronic pain, which is mainly due to malignancy and also due to antineoplastic treatments (Portenoy & Dhingra, 2011). It is associated with generalized sympathetic hyperactivity, which results in diaphoresis, hypertension, and tachycardia (Turk & Okifuji, 1999). Chronic pain occur due to nociceptive somatic pain due to bone metastases and soft tissue injury, nociceptive visceral pain due to malignancy, neuropathic pain due to malignancy and also due to antineoplastic therapies like chemotherapy, hormonal treatments, immunotherapy, radiation therapy, and so on.

Treatment of Cancer Pain with Natural Remedies

Natural drugs are well known for their diverse biological activities. There are numerous literatures stating

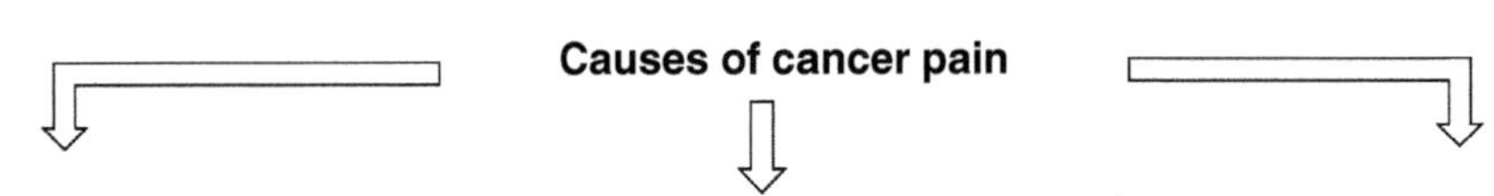

Malignancy related causes
- Bone metastases
- Soft tissue metastases
- Visceral metastases
- Leptomeningeal metastases
- Epidural spinal cord compression
- Malignant bowel obstruction
- Pathologic fracture
- Hemorrhage into a tumor
- Tumor related neuropathic pain

Antineoplastic therapies related causes
- Side effects from chemotherapy, immunotherapy, hormonal therapy, and radiation therapy
- Postprocedural and postsurgical pain

Other comorbidities related causes
- Immobility
- Constipation
- Thrombophlebitis
- Unaddressed psychococial and psychiatric issues

FIGURE 8.2 **Causes of cancer** (Twycross et al., 1996).

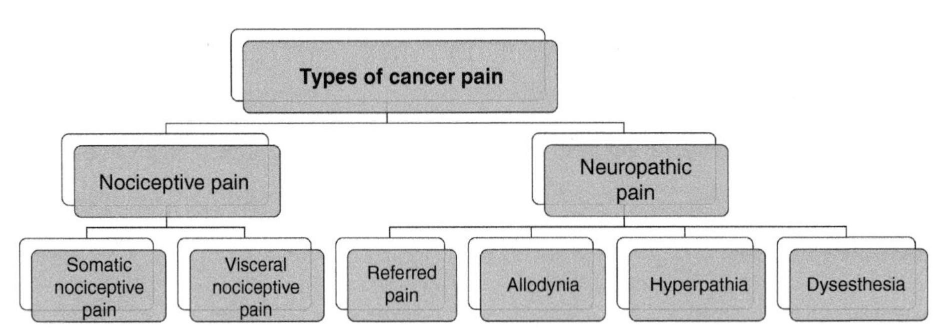

FIGURE 8.3 **Types of cancer pain.**

analgesic activities of the compounds obtained from natural sources. Different scientific studies are reported which proves their antinociceptive activity. Still, very less number of drugs obtained from the natural sources has been established in management of the pain related with the cancer. Except opioids, comparatively very less evidences are available for the use of natural remedies in treatment of cancer pain. Some meta-analysis are reported which have reviewed the use of herbal medicines and phytomedicines in management of cancer pain (Harrison, Heritier, Childs, Bostwick, & Dziadzko, 2015; Lee et al., 2015).

There are controversies in using the traditional medicines, herbal drugs, and phytochemicals in treatment of cancer pain. Researchers are trying to discover the use of the natural drugs in cancer pain by exploring different mechanistic approaches. Some toxins have also showed promising effect in cancer pain treatment. Various clinical trials are reported for use of natural drugs and their formulations in management of cancer pain. Many of the natural drugs are used as supportive treatment to lessen the symptoms related with cancer pain.

Natural Opioids

Natural opioids are the alkaloids obtained from the resin of the plant opium poppy (*Papaver somniferum*, family Papaveraceae). Opioids plays key role in cancer pain management. Opioid analgesics are also mentioned in many major guidelines related with the management of cancer related pain (Jacox, Carr, Payne, & Berde, 1994; WHO, 1996; Miaskowski et al., 2005). Morphine and codeine are the two widely used natural opioids for management of cancer pain.

Morphine

Morphine is an isoquinoline alkaloid obtained from opium poppy (Fig. 8.4).

Many years of clinical use of it shows that oral morphine is the most effective drug for treatment of pain associated with cancer. Oral morphine remains the gold standard for treating moderate to severe cancer pain.

Morphine binds to opioid receptors to produce pain relief. Three different receptors have been identified which includes Mu receptors (subdivided into μ1, μ2, and μ3), kappa receptors and delta receptors. Activation of which leads to relief from pain.

A recent review published in Cochrane Library by Wiffen and McQuay (2007) have explained the development of morphine in treatment of cancer related pain. Since 1950s, morphine is used orally for controlling cancer pain. It was first recommended in England for the treatment of cancer pain in the form of "Brompton cocktail", which contained cocaine and alcohol in addition to morphine or diamorphine. Further, it was found that oral morphine alone can show effective pain relief.

World Health Organization (WHO) in 1986 published a guideline in which they have recommended taking of oral solution of morphine after every 4 h (WHO, 1986) for management of cancer pain. Modified release tablets of morphine were formulated afterward, which extended the dosage interval to 12 h. Now a wide range of formulations and dosages (10 to 150 mg) of morphine are available giving flexibility in deciding the dose regimen for the management of mild to severe cancer pain (Grahame-Smith & Aronson, 1992).

Codeine

Like morphine, codeine is also an isoquinoline alkaloid obtained from opium poppy. Codeine is the most widely used naturally occurring opioid for its medicinal use. Codeine is a prodrug, which gets metabolized into morphine in the liver. It can also be synthesized from morphine (Fig. 8.5).

Codeine is manly available in the form of tablets and syrup. It is also available as intramuscular and subcutaneous injections. Codeine have different fate in different individuals because of the different pattern of its metabolism, which varies from individual to individual. In many of the people, 5 to 10% of codeine is metabolized

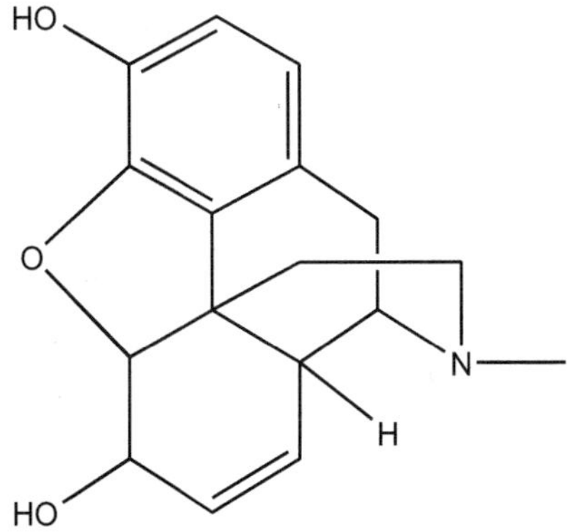

HO
O
N
H
HO

FIGURE 8.4 **Structure of morphine.**

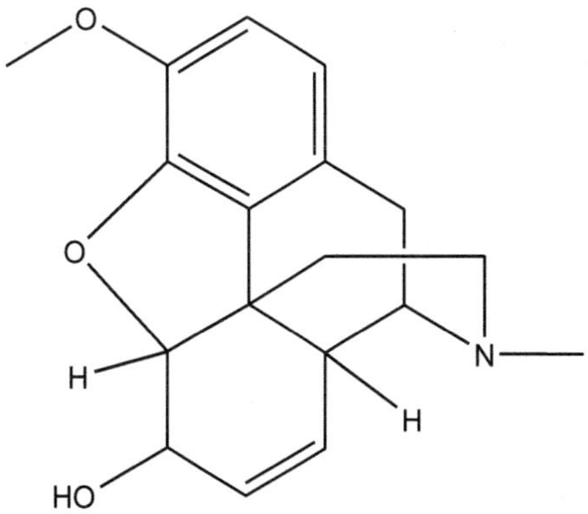

O
O
H
N
H
HO

FIGURE 8.5 **Structure of codeine.**

to morphine hence dose of 30 mg of codeine is considered equivalent to that of 3 mg dose of morphine. The ability to metabolize codeine is very less in Asians (2%) and Arabs (1%), which makes it codeine is a relatively ineffective analgesic in these populations.

CANNABIS (MARIJUANA)

Cannabis, which is also known as marijuana, is flowering tops of *Cannabis sativa* (family Cannabaceae). Cannabis has been used in medicine for thousands of years. Cannabis is constituted of three different bioactive molecules, which includes flavonoids, terpenoids, and cannabinoids. Cannabinoids mimic the effects of the endogeuous cannabinoids, which may prove beneficial in the management of cancer related pain. They also can show synergistic effect when used with opioid analgesics. THC (Δ9-tetrahydrocannabinol) is one of the well-studied cannabinoid. Small modifications in the chemical structures of cannabinoids can dramatically change their potency (Razdan, 1986) (Fig. 8.6).

Cannabis shows the activity by binding to specific receptors called cannabinoid receptors. These receptors forms the endogenous cannabinoid system. There are two kinds of cannabinoid receptors, receptor 1 and 2 (CB1 and CB2). They inhibit adenylate cyclase and calcium channels and activate inward rectifying potassium channels (McAllister & Glass, 2002).

Several clinical trials examining the use of cannabinoid receptor agonists to relieve chronic cancer pain have been published. Cannabinoids have been studied specifically for the neuropathic pain associated cancer showing significant relief from pain (Manzanares, Julian, & Carrascosa, 2006). In the central nervous system, cannabinoid 1 receptors are abundant in areas of the brain that modulate nociception (Martin & Rashidian, 2014). Cannabinoids also inhibit the release of inflammatory modulators by acting on mast cell receptors and also enhance the release of analgesic opioids to reduce the inflammation (Facci et al., 1995; Ibrahim et al., 2005).

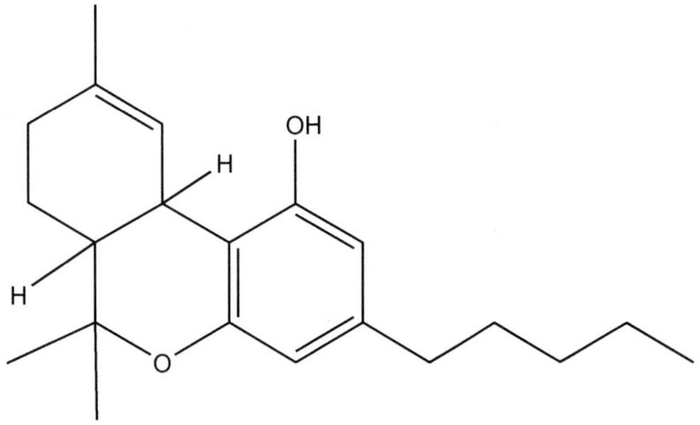

FIGURE 8.6 **Structure of Δ9-tetrahydrocannabinol.**

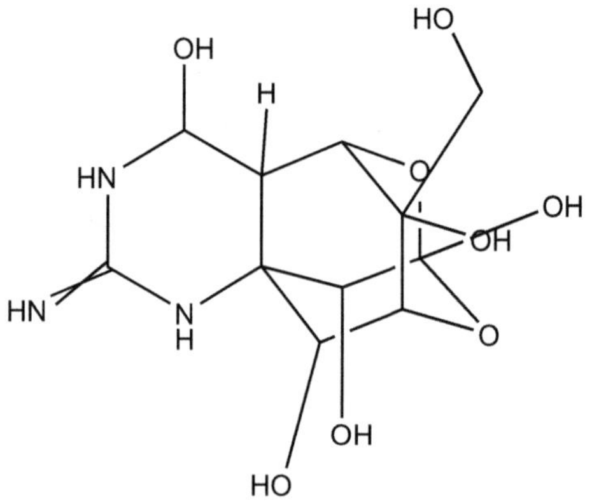

FIGURE 8.7 **Structure of Tetrodotoxin.**

Cannabinoids are also believed to have a synergistic analgesic effect with opioids via unknown mechanisms (Abrams & Guzman, 2015). Cannabinoids may function to suppress spinal and thalamic nociceptive neurons (Walker, Strangman, & Huang, 2000).

Tetrodotoxin

Tetrodotoxin is a naturally occurring sodium channel blocker. It is found in several species of tetraodon puffer fish (family Tetraodontidae). Tetrodotoxin is also found in various other marine animals like globefish, starfish, sunfish, stars, frogs, crabs, snails, Australian blue-ringed octopus, and so on (Fig. 8.7).

Tetrodotoxin has been in use by neuroscientists for decades. It is guanidinium toxin having strong analgesic activity with tolerable safety profile (Omana-Zapata, Khabbaz, Hunter, Clarke, & Bley, 1997; Marcil et al., 2006). Sodium channels are found on most nociceptive pain fibers. Tetrodotoxin selectively blocks the sodium (Na^+) channels found on nociceptive pain fibers. It is supposed that it stabilizes the neuronal membranes by inhibiting the Na^+ ionic fluxes, which is necessary for initiation, as well as conduction of impulses (Amir et al., 2006).

Tetrodotoxin was originally developed at Wex Pharmaceuticals. It is in Phase III clinical trials for the treatment of cancer related pain (WEX Pharmaceuticals, 2016). Another clinical trial has demonstrated that parenteral tetrodotoxin can be effectively used in reducing the dose of opioids and giving the relief from pain related with cancer (Hagen et al., 2008).

Role of Vitamins in Cancer Related Pain

Vitamins cover major part of nutrition playing vital role in different biological activities, as well as low levels of different vitamins are related with various diseases. Scientific reports show that vitamin C and vitamin D have a correlation with cancer pain.

Intravenous administration of vitamin C in cancer patients is reported to decrease the cancer-and chemotherapy-related pain (Carr, Vissers, & Cook, 2014). There are studies reporting use of high-dose of vitamin C in patients with advanced cancer indicated reduced pain and the necessity of analgesics in patients with different types and stages of cancer pain (Cameron & Campbell, 1974).

Palliative cancer patients are commonly observed with vitamin D deficiency, which has been connected with increased risk for pain (Bergman, Sperneder, Höijer, Bergqvist, & Björkhem-Bergman, 2015). Studies show that cancer patients generally have lower vitamin D levels than healthy controls (Dev et al., 2011). There are case reports stating the significance of vitamin D supplements in reducing the dose of opioid, as well as in decreasing the pain (Björkhem-Bergman & Bergman, 2016). Vitamin D supplements may be a useful adjunct for management of cancer related pain. A phase II clinical trial showed that treatment of vitamin D deficiency in patients with metastatic prostate cancer may improve bone pain (van Veldhuizen, Taylor, Williamson, & Drees, 2000).

SUMMARY

Among different consequences of cancer, pain is one of the most notorious indications. It has become crucial to manage the cancer related pain as it directly affects the quality of the life of the patient. Different strategies are adapted by the clinicians for cancer pain management. WHO has specifically designed ladder to guide the cancer pain management. Opioids have key role in the controlling the cancer pain. Morphine, a naturally occurring opioid is considered as gold standard for cancer pain management. It has guided the development of other semisynthetic and synthetic opioids and their use in cancer pain. Among other natural drugs, cancer pain is one of the important indications for medicinal use of cannabis. Tetrodotoxin, which is specific sodium channel blocker, has open sodium channel as a new target for treating the cancer pain.

An extensive research is required to explore the use of natural drugs in cancer pain management.

References

Abrams, D. I., & Guzman, M. (2015). Cannabis in cancer care. *Clinical Pharmacology & Therapeutics, 97*(6), 575–586.

Ahles, T. A., Ruckdeschel, J. C., & Blanchard, E. B. (1984). Cancer related pain–I. Prevalence in an outpatient setting as a function of stage of disease and type of cancer. *The Journal of Psychosomatic Research, 28*, 115–119.

Amir, R., Argoff, C. E., Bennett, G. J., Cummins, T. R., Durieux, M. E., Gerner, P., & Strichartz, G. R. (2006). The role of sodium channels in chronic inflammatory and neuropathic pain. *The Journal of Pain, 7*(5), S1–S29.

Bergman, P., Sperneder, S., Höijer, J., Bergqvist, J., & Björkhem-Bergman, L. (2015). Low vitamin d levels are associated with higher opioid dose in palliative cancer patients—results from an observational study in Sweden. *PloS One, 10*(5), e0128223.

Björkhem-Bergman, L., & Bergman, P. (2016). Vitamin D and patients with palliative cancer. *BMJ Supportive & Palliative Care*, bmjspcare-2015-000921.

Breivik, H., Cherny, N., Collett, B., De Conno, F., Filbet, M., Foubert, A. J., & Dow, L. (2009). Cancer-related pain: a pan-European survey of prevalence, treatment, and patient attitudes. *Annals of Oncology, 20*(8), 1420–1433.

Brescia, F. J., Portenoy, R. K., Ryan, M., Krasnoff, L., & Gray, G. (1992). Pain, opioid use, and survival in hospitalized patients with advanced cancer. *Journal of Clinical Oncology, 10*(1), 149–155.

Cameron, E., & Campbell, A. (1974). The orthomolecular treatment of cancer II. Clinical trial of high-dose ascorbic acid supplements in advanced human cancer. *Chemico-Biological Interactions, 9*(4), 285–315.

Carr, A. C., Vissers, M. C., & Cook, J. S. (2014). The effect of intravenous vitamin C on cancer-and chemotherapy-related fatigue and quality of life. *Frontiers in Oncology, 16*(4), 283.

Davis, M. P. (2012). Drug management of visceral pain: concepts from basic research. *Pain Research and Treatment, 2012*(2012), 1–18.

Dev, R., Del Fabbro, E., Schwartz, G. G., Hui, D., Palla, S. L., Gutierrez, N., & Bruera, E. (2011). Preliminary report: vitamin D deficiency in advanced cancer patients with symptoms of fatigue or anorexia. *The Oncologist, 16*(11), 1637–1641.

Facci, L., Dal Toso, R., Romanello, S., Buriani, A., Skaper, S. D., & Leon, A. (1995). Mast cells express a peripheral cannabinoid receptor with differential sensitivity to anandamide and palmitoylethanolamide. *Proceedings of the National Academy of Sciences, 92*(8), 3376–3380.

Grahame-Smith, D. G., & Aronson, J. K. (1992). *Oxford textbook of clinical pharmacology and drug therapy*. Oxford University Press.

Greenwald, H. P., Bonica, J. J., & Bergner, M. (1987). The prevalence of pain in four cancers. *Cancer, 60*(10), 2563–2569.

Grond, S., Zech, D., Diefenbach, C., Radbruch, L., & Lehmann, K. A. (1996). Assessment of cancer pain: a prospective evaluation in 2266 cancer patients referred to a pain service. *Pain, 64*(1), 107–114.

Hagen, N. A., du Souich, P., Lapointe, B., Ong-Lam, M., Dubuc, B., & Walde, D. Canadian Tetrodotoxin Study Group. (2008). Tetrodotoxin for moderate to severe cancer pain: a randomized, double blind, parallel design multicenter study. *Journal of Pain and Symptom Management, 35*(4), 420–429.

Harrison, A. M., Heritier, F., Childs, B. G., Bostwick, J. M., & Dziadzko, M. A. (2015). Systematic Review of the Use of Phytochemicals for Management of Pain in Cancer Therapy. *BioMed Research International, 2015*, 1–8.

Ibrahim, M. M., Porreca, F., Lai, J., Albrecht, P. J., Rice, F. L., Khodorova, A., ... & Malan, T. P. (2005). CB2 cannabinoid receptor activation produces antinociception by stimulating peripheral release of endogenous opioids. *Proceedings of the National Academy of Sciences of the United States of America, 102*(8), 3093–3098.

Jacox, A., Carr, D. B., Payne, R., & Berde, C. B. (1994). Management of cancer pain. Clinical practice guideline no. 9. AHCPR publication no. 94-0592. Agency for Health Care Policy and Research, US Department of Health and Human Services. Public Health Service, Rockville, MD.

Lee, J. W., Lee, W. B., Kim, W., Min, B. I., Lee, H., & Cho, S. H. (2015). Traditional herbal medicine for cancer pain: a systematic review and meta-analysis. *Complementary Therapies in Medicine, 23*(2), 265–274.

Manzanares, J., Julian, M. D., & Carrascosa, A. (2006). Role of the cannabinoid system in pain control and therapeutic implications for the management of acute and chronic pain episodes. *Current Neuropharmacology, 4*(3), 239–257.

Marcil, J., Walczak, J. S., Guindon, J., Ngoc, A. H., Lu, S., & Beaulieu, P. (2006). Antinociceptive effects of tetrodotoxin (TTX) in rodents. *British Journal of Anaesthesia, 96*(6), 761–768.

Martin, A., & Rashidian, N. (2014). *A New Leaf: The End of Cannabis Prohibition*. New Press.

McAllister, S. D., & Glass, M. (2002). CB 1 and CB 2 receptor-mediated signalling: a focus on endocannabinoids. *Prostaglandins, Leukotrienes and Essential Fatty Acids (PLEFA)*, *66*(2), 161–171.

Miaskowski, C., Cleary, J., Burney, R., Coyne, P., Finley, R., Foster, R., & Weisman, S. J. (2005). *Guideline for the management of cancer pain in adults and children*. Glenview, IL: American Pain Society, 3.

Omana-Zapata, I., Khabbaz, M. A., Hunter, J. C., Clarke, D. E., & Bley, K. R. (1997). Tetrodotoxin inhibits neuropathic ectopic activity in neuromas, dorsal root ganglia and dorsal horn neurons. *Pain*, *72*(1), 41–49.

Portenoy, R. K., & Dhingra, L. K. (2011). Overview of cancer pain syndromes. In Abrahm, J. (Ed.), UpToDate. Waltham, MA: UpToDate; 2013.

Razdan, R. K. (1986). Structure-activity relationships in cannabinoids. *Pharmacological Reviews*, *38*(2), 75–149.

Turk, D. C., & Okifuji, A. (1999). Assessment of patients' reporting of pain: an integrated perspective. *The Lancet*, *353*(9166), 1784–1788.

Twycross, R., Harcourt, J., & Bergl, S. (1996). A survey of pain in patients with advanced cancer. *Journal of Pain and Symptom Management*, *12*(5), 273–282.

van den Beuken-van Everdingen, M. H. J., De Rijke, J. M., Kessels, A. G., Schouten, H. C., Van Kleef, M., & Patijn, J. (2007). Prevalence of pain in patients with cancer: a systematic review of the past 40 years. *Annals of Oncology*, *18*(9), 1437–1449.

van den Beuken-van, M. H., de Rijke, J. M., Kessels, A. G., Schouten, H. C., van Kleef, M., & Patijn, J. (2009). Quality of life and non-pain symptoms in patients with cancer. *Journal of Pain and Symptom Management*, *38*(2), 216–233.

van Veldhuizen, P. J., Taylor, S. A., Williamson, S., & Drees, B. M. (2000). Treatment of vitamin D deficiency in patients with metastatic prostate cancer may improve bone pain and muscle strength. *The Journal of Urology*, *163*(1), 187–190.

Ventafridda, V., & Stjernsward, J. (1996). Pain control and the World Health Organization analgesic ladder. *JAMA*, *275*(11), 835–836.

Walker, J. M., Strangman, N. M., & Huang, S. M. (2000). Cannabinoids and pain. *Pain Research & Management: the Journal of the Canadian Pain Society (Journal de la Societe Canadienne Pour le Traitement de la Douleur)*, *6*(2), 74–79.

WEX Pharmaceuticals (2016). Available from: http://www.wextech.ca/clinical_trials.asp?m=1&s=0&p=0

Wiffen, P. J., & McQuay, H. J. (2007). Oral morphine for cancer pain. *Cochrane Database System Review*, *4*(4), .

Woolsey, R. M., & Martin, D. S. (2003). The neurologic manifestations of spinal cord disease. In V. W. Lin, D. D. Cardenas, N. C. Cutter et al., (Eds.), *Spinal cord medicine: principles and practice*. New York, NY: Demos Medical Publishing.

World Health and Organization. (1986). *Cancer pain relief*. Geneva: World Health Organization.

World Health and Organization. (1996). *Cancer pain relief: with a guide to opioid availability*. Geneva: World Health Organization.

Zech, D. F., Grond, S., Lynch, J., Hertel, D., & Lehmann, K. A. (1995). Validation of World Health Organization Guidelines for cancer pain relief: a 10-year prospective study. *Pain*, *63*(1), 65–76.

CHAPTER

9

Capsicum: A Natural Pain Modulator

Y.A. Kulkarni, S.V. Suryavanshi*, S.T. Auti*, A.B. Gaikwad***

***Shobhaben Pratapbhai Patel School of Pharmacy & Technology Management, SVKM's NMIMS, Mumbai, Maharashtra, India; **Department of Pharmacy, Birla Institute of Technology and Science, Pilani Campus, Pilani, Rajasthan, India**

INTRODUCTION

Pain is not only an obnoxious sensation, but also a complex sensory process essential for survival. Noxious stimuli (thermal, chemical, mechanical trauma, diseased condition, or electrical) causes cellular damage. In response to damage, cell releases chemical mediators (histamine, bradykinin, prostaglandins, etc.), which activate nociceptive receptors via cascade of reactions and the nociceptive signal will be modulated from the periphery to the brain at all levels of the central nervous system (CNS).

The International Association for the Study of Pain (IASP) defines pain as: "an unpleasant sensory and emotional experience associated with actual or potential tissue damage, or described in terms of such damage." Though pain and coupled responses can be unpleasant and often debilitating, it implicates identification and localization of noxious stimuli, initiate withdrawal responses that limit tissue injury thereby enhance wound healing.

Types of Pain

Pain can be classified according to several variables, including its duration (acute, chronic), its physiologic, or pathophysiologic mechanisms (nociceptive, neuropathic, physiologic), and its clinical milieu (e.g., postsurgical, malignancy related, neuropathic, degenerative, etc.).

Acute pain is limited to pain of less than 30 days duration, whereas chronic pain persists for more than 6 months. Subacute pain comprises the interval from the end of the first month to the beginning of the seventh month of continued pain (Cole, 2002). Acute pain is provoked by a specific disease or injury, serves a useful biologic purpose, is associated with skeletal muscle spasm and sympathetic nervous system activation, and is self-limited (Grichnik & Ferrante, 1991). Chronic pain, in contrast, may be considered a disease state. It is pain that survives the normal time of healing, if associated with a disease or injury. Chronic pain may arise from psychological states, serves no biologic purpose, and has no recognizable end-point (Henry, 2008).

Nociceptive pain is experienced due to activation of nociceptors in peripheral tissues resulting from cellular damage due to traumatic or disease related injuries. Nociceptive pain has also been termed as *inflammatory pain*; as inflammatory mediators play role in its initiation and development (Vadivelu, Whitney, & Sinatra, 2009). Pain after surgery, pain associated with sports injury, sprains are typical examples of nociceptive pain.

Neuropathic pain results from dysfunction of the nervous tissue or nervous system lesions like in diabetic neuropathy (Nicholson, 2006). Dysfunction of nerve tissue alters physiologic nociceptive pathways. For example, damage to inhibitory pathways or overstimulation of nociceptive pathway can change balance between nonpainful and painful sensory stimuli respectively that causes pain without activation of primary afferent nociceptors (Nicholson, 2006).

Physiologic pain is a protective mechanism of an individual to tissue injury or harmful environment, characterized by discomfort due to trauma or noxious stimuli (mechanical, thermal, or chemical) of very short duration. Physiologic pain prevents or minimizes tissue injury by initiating withdrawal reflexes and thereby alerting individual regarding potential harmful environment (Vadivelu et al., 2009).

Nutritional Modulators of Pain in the Aging Population. http://dx.doi.org/10.1016/B978-0-12-805186-3.00009-6
Copyright © 2017 Elsevier Inc. All rights reserved.

Nociception and Nociceptors

Nociception is a dynamic phenomenon in which the nociceptive signal is modulated from peripheral nervous system to brain. The nociceptive pathways can be better understood following the integration and modulation of nociceptive signal at all level of CNS (Marchand, 2008).

Nociceptors are the relatively unspecialized, free, lightly myelinated, or unmyelinated nerve endings. Like other subcutaneous and cutaneous receptors, they detect noxious stimuli and convert the noxious stimuli into electrical signal and trigger afferent action potential into nerve endings, which in turn initiate sensation of pain (Purves et al., 2001; Burgess & Perl, 1973). Nociceptors, similar to other somatic sensory receptors; originate from cell bodies that are located in the dorsal root ganglia (DRG) or trigeminal ganglia (Purves et al., 2001). The DRG or trigeminal ganglia have two axonal processes; one extends into peripheral while another extends into spinal cord or brainstem (Basbaum, Bautista, Scherrer, & Julius, 2009) (Fig. 9.1).

As nociceptors are the free axon terminals; according to the nerve fibers associated with them they are classified into four classes (Burgess & Perl, 1973). The somatic sensory nerve fibers Aα and Aβ (Table 9.1) are highly myelinated, conduct impulse with rapid velocity. These nerve fibers are responsible for the nonnoxious (nonpainful) impulse. In contrast, nerve fibers associated with nociceptiors are lightly myelinated or unmyelinated and hence the conduction velocity of these fibers is relatively slow (Dray, 1995). Further, the latter two classes assigning pain subdivided into either the lightly myelinated Aδ afferents which convey faster impulses or into the unmyelinated C fibers, which conduct slow pain (Patel, 2010).

Generally, the Aδ fibers respond either to extremely noxious mechanical or to mechanothermal stimuli. On other hand unmyelinated C fibers respond to mechanical, thermal, and chemical stimuli and hence said to be polymodal (Purves et al., 2001). Based on these properties of afferent nerves nociceptors in the skin can be classified into three major classes: Aβ mechanothermal

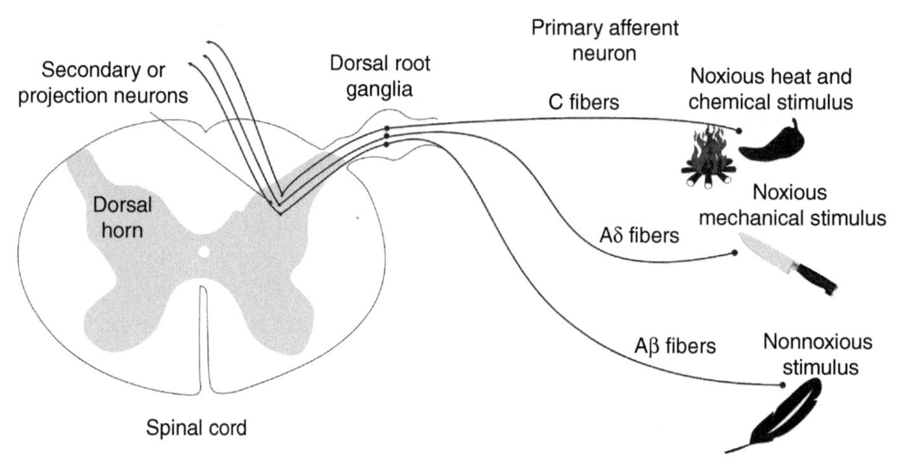

FIGURE 9.1 **Sensory afferent nerve fibers.**

TABLE 9.1 Properties of Primary Afferent Fibers

	Aα Fibers	AβFibers	AδFibers	C Fibers
Myelination	Highly myelinated	Highly myelinated	Lightly myelinated	Unmyelinated
Fiber diameter	Large (12–20 μm)	Large (6–11 μm)	Small (1–5 μm)	Very Small (0.3–1.5 μm)
Conduction velocity	Very High (72–120 m/s)	High (30–70 m/s)	Medium (4–30 m/s)	Slow (0.5–2 m/s)
Receptor type	Proprioceptors Baroreceptors	Proprioceptors Baroreceptors	Nociceptors Thermoreceptors Proprioceptors	Nociceptors Thermoreceptors Proprioceptors
Receptor activation thresholds	Low	Low	Both high and low	High
Sensation on stimulation	Non noxious Light touch	Non noxious Light touch	Short duration, Rapid localized pain	Slow, diffuse, dull pain

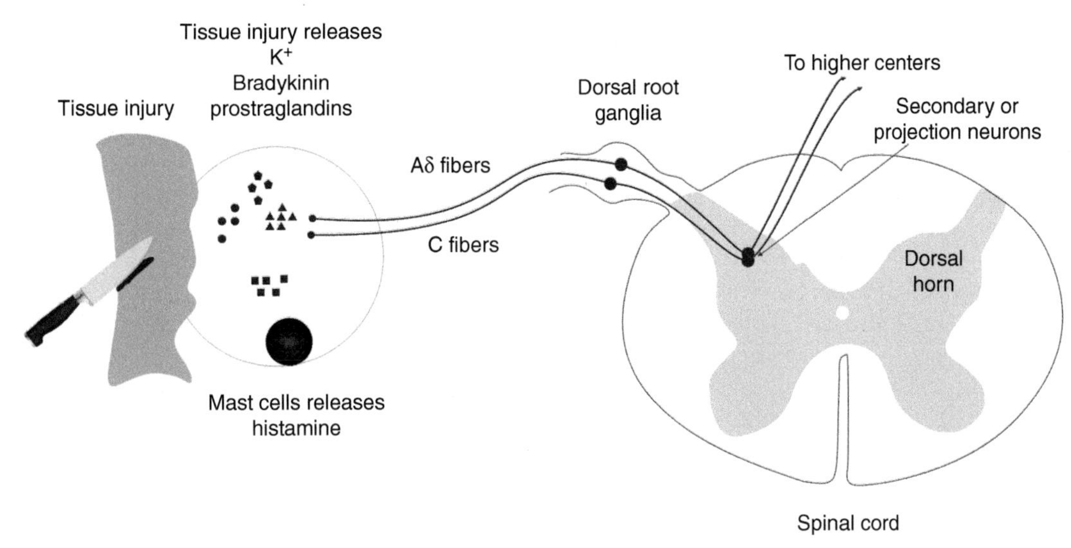

FIGURE 9.2 **Activation of nociceptors.**

nociceptors; Aδ mechanosensitive nociceptors; and C fibers polymodal nociceptors (Burgess & Perl, 1973; Purves et al., 2001).

Response of Nociceptors to Noxious Stimuli

Activation of nociceptors takes place only when an adequate stimulus of sufficient amplitude and duration depolarizes peripheral nerve terminals. In response to tissue injury peripheral nerve terminals releases a variety of molecules (Fig. 9.2) that modifies concentration dependent change in local tissue environment and pain sensation (Dray, 1995).

Stimulation of nociceptors by mechanical, chemical, or thermal stimulus will bring about depolarization of in the primary somatosensory neuron and signal will be transmitted to the dorsal horn of the spinal cord. Subsequently, the primary neuron will formulate a synapse with the projection neuron. Immediately the projection neurons will send signals to higher centers through the medial (spinoreticular) and lateral (spinothalamic) tracts to produce second synapse with tertiary neurons in the thalamus (Fig. 9.3) (Dray, 1995). Further, the tertiary neurons send signals to primary and secondary somatosensory cortices and limbic system including insula and cortex.

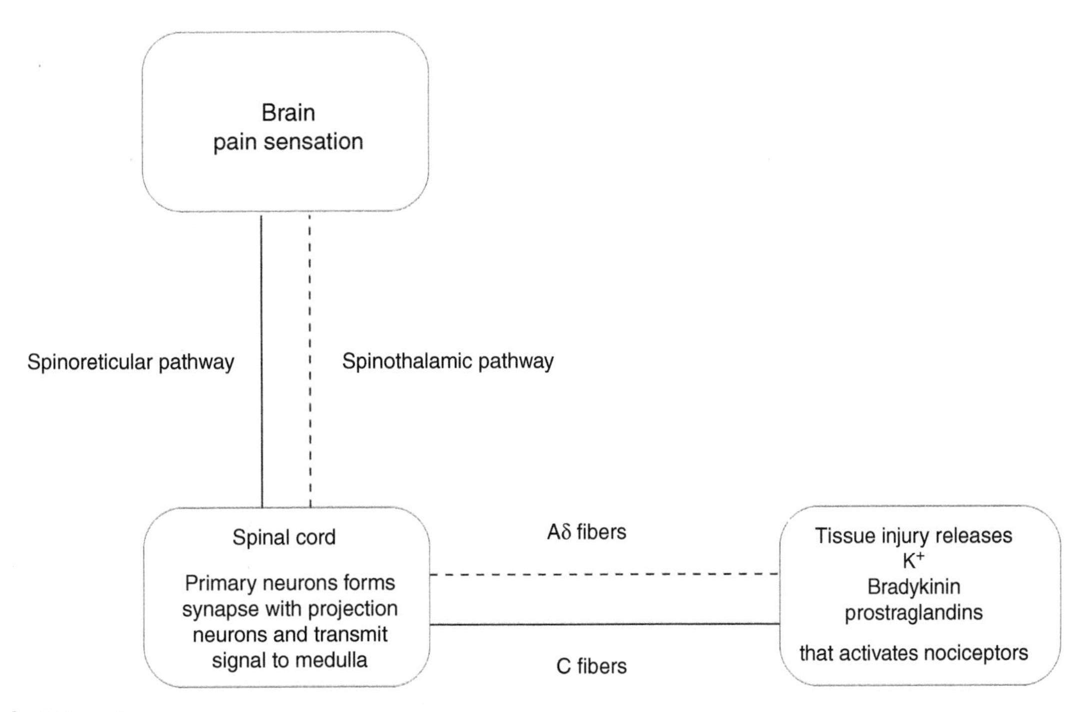

FIGURE 9.3 **Pain pathways.**

In association with typical spinothalamocortical nociceptive projections, another ascending nociceptive pathway which originates at dorsal horn of a spinal cord and projects further to brainstem and then to various brain structures. The dorsocaudal pathway also originates from the dorsal horn of the spinal cord and projects further to subnucleus reticularis dorsalis (SRD), then to the ventromedian nucleus (VMN) of the thalamus, and finally to the dorsolateral frontal lobes (Monconduit, Bourgeais, Bernard, Le Bars, & Villanueva, 1999; Rainville, 2002).

Another ascending pathway originates at the spinal cord and projects through to the parabrachial (Pb) nucleus, hypothalamus, and finally reaches to the amygdala (Bernard, Bester, & Besson, 1995; Bester, Chapman, Besson, & Bernard, 2000). Research findings from research done by Bourgeais et al. (2001) suggest that Pb nucleus convey nociceptive information from the dorsal horn of a spinal cord to the intralaminar nucleus of thalamus finally to the frontal cortices (Bourgeais, Monconduit, Villanueva, & Bernard, 2001; Bourne, Machado, & Nagel, 2014).

PAIN MODULATION

There is a difference between the objective perception of pain and subjective response to the pain. In short, the pain modulation is the pain suppression. For instance, during boxing fight the boxers experiences little or almost no pain with respect to severe injuries. This dissociative experience between pain and injury implies that body-modulate pain in association with some endogenous mechanisms present in it. The pain modulation is an important advantage for survival which is achieved by different mechanisms namely descending inhibitory nerve system, segmental inhibition also known as gate theory of pain control, and endogenous opioid and cannabinoid receptor dependent system (Price, 1999; Patel, 2010).

In addition to the ascending pathways, the periacqueductal gray area (PAG) plays an important role in descending pathway and thereby modulation of spinal nociceptive activity (Bourne et al., 2014). Some studies in the rats, monkeys, cats, and rabbits indicate that the rostral anterior cingulate cortex area (rACC) may be involved in modulation of stimulation produced pain avoidance (Mayer & Saper, 2000; Mantyh, 1982). Melzack and Wall (1965) proposed a theory known as gate theory of pain control. According to that theory, the pain perception can be inhibited or totally blocked in the dorsal horn of spinal cord across the synapse between Aδ and/or C nerve fibers and the cells at pain site (Johansen, Fields, & Manning, 2001). Another way of pain modulation is inhibition of opioid and/or cannabinoid receptors by endogenous compounds, such as Enkephalins, endorphins, and dynorphin. These endogenous compounds possibly act through descending modulatory processes at periaqueductal gray (PAG) matter, ventral medulla, amygdala, and spinal cord (Melzack & Wall, 1967; Richardson, 2000). From the aforementioned studies, it can be concluded that the higher order cerebral structures are involved in regulation pain perception and thereby behavior by integrating nociceptive information received from dorsal horn of the spinal cord (Rainville, 2002).

Herbal Drugs in Pain Modulation

Many herbal medicines have been used for centuries for pain relief and treatment in various traditional systems of medicines in all over the world. Over the past several decades, herbal medicines have became very popular and use of herbals in treatment of various diseases has gradually increased in various countries (Parthasarathy, Chempakam, & Zachariah, 2008). Despite the increasing popularity, both the public and the experts are incredulous about the use of the natural products (Walsh & Hoot, 2001). The reasons behind this incredulity include the lack of proper documentation regarding the proper source and formulations used; batch-to-batch consistency, standardization of the composition, mechanisms of action; and safety of herbal products. For this reason now, it is requisite to document and share best practices about herbal drugs. This chapter focuses on the *Capsicum* especially emphasizing on its pharmacology and its pungent active principle capsaicin as pain modulator.

Genus *Capsicum*

Capsicum, also known as peppers, is a genus of flowering plants native to tropical America and belongs to the nightshade family Solanaceae. The original geographic distribution of *Capsicum* is very difficult to determine as the humans have been affecting spreading since primitive time (Walsh & Hoot, 2001).

Capsicum is an annual, perennial flowering shrub widely known for its fruit, commonly used fresh or cooked; as a dry powder for its flavor, aroma, and color or processed into oleoresins. *Capsicum* oleoresin is prepared commercially by solvent extraction of dried ripe fruit and subsequent solvent evaporation (Wesolowska, Jadczak, & Grzeszczuk, 2011).

At present, this genus is believed to consist of 27 species, 5 of which are domesticated and used as fresh vegetables and spices: *Capsicum annuum*, *Capsicum baccatum*, *Capsicum chinense*, *Capsicum frutescens*, and *Capsicum pubescens*, along with approximately 3000 varieties (Ibiza, Blanca, Cañizares, & Nuez, 2012).

Capsicum exhibits extensive morphological variation, especially in fruit size, shape, and color. Inflorescences range from single to seven flowers at single node. The calyx may vary from long, spine like projections to truncate sepals to green sepals. The corolla is infrequently campanulate with variable coloration between different species. Pubescence of stems and leaves vary from glabrous to pubescent. Seeds are cream colored to black seeds (Walsh & Hoot, 2001).

Chemical Constituents in *Capsicum*

Capsicum mainly contains active pungent principles; a chemical group of nonvolatile alkaloid compounds collectively called as capsaicinoids. All the capsaicinoids are acid amides with vanillylamide and C_9–C_{11} branched chain fatty acid (Wesolowska et al., 2011; Huang, Xue, Jiang, & Zhu, 2013). Capsaicin, ($C_{18}H_{27}NO_3$, *trans*-8-methyl-*N*-vanillyl-6-nonenamide) a colorless, crystalline compound is found most abundantly (46%) amongst other capsaicinoids in *Capsicum* (Fig. 9.4). Other capsaicinoids include dihydrocapsaicin (41%), nordihydrocapsaicin (7%), norcapsaicin (7%), homocapsaicin (3%), homodihydrocapsaicin (2%), and others (Wesolowska et al., 2011).

The most important differences between the capsaicinoids are: their relative pungency, the length of the branched chain, the branching point and the number of unsaturation in side chain. Generally, capsaicin and dihydrocapsaicin are almost 10 times more pungent than other capsaicinoids (Wesolowska et al., 2011).

Along with capsaicinoids, *Capsicum* also contains ascorbic acid, fixed oil, thiamine, and carotenoid pigments (Santos et al., 2012). Carotenoids in *Capsicum* are responsible of red color of mature fruits including capsanthin, capsorubin, and β-carotene. From these carotenoids capsanthin and capsorubin are chemically fatty acid esters and not found in other plant of animal species (Moscone et al., 1993). The major pigments in *Capsicum* include capsanthin (31.7% of total carotenoids), β-carotene (12.3%), and capsorubin (7.5% of total carotenoids) in red ripe fruit (Govindarajan & Salzer, 1986) (Fig. 9.5).

Capsicum and Traditional Uses

In folk medicine, *Capsicum* has been used as stomachic, carminative, aphrodisiac, digestive, antispasmodic, counterirritant, astringent, depurative, rubefacient, and antiseptic (Duke, 2002). *Capsicum* has been used for diarrhoea, toothache, respiratory complaints, cramps, flatulence, to treat neuralgia, fresh burns, and arthritic pain (McKenna, Jones, & Hughes, 2002).

In India, *Capsicum annum* has been used for treatment of lumbago in combination with garlic, storax, and pepper in the form of plasters. It has been used in combination with *Cinchona* bark to treat rheumatism, snake bite and gout. The *Capsicum* tincture has been used for flatulence or poor appetite (Nadkarni, 2007). *Capsicum* has also been used in brain complaints, delirium, chronic ulcers, muscular pain, loss of consciousness, cholera, dyspepsia, jaundice, and typhoid fever (Kirtikar & Basu, 2005)

Capsaicin and Pain Modulation

The Overview of TRP Family

Transient receptor potential (TRP) channel is one of the largest families of ion channels and it have been classified into six subfamilies depending upon amino acid sequence homology; TRPM (Melastatin), TRPC (Canonical), TRPA (Ankyrin), TRPP (Polycystin), TRPV (Vanilloid), and TRPML (Mucolipin) (Fields, 2004; Clapham, 2003; Corey, 2003; Montell, Birnbaumer, & Flockerzi, 2002a). All the members of TRP channels are topologically similar to voltage gated ion channels and are permeable to cations. These channels have six transmembrane protein (Fig. 9.6) domains with intracellular N and C terminals (Fields, 2004). They have pore loop between 5th and 6th transmembrane protein. Although the TRP channels are structurally similar to voltage

Capsaicin
Dihydrocapsaicin
Homocapsaicin
Homodihydrocapsaicin
Norcapsaicin
Nordihydrocapsaicin

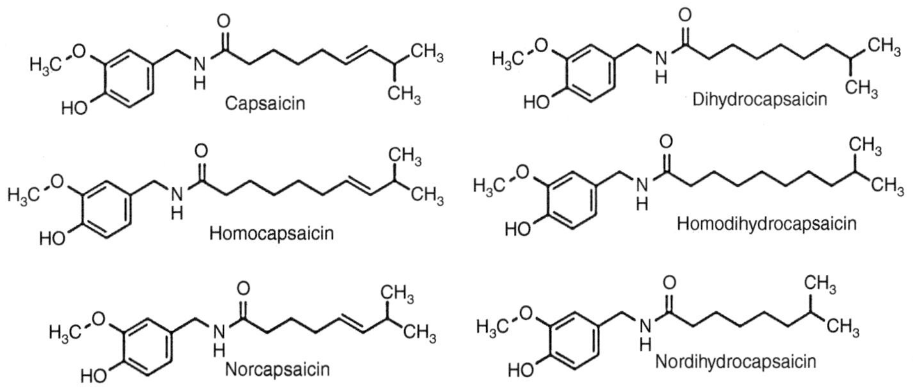

FIGURE 9.4 **Active constituents of *Capsicum*.**

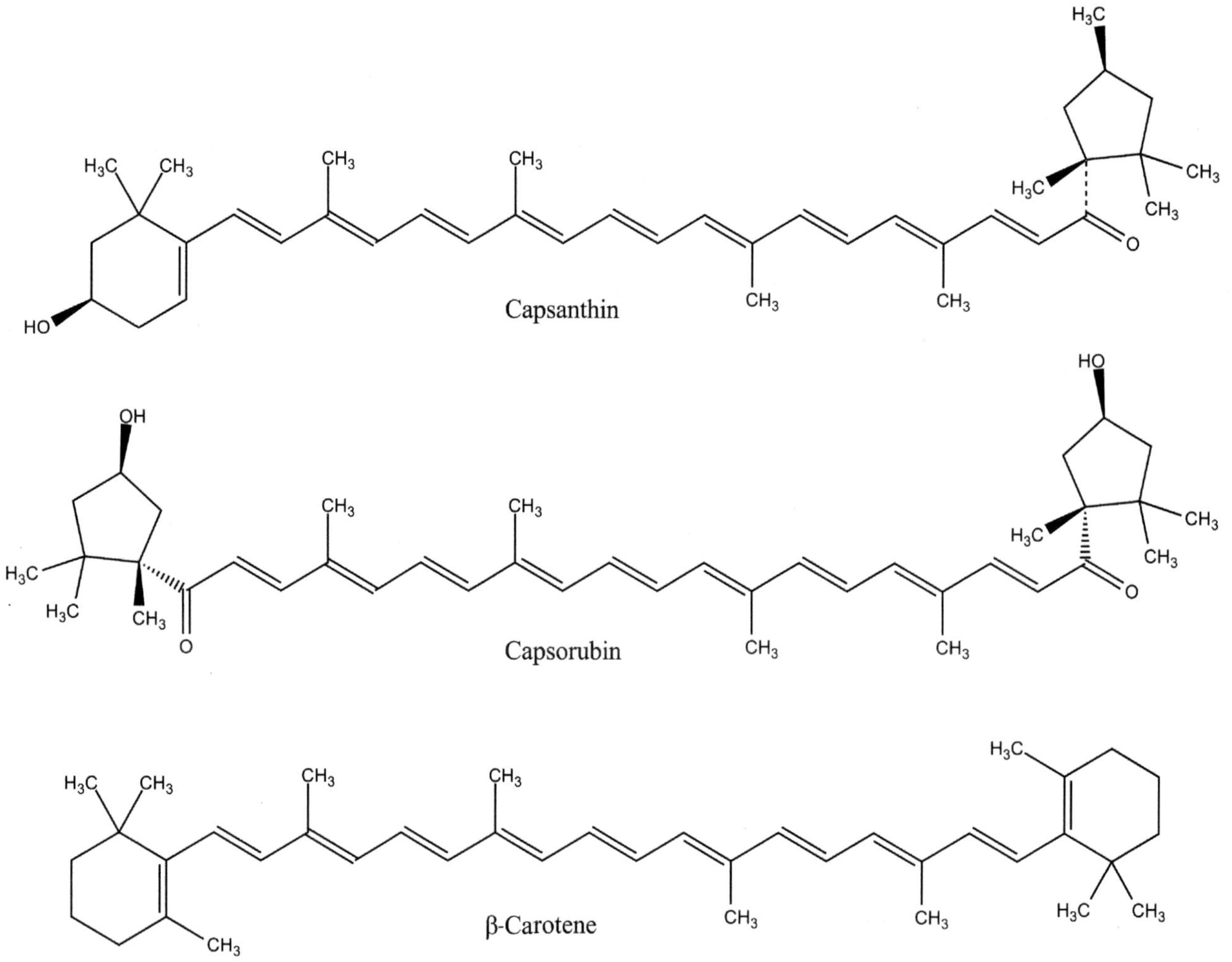

Capsanthin

Capsorubin

β-Carotene

FIGURE 9.5 **Structures of major carotenoids in *Capsicum*.**

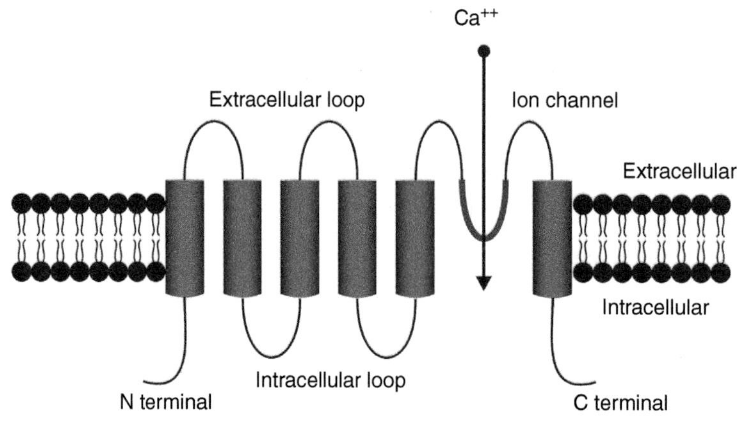

FIGURE 9.6 **Structure of TRPV receptor.**

gated ion channels they are markedly diverse in nature as they lack the voltage sensor and are weakly voltage dependent (Montell et al., 2002b; Männikkö, Elinder, & Larsson, 2002). TRP channels are activated by variety of stimulus, such as thermal, mechanical, chemical, oxidative stress, low pH and endogenous lipids derived from dopamine and regulated by transcription, glycosylation, alternative splicing, and phosphorylation (Nilius et al., 2005).

TRPV (CAPSAICIN) RECEPTORS

TRPV1 (capsaicin) receptor is the founding member of the TRPV subfamily. Recent study describes six different thermosensitive channels namely TRPV2, TRPV3, TRPV4, TRPM8, and TRPA1 from same family (Nilius et al., 2005; Tominaga, 2007). TRPV1 receptors are activated by low pH, capsaicin, heat, and lipids derived from dopamine; followed by integration of noxious and physical stimuli to transduce and modulate acute and chronic pain (Levine & Alessandri-Haber, 2007). Caterina et al. (1997) confirmed the role of capsaicin receptors in modulation and transduction of chronic pain and its promising potential in treatment of acute and chronic pain

TRPV1 receptors are exclusively activated by capsaicin. The application of capsaicin produces concentration and mode of administration dependent analgesic and/or hyperalgesic effects (Caterina et al., 1997; Szallasi, Cortright, Blum, & Eid, 2007; Numazaki & Tominaga, 2004; Ossipov, 2012). Intravenous and intradermal injection of high concentration capsaicin leads to degeneration of primary neurons in rats and epidermal nerve fibers in human and reduce postoperative pain (Jancsó, Kiraly, Such, Joo, & Nagy, 1986; Nagy, Iversen, Goedert, Chapman, & Hunt, 1983; Simone, Baumann, & LaMotte, 1989; Pospisilova & Palecek, 2006; Caterina et al., 2000). Experiments on mice lacking TRPV1 receptors demonstrated that capsaicin showed attenuation in thermal hypersensitivity, induction in pain and normal responses to noxious pain (Ahern, Brooks, Miyares, & Wang, 2005).

Capsaicin Receptors and Pain

Studies on TRPV1–null mice demonstrated extracellular cations (Na^{+}, Mg^{++}, and Ca^{++}), which potentiate capsaicin receptors via electrostatic interactions and phospholipase C–mediated cation effects (Caterina et al., 2000). Cations contribute to bradykinin-evoked activation of TRVP1 receptors and thereby contribute inflammatory pain signaling (Choi, Lim, Yoo, Kim, & Hwang, 2016; Voets, Talavera, Owsianik, & Nilius, 2005; de Novellis et al., 2011)

During neuropathic pain, excitatory signal is transmitted through amygdala medial prefrontal cortex neuron in prelimbic and infralimbic cortex and the TRVP1 receptors present on glutamatergic fibers are expressed to enhance extracellular glutamate levels (Voets et al., 2005). This contributes to processing of noxious stimuli. Further, *N*-arachidonoyl-serotonin; a typical TRVP1 receptor antagonist and fatty acid amide hydrolase inhibitor, normalize the imbalance between excitatory and inhibitory responses lead to modulation in pain (Mohapatra & Nau, 2003) (Fig. 9.7).

Another mechanism of Capsaicin to activate TRVP1 receptor is via phoshorylation of receptor by protein kinases, thereby activation of calcium and calmodulin dependent protein kinase II and finally cleavage of

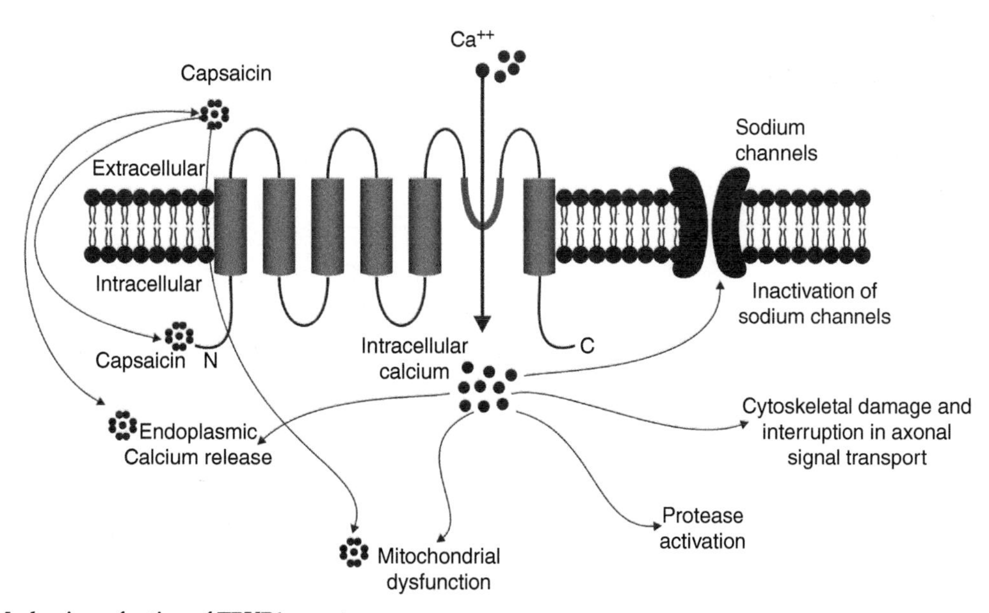

FIGURE 9.7 **Mechanism of action of TRVP1 receptors.**

phophatidylinositol 4,5-biphosphate by phospholipase C (Premkumar & Ahern, 2000; Szallasi & Blumberg, 1999). When capsaicin receptor activates TRVP1 receptors, they undergo long refractory state and hence neurons become resistant to various mechanical, proinflammatory, and endo/exogenous pain stimuli and thereby pain relief (Liu & Simon, 1996). At the molecular level, activation of TRVP1 receptors by capsaicin results in calcium dependent conformational changes in the receptor proteins and receptors undergo refractory state closing the channel pore (Lundberg, 1996).

TRVP1 receptors upon excitation release numerous sensory neuropeptides depending on the concentration of capsaicin (Gamse, Petsche, Lembeck, & Jancso, 1982). Simultaneously it also blocks the axoplasmic transport of somatostatin and substance P in sensory neuron and inhibits restoration of neuropeptides thereby depletion of neuropeptides (Anand & Bley, 2011). This was thought to be mechanism of capsaicin induced pain relief, but capsaicin produce analgesia by defunctionalization of nociceptive nerve fibers by inability to transport neurotrophic factors and loss of membrane potential, along with depletion of neuropeptides (Backonja et al., 2008). Capsaicin, on repeated application; damage cutaneous autonomic nerve fibers and dermal sensory nerve endings possibly by calcium overload and glutamate release causing pain relief (Chard, Bleakman, Savidge, & Miller, 1995; Sikand & Premkumar, 2007; Nolano et al., 1999; Sharma, Vij, & Sharma, 2013).

There are several endogenous agonists of the TRVP1 receptor that have structural similarity to capsaicin, such as lipoxygenase products of arachidonic acid, unsaturated *N*-acyldopamines and anandamide (collectively called endovanilloids). All endovanilloids activates TRVP1 receptors and maintain desensitization of receptors induced by capsaicin. This helps in prolongation of analgesic effect at inflamed tissue (Baamonde, Lastra, Juarez, Hidalgo, & Menéndez, 2005; Wang, Svensson, Sessle, Cairns, & Arendt-Nielsen, 2010).

CAPSICUM AND PAIN THERAPEUTICS

Acute and Chronic Pain

For pain relief, US FDA has approved 8% capsaicin dermal patch; which contains synthetic capsaicin 640 mcg/cm^2 and total dose of 179 mg in one patch (Derry & Moore, 2012). Frerick et al. (2003) investigated the effect of *Capsicum* plaster in chronic low back pain by conducting a double-blind, randomized, multicentre study. A compound pain subscore of the Arhus low back rating scale was measured as an outcome measure. One 12 × 18 cm *Capsicum* plasters containing ethanolic extract of cayenne pepper equivalent to 22 μg/cm^2 capsaicin were applied for 4–8 h once a daily for 3 weeks. There was 42% reduction in compound pain subscore. *Capsicum* plaster offers significant pain relief in chronic low back pain.

A nonpungent capsaicinoid other than capsaicin found in very low amount in *Capsicum* is *N*-palmitoyl-vanillamide (palvanil). It rapidly desensitizes transient TRPV1 receptors similar to that of capsaicin and produce analgesic effect when administered locally. Luongo, Bellini, De Chairo, and Di Marzo (2012) evaluated varying doses of palvanil in mice with spread nerve injury (SNI) against carrageenan-induced oedema, formalin-induced nocifensive behavior, thermal hyperalgesia, and mechanical allodynia. Palvanil (0.5–2.5 mg/kg) reduced formalin-induced nocifensive behavior, significantly inhibited SNI-induced thermal hyperalgesia and mechanical allodynia, thermal hyperalgesia, and carrageenan-induced oedema.

Backonja, Malan, Vanhove, and Tobias (2010) conducted a double-blind, multicenter and parallel-group trial, on 402 patients with 18–90 age groups and had postherpetic neuralgia for at least 6 months and numeric pain rating scale (NPRS) score 3–9. A high dose 8% (640 μg/cm^2) and low dose control 0.04% (3.2 μg/cm^2) capsaicin patches were assigned to patients for 60 min. The percentage change in NPRS score were analyzed from 2–8 weeks. The study confirmed rapid and sustained pain relief of 8% capsaicin patch compared to control patch. No adverse events were reported except for local reactions, such as short-lasting erythema at the site of application. Kulkantrakorn, Lorsuwansiri, and Meesawatson (2013) confirmed that low dose of capsaicin (0.075% cream and 0.025% gel) have no clinical use in pain reduction.

Neuropathic Pain

Postmastectomy is a type of neuropathic pain may be associated with intercostobrachial nerve damage. Watson and Evans (1992) conducted a randomised trial in patients with postmastectomy pain symdrome using 0.075% capsaicin and vehicle (Placebo). Topical application of 0.075% capsaicin produces significant difference visual analogue scale (VAS) compared to placebo. Capsaicin produced more than 50% improvement in 62% patients. Hence, capsaicin can produce significant reduction in stabbing pain but no significant improvement in constant pain reduction.

Morton's neuroma is a benign neuroma of an intermetatarsal plantar nerve, characterized by thickening of nerve tissue at metatarsal spaces, burning sensation, and pain. A pilot study done by Diamond, Richard, and Miller (2006) in patients with Morton's neuroma confirmed that, 100 μg in 0.5 mL pure capsaicin injection (ALGRX 4975) in to intermetatarsal space followed by lignocaine injection after 10 min relieves pain for 3 weeks.

Irving et al. (2011) conducted multicenter trial for 8% capsaicin dermal patch for the treatment of postherpetic neuralgia. Capsaicin 8% dermal patch showed more than 30% reduction in mean NPRS when compared to capsaicin (0.04%) control patch.

Maihofner and Heskamp (2013) conducted prospective, noninterventional study in 1044 patients suffering with peripheral neuropathic pain by applying single dose of 8% capsaicin cutaneous patch for 12 weeks. The average NPRS, neuropathy symptoms, quality of life, sleep parameters, pain attacks, working-capacity, and concomitant neuropathic pain parameters were evaluated. The pain intensity was reduced in almost 80% patients with significant improvement in sleep quality, sleep duration, and pain attacks. 10% patients showed mild ADRs mainly at the site of application (erythema and pain). Patients (1.6%) showed serious ADRs, such as subarachnoidal hemorrhage due to ruptured cerebral aneurysm.

A metaanalysis of clinical trial database for capsaicin 8% (Qutenza) patch was done by Mou et al. (2013). They included trials conducted for Human Immunodeficiency Virus -Assisted Neuropathy (HIV-AN), postherpetic neuralgia, and peripheral neuropathy. The results confirmed that the capsaicin 8% patch reduces pain intensity more than 30% in HIV-AN, peripheral neuropathy, and postherpetic neuralgia.

HIV infection frequently report neurologic complication called distal sensory polyneuropathy (HIV-DSP). This complication is characterized by predominant symmetrical signs of loss of ankle reflexes and distal sensory loss. Symptoms includes allodynia, distal painful dysesthesias, severe burning pain, and lack of sensation usually begin in the feet and progress bilaterally to the legs and arms depending on severity of HIV-DSP. Recent randomized trials confirmed capsaicin 8% wt./wt. control patch decrease in NPRS score providing significant pain relief (Brown et al., 2013; Simpson, Brown, Tobias, & Vanhove, 2014).

Musculoskeletal Pain

TRPV1 receptors exert dissimilar effects on every modality of pain; the inactivation of TRPV1 receptors is one of the advancement to analgesic drug development.

A clinical trial conducted by Wang, Svensson, Sessle, Cairns, and Arendt-Nielson (2010) suggests that peripheral glutamate may interact with capsaicin receptor mechanisms and modulate the sensitization and activation of nociceptive processes in muscles and produce analgesic and rubefacient effect.

Abdelhamid, Kovács, Honda, Nunez, and Larson (2013) compared the effect of TRPV1 receptors on musculoskeletal nociception on the basis of thermal and tactile nociception in mice. Systemic injection of capsaicin showed no tactile response but induced a transient hypothermia and hyperalgesia in mice, probably by agonistic action of capsaicin at TRPV1 sites.

Osteoarthritic Pain

The osteoarthritic pain is the product of release of substance P, which initiates inflammatory responses and pain. Therefore, a potent inhibitor of substance P, such as capsaicin may reduce osteoarthritic pain.

Deal et al. (1991) conducted double blind trial in 31 with rheumatoid arthritis and 70 patients with osteoarthritis. A 0.025% capsaicin cream was applied to patients at affected area 4 times a day for 4 weeks. Pain relief was assessed by visual analog scale (VAS). Capsaicin treated patients showed significant pain relief as compared to placebo. After weeks, 80% patients experienced reduction in pain.

McCleane (2000) investigated the analgesic efficacy of topical capsaicin in combination with glyceryl trinitrate in patients with osteoarthritic pain. Patients were topically applied over affected joints with one of creams containing placebo, 1.33% glyceryl trinitrate, 0.025% capsaicin, or 1.33% glyceryl trinitrate and 0.025% capsaicin for 6 weeks. The analgesic efficacy was measured by visual analogue score (VAS). Results confirmed that topical application of capsaicin (0.025% cream) can moderately reduce osteoarthritis pain and this action can be improved with the addition of glyceryl trinitrate as glyceryl trinitrate reduces discomfort of application when compared with capsaicin cream alone.

Cantillon et al. (2005) performed trial on 16 osteoarthritic patients. Patients received 10, 100, 300, and 1000 μg injection of pure capsaicin injections (Adlea) at affected joints followed by lignocaine injection. Pure capsaicin provides long-lasting pain relief and reduces pain in end stage osteoarthritis. These reports were supported Remadevi & Szallisi (2008).

The metaanalysis of randomized trials of topical capsaicin in treatment of osteoarthritis done by Laslett and Jones (2014) confirms that the low dose topical capsaicin application 4 times daily can moderately reduce pain intensity in osteoarthritis and it is well tolerated in patients with no major side effects.

Cancer Pain

In recent years numerous theories and experimental evidences have been put forth to establish anticancer activity of capsaicin. Evidences confirm that these effects are not mediated through activation of TRVP1 receptors (Raisinghani, Pabbidi, & Premkumar, 2005). However, it inhibits cancer pain probably by TRVP1 mediated increase intracellular calcium levels and initiating apoptotic cascade by activation of caspase and loss of mitochondrial membrane permeability (Lin, Lu, Wang, Chan, & Chen, 2013). It is confirmed that capsaicin inhibit activation of tumor necrosis factor-alpha (TNF-α) and nuclear factor-kappa (NF-κ) in prostatic cancer thereby reducing inflammation and pain (Mori et al., 2006).

Gastric Pain

The gastro intestinal tract is innervated by dense supply of nerve fibers containing TRVP1 receptors. These TRVP1 receptors may be involved in gastro-protection and modulation of gastric pain (Hayman & Kam, 2008). Mózsik, Szolcsányi, and Rácz (2005) evaluated gastroprotective effect of capsaicin in healthy human subjects against ethanol-indomethacin induced gastric mucosal damage. Capsaicin reduces pain due to gastropathy associated with ethanol and indomethacin probably through release of calcitonin gene-related protein (CGRP) and nitric oxide. Capsaicin shows dose dependent reduction in gastric acid secretion and also increase gastric emptying time (Deng et al., 2016).

Burning mouth syndrome represented by burning pain in tongue or oral mucosa along with altered taste sensation. It is considered that it may be associated with cranial nerve dysfunction. A clinical trial conducted by Grushka, Epstein, and Gorsky (2002) using 0.25% oral capsaicin demonstrated improvement in analgesic activity, nevertheless gastric irritation was reported in around one third patients.

Pruritus

Pruritus is a condition characterized by skin irritation, redness, and desire for itching. Tarng, Cho, Liu, and Huang (1996) conducted crossover study of patient having regular haemodialysis confirmed that, topical capsaicin (0.025%), when compared with placebo produce antipruritic effect which last upto 8 weeks after treatment.

Marketed Formulations

Capsicum is described in ancient documents for its analgesic activity. There has renewed interest in formulation and development of single capsaicin preparations or capsaicin in combination with other drugs for treatment of acute and chronic pain, neuropathic pain, musculoskeletal pain, osteoarthritic pain, or gastric pain. Many formulations, such as dermal patch, creams, ointments, topical gels, and plasters containing capsaicin are available in the market. Although these formulations have mild ADRs and have problems of patient compliance; these are promising alternative for both opium analgesics and nonsteroidal antiinflammatory drugs, which have serious adverse drug events, such as habituation and gastric mucosal damage respectively (Table 9.2).

TABLE 9.2 Some Formulations Marketed Worldwide are Given as:

Sr. No	Trade name	Active ingredients	Company
Topical gel			
1	Topac fast	Capsaicin 0.025%; Diclofenac Sodium 1%; Menthol 5%, Methyl Salicylate 5%	Abott
2	Diclomax power	Capsaicin 0.025%; Diclofenac Sodium 1.16%; Menthol 5%; Methyl Salicylate 10%; Linseed oil 3%	Torrent Pharmaceuticals
3	Voveran thermagel	Capsaicin 0.025%; Diclofenac Sodium 1%; Menthol 5%; Methyl Salicylate 5%	Novartis
4	Divexx gel	Capsaicin 0.022%; Diclofenac Sodium 1%; Menthol 5%; Methyl Salicylate 10%	Zuventis Healthcare
Topical cream			
1	Capzasin-P	Capsaicin 0.035%	Sanofi
2	Zostrix HP	Capsaicin 0.075%	Hi-Tech Pharmacal Co.
3	Qualitest trixaicin cream	Capsaicin (0.025%)	Qualitest Pharmaceuticals
4	Doloracin RX cream	Lidocaine (2%); menthol (5%); capsaicin (0.035%) Methyl salicylate (20%)	Two Hip Consulting LLC.
Patches			
1	Qutenza patch	Capsaicin (8%)	NeurogesX. Inc.
2	Anodyne RX patch	Menthol (5%); Lidocaine (2.5%); Capsaicin (0.05%)	Genpak solutions LLC.
3	Renovo patch	Capsaicin (0.0375%); Menthol (5%)	TMIG Inc.
4	Silvera pain relief patches	Lidocaine (1%); menthol (5%); capsaicin (0.0375%)	Home Aide Diagnostics Inc.

SUMMARY

Pain is unwanted sensation that initiates withdrawal responses and limit tissue injury. Capsicum has been used as counter irritant for treatment of neuralgia, lumbago, and rheumatism since ancient time. It has been reported that analgesic and antiinflammatory of capsicum is due to activation of TRVP1 receptors by its active pungent principle capsaicin. TRVP1 receptors upon activation by capsaicin release various neuropeptides (substance P, bradykinin, etc.), chemical mediators (Prostraglandins, Hisamine, etc.) and intracellular calcium; thereby, defunctionalization of sensory neuron and further analgesic effect. Capsaicin and its non-pungent analogue *N*-palmitoyl-vanillamide (palvanil) shows excellent analgesic effects in acute and chronic types of pain with few mild adverse effects, such as skin erythema at the site of application. It has been confirmed that the adverse events of capsaicin can be minimized using capsaicin in combination with local anesthetics, such as lignocaine.

A pure capsaicin injection is in the third phase of clinical trials and it is showing excellent results against neuropathic pain, Morton's neuroma. It has been confirmed that capsaicin 8% patch is very effective against HIV assisted neuropathy, peripheral neuropathy, and postherpetic neuralgia. The single dose high dose capsaicin patch reduces the risk of adverse events with great efficacy.

Capsaicin is also effective in musculoskeletal pain as it specifically activates TRVP1 receptors and desensitizes sensory nerves through hyperalgesia and hypothermia. In osteoarthritic pain an inflammatory neuropeptide substance P levels are increased. Capsaicin 0.025% capsaicin shows very prominent reduction musculoskeletal pain as it inhibits Substance P levels. Capsaicin also reduces gastric pain and burning mouth syndrome caused due to mucosal damage. There are many marketed formulations are available to treat various types of pain.

LIST OF ABBREVIATIONS

CGRP	Calcitonin gene-related protein
CNS	Central nervous system
DRG	Dorsal root ganglia
HIV	Human immunodeficiency virus
HIV-AN	Human immunodeficiency virus-assisted neuropathy
HIV–DSP	Human immunodeficiency virus-distal sensory polyneuropathy
IASP	International Association for the Study of Pain
NF-κ	Nuclear factor-kappa
NPRS	Numeric pain rating scale
Pb	Parabrachial nucleus
PAG	Periacqueductal gray area
rACC	Rostral anterior cingulate cortex area
SNI	Spread nerve injury
SRD	Subnucleus reticularis dorsalis
TRP	Transient receptor potential
TNF-α	Tumor necrosis factor-alpha
US FDA	United States Food and Drug Administration
VMN	Ventromedian nucleus

References

Abdelhamid, R. E., Kovács, K. J., Honda, C. N., Nunez, M. G., & Larson, A. A. (2013). Resiniferatoxin (RTX) causes a uniquely protracted musculoskeletal hyperalgesia in mice by activation of TRPV1 receptors. *The Journal of Pain, 14*(12), 1629–1641.

Ahern, G. P., Brooks, I. M., Miyares, R. L., & Wang, X. B. (2005). Extracellular cations sensitize and gate capsaicin receptor TRPV1 modulating pain signaling. *The Journal of Neuroscience, 25*(21), 5109–5116.

Anand, P., & Bley, K. (2011). Topical capsaicin for pain management: therapeutic potential and mechanisms of action of the new high-concentration capsaicin 8% patch. *British Journal of Anaesthesia, 107*(4), 490–502.

Baamonde, A., Lastra, A., Juarez, L., Hidalgo, A., & Menéndez, L. (2005). TRPV1 desensitisation and endogenous vanilloid involvement in the enhanced analgesia induced by capsaicin in inflamed tissues. *Brain Research Bulletin, 67*(6), 476–481.

Backonja, M., Wallace, M. S., Blonsky, E. R., Cutler, B. J., Malan, P., & Rauck, R. NGX-4010 C116 Study Group. (2008). NGX-4010, a high-concentration capsaicin patch, for the treatment of postherpetic neuralgia: a randomised, double-blind study. *The Lancet Neurology, 7*(12), 1106–1112.

Backonja, M. M., Malan, T. P., Vanhove, G. F., & Tobias, J. K. (2010). NGX-4010, a high-concentration capsaicin patch, for the treatment of postherpetic neuralgia: a randomized, double-blind, controlled study with an open-label extension. *Pain Medicine, 11*(4), 600–608.

Basbaum, A. I., Bautista, D. M., Scherrer, G., & Julius, D. (2009). Cellular and molecular mechanisms of pain. *Cell, 139*(2), 267–284.

Bernard, J. F., Bester, H., & Besson, J. M. (1995). Involvement of the spino-parabrachio-amygdaloid and -hypothalamic pathways in the autonomic and affective emotional aspects of pain. *Progress in Brain Research, 107*, 243–255.

Bester, H., Chapman, V., Besson, J. M., & Bernard, J. F. (2000). Physiological properties of the lamina I spinoparabrachial neurons in the rat. *Journal of Neurophysiology, 83*(4), 2239–2259.

Bourgeais, L., Monconduit, L., Villanueva, L., & Bernard, J. F. (2001). Parabrachial internal lateral neurons convey nociceptive messages from the deep laminas of the dorsal horn to the intralaminar thalamus. *The Journal of Neuroscience, 21*(6), 2159–2165.

Bourne, S., Machado, A. G., & Nagel, S. J. (2014). Basic anatomy and physiology of pain pathways. *Neurosurgery Clinics of North America, 25*(4), 629–638.

Brown, S., Simpson, D. M., Moyle, G., Brew, B. J., Schifitto, G., Larbalestier, N., & Tobias, J. K. (2013). NGX-4010, a capsaicin 8% patch, for the treatment of painful HIV-associated distal sensory polyneuropathy: integrated analysis of two phase III, randomized, controlled trials. *AIDS Research and Therapy, 10*(1), 1.

Burgess, P. T., & Perl, E. R. (1973). Cutaneous mechanoreceptors and nociceptors. In *Somatosensory system* (pp. 29–78). Berlin, Heidelberg: Springer.

Cantillon, M., Vause, E., Sykes, D., Russell, R., Moon, A., & Hughes, S. (2005). Preliminary safety, tolerability and efficacy of ALGRX 4975 in osteoarthritis (OA) of the knee. *The Journal of Pain, 6*(3), S39.

Caterina, M. J., Schumacher, M. A., Tominaga, M., Rosen, T. A., Levine, J. D., & Julius, D. (1997). The capsaicin receptor: a heat-activated ion channel in the pain pathway. *Nature, 389*(6653), 816–824.

Caterina, M. J., Leffler, A., Malmberg, A. B., Martin, W. J., Trafton, J., Petersen-Zeitz, K. R., & Julius, D. (2000). Impaired nociception and pain sensation in mice lacking the capsaicin receptor. *Science, 288*(5464), 306–313.

Chard, P. S., Bleakman, D., Savidge, J. R., & Miller, R. J. (1995). Capsaicin-induced neurotoxicity in cultured dorsal root ganglion neurons: involvement of calcium-activated proteases. *Neuroscience, 65*(4), 1099–1108.

Choi, S. I., Lim, J. Y., Yoo, S., Kim, H., & Hwang, S. W. (2016). Emerging role of spinal cord TRPV1 in pain exacerbation. *Neural Plasticity, 2016*, 1–11.

Clapham, D. E. (2003). TRP channels as cellular sensors. *Nature, 426*(6966), 517–524.

Cole, E. B. PAIN. (2002). Pain management: classifying, understanding, and treating pain. *Hospital Physician, 23*.

Corey, D. P. (2003). New TRP channels in hearing and mechanosensation. *Neuron, 39*(4), 585–588.

de Novellis, V., Vita, D., Gatta, L., Luongo, L., Bellini, G., De Chiaro, M., & Di Marzo, V. (2011). The blockade of the transient receptor potential vanilloid type 1 and fatty acid amide hydrolase decreases symptoms and central sequelae in the medial prefrontal cortex of neuropathic rats. *Molecular Pain, 7*(1), 1.

Deal, C. L., Schnitzer, T. J., Lipstein, E., Seibold, J. R., Stevens, R. M., Levy, M. D., ..., & Renold, F. (1991). Treatment of arthritis with topical capsaicin: a double-blind trial. *Clinical Therapeutics, 13*(3), 383–395.

Deng, Y., Huang, X., Wu, H., Zhao, M., Lu, Q., Israeli, E., & Shoenfeld, Y. (2016). Some like it hot: the emerging role of spicy food (capsaicin) in autoimmune diseases. *Autoimmunity Reviews, 15*(5), 451–456.

Derry, S., & Moore, R. A. (2012). Topical capsaicin (low concentration) for chronic neuropathic pain in adults. *Cochrane Database Systems Review, 12*(9), CD010111.

Diamond, E., Richards, P., & Miller, T. (2006). (760): ALGRX 4975 reduces pain of intermetatarsal neuroma: preliminary results from a randomized, double-blind, placebo-controlled, phase II multicenter clinical trial. *The Journal of Pain, 7*(4), S41.

Dray, A. (1995). Inflammatory mediators of pain. *British Journal of Anaesthesia, 75*(2), 125–131.

Duke, J. A. (2002). *Handbook of medicinal herbs*. New York, Washington, USA: CRC Press.

Fields, H. (2004). State-dependent opioid control of pain. *Nature Reviews Neuroscience, 5*(7), 565–575.

Frerick, H., Keitel, W., Kuhn, U., Schmidt, S., Bredehorst, A., & Kuhlmann, M. (2003). Topical treatment of chronic low back pain with a capsicum plaster. *Pain, 106*(1), 59–64.

Gamse, R., Petsche, U., Lembeck, F., & Jancso, G. (1982). Capsaicin applied to peripheral nerve inhibits axoplasmic transport of substance P and somatostatin. *Brain Research, 239*(2), 447–462.

Govindarajan, V. S., & Salzer, U. J. (1986). Capsicum—Production, technology, chemistry, and quality. Part III. Chemistry of the color, aroma, and pungency stimuli. *Critical Reviews in Food Science and Nutrition, 24*(3), 245–355.

Grichnik, K. P., & Ferrante, F. M. (1991). The difference between acute and chronic pain. *The Mount Sinai Journal of Medicine, New York, 58*(3), 217–220.

Grushka, M., Epstein, J. B., & Gorsky, M. (2002). Burning mouth syndrome. *American Family Physician, 65*(4.).

Hayman, M., & Kam, P. C. (2008). Capsaicin: a review of its pharmacology and clinical applications. *Current Anaesthesia and Critical Care, 19*(5), 338–343.

Henry, J. L. (2008). Pathophysiology of chronic pain. Available from: http://fhs.mcmaster.ca/paininstitute/documents/pathophysiology_of_chronic_pain.pdf

Huang, X. F., Xue, J. Y., Jiang, A. Q., & Zhu, H. L. (2013). Capsaicin and its analogues: structure-activity relationship study. *Current Medicinal Chemistry, 20*(21), 2661–2672.

Ibiza, V. P., Blanca, J., Cañizares, J., & Nuez, F. (2012). Taxonomy and genetic diversity of domesticated Capsicum species in the Andean region. *Genetic Resources and Crop Evolution, 59*(6), 1077–1088.

Irving, G. A., Backonja, M. M., Dunteman, E., Blonsky, E. R., Vanhove, G. F., Lu, S. P., & Tobias, J. (2011). A Multicenter, randomized, double-blind, controlled study of NGX-4010, a high-concentration capsaicin patch, for the treatment of postherpetic neuralgia. *Pain Medicine, 12*(1), 99–109.

Jancsó, G., Kiraly, E., Such, G., Joo, F., & Nagy, A. (1986). Neurotoxic effect of capsaicin in mammals. *Acta Physiologica Hungarica, 69*(3–4), 295–313.

Johansen, J. P., Fields, H. L., & Manning, B. H. (2001). The affective component of pain in rodents: direct evidence for a contribution of the anterior cingulate cortex. *Proceedings of the National Academy of Sciences, 98*(14), 8077–8082.

Kirtikar, K. R., & Basu, B. D. (2005). *Indian Medicinal Plants*. Dehradun: International Book Distributors, pp. 1769–1773.

Kulkantrakorn, K., Lorsuwansiri, C., & Meesawatsom, P. (2013). 0.025% Capsaicin gel for the treatment of painful diabetic neuropathy: a randomized, double-blind, crossover, placebo-controlled trial. *Pain Practice, 13*(6), 497–503.

Laslett, L. L., & Jones, G. (2014). Capsaicin for osteoarthritis pain. In *Capsaicin as a Therapeutic Molecule* (pp. 277–291). Springer Basel.

Levine, J. D., & Alessandri-Haber, N. (2007). TRP channels: targets for the relief of pain. *Biochimica et Biophysica Acta (BBA)-Molecular Basis of Disease, 1772*(8), 989–1003.

Lin, C. H., Lu, W. C., Wang, C. W., Chan, Y. C., & Chen, M. K. (2013). Capsaicin induces cell cycle arrest and apoptosis in human KB cancer cells. *BMC Complementary and Alternative Medicine, 13*(1), 1.

Liu, L., & Simon, S. A. (1996). Capsaicin-induced currents with distinct desensitization and Ca^{2+} dependence in rat trigeminal ganglion cells. *Journal of Neurophysiology, 75*(4), 1503–1514.

Lundberg, J. M. (1996). Pharmacology of cotransmission in the autonomic nervous system: integrative aspects on amines, neuropeptides, adenosine triphosphate, amino acids and nitric oxide. *Pharmacological Reviews, 48*(1), 113–178.

Luongo, L., Costa, B., D'Agostino, B., Guida, F., Comelli, F., Gatta, L., & Maione, S. (2012). Palvanil, a non-pungent capsaicin analogue, inhibits inflammatory and neuropathic pain with little effects on bronchopulmonary function and body temperature. *Pharmacological Research, 66*(3), 243–250.

Maihofner, C., & Heskamp, M. L. (2013). Prospective, non-interventional study on the tolerability and analgesic effectiveness over 12 weeks after a single application of capsaicin 8% cutaneous patch in 1044 patients with peripheral neuropathic pain: first results of the QUEPP study. *Current Medical Research and Opinion, 29*(6), 673–683.

Männikkö, R., Elinder, F., & Larsson, H. P. (2002). Voltage-sensing mechanism is conserved among ion channels gated by opposite voltages. *Nature, 419*(6909), 837–841.

Mantyh, P. W. (1982). Forebrain projections to the periaqueductral gray in the monkey, with observations in the cat and rat. *Journal of Comparative Neurology, 206*(2), 146–158.

Marchand, S. (2008). The physiology of pain mechanisms: from the periphery to the brain. *Rheumatic Disease Clinics of North America, 34*(2), 285–309.

Mayer, E. A., & Saper, C. B. (2000). Pain modulation: expectation, opioid analgesia and virtual pain. *The Biological Basis for Mind Body Interactions, 122*, 245.

McCleane, G. (2000). The analgesic efficacy of topical capsaicin is enhanced by glyceryl trinitrate in painful osteoarthritis: a randomized, double blind, placebo controlled study. *European Journal of Pain, 4*(4), 355–360.

McKenna, D. J., Jones, K., & Hughes, K. (2002). *Botanical medicines: the desk reference for major herbal supplements*. Binghamton, New York, USA: The Haworth Press.

Melzack, R., & Wall, P. D. (1965). Pain mechanisms: a new theory. *Science, 150*(3699), 971–979.

Melzack, R., & Wall, P. D. (1967). Pain mechanisms: a new theory. *Survey of Anesthesiology, 11*(2), 89–90.

Mohapatra, D. P., & Nau, C. (2003). Desensitization of capsaicin-activated currents in the vanilloid receptor TRPV1 is decreased by the cyclic AMP-dependent protein kinase pathway. *Journal of Biological Chemistry, 278*(50), 50080–50090.

Monconduit, L., Bourgeais, L., Bernard, J. F., Le Bars, D., & Villanueva, L. (1999). Ventromedial thalamic neurons convey nociceptive signals from the whole body surface to the dorsolateral neocortex. *The Journal of Neuroscience, 19*(20), 9063–9072.

Montell, C., Birnbaumer, L., & Flockerzi, V. (2002a). The TRP channels, a remarkably functional family. *Cell, 108*(5), 595–598.

Montell, C., Birnbaumer, L., Flockerzi, V., Bindels, R. J., Bruford, E. A., Caterina, M. J., Clapham, D. E., & Kojima, I. (2002b). A unified nomenclature for the superfamily of TRP cation channels. *Molecular Cell, 9*(2), 229–231.

Mori, A., Lehmann, S., O'Kelly, J., Kumagai, T., Desmond, J. C., Pervan, M., & Koeffler, H. P. (2006). Capsaicin, a component of red peppers, inhibits the growth of androgen-independent, p53 mutant prostate cancer cells. *Cancer Research, 66*(6), 3222–3229.

Moscone, E. A., Lambrou, M., Hunziker, A. T., & Ehrendorfer, F. (1993). Giemsa C-banded karyotypes in *Capsicum* (Solanaceae). *Plant Systematics and Evolution, 186*(3–4), 213–229.

Mou, J., Paillard, F., Turnbull, B., Trudeau, J., Stoker, M., & Katz, N. P. (2013). Efficacy of Qutenza®(capsaicin) 8% patch for neuropathic pain: a meta-analysis of the Qutenza Clinical Trials Database. PAIN®. *Pain, 154*(9), 1632–1639.

Mózsik, G., Szolcsányi, J., & Rácz, I. (2005). Gastroprotection induced by capsaicin in healthy human subjects. *World Journal of Gastroenterology: WJG, 11*(33), 5180–5184.

Nadkarni, K. M. (2007). The Indian Materia Medica. Bombay, Popular Prakashan. pp. 579–581.

Nagy, J. I., Iversen, L. L., Goedert, M., Chapman, D., & Hunt, S. P. (1983). Dose-dependent effects of capsaicin on primary sensory neurons in the neonatal rat. *The Journal of Neuroscience, 3*(2), 399–406.

Nicholson, B. (2006). Differential diagnosis: nociceptive and neuropathic pain. *The American Journal of Managed Care, 12*(Suppl. 9), S256–S262.

Nilius, B., Talavera, K., Owsianik, G., Prenen, J., Droogmans, G., & Voets, T. (2005). Gating of TRP channels: a voltage connection? *The Journal of Physiology, 567*(1), 35–44.

Nolano, M., Simone, D. A., Wendelschafer-Crabb, G., Johnson, T., Hazen, E., & Kennedy, W. R. (1999). Topical capsaicin in humans: parallel loss of epidermal nerve fibers and pain sensation. *Pain, 81*(1), 135–145.

Numazaki, M., & Tominaga, M. (2004). Nociception and TRP channels. *Current Drug Targets-CNS and Neurological Disorders, 3*(6), 479–485.

Ossipov, M. H. (2012). The perception and endogenous modulation of pain. *Scientifica,* 2012, 1–25 (Article ID 561761, Hindawi Publishing Corporation).

Parthasarathy, V. A., Chempakam, B., & Zachariah, T. J. (Eds.). (2008). *Chemistry of spices.* CABI.

Patel, N. B. (2010). Physiology of pain, chapter 3. In A. Kopf & N. B. Patel (Eds.), *Guide to pain management in low-resource settings.* Seattle, WA: IASP Press.

Pospisilova, E., & Palecek, J. (2006). Post-operative pain behavior in rats is reduced after single high-concentration capsaicin application. *Pain, 125*(3), 233–243.

Premkumar, L. S., & Ahern, G. P. (2000). Induction of vanilloid receptor channel activity by protein kinase C. *Nature, 408*(6815), 985–990.

Price, D. D. (1999). Psychological mechanisms of pain and analgesia. *Hippocampus, 19,* 893–901.

Purves, D., Augustine, G. J., Fitzpatrick, D., Katz, L. C., LaMantia, A. S., McNamara, J. O., & Williams, S. M. (2001). *Neuroscience.* Sunderland, MA: Sinauer Associates, Inc.

Rainville, P. (2002). Brain mechanisms of pain affect and pain modulation. *Current Opinion in Neurobiology, 12*(2), 195–204.

Raisinghani, M., Pabbidi, R. M., & Premkumar, L. S. (2005). Activation of transient receptor potential vanilloid 1 (TRPV1) by resiniferatoxin. *The Journal of Physiology, 567*(3), 771–786.

Remadevi, R., & Szallisi, A. (2008). Adlea (ALGRX-4975), an injectable capsaicin (TRPV1 receptor agonist) formulation for longlasting pain relief. *IDrugs: the Investigational Drugs Journal, 11*(2), 120–132.

Richardson, J. D. (2000). Cannabinoids modulate pain by multiple mechanisms of action. *The Journal of Pain, 1*(1), 2–14.

Santos, M. M. P., Vieira-da-Motta, O., Vieira, I. J. C., Braz-Filho, R., Gonçalves, P. S., Maria, E. J., & Souza, C. L. M. (2012). Antibacterial activity of *Capsicum annuum* extract and synthetic capsaicinoid derivatives against *Streptococcus* mutans. *Journal of Natural Medicines, 66*(2), 354–356.

Sharma, S. K., Vij, A. S., & Sharma, M. (2013). Mechanisms and clinical uses of capsaicin. *European Journal of Pharmacology, 720*(1), 55–62.

Sikand, P., & Premkumar, L. S. (2007). Potentiation of glutamatergic synaptic transmission by protein kinase C-mediated sensitization of TRPV1 at the first sensory synapse. *The Journal of Physiology, 581*(2), 631–647.

Simone, D. A., Baumann, T. K., & LaMotte, R. H. (1989). Dose-dependent pain and mechanical hyperalgesia in humans after intradermal injection of capsaicin. *Pain, 38*(1), 99–107.

Simpson, D. M., Brown, S., Tobias, J. K., & Vanhove, G. F. NGX-4010 C107 Study Group. (2014). NGX-4010, a capsaicin 8% dermal patch, for the treatment of painful HIV-associated distal sensory polyneuropathy: results of a 52-week open-label study. *The Clinical Journal of Pain, 30*(2), 134–142.

Szallasi, A., & Blumberg, P. M. (1999). Vanilloid (capsaicin) receptors and mechanisms. *Pharmacological Reviews, 51*(2), 159–212.

Szallasi, A., Cortright, D. N., Blum, C. A., & Eid, S. R. (2007). The vanilloid receptor TRPV1: 10 years from channel cloning to antagonist proof-of-concept. *Nature Reviews Drug Discovery, 6*(5), 357–372.

Tarng, D. C., Cho, Y. L., Liu, H. N., & Huang, T. P. (1996). Hemodialysis-related pruritus: a double-blind, placebo-controlled, crossover study of capsaicin 0.025% cream. *Nephron, 72*(4), 617–622.

Tominaga, M. (2007). Nociception and TRP channels. In *Transient Receptor Potential (TRP) Channels* (pp. 489–505). Berlin, Heidelberg: Springer.

Vadivelu, N., Whitney, C. J., & Sinatra, R. S. (2009). Pain pathways and acute pain processing. In R. S. Sinatra, O. A. de Leon-Casasola, E. R. Viscusi, & B. Ginsberg (Eds.), *Acute pain management* (pp. 3–20). New York: Cambridge University Press.

Voets, T., Talavera, K., Owsianik, G., & Nilius, B. (2005). Sensing with TRP channels. *Nature Chemical Biology, 1*(2), 85–92.

Walsh, B. M., & Hoot, S. B. (2001). Phylogenetic relationships of Capsicum (Solanaceae) using DNA sequences from two noncoding regions: the chloroplast atpB-rbcL spacer region and nuclear waxy introns. *International Journal of Plant Sciences, 162*(6), 1409–1418.

Wang, K., Svensson, P., Sessle, B. J., Cairns, B. E., & Arendt-Nielsen, L. (2010). Interactions of glutamate and capsaicin-evoked muscle pain on jaw motor functions of men. *Clinical Neurophysiology, 121*(6), 950–956.

Watson, C. P. N., & Evans, R. J. (1992). The postmastectomy pain syndrome and topical capsaicin: a randomized trial. *Pain, 51*(3), 375–379.

Wesolowska, A., Jadczak, D., & Grzeszczuk, M. (2011). Chemical composition of the pepper fruit extracts of hot cultivars *Capsicum annuum* L. *Acta Scientiarum Polonorum Hortorum Cultus, 10*(1), 171–184.

SECTION C

ROLE OF PAIN: DIET, FOOD AND NUTRITION IN PREVENTION AND TREATMENT

CHAPTER

10

Honey—A Natural Remedy for Pain Relief

N.M. Lazim, A. Baharudin

Department of Otorhinolaryngology, Head and Neck Surgery, School of Medical Sciences, Universiti Sains Malaysia, Kubang Kerian, Kelantan, Malaysia

INTRODUCTION

Honey has been used as food and medicinal products since the ancient time. It is the natural substance produced by the honey bees *Apis mellifera*, from the nectar or blossom or exudates of trees and plants giving nectar honey or honeydew respectively (Suarez, Tullipani, Romadini, Bertoli, & Battino, 2010). As the only available natural sweetener, honey was an important food for *Homo sapiens* from the very beginning. Indeed, the relationship between bees and humans started as early as stone-age. The first written reference to honey was found on a Sumerian tablet dating back 2100–2000 BC, mentioning the use of honey as drugs and ointment. Other documentation on honey also written in many of religious text including the Quran (Taghavizad, 2011). The ancient Egyptians, Greeks, and Romans used honey as a gift to their Gods, as well as an ingredient in the embalming fluid. The great Aristotle had written about the bee as early as in the 4th century BC and in England during the Saxon rule, that honey was used as part of payments from the tenant to the landlords. The archaeologist discovered crystallized honey among the artifacts and furnitures in the Egyptian tomb in the valley of the king's belonging in the 18th century and it is still edible despite the fact that it has crystallized.

Honey contains numerous beneficial nutrients and phytochemicals. It has been extensively used in the traditional folk medicine and apitherapy. Its myriads advantages and benefits have been echoed both by common people and scientists. For a long time in human history it was an important source of carbohydrate and the only widely available natural sweetener. Honey has been used in almost every cultures, civilization, and religion across the globe. The local population in nearly every continents, have used honey in their daily lives either as a medicinal products or it form parts of their supplementary diet. If consumed orally, honey can prevent bacterial infections, reduce ailments, enhance healing, as well as promote body's own physical immunity. It has been shown that honey reduces skin inflammation, edema, and exudation, diminished scar tissues and stimulates tissue regeneration (Molan, 2001). Its medicinal properties also includes as a remedy for burns, cataracts, ulcers, and wound healing. It can alleviate the symptoms of reflux, gastroenteritis, allergies, cold, cellulitis, and many more. Honey contains an array of chemicals which may act alone or in combination in producing the antioxidant, antiinflammatory, antibacterial, and antimutagenic activity. Current research also has focused on the antinociceptive effect of honey. The belief that honey could be used as a nutrient, a drug and an ointment has continued to the present time.

At present, there are wide ranges of honey available globally. Numerous retailed honey, with different brands and different cost available for the people to choose from. This honey differs in its quality according to the geographical distribution and the way they are processed. Different flora and fauna across the continents gives specific unique characters to certain honey. Honey bees (*Apis mellifera*) collect the nectar and pollen from the trees and flowers which then are stored in their hives. Three distinct genetic subspecies of honey bees have been identified which originated from Africa, Eastern Europe, and Western Europe. Some however, believed that the first colony of honey bees originated from Africa. The Chinese is the first who procure the beehives. Most of the honey derived their names from the tree that the honeybees formed their hives. Two well known honey types in New Zealand are manuka (*Leptospermum scoparium*) and kanuka honey (*Kunza ericoides*) (Lu et al., 2013). Manuka honey that was well known in

Nutritional Modulators of Pain in the Aging Population. http://dx.doi.org/10.1016/B978-0-12-805186-3.00010-2
Copyright © 2017 Elsevier Inc. All rights reserved.

New Zealand was found on the manuka trees which are rich at the mountainous area of New Zealand as well as Australia. Other well known types of honey in Australia and New Zealand includes kanuka honey, kamahi, rewarewa, clover (*Trifolium* spp.) and royal jelly. In South East Asia, specifically in Malaysia, Tualang, honey also get its name from a Tualang tree and is becoming popular not only among the locals for its medicinal value but also among clinicians and researchers. These researchers have made multiple publications of Tualang honey highlighting its positive effects and some of which is equivalent to manuka honey of New Zealand. Other honey types include, cedar honey, acacia honey, Jerry bush, Kelulut, and Gelam.

The honey which contains high and potent antibacterial properties has higher market price and is highly sought. The antibacterial property of honey is attributed to the hydrogen peroxide, phenolic acid, high osmolarity, its high viscosity, and nonperoxide components, such as methylglyoxal (Mandal & Mandal, 2011). Since there is a high demand for honey, the adulteration of honey is becoming a major issue to the consumer and the honey producer. It is important to confirm the authenticity of honey as the adulteration of honey has increased dramatically in recent years. Certain honey contains unique chemical components that allows for labelling fingerprinting in order to identify their floral origin. There are several novel and fast methods used for the purpose of authentication of the honey, which includes nuclear magnetic resonance (NMR) spectroscopy (Arvanitoyannis, Chalhoub, Gotsiou, Lydakis-Simantiris, & Kefalas, 2005). The application of high resolution NMR combining with appropriate data processing procedures and multivariate analysis method will aid the development of an effective model for honey adulteration detection (Bertelli et al., 2010). Minerals and trace elements are also useful to determine the botanical origins of the honey. A study by Kato et al. (2016) documented that leptosperin has been specifically identified in manuka honey and this substance is temperature stable which can be used to identify the true types of honey.

Nevertheless, not all honey are safe to consume orally. Some honey may contain hazardous substances for instance metal traces, bacterial spores, and other harmful components. Bad honey intoxication has been documented in the literatures. This is mainly due to a component called grayanatoxin that contains in certain types of honey. A study done by Yaylaci et al. (2015) documented that mad honey consumption can affect the cardiovascular system, as well as the neurological system. Patient may presents with manifestation of bradycardia, hypotension, and atrioventricular block. Chen et al. (2013) also reported a case of mad honey poisoning where a patient presented with signs and symptoms of myocardial infarction with ST elevation on the echocardiogram and it was successfully treated with intravenous atropine. Pesticides can also be found in some honey from certain geographical areas. Several tracers of pesticides can be detected using for instance the spectrometry coupled with liquid or gas chromatography (Souza, Rocha Guidi, de Abreu Gloria, & Fernandes, 2016). The geographical location also determines the safety content of specific honey. A study in Slovakia by Kovacik, Gruz, Biba, and Hedbavny (2016) of three types of honey that originated near an industrial town showed that these types of honey have different concentration of toxic metals. Higher metals are found in the forest honey followed by rapeseed and black locust honey.

Honey Types and its Components

At present, there are numerous types of honey available globally. Different flora gives different types of honey with different composition. Unifloral honey is said to be more valuable than polyfloral honey. Imperatively, this unifloral honey differs in their physical properties based on their geographical distributions. Melissopalynology is the science that studies the quantity and quality of the honey sediments to determine their botanical and geographical origin (Terrab, Gonzale, & Gonzale, 2003). Nowadays, this study is complemented with sensory and physico-chemical analysis and requires a high degree of expertise (Jandric et al., 2015). The physicochemical studies began in 1970 and recently more researches have been performed in order to identify the chemical components of honey, which originated from the nectar or produced by the bees through biochemical transformation of the nectar composition. Examples of such physicochemical parameters include pH, moisture, proline, sugar composition, color properties, and mineral contents. All these informations could be used as a marker for floral origin of honeys (Suarez et al., 2010). Wang and Li (2011) revealed the chemical components and markers of different honey to identify their botanical and biographical origin. These components include the flavanoids, pollen aromatic compounds, oligosaccharide, trace elements, amino acids, and proteins.

Honey is mainly made up of carbohydrates, which constitute about 95% of its dry weight. It is a highly complex mixture of sugars most of which are digestible in the small intestine. The sugar components are mainly monosaccharides, which are fructose and glucose. The nonsugar counterparts of honey are protein, enzymes, amino acids, pollens, pigments, wax, and plant secondary metabolites (Bong, Loomes, Schlothauer, & Stephens, 2016). The flavanoids component in the manuka honey includes pinobanksin, pinocembrin and chrysin, luteolin, quercetin, kaemferol, and galangin. The additional composition of honey includes isomaltose, nigerose, turanose, maltulose, kojibiose, gentibiose, maltotriose, panose, erlose, and many more (Suarez et al., 2010). These are the disaccharides and oligosaccharides or high sugars and are formed during the ripening and storage process with the action of invertase, a bee enzyme. The composition of honey varies according to its source, the harvest season, the plants from which the nectar is gathered and the modalities of honey collection and storage (Werner & Laccourreye, 2011). In general, the dark colored honey is associated with high phenolic content and antioxidant activity.

Manuka honey aka red tea tree is well known in Australia and New Zealand and it is renowned for high antibacterial activity. The other honey that has been recognized in this oceania region are kanuka (*Kunzea ericoides*), clover (*Trifollium* spp.), rata, and kamahi. These four types of honey have different floral origins (Jandric et al., 2015). They have been shown to have multiple valuable properties and advantages both in clinical usage and research purposes. It has potent antibacterial activity, even to the antibiotic resistant bacteria due to its unique properties (Kato et al., 2016). The manuka honey is unique, as it does not depend on the hydrogen peroxide for its antibactericidal activity. In fact, this honey depends on the methylglyoxal which originates from dihydroxyacetone that is present in nectar in manuka flowers (Adams, Manley-Harris, & Molan, 2009).

Acacia honey originates from the black locust tree, which is native to North America and it is also found in Eastern Europe. It has pale color and is slow to crystallize due to high fructose concentration. It has also been shown to contain strong antibacterial and antioxidant properties. It has vitamins, minerals, flavanoids, and phenolic. Majtan, Kumar, Majtan, Walls, and Klaudiny (2010) documented that acacia honey stimulates keratinocytes to produce matrix metallopeptidase-9 (MMP-9), tumor necrosis factor alpha (TNFα), interleukin beta (IL-β), and tumor growth factor beta (TGFβ). It may also have positive effect in combatting neurological diseases and cancers (Muhammad et al., 2016). The rare type of Polish honey includes sour cherry, coriander, thymus, savory, cornflour, and willow honey (Kus, Szweda, Jerkovic, & Tuberoso, 2016). Polish honey like cornflower, thyme, and buckwheats honey have been studied in contrast to the manuka honey and they found that some of the honey has higher antibacterial properties with the most active honey were darker honey with strong yellow color component. Fir honeydew honey contains the flavanoids apigenin and kaemferol, which inhibited TNFα induced production of MMP-9 from keratinocytes (Majtan et al., 2013).

Africa is well known for its floral biodiversity and its honey also has been investigated for its neutracetical properties. These honey ranges from Pincushion honey (unique to Cape Peninsula), Fynbos honey (*Erica* species), and blossoms of *Leucospermum cordifolium* (Basson & Grobler, 2008). Turkish honey also varies which includes chestnut, heather, chaste tree, rhododendron, common eryngo, lavender, Jerusalem tea, astragalaus, clover, and acacia (Can et al., 2015). The dark colored honey, such as the oak, chester, and heather has higher therapeutic potentials. Estevinho, Feas, Seijas, and Vazquez-Tato (2012) studied 75 organic honey sample from a Montes region of Portugal and found that this honey type are free from contaminants like *salmonella* and sulfite reducing *clostridia* and fecal *colliforms*. However, they detect a low account of the yeast and molds. Gomes, Feas, Iglesias, and Estevinho (2011) also studied the northeast Portugal organic honey and documented that the monofloral lavender honey exceeded the international physicochemical standards and showed low microbioligal counts, such as yeast, mould, and aerobics mesophiles. In South East Asia, Malaysian honey is mainly produced by bees, such as *Apis dorsata* and *Apis meliferra*. The honey gets the name from the tree, which houses the hives of the bees, such as Tualang (*Kompasia excelsa*), and Gelam (*Leptospermum flavescens*) or the main source of nectar such as coconut trees (*Cocos nucifera*). Tualang honey has a dark brown apperance and is more acidic than other local Malaysian honeys, such as Kelulut Hitam, Kelulut Putih, and Gelam (Ghazali, 2009). It also contains more flavanoids and phenolic acids than manuka honey and other local Malaysian honeys (Kishor, Halim, Syazana, & Sirajudeen, 2011).

Specific Properties of Honey

The properties of different honeys vary greatly on the particular floral nectar gathered by the honeybees and different proteins secreted from the cephalic glands of the honeybees (Rossano et al., 2012). Honey freshness will depend on the hydroxymethylfurfuraldehyde (HMF) content. HMF is formed by the breakdown of fructose in the presence of an acid. It is derived from furan and contains both aldehyde and alcohol functional groups. It occurs naturally in most honeys and usually increases with duration of storage and heat treatment of honey. The normal range is 2.1–19.8 mg/kg and is influenced by honey quality and the extent of heat processing (Oroian, Paduret, Amariei, & Gutt, 2016). The lower HMF value indicates that the honey is fresh and not subjected to the excessive heating process.

Honey contains protein, enzymes, and amino acids. Different protein content has been reported in honey that originated from different floral sources. The protein content in a specific honey can be measured for example by using electrophoresis. The three main honey enzymes are diastase, invertase, and glucose oxidase with different function and biological activity. Proline is the main amino acid, which constitutes about 50% of the total free amino acids. Besides proline, there are 26 other amino acids with varying concentrations depending on their origin either from nectar or honeydew. In addition, pollen is the main source of honey amino acid (Suarez et al., 2010). Apalbumin I or the major royal jelly (RJ) protein is an authentic and regular component of honey (Bilikova, Kristof Karakova, Yamaguchi, & Yamaguchi, 2015). It is responsible for the immunostimulatory effects and antibacterial properties of honey. Other important contents of honey include vitamins, minerals, and trace element and polyphenolic. The polyphenolic composition of honey is important in determining its basic appearance, functional properties and floral origins. The main ones are benzoic acid, cinnamid acid, and flavanoid (Suarez et al., 2010). Nonaromatic organic acids contributes to <0.5 % of honey constituents and responsible for the organoleptics, physical, and chemical properties of honey (Mato, Huidobro, Simal-Lozano, & Sancho, 2003). At present there are 30 nonaromatic organic acids have been identified and they may have significant role as an antibacterial and antioxidant activity of honey. They also can be used to study the origin of honey.

The rheological properties of honey which includes temperature, chemical composition, water content, and shear rate are also very important determinants of functioning honey. These factors are correlated with its chemical composition thus influence its biological effects. The water content is a quality parameter of honey shelf life. Differences of water content of specific honey affects its degree of viscosity and crystallization. The viscosity of honey decreases exponentially with the increase in the water content.

Medicinal Value of Honey

Honey is not only used as nutrition but also used in wound healing and as an alternative treatment for clinical conditions ranging from gastrointestinal tract (GIT) problems to ophthalmic conditions (Khan, Ul Abadin, & Raufe, 2007). During the early part of 20th century, researchers began to document the wound healing properties of honey. The introduction of antibiotics in 1940, temporarily stymied the use of honey. Nevertheless, concerns regarding antibiotic resistance and renewed interest in natural remedies has promoted a resurgence of interest in antimicrobial and wound healing properties of honey. The properties of honey that make it effective against bacterial growth are (1) high sugar content, (2) low moisture content, (3) gluconic acid that creates an acidic environment, and (4) hydrogen peroxide. Another effect of honey on wounds that has been noted is that it reduces inflammation, hastens subsidence of passive hyperaemia, and also reduces oedema (Khan et al., 2007).

Many studies have shown that honey is an effective broad-spectrum antibacterial agent. Honey antimicrobial action explains the external and internal uses of honey. Honey has been used to treat adult and neonatal postoperative infection, burns, necrotizing fasciitis, infected and nonhealing wounds and ulcers, boils, pilonidal sinus, venous ulcers, and diabetic foot ulcers (Al-Waili, Salom, Butler, & Al Ghamdi, 2011). These effects are ascribed to honey's antibacterial action, which is due to acidity, hydrogen peroxide content, osmotic effect, nutritional and antioxidants content, stimulation of immunity, and to unidentified compounds. When ingested, honey also promotes healing and shows antibacterial action by decreasing prostaglandin levels, elevating nitric oxide levels, and exerting prebiotic effects. Prostaglandins are mediators of inflammation and pain. Honey decreased plasma prostaglandins concentrations in healthy individuals. Its inhibitory effect was increased with time. The site of actions could be at cyclooxygenase-1 or -2 or both. The inhibition of prostaglandins by honey therefore might reduce edema and inflammation (Al-Waili et al., 2011). These factors play major role in controlling inflammation and promoting healing processes and pain relief. Its effect on inflammation, wound healing and antibacterial activity will help in our understanding of its role on pain relief.

Antibacterial and Antiinflammatory Effects of Honey

Antibacterial properties of honey is contributed by numerous factors namely the acidity, high osmotic pressure, presence of lysozymes, polyphenols, phenolic acids, flavanoids, and the recently identified methylgloxal. The pH of honey has been documented in a range of 6–7. Honey low pH can enhance offloading oxygen from hemoglobin in the capillaries. This provides more oxygenation to the tissues. This acidification of wounds ultimately promotes healing. In addition, the acidity also suppresses the protease activity in wounds. Increase of protease in wounds can either slow or stop healing by destroying the growth factors and the protein fiber and fibronectin in wound, which is necessary for the activation of fibroblast and migration of epithelial cells. The water content and the acidity of honey also differ and contributes to its antibacterial effect.

Hydrogen peroxide content is vital in determining the antibacterial effect of honey. It is made naturally in honey by the presence of an enzyme, glucose oxidase. Glucose oxidase is added to the nectar by the bees so as to prevent spoilage of unripe honey. During honey ripening, glucose oxidase is inactivated but it regains activity upon dilution of honey. However, other components have also been identified contributing to the antibacterial of honey, which are methylglyoxal and bee-defensin-1 (Kwakman & Zaat, 2012). Methylglyoxal is a nonperoxide components and possesses strong antibactericidal activity. It exists as reagent and can be added to honey to enrich its antibactericidal effects (Kato et al., 2016). Manuka honey contains high methylglyoxal components. This methylglyoxal may interact with apalbumin and mediate immunostimulation which results in antiinflammation and antibacterial of honey.

Despite recent advances in antimicrobial chemotherapy and burn wound management, infection continues to be an important problem in the treatment of burns. A variety of topical agents, such as silver sulphadiazine, silver nitrate, and sulphamylon, as well as systemic agents, such as penicillins, monobactams, cephalosporins, and aminoglycosides, also have been used, but none has completely eliminated the problem of infection. Honey is the most famous rediscovered remedy that has been used to promote wound and burn healing and also to treat infected wounds. The antimicrobial activity of bee honey has been attributed to several properties of honey, including its osmotic effect, its naturally low pH, and the production of hydrogen peroxide, and also the presence of phenolic acids, lysozyme, and flavanoids. Honey also has been shown to have more inhibitory effect (85.7%) on isolated Gram-negative bacteria (*Pseudomonas aeruginosa*, *Enterobacter* spp., and *Klebsiella*) than commonly used antibiotics (Abd-El Aal, El-Hadidy, El-Mashad, & El-Sebaie, 2007). In addition, it also possesses an inhibitory effect on all methicillin-resistant *Staphylococcus aureus* (100%). A synergistic effect of honey was observed when it was added to antibiotics for Gram-negative bacteria and also for coagulase-positive Staphylococci. Nitric oxide and prostaglandin might also explain some of the activities promoted by honey. Honey combats bacteria by direct and indirect action. Direct action is based on direct inhibition or killing of bacteria by specific honey components, and indirect action honey induces the antibacterial reaction of the whole organism toward bacteria (Al-Waili et al., 2011).

Honey has an antioxidant, antibacterial, and antiinflammatory properties. It can be used as a wound dressing to promote rapid and improved healing. These effects are due to honey's antibacterial action, secondary to its high acidity, osmotic effect, antioxidant content, and hydrogen peroxide content. The use of honey leads to improved wound healing in acute cases, pain relief in burn patients and decreased inflammatory response in such patients (Yaghoobi, Kazerouni, & Kazerouni, 2013). The antiinflammatory effect has been observed by microscopic examination of wound tissues after applying honey on wounds in animal models (reduction in the number of white blood cells was observed). Therefore, the antiinflammatory action of honey reduces edema and exudates, which can subsequently improve wound healing. This effect also reduces pain caused by pressure on nerve endings and reduces the amount of prostaglandin produced in inflammatory process. The antiinflammatory effects of honey have been observed in animal models, as well as in clinical settings. The evidence from animal studies may be more convincing. Animals do not show placebo effect and are free from bias as they are incapable of having behavioral influences on the healing process. Honey's antiinflammatory action and stimulatory effects on granulation and epithelialisation, help in rapidly reducing pain and edema (Yaghoobi et al., 2013).

Honey Wound Healing Property

The numerous components in honey may interact in a complex way in producing and promoting wound-healing process. The phenolic and flavanoids are equally important bioactive ingredients and play significant roles. Honey is hygroscopic and is used as an effective wound dressing in cases of burns, diabetic foot, postsurgical open wounds with encouraging results. It provides rapid autolytic debridement and wound deodorization which ultimately enhances healing process. Numerous researches have also indicated that honey possess strong antiinflammatory activity and stimulate immune responses within a wound. This leads to reduce infection rate and enhances wound healing in burns, ulcers, and other cutaneous wounds (Lusby, Coombes, & Wilkinson, 2002). Efem, Udoh, and Iwara (1992) observed that unhealed wound that failed conventional medical treatment responded well with the topical application of honey. Wounds that were sterile at the outset remained sterile until healed, while infected wounds and ulcer became sterile within 1 week of topical application of honey. Imperatively, honey debrided wounds rapidly, replacing sloughs with granulation tissue. In addition, it also promoted rapid epithelialization and absorption of oedema from around the ulcer margins. A study by Mat Lazim, Abdullah, and Salim (2013) documented that application of Tualang honey to the tonsillar fossa, as well as oral consumption of honey for 7 days following tonsillectomy enhances the healing process significantly. The group who received Tualang honey displayed accelerated reepithelialization of the tonsillar fossa compared to the control group.

Clinical observations indicate that honey may initiate or accelerate the healing of chronic wounds (Tonks et al., 2003). The three phases of wound healing are classically defined as inflammatory, proliferative, and remodeling. The richest amount of data demonstrates the ability of honey to modulate the inflammatory phase. Initially, it was shown that honey had antiinflammatory properties in guinea pigs. Additionally, it has been shown that honey improves tissue granulation and epithelialisation in the proliferative phase while decreasing total wound healing time (Lee, Sinno, & Khachemoune, 2011).

Immunomodulation Effects of Honey

Certain components of honey have been proven to possess strong immunomodulation effects. Apisimin is protein secreted from the hypopharyngeal and mandibular glands of the honeybees. It may have immunostimulatory effects by stimulating the release of TNFα from the monocytes. Arabinogalactan proteins (AGPs) on the other hand are also immunostimulatory and derived from the plants. It has been documented to exist in the majority of the New Zealand honey, which include manuka, kanuka, kowhai, and clover honey. Gannabathula, Krissansen, Skinner, Steinhorn, and Schlothauer (2015) documented that both apisimin and AGPs have the ability to enhance the stimulation of monocytes in producing TNFα. The other component in honey that may possess the immunostimulatory effects is apalbumins. All these three components may act synergistically in promoting release of TNFα and mediate the immunostimulation. TNFα has a vital role in sustaining the inflammatory response and results in overall antimicrobial and enhance wound healing.

Honey and its components are able to either stimulate or inhibit the release of certain cytokines for instance, TNFα, IL-1β, and IL-6 from human monocytes and macrophages, depending on the wound condition. Similarly, honey will either reduce or activate the production of reactive oxygen species from neutrophils, which also depends on the wound microenvironment. The honey-induced activation of both types of immune cells could promote debridement of a wound and speed up the repair process. Similarly, human keratinocytes, fibroblasts, and endothelial cell responses (e.g., cell migration and proliferation, collagen matrix production, chemotaxis) are positively affected in the presence of honey. Thus, honey may accelerate reepithelialization and wound closure. The immunomodulatory activity of honey is highly complex because of the involvement of multiple quantitatively variable compounds among honey of different origins. The identification of these individual compounds and their contributions to wound healing is crucial for a better understanding of the mechanisms behind honey-mediated healing of chronic wounds (Majtan, 2014).

Antinociceptive Effects of Honey

At present there are not many studies conducted to elucidate the effects of honey on pain. The documentation on the details mechanism of how honey may reduce pain is also scarce. Nevertheless, several biomarkers identified in honey may contribute to its antinociceptive effects. These biomarkers also potentiate the immunomodulation effects of honey. Such biomarkers include cytokines, TNFα, histamine, and nitrous oxide. These substances have been identified in the majority of honey and may play significant role in pain mediation. The mechanisms of immunomodulation and antiinflammatory of honey are complex process with the involvement of numerous bioactive components and overlapped functional activities. It involves the interplay of numerous protein and nonprotein factors which possess a pro- or antiinflammatory actions.

Pain is generated by multiple ways either by central mechanism or peripheral mechanism. Peripheral nociceptors are sensitized during inflammation and peripheral nerve fibers developed discharges during any nerve injury or with presence of any diseases. Consequently a complex neuronal response is evoked in the spinal cord where neurons becomes hyperexcitable and thus new balance is set between the excitation and the inhibition. Most of the nociceptors respond to noxious mechanical, thermal, and chemical stimuli. This pain will be conveyed through the pain fibers into the spinal cord.

Pain Relief in Postoperative Patients

Many studies have shown that honey has the ability to influence biological systems including pain transmission. The mechanism involves autonomic receptors in the antinociceptive and antiinflammatory effects of honey although the level of involvement depends on the different types of the receptors (Owoyele, Oladejo, Ajomale, Ahmed, & Mustapha, 2014). In addition, honey could decrease prostaglandin ADI3E2, prostaglandin alpha 2, and thromboxane B2 in blood and hence contributes to pain relief (Amani, Kheiri, & Ahmadi, 2015).

Tonsillectomy is one of the most common surgeries in the world and the most common problem is posttonsillectomy pain and bleeding. Pain following tonsillectomy is mainly the result of the disruption of the mucosa and irritation of open nerve endings of the glossopharyngeal and vagus nerves, as well as of spasms of the exposed pharyngeal and palatal muscles due to mechanical or thermal damage to the surrounding tissue. Oral flora may also increase throat pain by inducing inflammation and infection (Hwang, Song, Jheong, Lee, & Kang, 2014). The relief of postoperative pain helps increase early food intake and prevent secondary dehydration. Furthermore, postoperative pain and wound healing following tonsillectomy can result in dissatisfaction for the patient (Hwang et al., 2014).

Several different treatment techniques have been developed for use during and after surgery, including steroids, analgesics, antibiotics, and antinausea medications, and have been shown to have some positive outcomes in randomized trials. Injection of epinephrine and bupivacaine into the peritonsillar region had also been done and reported to have variable outcomes (Bameshki, Razban, Khadivi, Razavi, & Bakhshaee, 2013). Considering the inconsistent results of previous studies and the low cost of honey, many studies had been done to determine the effect of honey on decreasing pain and bleeding after tonsillectomy.

A study by Ozlugedik et al. (2006) demonstrated that oral administration of honey following pediatric tonsillectomy can relieve postoperative pain and decrease the need for analgesics in first 2 days after surgery. Another study conducted by Boroumand et al. (2013) has shown that the patients who received acetaminophen plus honey versus control group (who received only acetaminophen), had significantly less pain severity and analgesic consumption within the first 3 postoperative days. They recruited 104 patients, who were older than 8, and were scheduled for tonsillectomy, were divided into two equal groups, honey and placebo. Standardized general anesthesia, and postoperative usual analgesic, and antibiotic regimen were administrated for all patients. Acetaminophen plus honey for the honey group, and acetaminophen plus placebo for the placebo group were given daily. They began to receive honey or placebo when the patients established oral intake. The difference between acetaminophen and acetaminophen plus honey groups was statistically significant both for visual analogue scale (VAS), and number of painkillers taken within the first 3 postoperative days (Boroumand et al., 2013).

Many researches have been performed to investigate different analgesics' effects on post tonsillectomy pain, especially together with acetaminophen. In many studies, relief of early postoperative pain, in first hours of operation, was investigated. On the other hand, many studies look into postoperative pain after recovery room (Boroumand et al., 2013). In a study by Salonen, Kokki, and Nuutinen (2002) it was shown that ketoprofen combined with paracetamol–codeine seems to provide sufficient analgesia during the first 10 days after surgery. A systematic review by Hamunen and Kontinen (2005) revealed that no analgesic in single prophylactic dosage is enough to provide analgesia during the day of operation, thus, repeated administration, and also in combination with NSAIDS, and titrated opioids are needed to reach optimal result, and guarantee freedom from pain. It also recommended the use of oral acetaminophen rather than rectal form. In a study by Ozlugedik et al. (2006) the post tonsillectomy effect of honey in pain killing was surveyed for 14 days, and it was reported that pain scores in first 2 days after the operation were significantly less in honey group, compared to Boroumand et al. (2013) study which shows this difference from the first to the third day after tonsillectomy. They also reported the reduction in taking analgesics from the first to 8th day post tonsillectomy. Similarly, Boroumand et al. (2013) study shows significant difference of using analgesics in all 5 days of study and by using honey, the need for using analgesics decreased. All these studies showed that oral administration of honey after wake up, following tonsillectomy or adenotonsillectomy can reduce postoperative pain in pediatric patients, and may substantially decrease the need for analgesics.

A metaanalysis was further done by Hwang et al. (2014) to determine the role of honey in postoperative pain relief. Studies comparing postoperative oral administration of honey with administration of placebo where the outcomes of interest were pain and wound healing on postoperative days were included. Baseline study characteristics, study quality, numbers of patients in steroid-treated and control groups, and treatment outcomes were extracted. Sufficient data for metaanalysis were retrieved from 4 trials with a total of 264 patients. Patient-reported pain scores and quantities of administered analgesics during the first 5 postoperative days were analyzed. The pain score was significantly decreased in the honey-treated patients in comparison with the placebo-treated patients on postoperative day 1 only, but the analgesic intake of the honey-treated patients on the first 5 postoperative days was significantly less than that of the placebo-treated patients. In addition, honey significantly increased tonsillectomy bed wound healing in comparison with placebo during the first 2 weeks after surgery. This meta-analysis shows that postoperative administration of honey after tonsillectomy significantly reduces pain and promotes wound healing.

Pain following tonsillectomy is caused by postoperative inflammation, nerve irritation, and pharyngeal spasm. It is considered that the tonsillary fossa is healed in the form of an open wound after tonsillectomy. Therefore, it could be expected that honey accelerates the recovery of wounds and decreases postoperative pain. However, it is not possible to keep honey in continuous contact with the tonsillary fossa as it is a wound dressing. As a result, some studies proposed that oral administration of honey in wound healing is much more effective than topical application (Amani et al., 2015). Abdullah, Lazim, and Salim (2015) evaluated the effect of Tualang honey on post tonsillectomy pain by assessing the pain score, frequency of awakening at night and additional analgesia requirement from postoperative first to 7th day. Pain was assessed using ten points of visual analog score (VAS) for children of more than 7 years and facial pain scale for patients less than 7 years old. The assessment was done and documented by their parents. Patients were randomized into two groups. Treatment group received topical Tualang honey intraoperatively followed by oral consumption of Tualang honey three times daily for seven days with intravenous sultamicillin 3 times daily for first and second day followed by oral sultamicillin twice daily for 5 days. Control group received intravenous sultamicillin for 2 days followed by oral sultamicillin twice daily for 5 days. The results showed that there is no significant difference in post tonsillectomy pain between the two study groups. However, in Tualang honey-antibiotic group, the score was less than the antibiotic only group since postoperative day 1. The total pain score reduced gradually from day 1 to day 7 postoperatively in both groups. The antibiotic only group exhibits much higher score at early postoperative periods. It was postulated that this could be due to the soothing effects of topical application of honey intra operatively. By day 6–7 postoperatively, all pain score was zero in both groups, which could be explained by healing of tonsillar fossae with time.

Pain Relief in Radiation Induced Mucositis

Radiation-induced mucositis and associated pain are the major and most important causes of morbidity and treatment gaps during the standard management. Pain imparts additional morbidity and economic burden to patients in the form of requiring parenteral analgesia, interruption of radiation therapy (RT) and/or hospitalization, parenteral, or tube feeding, all of which have a negative impact on quality of life. There are various drugs tried for prevention and treatment of pain, but none have achieved satisfactory level. Topical application of honey to the oral cavity and pharynx results in reduction of pain to significantly low levels resulting in lesser analgesic use, treatment gaps, and weight loss hence overall improving their compliance and tolerability toward radiation schedule. This has helped in completing the radiation treatment protocol within the stipulated time period, hence causing the maximum possible effect achieved by RT on the tumor. Prophylaxis and management of radiation-induced mucositis by honey has been studied in the past in phase-II randomized controlled trials, and it has shown encouraging results (Samdariya, Lewis, Kauser, Ahmed, & Kumar, 2015).

A metaanalysis study of honey to determine its efficacy in the management of oral mucositis during radiotherapy in patients with head and neck cancer had been done (Cho, Jeong, Lee, Lee, & Hwang, 2015). Nine studies comprising 476 patients were included in the metaanalysis. The incidence of moderate to severe mucositis and the mean mucositis grade during the first 3 weeks of therapy were significantly lower in the honey group than the control group. Additionally, the onset of mucositis was significantly later in the honey group than the control. Although there were no significant differences in the incidences of microbial colonization and pain experienced between the two groups, the incidence of weight loss was significantly lower in the honey group than control group. The metaanalysis showed that oral administration of honey after radiotherapy could prevent moderate to severe mucositis and associated weight loss (Cho et al., 2015).

The philosophy of using honey in radiation mucositis was derived from basic research and clinical observation of rapid epithelialization in tissue injuries. Coating a wound with honey retards tissue oxygenation by sealing the damaged mucosa from air (oxygen). This could dampen pain within 30 s after application. Important factors that influence the effectiveness of honey are its hygroscopic nature, acidic pH prevents bacteria growth when applied to the mucosa, inhibin (hydrogen peroxide) converted from glucose oxydase and gluconic acid, enzymes (growth factors) and tissue-nutritive minerals and vitamins help repair tissue directly. In addition, the reduction of radiation-induced mucositis in honey-treated patients might be due to the bacteriostatic effect of viscid honey (Jayachandran & Balaji, 2012).

Mechanisms of Pain Relief

Honey stimulates an array of antiinflammatory factors from the monocytes and macrophages that includes prostaglandin E2, cytokines, such as interleukin (IL)-10, interleukins-1, transforming growth factor β and so forth. Several of these markers may have direct or indirect effect on the pain pathway and contributes to the antinociceptive effect of honey. The known mediators for pain are prostaglandin, serotonin, histamine, thromboxane, bradykinin, and substance P. Additional mediators include cytokines complement 3a and 5a, platelet activating factor, neutrophil chemotactic factor, fibrinopeptides, and leukotrienes. These mediators like cytokines IL-6, IL-IB, IL-10, tumor necrosis factor alfa and angiogenic factors like VEGF and FGF2 may also be involved in the generation of pain (Lipnik-Stangelj, 2013). There might be several pathways for the pain relief:

Opioid Receptor Activation

Opioid system are vital in the modulation of pain perception and nociception. Generally, there are four types of opiod receptors that are mu (μ), kappa (κ), delta and opiod receptor like 1 (orl-1). The μ receptors are the most important clinically and has been extensively studied in relation to the development of analgesia (Pasternak & Pan, 2011). This opioid systems, can be activated or inhibited either by endogenous or exogenous opioid peptides. Opioids can directly bind to presynaptic μ-opioid receptors causing inhibition of pain transmission via the 1st order (afferent sensory) nerve fibers entering the spinal cord. In addition, the opioid indirectly inhibit the second order ascending neurons within the spinal cord by modulating the release of serotonin

(5-HT) and substance P from the activated descending nerve fibers within the medulla that control endorphin containing neurons within the dorsal horn. The net effect of the direct and indirect effects of opioids on the nerve within the dorsal horn is inhibition of pain transmission to the brain and a decrease in the pain perception and experiences by patient.

Thromboxane and prostaglandin are the major players in the pain pathway. They are called prostanoids generated from arachidonic acid. They also are proinflammatory mediators. Their biosyntesis is blocked by analgesic for example the NSAIDs. The metabolism of arachidonic acid through the cyclo-oxygenase pathway (COX) results in numerous prostaglandins and thromboxanes. Certain prostaglandins may have different effect on different tissues and its action also depends on the availability and activation of specific receptors. Prostaglandin E2 (PGE2) can either be a proinflammatory or antiinflammatory. In low dose PGE2 is responsible for the experience of pain where it acts at the prostaglandin E3 (EP3) receptor types. Hyperalgesia is however attributed to the prostaglandin E1 (EP1) receptor signaling in the peripheral sensory nerves system, as well as in central nervous system. The level of prostaglandin and the degree of sensitization of these receptors will determine the pain experienced by the patients.

Honey has been shown to have effects on the thromboxane and the prostaglandin levels both in the human and animal models. Al-Waili and Boni (2003) documented in their study that the plasma concentration of thromboxane was reduced by 7, 34, and 35% and that of PGE2 by 14, 10, and 19% at 1, 2, and 3 h respectively after ingestion of 70 g of honey. This is a strong finding that justifies the antinociceptive effect of honey. Honey may have exert direct effects on the prostaglandin concentration in the blood or affects its receptor binding afinity.

Anti Inflammatory Mediators

Other possible explaination for the antinociceptive effects of honey is that it has been shown that it reduces the inflammatory mediators, such as the nitrous oxide, the histamines and TNFα. Nitrous oxide (NO) plays important role in mediating pain and this marker has been identified as a good target for pain management. It is a well-known analgesic used in labou pain. In addition, nitrous oxide and reactive nitrogen oxide species are involved in the perception and reduction of pain for instance in osteoarthritic pain (Abramson, 2008). Janicki and Jeske-Janicka (1998) documented that the NO are responsible for generation of pain throughout the central and peripheral nervous system, perivascular tissue, and peripheral nerve terminals. This NO may also be involved in the analgesic activity of the nonsteroidal antiinflammatory drugs (NSAIDs), opioids and other local anesthetics. Hamza et al. (2010) demonstrated that even though NO may have pronociception and antinociception, it may however, have the analgesic effect in the early stage of inflammation. Kassim, Achoui, Mansor, and Yusoff (2010) demonstrated on the animal model that *Gelam* honey has an inhibitory effects on the nitrous oxide and the prostaglandin E2 thereby reducing pain and oedema in the inflammatory tissues. Aziz, Ismail, Hussin, and Mohamad (2014) stated that phenolic and flavanoids compounds in Tualang honey contributes to its antioxidant activity and might have a role in its antinociceptive effects. Other research however, highlight that honey increases the nitrous oxide in the body, hence contributing to the reduction of pain perception by patient.

Autonomic Receptor Activation

Latest evidence from the literatures documented that the role of autonomic receptor regulations are involved in mediating the pain. In normal individual, activation of the sympathetic nervous system in the brain suppresses pain by inhibiting the nociceptive transmission in the spinal cord. Honey may exert direct effects on the symphathetic nervous system thereby reducing the pain perception. In addition, it may stimulate the production of certain bioactive substance that potentially enhances the sympathetic activity.

This is supported by Owoyele, Oladejo, Ajomale, Ahmed, and Mustapha (2014) in their animal studies that demonstrate honey may reduce pain perception by incorporating activity that reduce pain as shown by procedures of stellate ganglion block and lumbar symphatectomy. This autonomic receptor may also mediate the visceral pain. Sympathectomy or symphatetic nerve block for instance lessen the pain experienced by patients. However, even subtle changes in pathophysiology can dramatically change the effect of sympathethic nervous system on pain and vice versa (Schlereth & Birklein, 2008).

Central Pathway Mechanism

Beretta, Caneva, and Facino (2007) documented that the substance in honey may act in combination with flavanoids which is a COX2 inhibitor, thereby antagonizing the NMDA receptor which in parts play a role in mediating the pain. NMDA receptor is a glutamate receptor, which is a major excitatory neurotransmitter in the central nervous system (Vyklicky et al., 2013). This NMDA receptor activity can be modulated both positively and negatively. Lipnik-Stangelj (2013) also documented that activation of the *N*-methyl-D-aspartate (NMDA) receptors lead to hyperalgaesia. It may be also associated with neuropathic pain and reduced functionality of opioid receptors (Gustin et al., 2010). Petrenko, Yamakura, Baba, and Shimoji (2003) stated that the NMDA receptors may also mediate peripheral sensitization and visceral pain.

There are multiple NMDA receptor subtypes namely NR1, NR2 (A, B, C, and D), and NR3 (A and B) of which NR2B is important for nociception.

Aziz et al. (2014) has investigated the role of the Tualang honey as a nociception in the male rat. They divided the subjects into five groups where they received either distilled water as a placebo, prednisolone, and honey. They concluded that the Tualang honey has an antinoceptive property. This is attributed to the antioxidant, the vitamin C that may have a role in mediating the level of glutamate receptors in the central nervous system. Tualang honey also contains flavanoids and other polyphenolic acids, which may act synergistically to reduce pain. Mohamad Zaid, Kassim, and Othman (2015) highlighted that Tualang honey contains high total phenolic compounds namely gallic, syringic, benzoic, *trans*-cinnamic, p-coumaric, and caffeic acids, as well as flavanoids like catechin, kaempferol, naringenin, luteolin, and apigenin. Manuka honey has rich antioxidant activity that is based on the iron binding capacity and free radical scavenging systems. Each of this phytochemical may directly or indirectly involve in modulating pain transmission at the central level.

CONCLUSIONS

In this age of health concern and optimization of medical resources, the research and development of effective and inexpensive treatments constitute a major concern for all clinicians. Medical practitioners have become increasingly concerned about adequate pain management because of the increasing number of complex outpatient procedures and ambulatory surgeries. Therefore, the therapeutic use of honey for wound healing, anti inflammation and pain relief provides a real medical benefit.

References

Abd-El Aal, A. M., El-Hadidy, M. R., El-Mashad, N. B., & El-Sebaie, A. H. (2007). Antimicrobial effect of bee honey in comparison to antibiotics on organisms isolated from infected burns. *Annals Burns Fire Disasters*, *20*(2), 83–88.

Abdullah, B., Lazim, N. M., & Salim, R. (2015). The effectiveness of Tualang honey in reducing post tonsillectomy pain. *Kulak Burun Bogaz Ihtis Derg*, *25*(3), 137–143.

Abramson, S. B. (2008). Nitric oxide in inflammation and pain associated with osteoarthritis. *Arthritis Research Therapy*, *10*, S2.

Adams, C. J., Manley-Harris, M., & Molan, P. C. (2009). The origin of methylglyoxal in New Zealand Manuka (*Leptospermum scoparium*) honey. *Carbohydrate Research*, *344*, 1050–1053.

Al-Waili, N. S., & Boni, N. S. (2003). Natural honey lowers plasma prostaglandin concentration in normal individuals. *Journal of Medcinal Food*, *6*, 129–133.

Al-Waili, N. S., Salom, K., Butler, G., & Al Ghamdi, A. A. (2011). Honey and microbial infections: a review supporting the use of honey for microbial control. *Journal of Medicinal Food*, *14*(10), 1079–1096.

Amani, S., Kheiri, S., & Ahmadi, A. (2015). Honey versus diphenhydramine for post tonsillectomy pain relief in paediatric cases: a randomized clinical trial. *Journal of Clinical Diagnostic Research*, *9*(3), SC01–SC04.

Arvanitoyannis, I. S., Chalhoub, C., Gotsiou, P., Lydakis-Simantiris, N., & Kefalas, P. (2005). Novel quality control methods in conjunction with chemometrics (multivariate analysis) for detecting honey authenticity. *Critical Reviews in Food Science and Nutrition*, *45*(3), 193–203.

Aziz, C. B., Ismail, C. A., Hussin, C. M., & Mohamad, M. (2014). The antinociceptive effect of tualang honey in male Sprague-Dawley rats: a preliminary study. *Journal of Traditional and Complementary Medicine*, *4*(4), 298–302.

Bameshki, A. R., Razban, M., Khadivi, E., Razavi, M., & Bakhshaee, M. (2013). The effect of local injection of epinephrine and bupivacaine on post-tonsillectomy pain and bleeding. *Iranian Journal of Otorhinolaryngology*, *25*(73), 209–214.

Basson, N. J., & Grobler, S. R. (2008). Antimicrobial activity of two South African honeys produced from indigenous *Leucospermum cordifolium* and *Erica* species on selected micro-organisms. *BMC Complementary and Alternative Medicine*, *8*, 41.

Beretta, G., Caneva, E., & Facino, R. M. (2007). Kynurenic acid in honey from arboreal plants: MS and NMR evidence. *Planta Medica*, *73*(15), 1592–1595.

Bertelli, D., Lolli, M., Papotti, G., Bortolotti, L., Serra, G., & Plessi, M. (2010). Detection of honey adulteration by sugar syrups using one dimensional and two-dimensional high-resolution nuclear magnetic resonance. *J of Agricultural Food Chemistry*, *58*(15), 8495–8501.

Bilikova, K., Kristof Krakova, T., Yamaguchi, K., & Yamaguchi, Y. (2015). Major royal jelly proteins as markers of authenticity and quality of honey/Glavni proteini matične mliječi kao markeri izvornosti i kakvoće meda. *Arhiv za Higijenu Rada i Toksikologiju*, *66*(4), 259–267.

Bong, J., Loomes, K. M., Schlothauer, R. C., & Stephens, J. M. (2016). Fluorescence markers in some New Zealand honeys. *Food Chemistry*, *192*, 1006–1014.

Boroumand, P., Zamani, M. M., Saeedi, M., Rouhbakhshfar, O., Hosseini Motlaqh, S. R., & Aarabi Moghaddam, F. (2013). Post tonsillectomy pain: can honey reduce the analgesic requirements? *Anaesthesiology Pain Medicine*, *3*(1), 198–202.

Can, Z., Yildiz, O., Sahin, H., Turumtay, E. A., Silici, S., & Kolayli, S. (2015). An investigation of Turkish honeys: their physico-chemical properties, antioxidant capacities and phenolic profiles. *Food Chemistry*, *180*, 133–141.

Chen, S. P. L., Lam, Y. H., Ng, V. C. H., Lau, F. L., Sze, Y. C., Chan, W. T., & Mak, T. W. L. (2013). Mad honey poisoning mimicking acute myocardial infarction. *Hong Kong Medical Journal*, *19*(4), 354–356.

Cho, H. K., Jeong, Y. M., Lee, H. S., Lee, Y. J., & Hwang, S. H. (2015). Effects of honey on oral mucositis in patients with head and neck cancer: a metaanalysis. *Laryngoscope*, *125*(9), 2085–2092.

Efem, S. E., Udoh, K. T., & Iwara, C. I. (1992). The antimicrobial spectrum of honey and its clinical significance. *Infection*, *20*(4), 227–229.

Estevinho, L. M., Feas, X., Seijas, J. A., & Vazquez-Tato, P. M. (2012). Organic honey from Tras-OS-Montes region (Portugal): chemical, palynological, microbiological, and bioactive compounds characterization. *Food and Chemical Toxicology*, *50*(2), 258–264.

Gannabathula, S., Krissansen, G. W., Skinner, M., Steinhorn, G., & Schlothauer, H. (2015). Honeybee apisimin and plant arabinogalactanin honey costimulate monocytes. *Food Chemistry*, *168*, 34–40.

Ghazali, F. C. (2009). Morphological characterization study of Malaysian honey-AVPSEM, EDX randomised attempt. *Annals of Microscopy*, *9*, 93–102.

Gomes, T., Feas, X., Iglesias, A., & Estevinho, L. M. (2011). Study of organic honey from the Northeast Portugal. *Molecules*, *16*(7), 5374–5386.

Gustin, S. M., Schwarz, A., Birbaumer, N., Sines, N., Schmidt, A. C., Veit, R., Larbig, W., Flor, H., & Lotze, M. (2010). NMDA receptor antagonist and morphine decrease CRPS-pain and cerebral pain representation. *Pain, 151*(1), 69–76.

Hamunen, K., & Kontinen, V. (2005). Systematic review on analgesics given for pain following tonsillectomy in children. *Pain, 117*(1–2), 40–50.

Hamza, M., Wang, X. M., Wu, T., Brahim, J. S., Rowan, J. S., & Dionne, R. A. (2010). Nitric oxide is negatively correlated to pain during acute inflammation. *Molecular Pain, 6*, 55.

Hwang, S. H., Song, J. N., Jeong, Y. M., Lee, Y. J., & Kang, J. M. (2014). The efficacy of honey for ameliorating pain after tonsillectomy: a meta-analysis. *European Archives of Otorhinolaryngology, 273*(4), 811–818.

Jandric, Z., Haughey, S. A., Frew, R. D., McComb, K., Galvin-King, P., Elliot, C. T., & Cannavan, A. (2015). Discrimination of honey of different floral origins by a combination of various chemical parameters. *Food Chemistry, 189*, 52–59.

Janicki, P. K., & Jeske-Janicka, M. (1998). Relevance of nitric oxide in pain mechanisms and pain management. *Current Review of Pain, 2*(4), 211–216.

Jayachandran, S., & Balaji, N. (2012). Evaluating the effectiveness of topical application of natural honey and benzydamine hydrochloride in the management of radiation mucositis. *Indian Journal of Palliative Care, 18*(3), 190–195.

Kassim, M., Achoui, M., Mansor, M., & Yusoff, K. M. (2010). The inhibitory effects of Gelam honey and its extracts on nitric oxide and prostaglandin E(2) in inflammatory tissues. *Fitoterapia, 81*(8), 1196–1201.

Kato, Y., Araki, Y., Juri, M., Ishisaka, A., Nitta, Y., Niwa, T., Kitamoto, N., & Takimoto, Y. (2016). Competitive immunochromatographic assay for leptosperin as a plausible authentication marker of manuka honey. *Food Chemistry, 194*, 362–365.

Khan, F. R., Ul Abadin, Z., & Rauf, N. (2007). Honey: nutritional and medicinal value. *International Journal of Clinical Practice, 61*(10), 1705–1707.

Kishore, R. K., Halim, A. S., Syazana, M. S., & Sirajudeen, K. N. (2011). Tualang honey has higher phenolic content and greater radical scavenging activity compared with other honey sources. *Nutrition Research, 31*(4), 322–325.

Kovacik, J., Gruz, J., Biba, O., & Hedbavny, J. (2016). Contents of metals and metabolites in honey originated from the vicinity of industrial town Kosice (eastern Slovakia). *Environmental Science* and *Pollution Research International, 23*(5), 4531–4540.

Kus, P. M., Szweda, P., Jerkovic, I., & Tuberoso, C. I. (2016). Activity of Polish unifloral honeys against pathogenic bacteria and its correlation with colour, phenolic content, antioxidant activity and other parameters. *Letters in Applied Microbiology, 62*, 269–276.

Kwakman, P. H. S., & Zaat, S. A. J. (2012). Antibacterial component of honey. *IUBMB Life, 64*(1), 48–55.

Lee, D. S., Sinno, S., & Khachemoune, A. (2011). Honey and wound healing: an overview. *American Journal of Clinical Dermatology, 12*(3), 181–190.

Lipnik-Stangelj, M. (2013). Mediators of inflammation as targets for chronic pain treatment. *Mediators of Inflammation, 2013*, 783235.

Lu, J., Carter, D. A., Turnbull, L., Rosendale, D., Hedderley, D., Stephens, J., Gannabathula, S., Steinhorn, G., Schlothauer, R. C., Whitchurch, C. B., & Harry, E. J. (2013). The effect of New Zealand kanuka, manuka and clover honeys on bacterial growth dynamics and cellular morphology varies according to the species. *PLoS One, 8*(2), e55898.

Lusby, P. E., Coombes, A., & Wilkinson, J. M. (2002). Honey: a potent agent for wound healing? *Journal of Wound Ostomy and Continence Nursing, 29*(6), 295–300.

Majtan, J. (2014). Honey: an immunomodulator in wound healing. *Wound Repair Regeneration, 22*(2), 187–192.

Majtan, J., Kumar, P., Majtan, T., Walls, A. F., & Klaudiny, J. (2010). Effect of honey and its major royal jelly protein 1 on cytokine and MMP-9 mRNA transcripts in human keratinocytes. *Experimental Dermatology, 19*(8), e73–79.

Majtan, J., Bohova, J., Garcia-Villalba, R., Tomas-Barberan, F. A., Madakova, Z., Majtan, T., Majtan, V., & Klaudiny, J. (2013). Fir honeydew honey flavonoids inhibit TNF-α-induced MMP-9 expression in human keratinocytes: a new action of honey in wound healing. *Archives of Dermatological Research, 305*(7), 619–627.

Mandal, M. D., & Mandal, S. (2011). Honey: its medicinal property and antibacterial activity. *Asian Pacific Journal of Tropical Biomedicine, 1*(2), 154–160.

Mat Lazim, N., Abdullah, B., & Salim, R. (2013). The effect of Tualang honey in enhancing post tonsillectomy healing process. An open labelled prospective clinical trial. *International Journal of Pediatric Otorhinolaryngology, 77*(4), 457–461.

Mato, I., Huidobro, J. F., Simal-Lozano, J., & Sancho, M. T. (2003). Significance of nanoaromatic organic acids in honey. *Journal of Food Protection, 66*(12), 2371–2376.

Mohamad Zaid, S. S., Kassim, N. M., & Othman, S. (2015). Tualang honey protects against BPA-induced morphological abnormalities and disruption of ERα, ERβ, and C3 mRNA and protein expressions in the uterus of rats. *Evidence-Based Complementary and Alternative Medicine, 2015*, 202874.

Molan, P. C. (2001). Potential of honey in treatments of wounds and burns. *American Journal of Clinical Dermatology, 2*, 9–13.

Muhammad, A., Odunola, O. A., Ibrahim, M. A., Sallau, A. B., Erukainure, O. L., Aimola, I. A., & Malami, I. (2016). Potential biological activity of acacia honey. *Frontiers in Bioscience (Elite Ed)., 8*, 351–357.

Oroian, M., Paduret, S., Amariei, S., & Gutt, G. (2016). Chemical composition and temperature influence on honey texture properties. *Journal of Food Science and Technology, 53*(1), 431–440.

Owoyele, B. V., Oladejo, R. O., Ajomale, K., Ahmed, R. O., & Mustapha, A. (2014). Analgesic and anti-inflammatory effects of honey: the involvement of autonomic receptors. *Metabolic Brain Disease, 29*(1), 167–173.

Ozlugedik, S., Genc, S., Unal, A., Elhan, A. H., Tezer, M., & Titiz, A. (2006). Can postoperative pains following tonsillectomy be relieved by honey? A prospective, randomized, placebo controlled preliminary study. *International Journal of Pediatric Otorhinolaryngology, 70*(11), 1929–1934.

Pasternak, G., & Pan, Y. X. (2011). Mu opioid receptors in pain management. *Acta Anaesthesiology Taiwan, 49*(1), 21–25.

Petrenko, A. B., Yamakura, T., Baba, H., & Shimoji, K. (2003). The role of N-methyl-D-aspartae (NMDA) receptors in pain: a review. *Anesthesia and Analgesia, 97*(4), 1108–1116.

Rossano, R., Larocca, M., Polito, T., Perna, A. M., Padula, M. C., Martelli, G., & Riccio, P. (2012). What are the proteolytic enzymes of honey and what they do tell us? A fingerprint analysis by 2D zymography of unifloral honeys. *PLoS One, 7*(11), e49164.

Salonen, A., Kokki, H., & Nuutinen, J. (2002). The effect of ketoprofen on recovery after tonsillectomy in children: a 3-week follow-up study. *International Journal of Pediatric Otorhinolaryngology, 62*(2), 143–150.

Samdariya, S., Lewis, S., Kauser, H., Ahmed, I., & Kumar, D. (2015). A randomized controlled trial evaluating the role of honey in reducing pain due to radiation induced mucositis in head and neck cancer patients. *Indian Journal of Palliative Care, 21*(3), 268–273.

Schlereth, T., & Birklein, F. (2008). The sympathetic nervous system and pain. *NeuroMolecular Medicine, 10*(3), 141–147.

Souza, T. P. A., Rocha Guidi, L., de Abreu Gloria, M. B., & Fernandes, C. (2016). Pesticides in honey: a review on chromatographic analytical methods. *Talanta, 149*, 124–141.

Suarez, J. M. A., Tullipani, S., Romadini, S., Bertoli, E., & Battino, M. (2010). Contribution of honey in nutrition and human health. *Mediterranean Journal of Nutrition and Metabolism*, *3*, 15–23.

Taghavizad, R. (2011). The healing effect of honey as stated in Quran and Hadith. *Quran and Medicine*, *1*(2), 3–8.

Terrab, A., Gonzalez, A. G., Diez, M. J., & Heredia, F. J. (2003). Characterization of Morrocanunifloral honey using multivariate analysis. *European Food Research and Technology*, *218*, 88–95.

Tonks, A. J., Cooper, R. A., Jones, K. P., Blair, S., Parton, J., & Tonks, A. (2003). Honey stimulates inflammatory cytokine production from monocytes. *Cytokine*, *21*(5), 242–247.

Vyklicky, V., Korinek, M., Smejkalova, T., Balik, A., Krausova, B., Kaniakova, M., Lichnerova, K., Cerny, J., Krusek, J., Dittert, I., Horak, M., & Vyklicky, L. (2013). Structure, function and pharmacology of NMDA receptor channels. *Physiological Research*, *63*(Suppl. 1), S191–S203.

Wang, J., & Li, Q. X. (2011). Chemical composition, characterization, and differentiation of honey botanical and geographical origins. *Advances in Food and Nutrition Research*, *62*, 89–137.

Werner, A., & Laccourreye, O. (2011). Honey in otorhinolaryngology: when, why and how? *European Annals of Otorhinolaryngology, Head and Neck Diseases*, *128*(3), 133–137.

Yaghoobi, R., Kazerouni, A., & Kazerouni, O. (2013). Evidence for clinical use of honey in wound healing as an anti-bacterial, anti-inflammatory anti-oxidant and anti-viral agent: a review. *Jundishapur Journal of Natural Pharmaceutical*, *8*(3), 100–104.

Yaylaci, S., Ayyildiz, O., Aydin, E., Osken, A., Karahalil, F., Varim, C., Demir, M. V., Genc, A. B., Sahinkus, S., Can, Y., Kocayigit, I., & Bilir, C. (2015). Is there a difference in mad honey poisoning between geriatric and non geriatric patient groups? *European Review for Medical and Pharmacological sciences*, *19*(23), 4647–4653.

CHAPTER

11

Probiotics and Synbiotics for Management of Infantile Colic

H. Ahanchian*,**, A. Javid†

*Children's Health and Environment Program, Queensland Children's Medical Research Institute, University of Queensland, Brisbane, QLD, Australia; **Department of Allergy and Immunology, Mashhad University of Medical Sciences, Mashhad, Iran; †Department of Pediatrics, Mashhad University of Medical Science, Mashhad, Iran

INFANTILE COLIC

Infantile colic (IC) is defined as paroxysms of crying or fussing due to abdominal pain for 3 hours or more a day, occurring 3 days or more per week for 3 weeks,in a healthy infant age of 2 weeks–3 months (Kheir, 2014; Savino, 2007). IC is affecting up to 20% of infants and is a frustrating problem for parents and healthcare system (Wake et al., 2006). As IC usually begins at approximately 2 weeks of age and improves by month 4, it is a benign and self-limiting condition, albeit one that often puts stress on the parents' mental health.

Despite many recent studies the pathogenesis of IC remains unknown and likely it is multifactorial. Psychosocial theories, such as family tension, inadequate maternal–infant interactions, maternal anxiety and depression, and maternal smoking are some of the IC risk factors (Barr, 2000; Savino, Ceratto, De Marco, & Cordero di Montezemolo, 2014).

Gastrointestinal hypotheses include increased intraabdominal gas, hyperperistalsis, visceral pain, and immaturity of infant's nervous or digestive system (Barr, 2000; Savino, Garro, Nicoli, & Ceratto, 2015).

Despite many informed benign modalities no useful treatment for colic is available;

Support and reassurance suggested as the pillar of management (Adlerberth & Wold, 2009; Cohen-Silver & Ratnapalan, 2009; Garrison & Christakis, 2000; Lucassen & Assendelft, 2001).

In breast-fed infants using low allergic foods and omission of cow's milk protein from diet of mother maybe suggested (Cohen-Silver & Ratnapalan, 2009; Garrison & Christakis, 2000; Lucassen & Assendelft, 2001; Sung et al., 2014).

In bottle-fed infants, use of hypoallergenic formulas (based on hydrolyzed proteins + prebiotic oligosaccharides) was effective in some studies (Cohen-Silver & Ratnapalan, 2009; Garrison & Christakis, 2000; Savino et al., 2006b).

Drug treatment has little value in management of colic pain; some agents, such as Dicyclomine, Simethicone, and nutritional supplements may be helpful for some infants although few number of randomized controlled trials support their efficacy (Ghosh & Barr, 2004; Heine, 2013; Savino et al., 2006a).

Probiotic and synbiotic prescription for improvement colicky pain is suggested based on recent notable data (Kianifar et al., 2014; Saavedra, Abi-Hanna, Moore, & Yolken, 2004).

Although IC is self-limited and resolves after the first 3–4 months of life, it may increase the risk of maternal depression, (McMahon, Barnett, Kowalenko, Tennant, & Don, 2001) early breast feeding cessation (Howard, Lanphear, Lanphear, Eberly, & Lawrence, 2006), and shaken baby syndrome (Barr, 2012) and finding an effective treatment seems necessary.

GUT–BRAIN AXIS AND MICROBIOTA

The intestine of the newborn infant is basically sterile and early postnatal life serves as bacterial colonization period. The mother and the environment are the main sources of bacteria (Amaral et al., 2008; Gill et al., 2006).

Nutritional Modulators of Pain in the Aging Population. http://dx.doi.org/10.1016/B978-0-12-805186-3.00011-4
Copyright © 2017 Elsevier Inc. All rights reserved.

The human microbiome refers to the collection of genomes of these microbes (Turnbaugh et al., 2007).

The presence of these microbiota is essential for host physiology, such as gastrointestinal health, development of the immune system, and nutrient processing. Recently some studies reveal the necessity of gut microbiota for normal CNS function (Heijtz et al., 2011; Neufeld, Kang, Bienenstock, & Foster, 2011).

The gut microbiota consists of a multiplex community of bacteria. In recent studies using molecular and metagenomics tools, structure, and activity of gut microbiota has been better recognized. Many bacterial phyla exist in the gut, such as Bacteroides, Frimicutes, Protebacteria, Actinobacteria, Fusobacteria, and Verrucomicrobia (Eckburg et al., 2005). The two former accounting for at least 70–75% of microbiomes (Eckburg et al., 2005; Qin et al., 2010).

Bacterial composition consists of many factors. Prematurity, mode of delivery (Adlerberth & Wold, 2009), genetics, age, metabolism, diet, geographic region, probiotic, or antibiotic consumption and stress can all influence the microbiome complex (Bennet, Eriksson, & Nord, 2002; Cho et al., 2012; Karlsson et al., 2012). An adult human intestine contains approximately 100 trillion necessary bacteria (Gill et al., 2006) and by 2 years of age, the child's gut microbial composition begins to resemble an adult's microbiota (Barnes & Yeh, 2015).

Nowadays, several studies defend functional linking between the gastrointestinal tract and central nervous system (Mayer, 2011).The gut–brain axis (GBA) refers to biface relation between the central and the enteric nervous system. In the other words, correlation of emotional and/or cognitive centers of the brain and peripheral intestinal functions. This system includes the central nervous system (CNS), the autonomic nervous system (ANS), the enteric nervous system (ENS), and the hypothalamic pituitary adrenal (HPA) axis. (Fig. 11.1) (Carabotti, Scirocco, Maselli, & Severi, 2015).

The GBA is believed to be involved in the pathogenesis of several brain disorders such as autism (Cryan & Dinan, 2012), anxiety, depression (Park et al., 2013), and chronic pain (Amaral et al., 2008).

In this axis, information is transported between the gut and the brain through four major directions:

- Vagal and spinal afferent neurons by means of neurotransmitters
- Immune messages by means of cytokines
- Endocrine messages by means of gut hormones and
- Microbial factors (Collins, Surette, & Bercik, 2012; Cryan & Dinan, 2012; Holzer, Reichmann, & Farzi, 2012)

Although gut microbiota can enter the brain via the blood stream, some other probable mechanisms theorize that microbiota associate with immune mediators, gut hormones, and neurotransmitters.These four pathways are linked closely with each other (Holzer & Farzi, 2014).

In many of these communication tracts, the significant role of the biologically active gut peptides and neuropeptides are obvious.

To consider the regulatory gut microbiota on GBA, different approaches, such as manipulating the microbiota with antibiotics (Bercik et al., 2011), probiotic, synbiotic, and functional foods (Mayer, Tillisch, & Gupta, 2015), fecal microbial transplantation (Collins, Kassam, & Bercik, 2013), and germ free animal models (Sudo et al., 2004) have been applied and recent trials have shown that gut microbiota has an important role in gut–brain interactions (Carabotti et al., 2015).

There is increasing evidence suggestive of differences in intestinal microbiota among infants with colic and healthy controls (de Weerth, Fuentes, & de Vos, 2013). Most of these studies have used conventional culturing approaches. Reduction of biodiversity in the stools microbiota of colicky infants were found to have a lower amount of lactobacilli and higher counts of Gram-negative bacteria (de Weerth et al., 2013).

PROBIOTIC DEFINITION

The usage of fermented foods has a historical root. Ancient physicians of the Middle East prescribed yogurt for curing disorders of the stomach and intestines (Ahanchian, Jones, Chen, & Sly, 2012). In the Persian version of the Old Testament (Genesis 8:18) it states "Abraham owed his longevity to the consumption of sour milk" (Bottazzi & Reed, 1983).

In 1908, the popularity of probiotics and intestinal microbiota significantly increased when the Nobel Prize-winning Russian scientist Eli Metchnikoff suggested in that the long life of Bulgarian peasants resulted from their consumption of fermented milk products (Ahanchian et al., 2012).

In 2001, the Expert commission of international scientists supported by The Food and Agriculture Organization of the United Nations (FAO) and the WHO defined probiotics as "Live microorganisms which when administered in adequate amounts confer a health benefit on the host" (Hotel, 2001).

Besides probiotics, what are synbiotics and prebiotics?

Prebiotics are defined as "nondigestible food ingredients that beneficially affect the host by selectively stimulating the growth and/or activity of one or a limited number of bacteria in the colon, thus improving host health" (Gibson, Probert, Van Loo, Rastall, & Roberfroid, 2004). Lactobacilli and bifidobacteria are the usual genera that affected by prebiotics.

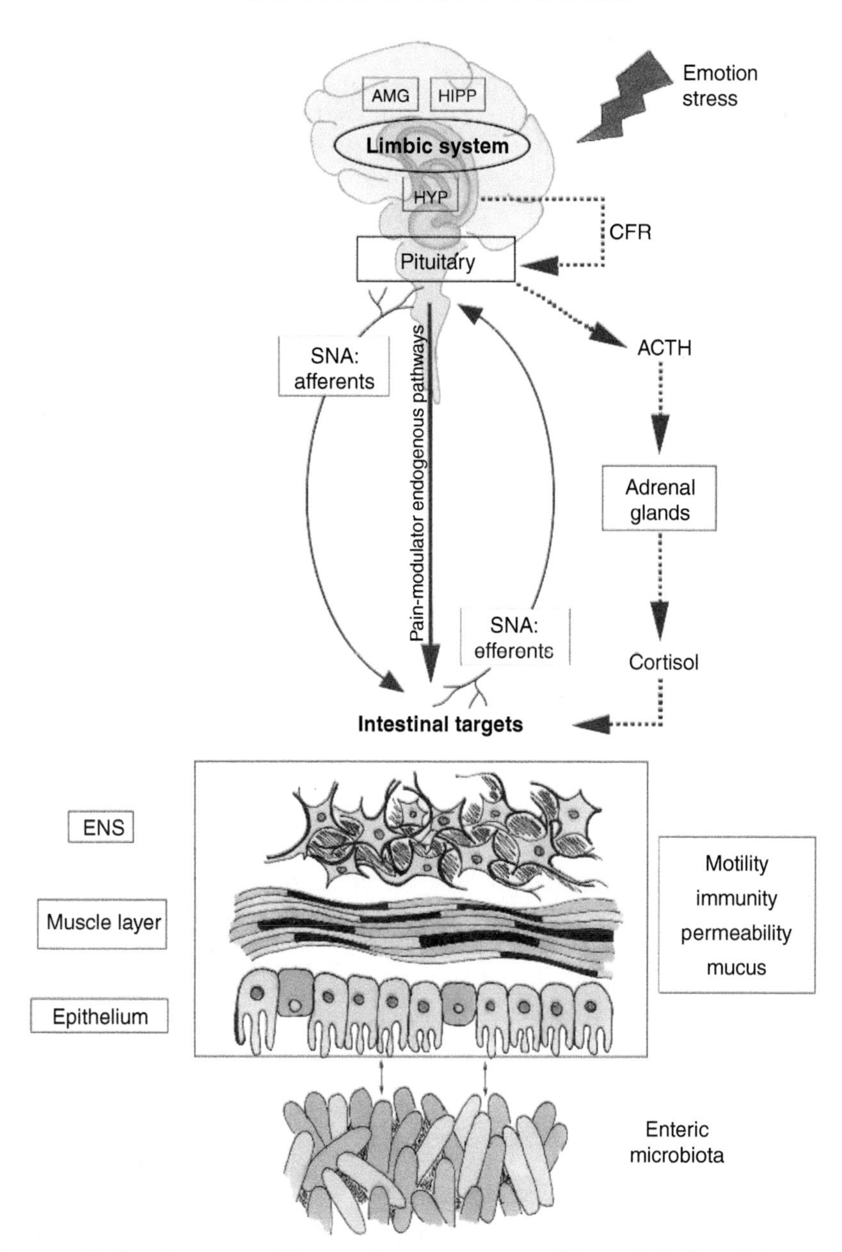

FIGURE 11.1 **Microbiome gut–brain axis structure.** The central nervous system and in particular hypothalamic pituitary adrenal (HPA) (axis dashed line) can be activated in response to environmental factors, such as emotion or stress.

Synbiotic refer to a products that contain both probiotic and prebiotic.

Previous studies have shown probiotics and synbiotics to be safe and well tolerated medications in the healthy children (Barnes & Yeh, 2015). Diarrhea, nausea, vomiting, and bloating are the most important reported side effects (Allen, Martinez, Gregorio, & Dans, 2011; Johnston, Goldenberg, Vandvik, Sun, & Guyatt, 2011).

Due to limited evidence about probiotic administration in high risk groups including preterm infants, immune deficient children, and children with catheters, using probiotics in these groups may be contraindicated (Enache-Angoulvant & Hennequin, 2005; Van den Nieuwboer et al., 2015).

PROBIOTICS FOR REDUCING COLIC AND PAIN

There is significant evidence that the composition of intestinal microbiota in colicky infants differs from control groups. In studies performed based on culturing approach, an imbalance in the intestinal microbiota has been reported as an independent risk factor for IC (Lehtonen, Korvenranta, & Eerola, 1994; Savino et al., 2005; Savino et al., 2009; Savino et al., 2004). Based on recent studies, increasing amounts of pathogenic bacteria and reduction of butyrate-producing bacteria or bifidobacteria leading to intestinal inflammation and pain (de Weerth et al., 2013). Some researchers suggest that Bifidobacterium and Lactobacillus may protect against crying and pain (Kianifar et al., 2014; Pärtty, Kalliomäki, Endo, Salminen, & Isolauri, 2012).

Roos et al. (2013), in an RCT compared the global microbial composition in fecal samples from colicky infants given *Lactobacillus reuteri* or placebo. They concluded that the increase of good bacteria (Bacteroidetes) in responder infants indicated that a decrease in colicky symptoms was linked to the changes of the microbiota (Roos et al., 2013).

Savino et al. (2010), in a trial of 46 breastfed colicky infants compared probiotic *L. reuteri* with placebo. Infants in the *L. reuteri*-treated-group showed significantly lower crying compared with the placebo group on day 7, 14, and 21. They suggested that gut microbiota changes induced by *L. reuteri* may be involved in clinical improvement (Savino et al., 2010).

Other researchers concluded that exclusively or predominantly breastfed infants with IC benefit from *L. reuteri* DSM 17938 compared with placebo (Szajewska, Gyrczuk, & Horvath, 2013).

Saavedra et al. (2004), showed that a formula containing two strains of probiotic including B. lactis and S. thermophilus reduced reporting of colic or irritability. Using a probiotic mixture might be more effective but as shown in other studies efficacy of the probiotic mixtures may be reduced by inhibitory effects between different probiotic strains.

A review article supports the profitable effects of probiotic supplementation in IC treatment. *L. reuteri* (strains-American Type Culture Collection Strain 55730 and DSM 17938) notably decreased the rate (min/day) of crying and pain, no short term side effects were identified (Anabrees, Indrio, Paes, & AlFaleh, 2013).

Prebiotics have been useful in management of IC in some studies but some trials failed to show any benefits (Ben et al., 2008). In 2008, a prospective controlled trial showed that a formula containing a mixture of galacto and FOS can reduce crying time. The authors commented that prebiotics can influence immune system not only via the intestinal microbiota but also by direct interaction with immune system (Moro et al., 2006).

Pärtty, Luoto, Kalliomäki, Salminen, and Isolauri, 2013 showed that early administration of prebiotics, probiotics, or placebo during the first 2 months of life to preterm infants provided relief to their crying and fussing and suggested that delayed colonization by *Bifidobacteria infantis* may has a relation to the risk of irritability in preterm infants.

The effects of synbiotics on infant colic is a new area of research. The therapeutic effects depend on the type, number, dosage and duration of intervention, study population, and environmental background (Ahanchian et al., 2012; Heydarian et al., 2010; Kianifar et al., 2015).

The prebiotic in the synbiotic improves the survival of probiotics and stimulates the beneficial bacteria. Mugambi, Musekiwa, Lombard, Young, and Blaauw, 2012, in a review of three studies using infant formula containing synbiotic concluded that synbiotics had no impact on incidence and frequency of colic, crying, and restlessness. The probiotic strains used in these studied were *Bifidobacteria longom* and *Bifidobacteria animalis* plus combination of galacto and fructooligosaccharide (FOS) as prebiotics.

Compared with this study, we used a of a mixture of higher dose (1×109) plus FOS alone:

Fifty breastfed infants aged 15–120 days with IC randomly assigned to receive either the synbiotic sachet containing 1 billion CFU of: Lactobacillus casei, L. rhamnosus, Streptococcus thermophilus, Bifidobacterium breve, L. acidophilus, B. infantis, L. bulgaricus, and fructooligosaccharide, or placebo daily for 30 days. The treatment success (reduction in the daily crying time >50%) was significantly higher in synbiotic group (82.6%) compared with placebo (35.7%) at day 7. At the end of 30 days, treatment success was 87% and 46% in synbiotic and placebo group, respectively. Symptom resolution (reduction in the daily crying time >90%) was also higher in synbiotic group (39%) compared with placebo (7%) at day 7 but not at day 30 (56% vs. 36%). We encountered no complication related to synbiotic use during the study (Kianifar et al., 2014).

CONCLUSIONS

Supplementation with the probiotic Lactobacillus reuteri, which appears to be safe and effective for the management of pain and fussiness in IC without causing adverse events. In the absence of other effective treatment modalities, probiotics, and synbiotics will have more important role in management of infant colic and pain.

For clear recommendations, higher quality, multicenter well-designed RCTs with longer follow-up, larger sample size, well-defined outcome measures, and different mixtures are needed to be able to determine the ideal effective product for treatment or even prevention of infant colic.

References

Adlerberth, I., & Wold, A. E. (2009). Establishment of the gut microbiota in Western infants. *Acta Paediatrica*, *98*(2), 229–238.

Ahanchian, H., Jones, C. M., Chen, Y. -S., & Sly, P. D. (2012). Respiratory viral infections in children with asthma: do they matter and can we prevent them? *BMC Pediatrics*, *12*(1), 147.

Allen, S. J., Martinez, E. G., Gregorio, G. V., & Dans, L. F. (2011). Probiotics for treating acute infectious diarrhoea. *Sao Paulo Medical Journal*, *129*(3), 185–1185.

Amaral, F. A., Sachs, D., Costa, V. V., Fagundes, C. T., Cisalpino, D., Cunha, T. M., . . . Nicoli, J. R. (2008). Commensal microbiota is fundamental for the development of inflammatory pain. *Proceedings of the National Academy of Sciences, 105*(6), 2193–2197.

Anabrees, J., Indrio, F., Paes, B., & AlFaleh, K. (2013). Probiotics for infantile colic: a systematic review. *BMC Pediatrics, 13*(1), 1.

Barnes, D., & Yeh, A. M. (2015). Bugs and guts practical applications of probiotics for gastrointestinal disorders in children. *Nutrition in Clinical Practice, 30*(6), 747–759.

Barr, R. G. (2000). Excessive crying. *Handbook of developmental psychopathology*. New York: Springer (pp. 327–350).

Barr, R. G. (2012). Preventing abusive head trauma resulting from a failure of normal interaction between infants and their caregivers. *Proceedings of the National Academy of Sciences, 109*(Suppl. 2), 17294–17301.

Ben, X. -M., Li, J., Feng, Z. -T., Shi, S. -Y., Lu, Y. -D., Chen, R., & Zhou, X. -Y. (2008). Low level of galacto-oligosaccharide in infant formula stimulates growth of intestinal Bifidobacteria and Lactobacilli. *World Journal Gastroenterology, 14*(42), 6564–6568.

Bennet, R., Eriksson, M., & Nord, C. E. (2002). The fecal microflora of 1–3-month-old infants during treatment with eight oral antibiotics. *Infection, 30*(3), 158–160.

Bercik, P., Denou, E., Collins, J., Jackson, W., Lu, J., Jury, J.,. McCoy, K. D. (2011). The intestinal microbiota affect central levels of brain-derived neurotropic factor and behavior in mice. *Gastroenterology, 141*(2), 599–609. e593.

Bottazzi, V., & Reed, G. (1983). Other fermented dairy products. *Biotechnology: Vol. 5. Food and feed production with microorganisms*. German Federal Republic: Verlag Chemie GmbH (pp. 315–363).

Carabotti, M., Scirocco, A., Maselli, M. A., & Severi, C. (2015). The gut-brain axis: interactions between enteric microbiota, central and enteric nervous systems. *Annals of Gastroenterology: Quarterly Publication of the Hellenic Society of Gastroenterology, 28*(2), 203.

Cho, I., Yamanishi, S., Cox, L., Methé, B. A., Zavadil, J., Li, K., & Teitler, I. (2012). Antibiotics in early life alter the murine colonic microbiome and adiposity. *Nature, 488*(7413), 621–626.

Cohen-Silver, J., & Ratnapalan, S. (2009). Management of infantile colic: a review. *Clinical Pediatrics, 48*(1), 14–17.

Collins, S. M., Surette, M., & Bercik, P. (2012). The interplay between the intestinal microbiota and the brain. *Nature Reviews Microbiology, 10*(11), 735–742.

Collins, S. M., Kassam, Z., & Bercik, P. (2013). The adoptive transfer of behavioral phenotype via the intestinal microbiota: experimental evidence and clinical implications. *Current Opinion in Microbiology, 16*(3), 240–245.

Cryan, J. F., & Dinan, T. G. (2012). Mind-altering microorganisms: the impact of the gut microbiota on brain and behaviour. *Nature Reviews Neuroscience, 13*(10), 701–712.

de Weerth, C., Fuentes, S., & de Vos, W. M. (2013). Crying in infants: on the possible role of intestinal microbiota in the development of colic. *Gut Microbes, 4*(5), 416–421.

Eckburg, P.B., Bik, E.M, Bernstein, C.N, Purdom, E., Dethlefsen, L., Sargent, M., . . . Relman, D. A. (2005). Diversity of the human intestinal microbial flora. *Science*, 308(5728), 1635–1638.

Enache-Angoulvant, A., & Hennequin, C. (2005). Invasive Saccharomyces infection: a comprehensive review. *Clinical Infectious Diseases, 41*(11), 1559–1568.

Garrison, M. M., & Christakis, D. A. (2000). A systematic review of treatments for infant colic. *Pediatrics, 106*(Suppl. 1), 184–190.

Ghosh, S., & Barr, R. G. (2004). Colic and gas. *Pediatric gastrointestinal disease. 4th ed. Hamilton, Ont: BC Decker Inc*, 210–224.

Gibson, G. R., Probert, H. M., Van Loo, J., Rastall, R. A., & Roberfroid, M. B. (2004). Dietary modulation of the human colonic microbiota: updating the concept of prebiotics. *Nutrition Research Reviews, 17*(02), 259–275.

Gill, S. R., Pop, M., DeBoy, R. T., Eckburg, P. B., Turnbaugh, P. J., Samuel, B. S., . . . Nelson, K. E. (2006). Metagenomic analysis of the human distal gut microbiome. *Science, 312*(5778), 1355–1359.

Heijtz, R. D., Wang, S., Anuar, F., Qian, Y., Björkholm, B., Samuelsson, A., . . . Pettersson, S. (2011). Normal gut microbiota modulates brain development and behavior. *Proceedings of the National Academy of Sciences, 108*(7), 3047–3052.

Heine, R. G. (2013). Cow's-milk allergy and lactose malabsorption in infants with colic. *Journal of pediatric gastroenterology and nutrition, 57*, S25–S27.

Heydarian, F., Kianifar, H. R., Ahanchian, H., Khakshure, A., Seyedi, J., & Moshirian, D. (2010). A comparison between traditional yogurt and probiotic yogurt in non-inflammatory acute gastroenteritis. *Saudi Medical Journal, 31*(3), 280–283.

Holzer, P., & Farzi, A. (2014). Neuropeptides and the microbiota-gut-brain axis. *Microbial Endocrinology: The Microbiota-Gut-Brain Axis in Health and Disease* (195–219): Springer.

Holzer, P., Reichmann, F., & Farzi, A. (2012). Neuropeptide Y, peptide YY and pancreatic polypeptide in the gut–brain axis. *Neuropeptides, 46*(6), 261–274.

Hotel, Amerian Córdoba Park (2001). Health and nutritional properties of probiotics in food including powder milk with live lactic acid bacteria. *Prevention, 5*(1), .

Howard, C. R., Lanphear, N., Lanphear, B. P., Eberly, S., & Lawrence, R. A. (2006). Parental responses to infant crying and colic: the effect on breastfeeding duration. *Breastfeeding Medicine, 1*(3), 146–155.

Johnston, B. C., Goldenberg, J. Z., Vandvik, P. O., Sun, X., & Guyatt, G. H. (2011). Probiotics for the prevention of pediatric antibiotic-associated diarrhea. *Cochrane Database Systems Review, 11*(11), .

Karlsson, C. L. J., Önnerfält, J., Xu, J., Molin, G., Ahrné, S., & Thorngren-Jerneck, K. (2012). The microbiota of the gut in preschool children with normal and excessive body weight. *Obesity, 20*(11), 2257–2261.

Kheir, A. E. M. (2014). Retraction: infantile colic, facts and fiction. *Italian Journal of Pediatrics, 40*, 9.

Kianifar, H., Ahanchian, H., Grover, Z., Jafari, S., Noorbakhsh, Z., Khakshour, A., . . . Kiani, M. (2014). Synbiotic in the management of infantile colic: a randomised controlled trial. *Journal of Paediatrics and Child Health, 50*(10), 801–805.

Kianifar, H. R., Farid, R., Ahanchian, H., Jabbari, F., Moghiman, T., & Sistanian, A. (2015). Probiotics in the treatment of acute diarrhea in young children. *Iranian Journal of Medical Sciences, 34*(3), 204–207.

Lehtonen, L., Korvenranta, H., & Eerola, E. (1994). Intestinal microflora in colicky and noncolicky infants: bacterial cultures and gas-liquid chromatography. *Journal of Pediatric Gastroenterology and Nutrition, 19*(3), 310–314.

Lucassen, P. L. B. J., & Assendelft, W. J. J. (2001). Systematic review of treatments for infant colic. *Pediatrics, 108*(4), 1047–1048.

Mayer, E. A. (2011). Gut feelings: the emerging biology of gut–brain communication. *Nature Reviews Neuroscience, 12*(8), 453–466.

Mayer, E. A., Tillisch, K., & Gupta, A. (2015). Gut/brain axis and the microbiota. *Journal of Clinical Investigation, 125*(3), 926.

McMahon, C., Barnett, B., Kowalenko, N., Tennant, C., & Don, N. (2001). Postnatal depression, anxiety and unsettled infant behaviour. *Australian and New Zealand Journal of Psychiatry, 35*(5), 581–588.

Moro, G., Arslanoglu, S., Stahl, B., Jelinek, J., Wahn, U., & Boehm, G. (2006). A mixture of prebiotic oligosaccharides reduces the incidence of atopic dermatitis during the first six months of age. *Archives of Disease in Childhood, 91*(10), 814–819.

Mugambi, M. N., Musekiwa, A., Lombard, M., Young, T., & Blaauw, R. (2012). Synbiotics, probiotics or prebiotics in infant formula for full term infants: a systematic review. *Nutrition Journal, 11*(1), 1.

Neufeld, K. -A. M., Kang, N., Bienenstock, J., & Foster, J. A. (2011). Effects of intestinal microbiota on anxiety-like behavior. *Communicative and Integrative Biology, 4*(4), 492–494.

Park, A. J., Collins, J., Blennerhassett, P. A., Ghia, J. E., Verdu, E. F., Bercik, P., & Collins, S. M. (2013). Altered colonic function and microbiota profile in a mouse model of chronic depression. *Neurogastroenterology and Motility, 25*(9), 733-e575.

Pärtty, A., Kalliomäki, M., Endo, A., Salminen, S., & Isolauri, E. (2012). Compositional development of Bifidobacterium and Lactobacillus microbiota is linked with crying and fussing in early infancy. *PloS One, 7*(3), e32495.

Pärtty, A., Luoto, R., Kalliomäki, M., Salminen, S., & Isolauri, E. (2013). Effects of early prebiotic and probiotic supplementation on development of gut microbiota and fussing and crying in preterm infants: a randomized, double-blind, placebo-controlled trial. *The Journal of Pediatrics, 163*(5), 1272–1277. e1272.

Qin, J., Li, R., Raes, J., Arumugam, M., Burgdorf, K. S., Manichanh, C., . . . Yamada, T. (2010). A human gut microbial gene catalogue established by metagenomic sequencing. *Nature, 464*(7285), 59–65.

Roos, S., Dicksved, J., Tarasco, V., Locatelli, E., Ricceri, F., Grandin, U., & Savino, F. (2013). 454 pyrosequencing analysis on faecal samples from a randomized DBPC trial of colicky infants treated with Lactobacillus reuteri DSM 17938. *PLoS One, 8*(2), e56710.

Saavedra, J. M., Abi-Hanna, A., Moore, N., & Yolken, R. H. (2004). Long-term consumption of infant formulas containing live probiotic bacteria: tolerance and safety. *The American Journal of Clinical Nutrition, 79*(2), 261–267.

Savino, F. (2007). Focus on infantile colic. *Acta Paediatrica, 96*(9), 1259–1264.

Savino, F., Cresi, F., Pautasso, S., Palumeri, E., Tullio, V., Roana, J., . . . Oggero, R. (2004). Intestinal microflora in breastfed colicky and non-colicky infants. *Acta paediatrica*, 93(6), 825–829.

Savino, F., Bailo, E., Oggero, R., Tullio, V., Roana, J., Carlone, N., . . . Silvestro, L. (2005). Bacterial counts of intestinal Lactobacillus species in infants with colic. *Pediatric allergy and immunology, 16*(1), 72–75.

Savino, F., Clara Grassino, E., Guidi, C., Oggero, R., Silvestro, L., & Miniero, R. (2006a). Ghrelin and motilin concentration in colicky infants. *Acta Paediatrica, 95*(6), 738–741.

Savino, F., Palumeri, E., Castagno, E., Cresi, F., Dalmasso, P., Cavallo, F., & Oggero, R. (2006b). Reduction of crying episodes owing to infantile colic: a randomized controlled study on the efficacy of a new infant formula. *European Journal of Clinical Nutrition, 60*(11), 1304–1310.

Savino, F., Cordisco, L., Tarasco, V., Calabrese, R., Palumeri, E., & Matteuzzi, D. (2009). Molecular identification of coliform bacteria from colicky breastfed infants. *Acta Paediatrica, 98*(10), 1582–1588.

Savino, F., Cordisco, L., Tarasco, V., Palumeri, E., Calabrese, R., Oggero, R., . . . Matteuzzi, D. (2010). Lactobacillus reuteri DSM 17938 in infantile colic: a randomized, double-blind, placebo-controlled trial. *Pediatrics, 126*(3), e526–e533.

Savino, F., Ceratto, S., De Marco, A., & Cordero di Montezemolo, L. (2014). Looking for new treatments of Infantile Colic. *Italian Journal of Pediatrics, 40*, 53.

Savino, F., Garro, M., Nicoli, S., & Ceratto, S. (2015). Infantile colic: looking to old data through new eyes. *Journal of Pediatric and Neonatal Individualized Medicine (JPNIM), 4*(2), e040230.

Sudo, N., Chida, Y., Aiba, Y., Sonoda, J., Oyama, N., Yu, X.-N., . . . Koga, Y. (2004). Postnatal microbial colonization programs the hypothalamic–pituitary–adrenal system for stress response in mice. *The Journal of physiology, 558*(1), 263–275.

Sung, V., Hiscock, H., Tang, M. L. K., Mensah, F. K., Nation, M. L., Satzke, C., . . . Wake, M. (2014). Treating infant colic with the probiotic Lactobacillus reuteri: double blind, placebo controlled randomised trial. *Bmj*, 348, g2107.

Szajewska, H., Gyrczuk, E., & Horvath, A. (2013). Lactobacillus reuteri DSM 17938 for the management of infantile colic in breastfed infants: a randomized, double-blind, placebo-controlled trial. *The Journal of Pediatrics, 162*(2), 257–262.

Turnbaugh, P. J., Ley, R. E., Hamady, M., Fraser-Liggett, C., Knight, R., & Gordon, J. I. (2007). The human microbiome project: exploring the microbial part of ourselves in a changing world. *Nature, 449*(7164), 804.

Van den Nieuwboer, M., Brummer, R. J., Guarner, F., Morelli, L., Cabana, M., & Claassen, E. (2015). Safety of probiotics and synbiotics in children under 18 years of age. *Beneficial Microbes, 6*(5), 615–630.

Wake, M., Morton-Allen, E., Poulakis, Z., Hiscock, H., Gallagher, S., & Oberklaid, F. (2006). Prevalence, stability, and outcomes of cry-fuss and sleep problems in the first 2 years of life: prospective community-based study. *Pediatrics, 117*(3), 836–842.

SECTION D

OBESITY AND MACRONUTRIENTS IN PAIN

CHAPTER

12

The Interrelationship of Obesity, Pain, and Diet/Nutrition

H.M. Rodgers

West Virginia University School of Medicine, Morgantown, WV, United States

Research in both human and animal models has demonstrated that there are differences in nociceptive sensitivity or pain threshold associated with specific physiological conditions, such as obesity (Mckendall & Haier, 1983; Rodgers, Liban, & Wilson, 2014). In addition to changes in pain threshold, obesity is often comorbid with chronic pain (Okifuji & Hare, 2015). There is a complex interaction of behavioral and physiological changes in obesity that may result in the differences in pain experienced by this population. With the growing obesity epidemic throughout the developed world, it is important to understand the relationship between pain and obesity and the role of dietary behavior/nutrition.

This chapter provides a brief overview of the literature on obesity including the known etiology and dietary behavior. Next, literature demonstrating the relationship between obesity and pain will be explored including chronic pain and nociceptive sensitivity. The potential modulators involved in the interrelationship of pain and obesity, such as hunger/satiety signals, diet, and vitamins will be addressed. Finally, a potential role for diet/nutrition in the prevention and treatment of pain in obesity will also be discussed.

OVERVIEW OF OBESITY: ETIOLOGY AND DIETARY BEHAVIOR

Rising obesity rates coupled with its significant health threat has made obesity an important and rapidly growing area of research. Obesity is a complex chronic condition resulting from an energy imbalance defined as occurring in individuals with a body mass index (BMI) greater than 30 kg/m^2 (Smith & Smith, 2016). The cause of this imbalance varies between individuals, and there may be several contributing factors within an individual. Thus, the etiology of obesity is complex and heterogeneous. Behavior/lifestyle issues (excessive energy intake and a lack of physical activity) and genetic susceptibility are considered to be the primary causal factors in obesity (Smith & Smith, 2016). Obesity is associated with altered physiology, therefore it is difficult to disentangle which physiological factors are contributors and which are consequences of obesity. For example, the alterations in hormones controlling appetite regulation could lead to changes in dietary behavior or could be the result of altered dietary behaviors (Lean & Malkova, 2015). Other factors including gene mutations, medication, environment, culture, and socioeconomic status may also play a role in the cause of obesity (Smith & Smith, 2016).

Dietary Behavior

Behavior is thought to be the primary cause of obesity, whereby there is a misbalance between energy intake and expenditure. This misbalance results when too many calories are consumed and insufficient physical activity occurs, leading to weight gain. The increasing obesity epidemic has been proposed to be the result of the creation of an obesogenic environment (high availability of cheap, convenient, and calorically-dense foods) that promotes poor dietary behavior (Allman-Farinelli, Partridge, & Roy, 2016). Dietary patterns associated with obesity are well documented. There are three main characteristic dietary behaviors associated with obesity, including: excess food consumption, consuming nutrient-poor energy-dense food, and altered meal timing.

Food consumption has increased in the last few decades as portion sizes have increased. Dietary data analyzed from over 39,000 American adults showed an

Nutritional Modulators of Pain in the Aging Population. http://dx.doi.org/10.1016/B978-0-12-805186-3.00012-6
Copyright © 2017 Elsevier Inc. All rights reserved.

increase in the quantity and energy density of food consumed from the 1970s to 2002 (Kant & Graubard, 2006). This increase parallels rising obesity rates during that time period. Obesity is often comorbid with binge eating disorder (BED) and food addiction. BED is a common eating disorder associated with obesity, particularly early onset and severe obesity. In BED, individuals regularly consume large quantities of food in a short period of time (Hudson, Hiripi, Pope, & Kessler, 2007). Food addiction or hedonic eating is a chronic condition often concomitant with obesity. Food addiction is characterized by increased consumption of food as a result of food cravings to reach a state of pleasure (von Deneen & Liu, 2011).

In addition to the increase in food intake, obesity is also associated with the consumption of calorically-dense food with a low nutritional quality. Dietary patterns showing regular consumption of foods high in both fat and sugar and low in fiber are associated with increased body mass and obesity (Allman-Farinelli et al., 2016; Langsetmo et al., 2010). Some examples of these foods include soft drinks, potato chips, French fries, hamburgers, hot dogs, bacon, doughnuts, and ice cream (Langsetmo et al., 2010). A longitudinal study has shown a positive correlation between consumption of energy-dense foods and weight gain whereas the opposite was true for consumption of fruits and vegetables (Mozaffarian, Hao, Rimm, Willett, & Hu, 2011). Obese individuals are more likely to pick a fast food restaurant over a more traditional sit down restaurant (Allman-Farinelli et al., 2016). Fast food, aside from being inexpensive and convenient is commonly high in fat and sugar content. Studies have shown dietary behaviors that included regular consumption of fast food predict increases in body mass over time in American females, and again the opposite was true for the consumption of fruit and vegetables (Allman-Farinelli et al., 2016). The poor nutritional quality of the obese diet may be partially responsible for the vitamin deficiencies associated with obesity (Smotkin-Tangorra et al., 2007).

Quantity and quality are not the only two issues associated with dietary patterns in obesity. A third characteristic is altered meal timing. Meal skipping (generally breakfast) has become a common dietary pattern especially among young adults (Allman-Farinelli et al. 2016). Timing of food intake is associated with the risk of obesity, wherein individuals who consume most of the days total energy intake in the evening are more likely to be obese (Wang et al., 2014).

OBESITY AND PAIN

Research has linked obesity with pain in two different ways. Obesity is associated with altered nociceptive sensitivity (pain threshold) and often comorbid with chronic pain (pain persisting for months or longer).

Chronic Pain and Obesity

Chronic pain is one of many co-morbid conditions found with obesity. One study in the elderly found that obese subjects were twice as likely to have chronic pain as normal weight subjects and severely obese subjects (BMI > 40 kg/m^2) were more than 4 times as likely (McCarthy, Bigal, Katz, Derby, & Lipton, 2009). Another study showed that obesity in early adulthood increases the risk of chronic lower back pain (Frilander et al., 2015). Back pain is a common form of chronic pain associated with obesity, and is especially frequent in those with abdominal obesity (Duruöz, Turan, Gürgan, & Deveci, 2012). In addition, obesity is frequently linked with osteoarthritis joint pain, including knees, hips, and hands (Thomazeau et al., 2014), chronic arm pain (Mork, Holtermann, & Nilsen, 2013), and chronic headaches (Scher, Stewart, Ricci, & Lipton, 2003). Obesity is also often comorbid with diabetes type 2 which can lead to diabetic neuropathy (Papanas & Ziegler, 2015).

Altered Pain Thresholds and Obesity

Research has also shown a significant association of obesity and altered nociceptive sensitivity. Evidence of altered pain thresholds comes from both human and animal models, however, the results are conflicting. Research using animal models of obesity has found pain perception differences in both dietary-induced models and genetic models of obesity. Dietary-induced obesity in nondiabetic rats displayed longer tail-flick latencies to noxious thermal stimuli suggesting a decrease in nociceptive sensitivity (Ramzan, Wong, & Corcoran, 2003). Another example of dietary-induced obesity and alterations in nociception was shown in rabbits. Diet-induced obese rabbits show a decreased in the pain response to formalin-induced tonic pain (Sinha et al., 2009). In a genetic model of obesity created by a mutation affecting leptin, genetically obese (*ob/ob*) mice show longer tail-flick latencies to thermal stimuli than lean mice across a range of noxious temperatures (Rodgers et al., 2014). This difference was found in both males and females and suggests decreased nociceptive sensitivity (analgesic response) or an increase in pain threshold. Examining the effects of age in the *ob/ob* model of obesity showed a modest effect, such that older obese mice displayed a greater analgesic response to noxious stimuli than younger obese mice (Rodgers et al., 2014). In contrast, a genetic model of obesity in rats showed an increase in pain sensitivity to both thermal and mechanical pain. In that study, female obese and diabetic Zucker (*fa/fa*) rats displayed shorter tail-flick and tail-pinch latencies than did lean controls (Roane & Porter, 1986). Shortened latencies on nociceptive tests suggest a hyperalgesic effect, indicating a lowered threshold or exaggerated response to normally painful stimulation. Another study showed that after carrageenan-induced inflammation male Zucker (*fa/fa*) rats had a lower threshold for mechanical and thermal pain, suggesting an analgesic response (Iannitti, Graham, & Dolan, 2012).

Studies of pain and obesity in humans have found similarly contrasting results. For example, Pradalier, Willer, Boureau, and Dry (1981) found nondiabetic obese women had lower thresholds for painful stimuli (percutaneous stimulation of the sural nerve) than did women of average weight. In contrast, another study showed pain thresholds were observed to be higher in obese subjects compared to lean subjects using electrical stimulation (Zahorska-Markiewicz, Kucio, & Pyszkowska, 1983). Tests of mechanical pain and obesity showed higher pain thresholds associated with increasing body weight (Khimich, 1997). Whereas, another study examining mechanical pain in obesity found obese participants had lower pain thresholds than the lean participants suggesting an increased sensitivity to pain (Mckendall & Haier, 1983). A recent study, using electrical stimulation examining pain in obesity before and after weight-loss surgery showed a higher pain threshold for obese participants that did not change with drastic weight loss (Dodet et al., 2013).

Evidence supports an alteration in nociceptive sensitivity in obesity. However, there is no clear agreement on whether there is increasing or decreasing sensitivity. Researchers studying pain in obesity suggest that the alterations in physiology in obesity are at least partially responsible for modulating the difference in pain threshold.

MODULATORS OF PAIN IN OBESITY

The association between pain and obesity has led to much speculation on the factors modulating this difference. There is a complex interrelationship between dietary behavior and altered physiology in obesity. This relationship is thought to lead to the changes in pain.

Obesity results from an energy imbalance that increases levels of adiposity. The increased adiposity leads to increased secretion of cytokines, which contribute to the dysfunction of many body systems (cardiovascular, immune, endocrine, nervous, and reproductive) and processes including the proinflammatory state associated with obesity (Redinger, 2007). Obesity affects glucose and lipid metabolism and is concomitant with diabetes type 2 mellitus and dyslipidemia (Redinger, 2007; Smith & Smith, 2016). Of particular relevance when considering pain and diet/nutrition are the alterations in obese physiology associated with vitamin D, leptin, ghrelin, endocannabinoids, and endogenous opioids. These are all altered in obesity, associated with dietary behavior and linked with pain.

Possibly as a consequence of the poor nutritional quality associated with the dietary behavior, one physiological difference in obesity is Hypovitaminosis D. Low serum vitamin D levels are correlated with high BMI, metabolic syndrome, and visceral adiposity in adults (Tosunbayraktar, Bas, Kut, & Buyukkaragoz, 2015). The inverse relationship of vitamin D and BMI is also found in the pediatric population. One study examined vitamin D levels in 217 obese children and adolescents and found over 50% were deficient in vitamin D and of those 21% were severely deficient (Smotkin-Tangorra et al., 2007). In patients with lower back pain, vitamin D, and BMI were found to be associated (Mattam & Sunny, 2016). In this study 80% of the patients with lower back had low levels of vitamin D and overweight/obese patients with lower back pain were more likely to have low levels of vitamin D than lean patients. Patients with osteoarthritis also show a correlation of low vitamin D levels and high BMI (Glover et al., 2015). The association of vitamin D and pain is well documented, especially in regards to chronic pain. Patients with lower back pain show significantly lower levels of vitamin D (Lodh et al., 2015). Low levels of vitamin D are also associated with chronic widespread pain (Kuru, Akyuz, Yagci, & Giray, 2015). Severe vitamin D deficiency has been shown to mimic chronic tension headache and generalized musculoskeletal pain in children (Prakash, Makwana, & Rathore, 2016). Hypovitaminosis D in postoperative patients is correlated with higher pain intensity scores (Lee, Chan, Samy, Chiu, & Gin, 2015) and higher required doses of analgesics in palliative cancer patients (Bergman, Sperneder, Höijer, Bergqvist, & Börkhem-Bergman, 2015).

Much of the research on obesity and its altered physiology have focused on the dysfunction in the systems regulating food intake. Some of the well documented signals involved in food intake include leptin, ghrelin, endocannabinoids, and endogenous opioids.

Leptin is produced predominantly by white adipose tissue and plays an important role in many physiological processes including body weight regulation through food intake and metabolism, where it acts as an anorexigenic agent (Lean & Malkova, 2015). Leptin also acts to regulate blood glucose levels through both appetite and fat storage, as well as through glucose storage in the liver independent of energy balance (Bates, Kulkarni, Seifert, & Myers, 2005). Leptin also has a role in hormone regulation via processes such as proopiomelanocortin (POMC) production (Inui, 1999). Circulating levels of leptin are positively correlated with body fat in humans and rodents (Maffei et al., 1995). Gene mutations in mice affecting leptin and leptin receptors often result in severe obesity (Lean & Malkova, 2015; Maffei et al., 1995). Obesity in humans is most commonly associated with leptin resistance, where despite high circulating levels of leptin there is a lack of responsiveness; thus it fails to decrease food intake (Lean & Malkova, 2015). Leptin resistance may be modulated through the intake of certain foods. Teasaponins, resveratrol, celastrol, caffeine, and taurine are associated with improved leptin signaling in neurons and vitamin A and D are associated with increased transport across the blood–brain barrier (Aragonès, Ardid-Ruiz, Ibars, Suárez, & Bladé, 2016).

There is evidence to suggest a role of leptin in pain, in addition to its other established physiological functions. Studies of leptin have shown an association with chronic pain and changes in pain threshold. Increased levels of leptin are correlated with increased reports of osteoarthritis shoulder pain (Gandhi, Takahashi, Rizeki, Dessouki, & Mahomed, 2012). Leptin has been linked with body pain in females. The study showed higher levels of pain in women correlated with increased leptin levels and BMI (Younger, Kapphahn, Brennan, Sullivan, & Stefanick, 2016). In lean mice, acute administration of leptin was shown to decrease thermal pain threshold, thus increasing pain sensitivity (Kutlu et al., 2003). Studies examining leptin and pain in obesity have shown inflammatory hyperalgesia in Zucker (*fa/fa*) rats, a model of obesity with a leptin receptor deficiency (Iannitti et al., 2012). Examining pain threshold in aged leptin deficient genetically obese (*ob/ob*) mice showed these mice had decreased responses to thermal pain (higher thresholds) and administration of leptin was able to partially normalize their analgesic response (Rodgers et al., 2014). These studies provide strong evidence that leptin is associated with increased pain. Both the endogenous opioid system and endocannabinoid system have been implicated as the underlying nociceptive pathway associated with leptin (Al'Absi, Lemieux, Nakajima, Hatsukami, & Allen, 2015; Cristino et al., 2016).

Another widely studied signal involved in food intake that is altered in obesity is ghrelin. Ghrelin is an orexigenic peptide secreted from the stomach (Lean & Malkova, 2015). While it has many physiological actions, it is widely known for its role in stimulating food intake via actions on neurons in the hypothalamus (Lean & Malkova, 2015). Serum ghrelin levels peak prior to food intake and decrease after food intake (Lean & Malkova, 2015). Although ghrelin is considered a short term regulator of feeding behavior, it may impact energy balance considering prolonged ghrelin administration increases adiposity (Tschöp, Smiley, & Heiman, 2000). A secondary role for ghrelin in feeding has been proposed in relationship with food addiction or hedonic eating because ghrelin activates brain regions important for reward processing (Wei et al., 2015). Ghrelin levels are reduced in obesity and show a negative correlation with high BMI (Tschöp et al., 2001). Furthermore, there is evidence to suggest the ghrelin response after a meal is altered in obesity (Lean & Malkova, 2015). Abnormal hunger scores are associated with obesity, interestingly, exogenous ghrelin administration normalizes the scores (Huda et al., 2009).

Recently numerous studies have linked ghrelin with pain. In a rat model of neuropathic pain, rats had a hyperalgesic response to mechanical and thermal stimuli and showed reduced levels of ghrelin (Zhou et al., 2014). Administration of ghrelin was shown to decrease the hyperalgesia and allodynia (Zhou et al., 2014). Similar results have been shown for thermal hyperalgesia and the administration of ghrelin using the same neuropathic pain rat model (Guneli et al., 2010). On tests of inflammatory pain, ghrelin has been shown to attenuate pain. This effect was reversed with administration of the opioid antagonist, naloxone (Sibilia et al., 2006). This study suggests the opioid system is mediating the effects of ghrelin on inflammatory pain. The interaction of the opioid system and ghrelin was further supported by the finding that administration of ghrelin decreased the analgesic effects of morphine administration (Zeng et al., 2013). Ghrelin has also been shown to play a role in the modulation of acute pain at the supraspinal level. On thermal tests of pain (tail-flick and hot-plate), administration of ghrelin had an analagesic effect in mice (Wei et al., 2013). Participation of the opioid system was shown by the ability of naloxone administration to reduce the antinociceptive effect of ghrelin (Wei et al., 2013). A similar antinociceptive effect was shown for the ghrelin receptor agonist, GHRP-2 on pain at the supraspinal level (Zeng et al., 2014).

The endocannabinoid system is an important neuromodulatory system altered in obesity. It is made up of endogenous cannabinoids (anandamide and 2-arachidonoylglycerol) and cannabinoid receptors (CB_1 and CB_2). The endocannabinoid system is well known for its role in mediating the effects of cannabis, which binds with the CB_1 receptor (Lu & Mackie, 2016). However, the endocannabinoid system is involved in many physiological processes, such as mood, memory, stress, addiction, appetite regulation, pain, and inflammation (Lu & Mackie, 2016). Alterations in the endocannabinoid system are associated with obesity. In humans, researchers have found an increase in both anandamide (AEA) and 2-arachidonoylglycerol (2-AG) associated with obesity and morbid obesity (Annuzzi et al., 2010; Matias et al., 2012). Levels of AEA directly correlated with BMI and waist circumference (Matias et al., 2012). Weight loss as a result of lifestyle changes significantly reduced the elevated AEA levels associated with obesity (Matias et al., 2012). The endocannabinoid system is also associated with pain modulation. It is known to be a key pain regulatory system with the ability to modulate pain at all stages during pain processing (Woodhams, Sager, Burston, & Chapman, 2015). The endocannabinoid system has a role in acute, chronic, and inflammatory pain (Woodhams et al., 2015). In obesity, the endocannabinoid system has been shown to modulate arthritis pain in obese rats (Croci & Zarini, 2007). Additionally, there is evidence that along with the opioid system, endocannabinoids mediate the effects of leptin on pain (Al'Absi et al., 2015; Cristino et al., 2016).

Endogenous opioids are neuropeptides well known for the role they play in analgesia. However, they have many other functions including effects on behavior, appetite regulation, mood, cognition, reproduction, and stress response (Eyvazzadeh et al., 2009). There are several families of endogenous opioids including endorphins, enkephalins, and dynorphins. These peptides bind with opioid receptors (mu, kappa, or delta) with varying selectivity and affinity. There is considerable evidence showing dysfunction in the opioid system associated with obesity. Increased levels of beta-endorphin have been found in obese women (Percheron et al., 1998). A relationship between body fat distribution and opioids within obesity exists. Increased levels of beta-endorphin were higher in those with abdominal obesity than those with peripheral obesity (Percheron et al., 1998). Levels of beta-endorphin in obese children are also elevated (Obuchowicz & Obuchowicz, 1997). The effects of weight loss on the beta-endorphin levels show that extensive weight loss after surgical intervention led to a significant reduction in the elevated beta-endorphin levels proportional to the amount of weight lost (Karayiannakis et al., 1998). As previously mentioned evidence is emerging showing the effects of leptin and ghrelin on pain are at least in part mediated through the opioid system.

TREATMENT AND PREVENTION OF PAIN IN OBESITY

The interrelationship of diet, pain, and obesity is complex making it difficult to disentangle their distinct roles. Obesity is associated with altered physiology, some directly relevant to dietary behavior (vitamin deficiencies) and others have a more complicated relationship where they could be the cause or the consequence of dietary behavior. Several studies have reported the effects of diet on the treatment of pain that are particularly pertinent in the obese population.

There is significant evidence for a role of Hypovitaminosis D in chronic pain and evidence of its role in chronic pain associated with obesity. Therefore, it would suggest that correcting that deficiency would have an effect on the pain experienced in this population. This supposition is at least in part supported in literature. While no studies have directly assessed the effect of increasing vitamin D on pain in the obese population, there are many studies demonstrating increasing vitamin D levels have positive effects on pain. Nursing home residents, another population that shows Hypovitaminosis D, when given vitamin D fortified foods showed decreases in pain scores (Costan, Vulpoi, & Mocanu, 2014). Vitamin D as a treatment for diabetic neuropathy (a common comorbid condition with obesity) showed positive results, a single injection of vitamin D in patients led to a decrease in pain symptoms (Basit et al., 2016). Vitamin D supplements given to osteoarthritis patients with Hypovitaminosis D over a period of 2 months restored vitamin D levels to normal in all but one patient and significantly decreased pain (Heidari, Javadian, Babaei, & Yousef-Ghahari, 2015). More studies are needed to elucidate the effects of vitamin D treatment on pain in the obese population, but it appears to a promising method of treatment.

Obesity and chronic pain are both increasing, however, it is unclear whether the chronic pain stems from greater body mass and therefore strain on joints and muscles or if other factors are involved. Osteoarthritis, a common form of chronic pain, is associated with obesity and can be found in the hands in addition to hips and knees of obese individuals. This supports the idea that more than just the mechanical strain of additional weight is responsible for the chronic pain in obesity (Thomazeau et al., 2014). One possibility is that the poor quality diet generally consumed in obesity is affecting pain. To examine the possibility that poor dietary behavior plays a role in modulating pain one study assessed the effects of an obesogenic diet on pain in mice. Mice were fed a nutritionally poor diet that was energy-dense, and high in fat and carbohydrates. On tests of mechanical and thermal pain mice fed the obesogenic diet were shown to have both increased pain thresholds and increased levels of circulating leptin and inflammatory cytokines (Totsch et al., 2016). In addition, on tests of chronic pain, hyperalgesia was increased and prolonged in the mice fed the obesogenic diet. This study provides evidence that suggests nutritional quality can affect nociception. More research needs to be done to assess if improving the nutritional quality of the diet would decrease the pain. The results of this study further suggest that consumption of good quality nutrition could help prevent the development of altered nociception and chronic pain.

Overall, the literature supports the importance of dietary behavior and good nutrition to decrease the risk for chronic pain or changes in nociceptive sensitivity suggesting that good nutrition would be a beneficial preventative measure. Furthermore, there is some evidence that proper nutrition and weight loss could help to normalize the altered pain experienced in the obese population. The altered physiology associated with obesity stems at least partially from dietary behavior. Food intake affects levels of leptin, ghrelin, endogenous opioids, and endocannabinoids, all of which can affect nociception. Ensuring proper levels of food intake of high nutritional quality may help reduce the risk or normalize the altered peptide levels and thus have a positive impact on pain. Additionally, good nutrition is needed to ensure adequate levels of vitamins, as vitamin deficiencies are also associated with pain. More research is needed to assess the roles of diet and nutrition in the treatment and prevention of pain in the obese population, but there is evidence that this may be a promising avenue of exploration.

References

Al'Absi, M., Lemieux, A., Nakajima, M., Hatsukami, D. K., & Allen, S. (2015). Circulating leptin and pain perception among tobacco-dependent individuals. *Biological Psychology*, *107*, 10–15.

Allman-Farinelli, M., Partridge, S. R., & Roy, R. (2016). Weight-Related Dietary Behaviors in Young Adults. *Current Obesity Reports*, *5*(1), 23–29.

Annuzzi, G., Piscitelli, F., Di Marino, L., Patti, L., Giacco, R., Costabile, G., Bozzetto, L., Riccardi, G., Verde, R., Petrosino, S., Rivellese, A. A., & Di Marzo, V. (2010). Differential alterations of the concentrations of endocannabinoids and related lipids in the subcutaneous adipose tissue of obese diabetic patients. *Lipids in Health and Disease*, *9*(1), 43.

Aragonès, G., Ardid-Ruiz, A., Ibars, M., Suárez, M., & Bladé, C. (2016). Modulation of leptin resistance by food compounds. *Molecular Nutrition and Food Research*.

Basit, A., Basit, K. A., Fawwad, A., Shaheen, F., Fatima, N., Petropoulos, I. N., Alam, U., & Malik, R. A. (2016). Vitamin D for the treatment of painful diabetic neuropathy. *BMJ Open Diabetes Research Care*, *4*(1), 10.

Bates, S. H., Kulkarni, R. N., Seifert, M., & Myers, M. G. (2005). Roles for leptin receptor/STAT3- dependent and independent signals in the regulation of glucose homeostasis. *Cell Metabolism*, *1*, 169–178.

Bergman, P., Sperneder, S., Höijer, J., Bergqvist, J., & Björkhem-Bergman, L. (2015). Low vitamin D levels are associated with higher opioid dose in palliative cancer patients results from an observational study in Sweden. *PLoS One*, *10*(5), .

Costan, A. R., Vulpoi, C., & Mocanu, V. (2014). Vitamin D fortified bread improves pain and physical function domains of quality of life in nursing home residents. *Journal of Medicinal Food*, *17*(5), 625–631.

Cristino, L., Luongo, L., Imperatore, R., Boccella, S., Becker, T., Morello, G., Piscitelli, F., Busetto, G., Maione, S., & Marzo, V. D. (2016). Orexin-A and endocannabinoid activation of the descending antinociceptive pathway underlies altered pain perception in leptin signaling deficiency. *Neuropsychopharmacology*, *41*(2), 508–520.

Croci, T., & Zarini, E. (2007). Effect of the cannabinoid CB1 receptor antagonist rimonabant on nociceptive responses and adjuvant-induced arthritis in obese and lean rats. *British Journal of Pharmacology*, *150*(5), 559–566.

Dodet, P., Perrot, S., Auvergne, L., Hajj, A., Simoneau, G., Declèves, X., Poitou, C., Oppert, J. M., Peo'Ch, K., Mouly, S., Bergmann, J. F., & Lloret-Linares, C. (2013). Sensory impairment in obese patients? Sensitivity and pain detection thresholds for electrical stimulation after surgery-induced weight loss, and comparison with a non-obese population. *The Clinical Journal of Pain*, *29*(1), 43–49.

Duruöz, M. T., Turan, Y., Gürgan, A., & Deveci, H. (2012). Evaluation of metabolic syndrome in patients with chronic low back pain. *Rheumatology International*, *32*(3), 663–667.

Eyvazzadeh, A. D., Pennington, K. P., Pop-Busui, R., Sowers, M., Zubieta, J., & Smith, Y. (2009). The role of the endogenous opioid system in polycystic ovary syndrome. *Fertility and Sterility*, *92*(1), 1–12.

Frilander, H., Solovieva, S., Mutanen, P., Pihlajamäki, H., Heliövaara, M., & Viikari-Juntura, E. (2015). Role of overweight and obesity in low back disorders among men: a longitudinal study with a life course approach. *BMJ Open*, *5*(8), .

Gandhi, R., Takahashi, M., Rizek, R., Dessouki, O., & Mahomed, N. N. (2012). Obesity-related adipokines and shoulder osteoarthritis. *The Journal of Rheumatology*, *39*(10), 2046–2048.

Glover, T. L., Goodin, B. R., King, C. D., Sibille, K. T., Herbert, M. S., Sotolongo, A. S., Cruz-Almeida, Y., Bartley, E. J., Bulls, H. W., Horgas, A. L., Redden, D. T., Riley, J. L., 3rd, Staud, R., Fessler, B. J., Bradley, L. A., & Fillingim, R. B. (2015). A Cross-sectional examination of vitamin D, obesity, and measures of pain and function in middle-aged and older adults with knee osteoarthritis. *The Clinical Journal of Pain*, *31*(12), 1060–1067.

Guneli, E., Onal, A., Ates, M., Bagriyanik, H. A., Resmi, H., Orhan, C. E., Kolatan, H. E., & Gumustekin, M. (2010). Effects of repeated administered ghrelin on chronic constriction injury of the sciatic nerve in rats. *Neuroscience Letters*, *479*(3), 226–230.

Heidari, B., Javadian, Y., Babaei, M., & Yousef-Ghahari, B. (2015). Restorative effect of vitamin D deficiency on knee pain and quadriceps muscle strength in knee osteoarthritis. *Acta Medica Iranica*, *53*(8), 466–470.

Huda, M. S., Dovey, T., Wong, S. P., English, P. J., Halford, J., Mcculloch, P., Cleator, J., Martin, B., Cashen, J., Hayden, K., Wilding, J. P., & Pinkney, J. (2009). Ghrelin restores 'lean-type' hunger and energy expenditure profiles in morbidly obese subjects but has no effect on postgastrectomy subjects. *International Journal of Obesity*, *33*(3), 317–325.

Hudson, J. I., Hiripi, E., Pope, H. G., & Kessler, R. C. (2007). The prevalence and correlates of eating disorders in the national comorbidity survey replication. *Biological Psychiatry*, *61*(3), 348–358.

Iannitti, T., Graham, A., & Dolan, S. (2012). Increased central and peripheral inflammation and inflammatory hyperalgesia in Zucker rat model of leptin receptor deficiency and genetic obesity. *Experimental Physiology*, *97*(11), 1236–1245.

Inui, A. (1999). Feeding and body-weight regulation by hypothalamic neuropeptides- mediation of the actions of leptin. *Trends in Neuroscience*, *22*, 62–67.

Kant, A. K., & Graubard, B. I. (2006). Secular trends in patterns of self-reported food consumption of adult Americans: NHANES 1971-1975 to NHANES 1999–2002. *The American Journal of Clinical Nutrition*, *84*(5), 1215–1223.

Karayiannakis, A. J., Zbar, A., Makri, G. G., Syrigos, K., Athanasiadis, L., Alexiou, D., & Bastounis, E. A. (1998). Serum beta-endorphin levels in morbidly obese patients: the effect of vertical banded gastroplasty. *European Surgical Research*, *30*(6), 409–413.

Khimich, S. (1997). Level of sensitivity of pain in patients with obesity [Abstract]. *Acta chirurgica Hungarica*, *36*, 166–167.

Kuru, P., Akyuz, G., Yagci, I., & Giray, E. (2015). Hypovitaminosis D in widespread pain: its effect on pain perception, quality of life and nerve conduction studies. *Rheumatology International*, *35*(2), 315–322.

Kutlu, S., Canpolat, S., Sandal, S., Ozcan, M., Sarsilmaz, M., & Kelestimur, H. (2003). Effects of central and peripheral administration of leptin on pain threshold in rats and mice. *Neuroendocrinology Letters*, *24*, 193–196.

Langsetmo, L., Poliquin, S., Hanley, D. A., Prior, J. C., Barr, S., Anastassiades, T., Towheed, T., Goltzman, D., Kreiger, N., & Group, T. C. (2010). Dietary patterns in Canadian men and women ages 25 and older: relationship to demographics, body mass index, and bone mineral density. *BMC Musculoskeletal Disorders*, *11*(1), 20.

Lean, M. E., & Malkova, D. (2015). Altered gut and adipose tissue hormones in overweight and obese individuals: cause or consequence? *International Journal of Obesity*, *40*(4), 622–632.

Lee, A., Chan, S. K., Samy, W., Chiu, C. H., & Gin, T. (2015). Effect of hypovitaminosis D on postoperative pain outcomes and short-term health-related quality of life after knee arthroplasty. *Medicine, 94*(42), .

Lodh, M., Goswami, B., Mahajan, R. D., Sen, D., Jajodia, N., & Roy, A. (2015). Assessment of vitamin D status in patients of chronic low back pain of unknown etiology. *Indian Journal of Clinical Biochemistry, 30*(2), 174–179.

Lu, H., & Mackie, K. (2016). An introduction to the endogenous cannabinoid system. *Biological Psychiatry, 79*(7), 516–525.

Maffei, M., Halaas, J., Ravussin, E., Pratley, R. E., Lee, G. H., Zhang, Y., Fei, H., Kim, S., Lallone, R., Ranganathan, S., Kern, P. A., & Friedman, J. M. (1995). Leptin levels in human and rodent: measurement of plasma leptin and *ob* RNA in obese and weight-reduced subjects. *Nature Medicine, 11*, 1155–1161.

Matias, I., Gatta-Cherifi, B., Tabarin, A., Clark, S., Leste-Lasserre, T., Marsicano, G., Piazza, P. V., & Cota, D. (2012). Endocannabinoids measurement in human saliva as potential biomarker of obesity. *PLoS One, 7*(7), .

Mattam, A., & Sunny, G. (2016). Correlation of vitamin D and body mass index with modic changes in patients with non-specific low back pain in a sub-tropical Asian population. *Asian Spine Journal, 10*(1), 14–19.

Mccarthy, L. H., Bigal, M. E., Katz, M., Derby, C., & Lipton, R. B. (2009). Chronic pain and obesity in elderly people: results from the Einstein aging study. *Journal of the American Geriatrics Society, 57*(1), 115–119.

Mckendall, M. J., & Haier, R. J. (1983). Pain sensitivity and obesity. *Psychiatry Research, 8*(2), 119–125.

Mork, P., Holtermann, A., & Nilsen, T. (2013). Physical exercise, body mass index and risk of chronic arm pain: longitudinal data on an adult population in Norway. *European Journal of Pain, 17*(8), 1252–1258.

Mozaffarian, D., Hao, T., Rimm, E. B., Willett, W. C., & Hu, F. B. (2011). Changes in diet and lifestyle and long-term weight gain in women and men. *New England Journal of Medicine, 364*(25), 2392–2404.

Obuchowicz, A., & Obuchowicz, E. (1997). Plasma beta-endorphin and insulin concentrations in relation to body fat and nutritional parameters in overweight and obese prepubertal children. *International Journal of Obesity and Related Metabolic Disorders, 21*(9), 783–788.

Okifuji, A., & Hare, B. D. (2015). The association between chronic pain and obesity. *The Journal of Pain Research, 8*, 399–408.

Papanas, N., & Ziegler, D. (2015). Risk factors and comorbidities in diabetic neuropathy: an update 2015. *The Review of Diabetic Studies, 12*(1–2), 48–62.

Percheron, C., Colette, C., Mariano-Goulart, D., Avignon, A., Capeyron, O., Boniface, H., Bressot, N., Monnier, L., et al. (1998). Relationship between insulin sensitivity, obesity, body fat distribution and beta-endorphinaemia in obese women. *International Journal of Obesity and Related Metabolic Disorders, 22*(2), 143–148.

Pradalier, A., Willer, J. -C., Boureau, F., & Dry, J. (1981). Relationship between pain and obesity: an electrophysiological study. *Physiology and Behavior, 27*, 9661–9964.

Prakash, S., Makwana, P., & Rathore, C. (2016). Vitamin D deficiency mimicking chronic tension-type headache in children. *BMJ Case Reports*, 1–4.

Ramzan, I., Wong, B. K., & Corcoran, G. B. (2003). Pain sensitivity in dietary-induced obese rats. *Physiology and Behavior, 54*, 433–435.

Redinger, R. N. (2007). The pathophysiology of obesity and its clinical manifestations. *Gastroenterology and Hepatology, 3*(11), 856–863.

Roane, D. S., & Porter, J. R. (1986). Nociception and opioid-induced analgesia in lean (Fa/−) and obese (fa/fa) zucker rats. *Physiology and Behavior, 38*, 215–218.

Rodgers, H. M., Liban, S., & Wilson, L. M. (2014). Attenuated pain response of obese mice (*B6.Cg-lep^{ob}*) is affected by aging and leptin but not sex. *Physiology and Behavior, 123*, 80–85.

Scher, I. A., Stewart, F. W., Ricci, A. J., & Lipton, B. R. (2003). Factors associated with the onset and remission of chronic daily headache in a population-based study. *Pain, 106*(1), 81–89.

Sibilia, V., Lattuada, N., Rapetti, D., Pagani, F., Vincenza, D., Bulgarelli, I., Locatelli, V., Guidobono, F., & Netti, C. (2006). Ghrelin inhibits inflammatory pain in rats: involvement of the opioid system. *Neuropharmacology, 51*(3), 497–505.

Sinha, R., Dhungel, S., Sinha, M., Paudel, B. H., Bhattacharya, N., & Mandal, M. B. (2009). Obesity attenuates formalin-induced tonic pain in British Angora rabbits. *Indian Journal of Physiology and Pharmacology, 53*, 83–87.

Smith, K. B., & Smith, M. S. (2016). Obesity statistics. *Primary Care: Clinics in Office Practice, 43*(1), 121–135.

Smotkin-Tangorra, M., Purushothaman, R., Gupta, A., Nejati, G., Anhalt, H., & Ten, S. (2007). Prevalence of vitamin D insufficiency in obese children and adolescents. *Journal of Pediatric Endocrinology and Metabolism, 20*(7), 817–823.

Thomazeau, J., Perin, J., Nizard, R., Bouhassira, D., Collin, E., Nguyen, E., Perrot, S., Bergmann, J. F., & Lloret-Linares, C. (2014). Pain management and pain characteristics in obese and normal weight patients before joint replacement. *Journal of Evaluation in Clinical Practice, 20*(5), 611–616.

Tosunbayraktar, G., Bas, M., Kut, A., & Buyukkaragoz, A. H. (2015). Low serum 25(OH)D levels are associated to higher BMI and metabolic syndrome parameters in adult subjects in Turkey. *African Health Sciences, 15*(4), 1161–1169.

Totsch, S. K., Waite, M. E., Tomkovich, A., Quinn, T. L., Gower, B. A., & Sorge, R. E. (2016). Total western diet alters mechanical and thermal sensitivity and prolongs hypersensitivity following complete freund's adjuvant in mice. *The Journal of Pain, 17*(1), 119–125.

Tschöp, M., Smiley, D. L., & Heiman, M. L. (2000). Ghrelin induces adiposity in rodents. *Nature, 407*(6806), 908–913.

Tschöp, M., Weyer, C., Tataranni, P. A., Devanarayan, V., Ravussin, E., & Heiman, M. L. (2001). Circulating ghrelin levels are decreased in human obesity. *Diabetes, 50*(4), 707–709.

von Deneen, K. M., & Liu, Y. (2011). Obesity as an addiction: why do the obese eat more? *Maturitas, 68*(4), 342–345.

Wang, J. B., Patterson, R. E., Ang, A., Emond, J. A., Shetty, N., & Arab, L. (2014). Timing of energy intake during the day is associated with the risk of obesity in adults. *Journal of Human Nutrition and Dietetics, 27*, 255–262.

Wei, J., Zhi, X., Wang, X., Zeng, P., Zou, T., Yang, B., & Wang, J. (2013). In vivo characterization of the effects of ghrelin on the modulation of acute pain at the supraspinal level in mice. *Peptides, 43*, 76–82.

Wei, X., Sun, B., Chen, K., Lv, B., Luo, X., & Yan, J. (2015). Ghrelin signaling in the ventral tegmental area mediates both reward-based feeding and fasting-induced hyperphagia on high-fat diet. *Neuroscience, 300*, 53–62.

Woodhams, S. G., Sagar, D. R., Burston, J. J., & Chapman, V. (2015). The role of the endocannabinoid system in pain. *Pain Control Handbook of Experimental Pharmacology*, 119–143.

Younger, J., Kapphahn, K., Brennan, K., Sullivan, S. D., & Stefanick, M. L. (2016). Association of leptin with body pain in women. *Journal of Women's Health*.

Zahorska-Markiewicz, B., Kucio, C., & Pyszkowska, J. (1983). Obesity and pain [Abstract]. *Human Nutrition. Clinical Nutrition, 37*(4), 307–310.

Zeng, P., Chen, J., Yang, B., Zhi, X., Guo, F., Sun, M., Wang, J. L., & Wei, J. (2013). Attenuation of systemic morphine-induced analgesia by central administration of ghrelin and related peptides in mice. *Peptides, 50*, 42–49.

Zeng, P., Li, S., Zheng, Y., Liu, F., Wang, J., Zhang, D., & Wei, J. (2014). Ghrelin receptor agonist, GHRP-2, produces antinociceptive effects at the supraspinal level via the opioid receptor in mice. *Peptides, 55*, 103–109.

Zhou, C., Li, X., Zhu, Y., Huang, H., Li, J., Liu, L., Hu, Q., Ma, T. F., Shao, Y., & Wu, Y. (2014). Ghrelin alleviates neuropathic pain through GHSR-1a–mediated suppression of the p38 MAPK/NF-κB pathway in a rat chronic constriction injury model. *Regional Anesthesia and Pain Medicine, 39*(2), 137–148.

CHAPTER

13

Effects of Obesity on Function and Quality of Life in Chronic Pain

L.I. Arranz

Department of Nutrition, Food Sciences and Gastronomy, Faculty of Pharmacy and Food Sciences, Univerisity of Barcelona, Barcelona, Spain

INTRODUCTION

Chronic pain is a sensory negative experience of possible injury in some part of the body that involves the nervous system and persists for weeks, months, or even years. Many people suffer from chronic pain and its prevalence is 30% in US adults being higher in females (Johannes et al., 2010). The most common types of chronic pain in adult patients are low back pain (LBP), arthritis, and fibromyalgia (FM), all of which are disabling in some degree (WHO, 2008). The situation may be even worse in people who have more than one chronic pain condition, leading to very poor functional capacity and decreased quality of life (QoL). The impact of disease on functional status and well-being is measured with health-related quality of life (HRQoL), which has been defined as the effect of medical conditions on well-being and physical and mental function, reflecting the functional effects of a disease as perceived by the patient.

On the other hand, obesity is an increasing global health issue, especially in developed countries, with serious repercussions due to the increased potential for development of comorbid conditions. Obesity is defined as body weight greater than normal as the result of an abnormal increase in body fat storage. It is usually categorized using body mass index (BMI) which is calculated as the body mass divided by the square of the body height, and is universally expressed in units of kilogram per square meter. As it is shown in Table 13.1 depending on these figures people may be classified as underweight, normal, overweight, or obese, although it is recommended to additionally use other measurements, such as waist circumference and waist-to-hip ratio to have proper information about fat stores.

Obesity classes II and III are considered severe and morbid obesity, respectively, and generally have much more health implications than just overweight. The two main causes to reach these conditions are high-energy food intake, especially through high fat intake, and low physical activity; however, there may be associated factors, such as lack of sleep, stress, metabolic disorders, and probably chronic inflammation. The direct health consequences of obesity are chronic diseases, such as diabetes mellitus type-2, dyslipidemia, coronary heart disease, osteoarthritis (OA), sleep apnea, certain types of cancers, and psychosocial problems. Moreover, obesity is a detrimental factor for other diseases. Chronic pain and limitations in everyday functioning of overweight and obese individuals are the cause and consequence of comorbidities due to a mechanical impairment of the musculoskeletal system, which is caused not only by an excessive weight, but also by an increased chronic inflammatory state (Seaman, 2013; Wright et al., 2010). Although it remains uncertain whether a common cause of obesity and chronic pain exists, some studies reflect similar or equal mechanisms or pathophysiologic processes, with systemic chronic inflammation as a possible key issue (Seaman, 2013) because it has been associated with increased joint inflammation and OA (Gandhi et al., 2010). Systemic inflammation is involved even in some rheumatic disorders, increasing bone loss and fracture risk, and it is also known that oxidized low-density lipoprotein (LDL) induces the production of proinflammatory factors and their receptors (Bultink et al., 2012). Moreover, this circle of chronic/acute and central/peripheral inflammation probably is related to the fact that a sedentary lifestyle contributes to obesity and, inversely, obesity exacerbates disability and consequently

Nutritional Modulators of Pain in the Aging Population. http://dx.doi.org/10.1016/B978-0-12-805186-3.00013-8
Copyright © 2017 Elsevier Inc. All rights reserved.

TABLE 13.1 International Classification of Adult Underweight, Overweight, and Obesity According to Body Mass Index (WHO, 2000)

Classification group		BMI (kg/m²)
Underweight		<18.50
Normal range		18.50–24.99
Overweight		25.00–29.99
Obesity	Class I	30.00–34.99
	Class II	35.00–39.99
	Class III	≥40.00

BMI, Body mass index

a sedentary lifestyle. The role a lack of physical activity plays in weight gain emphasizes the fact that among people with pain and disabling conditions, obesity rates are significantly higher (Piechota, Małkiewicz, & Karwat, 2005).

Pain and obesity both have a negative effect on the QoL and functional capacity of people of all ages and both sexes. Pain management is the key to obese patients becoming more active and achieving a better QoL (D'Arcy, 2011). Inversely, weight management also is a key factor for patients with chronic pain conditions who have obesity as comorbidity. These relationships have a lot of implications for patient life and this is the reason why their management is of a big importance. Moreover, body weight is negatively affected by other common conditions among chronic pain and obese patients. The evaluation of the possible positive role of nutrition management is an interesting aspect to improve patient functionality.

EFFECTS OF OBESITY ON FUNCTION AND QOL IN CHRONIC PAIN CONDITIONS

General Relationship Between Obesity and Pain, Quality of Life, and Disability

With the knowledge we have at the moment, it is important to understand how chronic pain is related to obesity, and vice versa. It is of a big relevance also to be aware in which extent both conditions affect patient functionality and QoL, and how to improve this. The consequences of chronic pain increase the risk of obesity and worsen the progress of an obese person, and at the same time, consequences of obesity negatively affect to chronic pain. Therefore, in order to avoid entering in a vicious circle in which global health, QoL, and functionality get worse, and this deterioration even leads to more pain and more obesity, it is needed to evaluate our patients globally taking into account all possible factors around this. To lose weight, reduce high levels of cholesterol, reduce abdominal fat, improve calorie and nutrient diet content, achieve an optimal sleep time, and ensure an individualized program of physical activity, are examples of essential strategies we should reach to improve obese chronic pain patient evolution in time.

Obesity and Pain

The relationship between obesity and pain is not likely to be direct and many interacting factors appear to contribute. As there is no single causative relationship, the link between them seems to be multifactorial, and additionally they are two different conditions adversely impacting each other. Obesity is expected to increase in many countries and therefore it can be expected that the presentation of obese patients with chronic pain will also rise in accordance with the future higher prevalence of obesity. Therefore, it is urgent to have a better understanding on how to manage both conditions in order to break the negative reciprocal impact. Based upon the existing research, there are several potential mechanisms that may link the two phenomena, including mechanical/structural factors, chemical inflammatory mediators, depression, sleep, and lifestyle. About the first one, it is known that the increased loading due to heavy weight on joints and the spine is one of the most discussed links between obesity and pain. Furthermore, significantly altered body mechanics and postures are very common in obese humans, suggesting that such changes may be involved in the link between obesity and pain. But there is something more than that. Research on potential chemical mediators linking obesity with pain is rapidly growing. Nowadays, we know that adipose tissue is not a passive storage unit for fat cells and that its metabolic activity may have health implications also for chronic pain through the increased levels of proinflammatory cytokines and adipokines. Research suggests that obesity may be characterized by a low-grade chronic inflammatory state as reflected by elevated levels in many inflammatory markers in the serum, such as interleukin-6 (IL-6) and C-reactive protein, and this systemic inflammation may be one of the main mediators between obesity and pain. Vitamin D is pointed as another possible mediator, as it seems that levels are reduced in obese patients and this could be related to poor skeletal mineralization and pain (Okifuji & Hare, 2015). It must be noted, as some authors point out, that while there exists much evidence to support an increased quantity of inflammatory cytokines in obese individuals and much theory in how inflammatory cytokines contribute to pain, there is as yet very little evidence to directly link obesity with pain through inflammatory cytokine production, and this perhaps is an exciting area for future study. This will also help in understanding the relationship between obesity, chronic pain, and metabolic syndrome. It is known that the prevalence of metabolic syndrome increases with increasing BMI and chronic pain, and so it may be that some confounding factor of metabolic syndrome relates obesity to pain. In this sense there is also a need to know more details about this link (McVinnie, 2013). In addition, when chronic pain and/or obesity are present it is very difficult for the patient to carry out a healthy lifestyle, mainly because physical activity is normally reduced and even affected by the usual lack of sleep.

Therefore, it is clear that there are also other factors to take into account around this relationship because they are detrimental for both pain and obesity. It is the case of the association between obesity and depression, which in turn could be mediated by the levels of weight and shape concern, binging eating disorder, and also by the poor sleep quality. In patients with a chronic pain condition FM overweight or even obesity is common and also some eating disorders probably due to the search for hedonic foods to briefly mitigate pain and also to compensate fatigue. Moreover, after this behavior, not controlling food intake, patients have a bad feeling about their incompetence to manage their basic impulses. And this has a negative effect on depression. Obviously, identification of the specific variables that mediate the effect of obesity on depression has implications for the clinical management of FM patients seeking treatment for weight loss. Some authors suggest that effectively treating sleep disturbances and the focus on stabilization of eating behavior in order to reduce or stop binge eating in obese patients with FM might have beneficial effects beyond weight reduction alone (Senna, Ahmad, & Fathi, 2013). For successful interventions it is necessary to give nutritional education to patients containing all the basic information about their diets, beneficial foods, and harmful habits. In this sense, it is useful also to target the negative self-image feelings to improve adherence to weight loss and even to depression treatments, creating a right self-perception that one can benefit from weight loss, first to improve health, and afterward pain and also body shape.

Food intake is also seriously affected by sleep time, nowadays it is known that sleep duration is a crucial factor affecting both body weight and feeding behavior. Some data show how individuals with lack or nonrestorative sleep have a higher energy intake especially from higher carbohydrate consumption per day. This may be due to a simple compensatory mechanism looking for more energy when people feel tired. Sleep duration is negatively associated with fat mass and QoL questionnaire, SF-36, total score (Poggiogalle et al., 2016).

Should there are those many factors affecting obesity and pain the treatment must deal with all of them as a whole in order to reverse the negative relationships among them. Although not all the mechanisms are perfectly known, it is reasonable that treating globally all these factors, obesity, metabolic syndrome, poor sleep, eating disorders, depression, and others in order to improve patients health.

Obesity, Functionality, and QoL

Obesity is the fifth leading global risk factor for mortality (WHO, 2009); it leads to an increase in morbidity and is associated with lower HRQoL and increased disability by increasing limitations on daily life activities. Obese people have fewer years of healthy life, report more health problems than normal-weight subjects, and have more chronic diseases that increase physical disability and reduce normal functioning. Overweight and obese individuals report more self-perceived pain on bodily pain subscales of HRQoL measurements compared to normal weight people (Wright et al., 2010; Yancy et al., 2002; Dixon, 2010).

Generally, it has been shown that an increase in body weight corresponds to deterioration in QoL scores, but specifically in the physical function and general health domains, and not in mental scores (Sirtori et al., 2012). Most studies show that higher degrees of obesity are associated with greater impairment and that weight reduction, even if modest, is associated with enhanced QoL (Fontaine & Barofsky 2001; Castres et al., 2010). Moreover, the number of comorbidities correlates with the degree of obesity, which also determines a worse HRQoL (Sendi et al., 2005). Additionally, it is important to note that this correlation is greater in women and elderly people (Oliva-Moreno & Gil-Lacruz, 2013).

Obese people face other problems that affect QoL, such as difficulties in mobility, pain, and sleep quality. Obesity is associated with insufficient sleep or poor sleep quality, and it appears overweight and obese individuals who eat less have better perceived general health (Wang et al., 2013). However, it is known that a chronic lack of sleep (quantitative or qualitative) is associated with weight gain, metabolic disorders, cardiovascular risk, worse immune function, higher systemic inflammation, and even psychiatric disorders (Chaput, Klingenberg, & Sjödin, 2010; Greer, Goldstein, & Walker, 2013; Touma & Pannain, 2011; Bollinger et al., 2010; Grandner et al., 2013; Krystal, 2012).

Effects of Obesity and Chronic Pain on Function and QoL

Obesity and chronic pain conditions are increasing morbidities that negatively affect function and well-being, and both have significant public health consequences. Excess body weight, especially obesity, contributes to chronic pain, probably as a result of two different mechanisms. The first mechanism is mechanical stress on the whole skeletal system and joints; the second is systemic proinflammatory status worsening widespread and local pain. Inversely, chronic pain contributes to obesity mainly through physical inactivity as the direct result of fear of movement or physical disability, causing deconditioning and increasing pain (Wright et al., 2010; Caldwell, Hart-Johnson, & Green, 2009).

Perhaps one of the most direct studies assessing the effect of BMI on patients with chronic pain evaluated pain severity, disability, depression, anxiety, and QoL in 372 patients receiving or seeking treatment for chronic pain (Marcus, 2004). The results showed that increased BMI was associated with comorbid pain disability, depression, and reduced physical function as measured by the SF-36 health survey. Moreover, other researchers have suggested that pain may mediate the relationship between increasing BMI and HRQoL, meaning that the effects of high BMI on HRQoL are magnified in the presence of pain, and highlighted that a change from high to normal BMI may improve HRQoL (Heo et al., 2003). Another study found that among patients with class II or III obesity, higher BMI alone was not directly associated with lower QoL; however, the presence of LBP in the context of obesity was significantly associated with reduced QoL, as measured by the EuroQoL questionnaire (Sendi et al., 2005).

An interesting study examined the relationship among obesity, body composition, foot pain, and disability. The results demonstrated that increasing BMI, specifically android distribution of fat mass, was strongly associated with foot pain and disability. In contrast, a beneficial effect of a gynoid distribution of fat was observed, suggesting that the mechanism of obesity's effect on disability might be the result of both a mechanical effect, by increasing the load on the skeletal system, and a systemic effect related to metabolic factors (Tanamas et al., 2012). It is important to consider that evidence exists regarding the beneficial effect of weight loss treatment, with either surgical intervention or lifestyle changes, such as exercise and diet, on HRQoL in obese patients with chronic pain (Janke, Collins, & Kozak, 2007).

While obesity and pain reduce functional capacity and QoL, making people less physically active and more depressed, this situation might lead to reduced sleep, more stress, a sedentary lifestyle, and consequently an increased chronic inflammation status (Dixon, Schachter, & O'Brien, 2001; Vorona et al., 2005). Also, obese people with chronic pain suffer more depressive symptoms than normal-weight or overweight people with pain (Wright et al., 2010). They have hedonic hunger triggered by physical pain and associated with depression and guilt, and experience emotional or "binge" eating, as well as altered dietary choices, in response to pain. Many studies have emphasized the fact that obese people with chronic pain have difficulty with physical activity because of physical disability, reduced self-efficacy due to pain, and avoidance of movement because of the fear of pain (Amy Janke & Kozak, 2012). Because of this pain, but also because of fear of movement, morbidly obese patients avoid physical activity, which interferes with activities of daily living and participation in social or recreational activities. Obese patients have been shown to engage in greater catastrophizing behavior (Somers et al., 2008), and those reporting poor self-rated health and a depressed mood might be at a higher risk for pain chronicity (Seaman, 2013; Lebovits et al., 2009). These events lead to a vicious circle: obesity leads to avoidance of activity, depression, lack of sleep, and an increase in pain that leads to fear of movement, resulting in further avoidance of physical exercise and worsening of obesity and pain.

There is no doubt that obesity and BMI have a negative impact on QoL in people with chronic pain conditions. This impact is especially significant in some populations, such as African Americans, children, and adolescents. In the case of African Americans, because they are more prone to obesity and chronic pain, the impact of both conditions on QoL is greater. Being African American is indirectly associated with lower physical function and more pain-related disability (Caldwell et al., 2009). In children and adolescents, cooccurring chronic pain and obesity significantly exacerbate the impact chronic pain would have alone on overall QoL. Compared with adults who have an increased BMI correlated with depression and reduced QoL for physical function, the impact on children and adolescents may be more extensive, affecting physical and psychosocial domains (Hainsworth et al., 2009).

There are so many chronic pain conditions, such as FM, OA, rheumatoid arthritis (RA), and LBP, where the triad obesity, pain and function, and QoL have been observed. In all of them the cooccurrence of obesity is frequent and exacerbates symptoms, reduces functionality and QoL scores and makes other life conditions worse, such as it is the case for sleep, physical activity, psychological, and emotional status, and so on (Arranz, Rafecas, & Alegre, 2014).

Fibromyalgia

FM is a common and increasingly diagnosed chronic pain condition with an unknown cause and a prevalence of around 2–4%, depending on the country. FM patients have widespread musculoskeletal pain and stiffness, general fatigue, sleep disorders, cognitive impairment, and other symptoms affecting their QoL. Recent reviews reveal that multidimensional treatment approaches are most preferable: medications, physical activity, relaxation techniques, and cognitive–behavioral therapy are among the most useful approaches used today to treat FM (Chakrabarty & Zoorob 2007; Carville et al., 2008). FM has an enormous impact on QoL, limiting daily life activities. The cooccurrence of FM and obesity is high, around 30% and even 45%, respectively, and it appears obesity plays a relevant role in the pathogenesis of FM, although this relationship has been analyzed for many authors and it is still uncertain (Yunus, Arslan, & Aldag, 2002; Bennett et al., 2007; Aparicio et al., 2011a; Arranz, Canela, & Rafecas, 2010; Okifuji et al., 2010; Arranz, Canela, & Rafecas, 2012; Gota, Kaouk, & Wilke, 2015).

It has been argued that obesity contributes to the presence of FM and increases its severity (D'Arcy, 2011). Obesity has been associated with greater pain sensitivity to tender point palpation, reduced physical strength, decreased flexibility, shorter sleep duration, and greater restlessness during sleep (Okifuji and Hare, 2011). The direct relationship among BMI, functional capacity, and QoL has been observed in these patients. Lower QoL and higher pain sensitivity have been observed in overweight and obese individuals compared with those of normal weight (Neumann et al., 2008). Additionally, obese female FM patients seem to have higher levels of anxiety and depression and worse QoL, cardiorespiratory fitness, agility, and flexibility than their normal-weight peers (Aparicio et al., 2011b). In our study with 103 females with FM, the results suggested a decrease in SF-36 scores for physical and social function, emotional role, and mental health in overweight and obese patients. An additional analysis was performed for adipose body mass and lean mass values, which were not equally related to the different domains of QoL, suggesting that these relationships should be studied in more depth (Arranz et al., 2012). Similar results were found in other studies, with lower SF-36 scores in higher BMI groups indicating poorer QoL in the subscales of physical function, pain index, general health perceptions, emotional role, and physical component, with no significant group differences in SF-36 scores in physical role, vitality, social function, mental health index, and mental component (Kim et al., 2012). Other authors found no associations between BMI and FM symptoms and total FM Impact Questionnaire score and its 10 subset scores, however found a significant correlation between BMI and disability (Gota et al., 2015).

As some authors have pointed out, weight loss may improve physical functioning in this chronic pain disorder (Yunus et al., 2002). In a 20-week intervention of behavioral weight loss treatment patients lost an average of 4.4% of their initial weight and improved FM symptoms, pain interference, body satisfaction, and QoL (Shapiro, Anderson, & Danoff-Burg, 2005). Depression, sleep quality, and tender point count of obese patients with FM also improved significantly with weight loss (Senna et al., 2012). Exercise, regardless of type, has benefits on FM symptoms and functional capacity; however, improvements usually are not maintained over time (Fontaine, Conn, & Clauw, 2011) because of attrition and fear of movement with avoidance of physical activity, which is frequent in FM patients (Sañudo et al., 2012; Nijs et al., 2013). Findings suggest that behavioral weight loss treatment and exercise would benefit the management of overweight/obese FM patients, and consequently this would improve other areas, such as poor mood.

Osteoarthritis

OA is the most common form of arthritis and a leading cause of disability among older people. Clinically, it is characterized by joint pain, tenderness, limitation of movement, and various degrees of local inflammation. The course of the disease varies; it often is progressive, and the condition generally is not reversible. The association between OA and obesity is well established; widely acknowledged as a risk factor for both the incidence and progression of OA, obesity also has a negative influence on disease outcomes, such as the need for surgery. Hence, weight loss, coupled with exercise, is recognized as an important approach in the management of obese patients with OA. Mechanisms for this association seem to be both biomechanical and also inflammatory, as some association has been observed between obesity and OA with metabolic abnormalities (Bliddal, Leeds, & Christensen, 2014).

There are different studies around this relationship. A high BMI has been shown to be a likely risk factor for development and progression of OA of the knees, the hips, and possibly the hands (Janke et al., 2007). There is strong evidence for the important relationship between the onset and progression of knee OA and BMI. Obesity is an independent risk factor for incident radiographic OA, and patients with the highest degree of obesity are at greater risk of developing both symptomatic and radiologic knee OA. However, the mechanisms for these relationships are not completely understood and the data seem to suggest that increased weight initiates a pathway of cartilage degeneration before OA symptoms emerge (Anandacoomarasamy et al., 2008; Anandacoomarasamy, Fransen, & March, 2009). Therefore, a possible mechanism by which increased adipose mass is associated with joint damage might be related to the metabolic effects of obesity on knee OA. It has been shown that serum leptin levels are associated with the prevalence and incidence of knee OA in females. Women with incident knee OA during a 10-year follow-up period had consistently higher serum leptin levels compared with women without knee OA (Karvonen-Gutierrez et al., 2013). A high BMI is present in most adults with knee OA, and it is a relevant determinant of pain and functional loss in these patients (Creamer, Lethbridge-Cejku, & Hochberg, 2000; Tukker, Visscher, & Picavet, 2009; Marks, 2007). It has been reported that patients with a high BMI and knee OA, specifically women, are at greater risk of having symptoms (Elbaz et al., 2011). Exercise adherence is associated with improved physical function in overweight and obese older adults with knee OA (van Gool et al., 2005). However, the combination of moderate exercise and modest weight loss is most beneficial for pain reduction and improvement of physical function in knee OA, even more than diet or exercise alone (Miller et al., 2003; Messier et al., 2004). Fear of movement was found to be increased in morbidly obese adults with knee pain (mixed conditions, such as postsurgical, acute, and chronic) compared with their nonobese counterparts. Therefore, obese patients might benefit from rehabilitation that reduces their fear of movement to optimize their participation in rehabilitation activities and achievement of functional improvement (Vincent et al., 2010).

Even small weight reductions (e.g., 10% of initial weight) have resulted in 28% improved function (Christensen et al., 2005). Results are even better with weight loss greater than 5% achieved within a period of 20 weeks (Christensen et al., 2007). When a formula-diet weight loss program was used, beneficial effects were found independent of type, with no difference between a 415- and 810-kcal/day diet (Riecke et al., 2010). Massive weight loss after gastric surgery leads to improvement in pain and function, and decreases low-grade inflammation (joint biomarkers), suggesting even structural effects on cartilage (Richette et al., 2011). Therefore, growing evidence indicates that regardless of the weight loss method, losing weight is beneficial and reductions of body fat can reduce the mechanical and biochemical stressors that contribute to joint degeneration and greater disability. This is a good review of the relevance of weight loss by different strategies for obese patients with OA; it highlights the importance of body fat reduction to achieve a reduction in mechanical and biochemical stress (Vincent et al., 2012a).

Behavior is a relevant issue to take into account. Better functional abilities or self-efficacy for pain, physical activity, and eating behavior seem to result in improved functional capacity in OA patients (Pells et al., 2008). Therefore, patient perceptions of their self-efficacy may be relevant, because it has been reported that borderline morbidly obese OA patients (BMI > 38 kg/m^2) have higher levels of pain catastrophizing than nonmorbidly obese patients. This finding is associated with more frequently reported pain, higher levels of binge eating, lower self-efficacy in controlling eating, and lower weight-related QoL (Somers et al., 2008). Additionally, a study of 105 overweight and obese patients with knee OA found that depression symptoms were associated with reported decreased function, increased knee stiffness, and more walking impairment compared with nondepressed patients (Possley et al., 2009). Therefore, a psychological and cognitive–behavioral approach is needed. Although knee OA is more prevalent in obese and overweight individuals, similar associations between hip OA and obesity are not apparent (Ackerman and Osborne, 2012). An Australian survey from 1157 individuals with knee and hip joint disease showed that hip OA pain was associated with greater BMI and that patients classified as obese had higher pain levels, worse physical function, markedly lower QoL, and greater disease severity. Compared with healthy controls, obese patients with hip OA had an extremely low HRQoL. Combined exercise and weight loss programs might be a potential approach to improve physical functioning, pain, QoL, and other related parameters in overweight patients with hip OA (Paans et al., 2009). Total hip arthroplasty confers pain reduction and improvement in QoL, irrespective of BMI (Stevens et al., 2012). However, although functional improvement occurs after hip replacement, available evidence indicates that obese patients are less likely to attain the same level of physical function over the long term. Therefore, it is important to include weight loss strategies in rehabilitation management after total hip arthroplasty to maintain benefits and avoid worsening of function (Vincent et al., 2012b).

In summary, for all obese patients with OA, weight loss should be as a first-line management approach, with a goal of rapid initial weight loss of approximately 10% of bodyweight. The challenge of how to maintain weight loss, probably with the achievement of long-term healthy habits, and the question of whether or not weight loss can alter progression of OA, are key areas for future research.

Rheumatoid Arthritis

RA is an autoimmune disease associated with significant disability, joint pain and destruction, and chronic systemic inflammation. Old age and female gender are risk factors for both the development and worse outcomes of RA (Symmons, 2002). With the prevalence of obesity increasing dramatically worldwide over the past several decades, an increasing body of literature has examined the impact of obesity in the context of RA. Obesity has been identified as a risk factor for RA (Anandacoomarasamy et al., 2008) and found to be independently associated with impaired QoL (García-Poma et al., 2007; Stavropoulos-Kalinoglou et al., 2009). In RA, the impact of BMI and body composition on disease outcomes, such as disability, is unclear. However, obesity has the potential to affect functional disability in RA in different ways: increasing BMI has been associated with more bodily pain and greater disability from the same amount of pain, obese patients may be less able to use physical therapy effectively because of their body weight, and obese patients may have an increased inflammatory burden due to the metabolic activity of adipose tissue (Stavropoulos-Kalinoglou et al., 2011). In a group of 1246 patients with early inflammatory polyarthritis, most of who fulfilled the criteria for RA, class II and III obesity was significantly associated with functional disability affecting daily life activities (Humphreys et al., 2013).

Nevertheless, there is contradictory data in early RA. Normal weight, which has health benefits for the general population, turned out to be a risk factor for radiographic joint damage in patients with RA (Westhoff, Rau, & Znk, 2007). In a recent large RA study, BMI was associated with an increased risk of comorbidity, substantial functional loss, increased pain, fatigue, and reduced general QoL. However, overweight and obesity paradoxically seemed to reduce the relative risk of all-cause and cardiovascular mortality across different age groups and durations of RA (Wolfe & Michaud, 2012). The key issue is that RA is associated with altered body composition but not necessarily with changes in BMI. The chronic inflammatory state of this disease triggers metabolic alteration, which in combination with an inactive lifestyle, frequently leads to degradation of free-fat mass (skeletal muscle, bone, organs, skin), especially muscle mass. Thus, the presence of reduced muscle mass (rheumatoid cachexia) in RA patients is frequent, and there is an increased accumulation of fat mass, probably as a consequence of the increased metabolic index and nutritional requirements related to chronic inflammation status and glucocorticoid treatments (Gómez-Vaquero et al., 2001). The association of RA with sarcopenia and increased fat mass has been shown to be greater in women than in men (Symmons, 2002; Giles et al., 2008) Moreover, BMI rates tend to be similar to those of the general population in some regions (Stavropoulos-Kalinoglou et al., 2011), and the prevalence of overweight and obesity in RA patients might vary depending on their geographic location (Ibn Yacoub et al., 2012), as well as the correlation of BMI with functional capacity (Ide et al., 2011). Additionally, it seems more important to take into account the association of metabolic alterations and central adiposity of patients with RA (Giles et al., 2008; Dao, Do, & Sakamoto, 2010) and, furthermore, its relationship to functional capacity and QoL. In fact, the seemingly paradoxical association between obesity and decreased mortality has also been observed in other chronic illnesses and among the elderly. This phenomenon is important to understand, since a low BMI and especially unintentional weight loss may have prognostic implications and predict the occurrence of many adverse outcomes. It seems that RA patients have a higher level of muscular fat mass and weight loss is negative when associated to lean mass loss, nevertheless future research is needed to understand the prognostic value of body composition alterations (George & Baker, 2016).

In a systematic review about effectiveness and safety of dietary interventions for RA authors concluded that the effects of dietary manipulation, including vegetarian, Mediterranean, and elemental eating plans, and elimination diets are still uncertain due to the absence of enough large trials with no risk of bias. At the moment, there is some evidence that fasting followed by a vegetarian eating plan and a Cretan Mediterranean-style eating plan improve pain, but not stiffness and physical function, when compared to an ordinary diet. Moreover, few studies provided long-term results or information on whether the experimental diet was used by patients after the intervention period. And additionally, it is of concern the finding that dietary manipulation may be associated with higher dropout rates, which may suggest difficulty following the diet. Some dietary manipulations may be associated with weight loss or the exacerbation of existing nutritional risks associated with RA and its medical treatments, therefore there is a need for more and better research on this field to reach a sound knowledge (Smedslund, Byfuglien, Olsen, & Hagen, 2010).

Taking into account all these data, we should not interpret that obesity or high BMI is biologically protective for RA. In fact, quite the opposite, adiposity likely carries, at least, the same risk in RA as in the general population. Weight loss through diet and exercise, reducing specifically fat mass and not lean body mass, may improve cardiovascular outcomes, as well as physical function and disability. In contrast, especial attention may be paid when there is unintentional weight loss and a low BMI, which in this case are markers of more inflammatory and destructive disease and a warning of increased mortality risk. In these patients dietary management should try to keep proper body composition, with a normal BMI, fat mass, and lean mass.

Low Back Pain

LBP is among the most common chronic pain conditions and causes significant personal suffering and public health consequences. This health problem may be triggered by physical injuries but worsened by overweight or obesity. Although a causal association between high BMI and suffering from LBP remains controversial (Janke et al., 2007; Anandacoomarasamy et al., 2008), it is apparent from some studies that obesity is associated with a higher LBP prevalence (Shiri et al., 2010; Heuch et al., 2010, 2013). Moreover, it has been observed that in older patients with chronic LBP, the obese ones had higher pain during walking and stair climbing and had lower lumbar strength compared with the overweight (Vincent et al., 2013), increased disability, reduced physical HRQoL, pain, and comorbidities (Fanuele et al., 2002). In obese subjects with LBP, weight loss after bariatric surgery significantly improved functional disability (Melissas, Volakakis, & Hadjipavlou, 2003; Melissas et al., 2005), or, at least in some studies, there was a positive trend for improvement in the physical component of QoL scores (Lidar et al., 2012). The association of overweight and obesity with LBP is stronger for women than for men (Shiri et al., 2010), and

BMI predicts recurrence of LBP among women (Heuch et al., 2013). This might be the result of hormone-related obesity, body fat mass distribution, or the proportion of lean body mass/fat mass. In men, a high BMI may reflect a high degree muscle mass, whereas in women, it may indicate a greater amount of adipose tissue. It also seems that metabolic syndrome might be more prevalent in LBP patients (women more than men) (Duruöz et al., 2012). In a recent investigation, BMI was associated with higher levels of back pain intensity and disability, with positive associations between higher levels of low back disability and total body, upper and lower limb, and fat mass (Urquhart et al., 2011). The study highlights the importance of body composition because greater fat, but not lean mass, was associated with high levels of LBP intensity and disability.

The effect of obesity on cognitive–behavioral pain treatment for LBP patients has been studied, with lower responses for obese than nonobese patients (Sellinger et al., 2010). Physiotherapy is another approach for managing LBP and improving QoL. A recent study showed that after a multimodal physiotherapy program, nonobese patients with LBP demonstrated greater improvement in disability, physical component, and QoL (Cuesta-Vargas & González-Sánchez, 2013). However, other studies reported that BMI does not seem to influence the overall recovery from LBP in patients undergoing physiotherapy (Mangwani et al., 2010). Fear of movement seems to be greater in obese LBP patients, and it predicts greater self-reported disability. It may be useful to assess fear of movement in LBP patient populations to identify individuals who are at increased risk for chronic disability and who might benefit from therapeutic strategies to overcome this fear (Vincent et al., 2011).

Recent findings in men aged 30–50 years (n=1385) imply that being overweight or obese in early adulthood, as well as during the life course increases the risk of radiating but not nonspecific LBP among men. Therefore, taking into account the current global obesity epidemic, emphasis should be placed on preventive measures starting at youth and, also, authors recommend that measures for preventing further weight gain during the life course should be implemented (Frilander et al., 2015).

OBESITY AND MACRONUTRIENTS IN PAIN

Diet, Macronutrients, and Other Related Factors Influencing Obesity and Pain

Diet is recognized as a relevant factor to keep a good health status but also to prevent or improve some diseases. Generally, obesity, cardiovascular, osteoporosis, cancer, deficiencies, and caries are commonly known diet-related diseases, because a dietary intervention involves an easily measurable improvement. However, there are other conditions, as chronic pain ones, where diet also plays a main role.

The fact that diet is relevant for pain treatment should be something logical and not surprising us. Physiologically, we all know that our body needs nutrients and other substances provided by diet to function properly and recover. Our nervous system requires nutrients, such as vitamins, minerals, omega-3 fatty acids, or some amino acids in order to function optimally. For example, our endogenous pain-relieving systems require serotonin which is synthesized from the essential amino acids L-tryptophan which in turn needs to be provided by diet. Other relevant example is the need to an adequate amount of omega-3 fatty acids due to their role in cell membranes and in the production of antiinflammatory eicosanoids. We must be aware that either our physiological or pathophysiological processes will not work properly if diet is not providing the right calories and nutrients content.

A healthy diet should be that rich in foods of all groups and full of micronutrients, that is, vitamins and minerals, and also with a balanced calorie and macronutrients content. The amount of carbohydrates, proteins, and fats should be adapted to individual needs; however, there are some general recommendations that serve as a reference. For example, Mediterranean Diet (MeDiet) has shown large benefits for cardiovascular disease but also for weight control and other proinflammatory and degenerative diseases. Therefore, a vegetable rich MeDiet supplemented with extra-virgin olive oil and nuts is a reference model due to its high content of α-linolenic acid, marine omega-3 fatty acids, and polyphenols (Martínez-González et al., 2015; Sala-Vila et al., 2016). Total content of polyphenols give this dietary model a high antioxidant capacity, results from the PREDIMED (acronym from the Spanish PREvención con DIeta MEDiterránea) study suggest that consumption of more polyphenols could exert a protective effect against some cardiovascular risk factors, such as plasma triglyceride and glucose concentration and diastolic blood pressure (Guo et al., 2016). Polyphenols in diet are usually provided from extra-virgin olive oil, vegetables and fruits, wine, and nuts. An interesting datum is that extra-virgin olive oil contains oleocanthol which is a substance with an ibuprofen-like activity, causing dose-dependent inhibition of cyclooxygenase 1 and 2 activities (Beauchamp et al., 2005). Nevertheless, although MeDiet is an excellent model, diets must be adapted to the real situation of people, especially to the place where individuals live in order to facilitate the use of local and easily available fresh foods. Whatever the local diet is, the goal should always be to improve people's health through a balanced and optimized calories, carbohydrates, proteins and fats content with the maximum vitamins, minerals and antioxidant substances density. The goal should be to take the lower calories with the higher nutritional value.

On the other hand, it is also known that hedonic eating has an analgesic effect and usually we find this in patient behavior. They sometimes eat whatever is pleasant for them in order to feel a little relief in their pain. This is a real effect, not depending on the sort of food but on the pleasure and emotion felt, however, it is ephemeral because it disappears when eating action ends. In this pain relief strategy there is a big nutritional and health risk. Patients who eat looking for a relief of pain, usually have a considerable affinity to sweet taste and fatty foods, therefore they are prone to consume too much sugar, fats, and calories, which in turn, would lead to weight gain and consequently to pain worsening. These behavioral mechanisms promote comorbid pain and obesity making treatment even more problematic (Amy Janke and Kozak, 2012). At this point, nutritional education is completely necessary to explain patients that this is a short-term strategy not leading to positive long-term effects neither on pain nor obesity, and also to show them how to eat properly and enjoy healthy foods and recipes.

In summary, diet should ensure:

- Nutritional requirements: an adequate intake of calories and all macro and micronutrients in order to keep a proper physiological functionality and body weight.
- Reduce inflammatory mediators: in order to avoid high levels of pain and metabolic disorders mediators, diet must be low in inflammatory foods, such as sugars, red meat, refined carbohydrates, and so on, and high in omega-3, through oily fish and nuts, and antioxidant substances, such as flavonoids present in vegetables. High-energy diets could also act as proinflammatory favoring obesity, metabolic disorders, and therefore worsening chronic pain conditions.
- Avoid possible triggers: gluten, lactose, fructose, and other substances present in diet might initiate or acute the emergence of pain symptoms in patients with untreated food intolerances. It is critical to diagnose them accurately trying also to distinguish primary and secondary food intolerances to just eliminate foods from diet when completely necessary.

There are other lifestyle factors affecting also to obesity and pain which at the same time are related in some way with diet or eating behavior. It is the case for physical exercise and sleep. To rest enough time with a good quality of sleep is relevant to a proper functionality and recovery of our organism. Pain usually disrupts sleep and not sleeping enough chronically affects and is directly related to pain. There is strong evidence of a link between sleep disturbance and chronic widespread pain (McBeth, Wilkie, Bedson, Chew-Graham, & Lacey, 2015). Moreover, also metabolism is affected by lack of sleep, favoring a proinflammatory status (Grandner et al., 2013), altering glucose tolerance and also satiety mechanisms (Touma & Pannain, 2011), and favoring a greater food intake, especially with hedonic foods (Greer et al., 2013). At the same time, whether patients feel more fatigued and painful are not motivated to make any physical activity avoiding it, entering in a vicious circle with all these factors worsening symptoms, body weight, and health.

Energy Intake

The complex relationship between nutrition and age-related health conditions is not fully understood, however, some studies point to some factors as important mediators. It is the case of calorie intake and energy restriction, micronutrients and antioxidants presence, and also macronutrient proportions. Under a nutritional point of view, calorie intake should be adequate to each person depending mainly on age, sex, body composition, and physical activity. Energy is needed by the body to stay alive, grow, keep warm, and move. The total energy our body expends is the sum of the basal metabolic rate (amount of energy expended while at complete rest), the thermic effect of food (energy required to digest and absorb food), and the energy expended in physical activity. When energy intake exceeds expenditure, there is a weight gain, and at the contrary, when energy intake is lower than expenditure, weight loss occurs. Therefore, to keep a healthy body weight and prevent overweight or obesity, it is necessary to balance the energy derived from food with that expended in physical activity. It seems theoretically simple, but not really in the practice.

Currently, in developed countries, there is a rise in chronic diseases, including obesity, type-2 diabetes, chronic pain conditions, heart and cerebrovascular diseases, cancer, and others. Major risk factors for the onset of some of the most prevalent chronic diseases are the consumption of diets rich in empty calories and poor in nutrients (e.g., vitamins, phytochemicals), physical inactivity, and smoking; unless there are substantial reductions in the underlying risk factors, the human and economic costs from cardiovascular disease, cancer, and diabetes are expected even to rise in the near future. In contrast to the detrimental effects of overeating energy-dense foods, a reduction in calorie intake without malnutrition defined as calorie restriction (CR), has a wide range of benefits. Moderate CR can prevent or reverse the damaging effects of overweight and obesity, type-2 diabetes, hypertension, chronic inflammation, and other age-associated metabolic diseases. Studies on rodents, monkeys, and preliminary studies on humans have shown that more severe CR has additional benefits (Omodei and Fontana, 2011). However, is it an adequate strategy to pain and obesity management?

In spite of data about the fact that reduced calorie content by general reduced food intake, obviously avoiding malnutrition, can ameliorate aging and aging-associated diseases in animal models and also in humans, there are other relevant points to be taken into account. Recent findings indicate that meal frequency and timing is crucial, with both intermittent fasting and adjusted diurnal rhythm of feeding improving health and function, in the absence of changes in overall intake. Lowered intake of particular nutrients rather than of overall calories is also key, with protein and specific amino acids playing prominent roles, and the promising key role played by the gut microbiota (Fontana & Partridge, 2015). Interesting data from a systematic review reveal that fasting has an antiinflammatory effect and relieves pain in patients with RA during the period of fasting, while short-term fasting followed by a vegetarian diet can lead to clinically relevant long-term improvement in patients with this chronic pain condition. Probably, fasting followed by vegetarian diets might be useful in the treatment of RA, however, more randomized long-term studies are needed to confirm this (Müller, de Toledo, & Resch, 2001).

Therefore, although there is widespread consensus in aging research that eating fewer calories results in a longer, healthier life, CR has the risk of missing essential nutrients and this can be detrimental to reproduction, bone structure and overall metabolic health. Intermittent fasting and time-restricted feeding could have some benefits, but it is also recognized that quality of calories eaten is more relevant than quantity, suggesting that balance of macronutrients plays a stronger role rather than total energy intake. In this sense, it is possibly more important what and how we eat than how much. Nevertheless, how calories and macronutrients, and the interplay of both, affect is a fundamental question still to resolve (Solon-Biet et al., 2014, 2015). At the moment, the more common sense recommendation is to keep the lower calorie intake needed to cover individual energy and nutrient requirements.

Fats: The Role of Omega-3 Fatty Acids

The presence of fats in our diet is necessary because they provide us some part of the energy we need and, moreover, because they provide some essential substances for our metabolism and functioning. It is recommended that around 30% of the energy we obtain from foods comes from fats. However, not only the total amount but also the kind of fats we eat is important for health. One sound advice is that of the American Heart Association's Nutrition Committee who strongly advises these fat guidelines for healthy people:

- Eating between 25% and 35% of your total daily calories as fats from foods, such as fish, nuts, and vegetable oils.
- Limiting the amount of saturated fats you eat to less than 7% of your total daily calories. That means if you need about 2000 cal/day, less than 140 calories (or 16 g) should come from saturated fats.
- Limiting the amount of trans-fats to less than 1% of your total daily calories. That means if you need about 2000 cal/day, less than 20 calories (or 2 g) should come from trans-fats.
- For good health, the majority of fats you eat should be monounsaturated or polyunsaturated.

In general terms, in order to achieve these recommended dietary intakes our diets should be richer in vegetables, lower on animal-based foods, except for fish, and lower in processed foods.

Polyunsaturated fats are simply fat molecules that have more than one unsaturated carbon bond (double bound) in their molecule. They are healthy fats, along with monounsaturated fat, and at the contrary that saturated and trans-fats which are unhealthy because can increase your risk for heart disease and other health problems. There are two main types of polyunsaturated fats: omega-3 (n–3) and omega-6 (n–6) fatty acids. Some of these polyunsaturated fats are classified as essential fatty acids (EFA) because our body can't synthesize them and has to get them from our diet. It is the case of alpha-linolenic acid (ALA), which is an omega-3 and the precursor of eicosapentaenoic acid (EPA), and docosahexaenoic acid (DHA), and linolenic acid, an omega-6 precursor of arachidonic acid (AA).

Omega-3 fatty acids are relevant to human nutrition and health. The three types of omega-3 involved in human physiology are ALA, EPA, and DHA. Omega-6 and omega-3 fatty acids are main constituents of cell membranes phospholipids. The human body contains trillions of cells in different systems and organs, each of which is formed by a lipid bilayer membrane composed of phospholipids and proteins. Besides this structural function, either n–6 and n–3 fatty acids are used by our organism to synthesize respective proinflammatory and antiinflammatory substances called eicosanoids which all of them have relevant regulatory functions. A right balance among them is needed in order to keep proper functioning (growth, immunity, cardiovascular health, blood pressure, etc.) and in general terms to keep a desirable health status. This will basically depend on our diet.

As we know, nutrition is an environmental factor of major importance. Whereas major changes have taken place in our food patterns over the past 10,000 years since the beginning of the Agricultural Revolution, our genes have not changed. The spontaneous mutation rate for nuclear DNA is estimated at 0.5% per million years.

Therefore, over the past 10,000 years, there has been time for very little change in our genes, perhaps 0.005%. In fact, surprisingly our genes today are very similar to the genes of our ancestors during the Paleolithic period 40,000 years ago, at which time our genetic profile was established. From a genetic point of view, humans today live in a nutritional environment that differs from that for which our genetic constitution was selected. Studies on the evolutionary aspects of diet indicate that major changes have taken place in our food intake, particularly in the type and amount of EFA, that is, polyunsaturated fatty acids (PUFA), and in the antioxidant content of foods (Simopoulos, 2002). And curiously, these are two relevant aspects (*n*–3 and antioxidants intake) for pro-inflammatory diseases, such as obesity and chronic pain which have also high oxidative stress levels.

In general terms, Western societies consume a diet with an omega-6 to omega-3 fatty acid ratio of about 10:1 or even 25:1, which is greater than the 1:1 ratio on which humans beings evolved and on which our genetic patterns were established. Current recommendation is to achieve a diet with omega-6 to omega-3 ratio must be less, or at least not more, than 4:1 in order to promote health and prevent heart disease, cancer and other pro-inflammatory diseases. A high n–6/n–3 ratio, as is found in today's Western diets, promotes the pathogenesis of many diseases, including cardiovascular disease, cancer, osteoporosis, and inflammatory and autoimmune diseases, whereas increased levels of omega-3 PUFA (a lower *n*–6/*n*–3 ratio), exert suppressive effects. Increased dietary intake of linoleic acid leads to oxidation of LDL, platelet aggregation, and interferes with the incorporation of EFA in cell membrane phospholipids. Both omega-6 and omega-3 fatty acids influence even gene expression. Omega-3 fatty acids have antiinflammatory effects, suppress interleukin 1beta , tumor necrosis factor-alpha , and interleukin-6 (IL-6), whereas omega-6 fatty acids do not. Because inflammation is at the base of many chronic diseases, such as chronic pain pathologic conditions and obesity, dietary intake of omega-3 fatty acids plays an important role in the manifestation of these diseases (Simopoulos, 2006), and should be taken into account in their management.

It is well established that *n*–3 are substrates for synthesis of novel series of lipid mediators (e.g., resolvins, protectins, and maresins) with potent antiinflammatory and proresolving properties, which have been proposed to partly mediate the protective and beneficial actions of *n*–3 (Lorente-Cebrián et al., 2015). Some studies have used omega-3 fatty acids as supplements with good results in chronic pain conditions or inflammatory diseases. Even recent evidence associates omega-3 fatty acids with pain reduction. Omega-3 fatty acids have antiinflammatory properties (Calder, 2013; Maskrey, Megson, Rossi, & Whitfield, 2013) and EPA and DHA, for example, are precursors of potent antiinflammatory lipid mediators, such as resolvins and protectins (Levy, 2010). In clinical and preclinical studies, *n*–3 intake contributed to the reduction of inflammatory pain associated, for example, with RA (Goldberg & Katz, 2007) neuropathic injury (Perez, Ware, Chevalier, Gougeon, & Shir, 2005), musculoskeletal injury (JoEriksen, Sandvik, & Bruusgaard, 1996), and inflammatory bowel disease (Belluzi et al., 2000). Even more relevant to pain management, some preclinical studies and a recent one suggest that the antinociceptive effects of *n*−3 may involve an opioidergic system (Escudero et al., 2015; Nakamoto et al., 2011), which is a promising data about the possible use of *n*–3 fatty acids in the long-term treatment of pain along with medicines when needed.

For example, supplementing patient knee OA diet with 1000 mg of fish oil (EPA 400 mg and DHA 200 mg) during 12 weeks and measuring knee pain and knee function, there was a significant efficacy improving knee performance. They also tested higher dose of 2000 mg of fish oil, however, it had not significant higher efficacy than 1000 mg, which is consistent with the fact that a proper intake must be balanced and aligned with an optimal omega-6/omega-3 ratio (Peanpadungrat, 2015). Indeed, dietary supplementation with omega-3 PUFA has proved efficacious in reducing joint pain, morning stiffness and nonsteroidal antiinflammatory drugs usage in RA patients. Although the mechanisms by which omega-3 PUFA exert their beneficial effects have not been completely described, it seems that actions of lipid mediators derived from n–3 include analgesic and bone-sparing properties, making them ideal therapeutic agonists for the treatment of inflammatory diseases, such as RA (Souza & Norling, 2016). It seems that there is also a role for *n*–3 in inflammatory bowel diseases which are also frequent in some patients suffering from chronic pain. Omega-3 fatty acids were associated with protection from ulcerative colitis, particularly DHA (John et al., 2010), and are susceptible agents to promote and maintain a beneficial gut microbiota in the colon (Peyrin-Biroulet et al., 2010). Regarding RA and considering current knowledge, *n*–3 fatty acids should be considered as potential therapeutic agents that contribute to improving the symptoms caused by RA. However, it is still unclear whether they should be used alone or concomitantly with other therapeutic strategies (such as nonsteroidal–antiinflammatory drugs). Although this fact should be considered carefully, currently ongoing studies and follow-ups will provide additional evidence to clarify the potential role of *n*–3 as therapeutic agents for this disease (Lorente-Cebrián et al., 2015).

The right balance of omega-6/omega-3 fatty acids is basic for health and an important determinant in decreasing the risk for coronary heart disease. It is known that both omega-6 and omega-3 fatty acids influence gene expression and that EPA and DHA n-3 fatty acids have the most potent antiinflammatory effects. Inflammation is at the base of many chronic diseases, including coronary heart disease, diabetes, arthritis, cancer, osteoporosis, mental health, dry eye disease and age-related macular degeneration. Dietary intake of omega-3 fatty acids may prevent the development of chronic diseases which are multifactorial. It is quite possible that the therapeutic dose of omega-3 fatty acids will depend on the degree or severity of disease resulting from the genetic predisposition (Simopoulos, 2008). Based on all the information available, it is obvious the essential need to increase the omega-3 and decrease the omega-6 fatty acid intake in order to have a balanced *n*-6/*n*-3 intake in our diets. At the moment, we must ensure that every chronic pain patient, obese or not, covers the basic nutritional needs of *n*-3 fatty acids through food intake and if necessary with some dietary supplements, as a baseline to apply other treatments.

Proteins: Minimum Requirements and Particular Role of L-Tryptophan

Protein and its building blocks, amino acids, play various functional, structural, metabolic, and developmental roles in the body. Adequate dietary protein is essential for overall human health, with recommendations differing throughout the human life. There are no true body stores for protein; therefore, insufficient protein intake to satisfy body requirements leads to a negative protein balance (i.e., protein synthesis lower than breakdown). During inadequate protein intake, an imbalanced protein metabolism generally occurs in the skeletal muscle, resulting in clinical manifestations, such as skeletal muscle atrophy, due to muscle mass loss, impaired muscle growth or regrowth, and functional decline (increased disability). Some populations, such as older adults, but also obese and chronic pain affected adults, are particularly vulnerable to insufficient protein because catabolism may be greater than anabolism due to impaired physiological mechanisms, low physical activity or even lower intake than recommended (Thalacker-Mercer & Drummond, 2014). In order to achieve the minimum requirements the recommended dietary intake for proteins is around 0.8 g/kg body mass/day, coming equally from vegetal and animal foods. This recommendation must be higher for athletes, but also for some population groups, such as the elderly or even some others. High-protein diets are those in which the level of daily protein intake is equal to or higher than 1.5 g protein/kg body weight/day. A report from the United States Institute of Medicine stated that there was insufficient scientific evidence to recommend an upper limit of protein intake, but it was found that the maximum amount of energy from this macronutrient should be within the range of 10–35% of the total energy requirements of an adult (Okręglicka, 2015).

Dietary intake of protein is a powerful independent stimulus of muscle protein synthesis and fundamental to maintaining skeletal muscle mass. Physical inactivity–induced muscle loss occurs as a result of a chronic negative protein balance driven by an unequal contribution of muscle protein synthesis and breakdown. Aside from the biological use of dietary protein and amino acids for skeletal muscle protein metabolism, amino acids are being characterized for their role in metabolism, for example, in insulin resistance. With the emergence of metabolomics, BCAAs have been identified as being related to and predictive of the development of type-2 diabetes mellitus in adults, children, and adolescents; findings that support earlier studies demonstrating higher levels of BCAAs, primarily leucine, in obese and insulin-resistant individuals. Nevertheless, whether dietary protein and amino acids play a causal role in the development of insulin resistance or are simply biomarkers for metabolic dysfunction remains to be determined (Thalacker-Mercer & Drummond, 2014). It has been shown that a high-protein diet (20% of energy) can help in combating dyslipidemia and thus reduce the risk of cardiovascular diseases, increase tissue sensitivity to insulin, and it may be also a potentially effective strategy for weight loss, metabolic syndrome, and hypertension. Maintaining a protein-rich diet for a long time does not seem to negatively affect the renal function in patients with no preexisting renal diseases (Okręglicka, 2015). Nevertheless, all this must be confirmed because the effects on health would be very different depending on the protein source. Diets with high content of animal-based foods would be rich in proteins but also rich in saturated fatty acids, which are associated with cardiovascular risk and obesity, among others, and poor in fiber. In any case, in the meantime we know more details about the involvement of some amino acids in metabolic disorders, and the proper amount of proteins, we should seek to grant an adequate intake in order to preserve skeletal muscle mass in obese and chronic pain patients who, in turn, are normally less physically active than the healthy population.

Obviously we all need the essential amino acids, provided through diet, to keep our physiological functions, however, regarding chronic pain and obesity the role of one of them, tryptophan, would be even more critical. L-Tryptophan (L-Trp) is an essential large neutral amino acid (aa) present in all living organisms. In humans, as it cannot be endogenously synthesized it is needed to supply it through diet. Foods with a higher content of L-Trp include both animal and vegetal origin, such as milk, cheese and other dairy products, eggs (white), meat, fish, crustaceous, potatoes, chickpeas, soybeans, cocoa beans, and nuts. Cereals also contain little amounts of

L-Trp. Therefore, a varied and balanced diet with enough calorie content will provide the daily L-Trp requirement. Nevertheless, this amino-acid is scarcely present in foods. For example, the frequency of L-Trp residues in proteins is around 1–2% which is lower than 5% of other amino-acids and 9% of leucine (the most abundant aa). The recommended dietary L-Trp daily dose for human adults ranges from 250 to 425 mg/day. Together with cysteine, L-Trp is the essential aa required in lesser amount in human diet (WHO, 2007). This seems a paradox due to the high amount of functions L-Trp has in our organism. It is also curious that it is the only aa which needs to be transported by albumin in plasma and that the pathways for intestinal absorption are accurately regulated suggesting all that a "right" amount is needed for human health but there is no need, or no way, to accumulate it.

Tryptophan is an intermediate of protein/peptide synthesis and turnover and also much more. After its absorption, it is transformed in a wide range of bioactive compounds influencing a big number of cell metabolic pathways and physiological responses related to inflammation, immune responses, excitatory neurotransmission, and many other functions. Among these compounds produced in the body, there is a relevant neurotransmiter, serotonin (or 5-hydroxy-tryptamine), which is known to regulate, in the human central nervous system, the main adaptative reactions and responses to environmental changes, such as mood-anxiety, cognition, nociception, impulsivity, aggresiveness, libido, feeding behavior, and body temperature. Serotonin also modulates the activity of the gut function, the immune inflammatory responses, the differentiation process of blood stem cells, and the hemodynamic function. Consequently, alterations related to L-Trp and serotonin can be found associated with a variety of metabolic diseases and syndromes, such as mood-affective disorders, autism, cognitive deficit, anorexia and bulimia nervosa, obesity, FM, chronic fatigue syndrome, and irritable bowel syndrome (IBS) (Palego, Betti, Rossi, & Giannaccini, 2016). Serotonin is also the precursor of two circadian regulators which are *N*-acetyl-5-hydroxy-tryptamine and melatonin, therefore any alteration at serotonin levels could affect to the amount and quality of sleep time, and lack of sleep is associated with more pain and obesity.

Recently emerging interesting aspect is the possible role of gut microbiome, that is, the collection of microorganisms and their genomes in the gut habitat, as a relevant factor to gut aa absorption, L-Trp fates and functions (Palego et al., 2016). We know that the brain-gut axis is a bidirectional communication system between the central nervous system and the gastrointestinal tract and that serotonin functions as a key neurotransmitter at both terminals of this network. Current evidence points to the microbial influence on tryptophan metabolism and the serotonergic system as an important node in regulating normal functioning of this axis. Several studies show evidence on direct and indirect microbial regulation of tryptophan metabolism, availability, and serotonin synthesis (O'Mahony, Clarke, Borre , Dinan, & Cryan, 2015). Microbiota is often altered when there are some food intolerances. There is some data about fructose malabsorption which is characterized by low L-Trp plasma levels and mild depressive symptoms, showing a relationship between gut dysfunction, L-Trp availability and mood. High intestinal fructose concentration seems to interfere with L-Trp metabolism, and it may reduce availability of tryptophan for the biosynthesis of serotonin (5-hydroxytryptamine) (Ledochowski, Widner, Murr, Sperner-Unterweger, & Fuchs, 2001). All these data suggest that we should pay special attention to chronic pain patients, with obesity or not, who complain of gastrointestinal discomfort, in order to treat food intolerances which may be affecting L-Trp availability and therefore altering some of its functions related to pain and even obesity.

Some studies suggested that depressed patients would be less capable of compensating dietary L-Trp variations compared to healthy subjects. Moreover, L-Trp depletion has also shown to affect gut motility in IBS (Kilkens, Honig, van Nieuwenhoven, Riedel, & Brummer, 2004), and an altered homeostasis of L-Trp versus other large neutral amino acids in plasma has been considered the origin of the "carbohydrate craving" syndrome linked to some types of obesity and feeding behavior disorders, often in comorbidity with depression and bipolar disorder (Kroes et al., 2014). This is aligned with the relationship observed between obesity and depression. It is also known that serotonin exhibits strong anorectic effect in the human brain. Indeed, the functions of serotonin in energy homeostasis range from central control of food intake to direct regulation of adipose tissue activity in the periphery. Evidences in support of serotonin as a metabolic regulator in the development of obesity are increasing, although, the majority of the data are still derived from animal studies and more human data is necessary (Namkung, Kim, & Park, 2015). Therefore, whether serotonin has a role in the physiological body weight regulation, any factor which could reduce its levels or L-Trp intake or absorption, should be avoided.

Carbohydrates: Healthy Intake, Fiber Content, and Food Intolerances

Carbohydrates are one of the main energy macronutrients along with fats. After digestion, they are converted into glucose which is used as energetic substrate by our cells. There are two types of carbohydrates: simple and complex. Simple carbohydrates include sugars, such as glucose, fructose, sucrose, lactose, and other mono- or disaccharides, either found naturally in foods, such as fruits, vegetables, milk, and milk products, or added during food processing and refining. Complex carbohydrates are larger molecules based on simple sugars, and are found in refined and whole grain breads and cereals (wheat, rye, barley, oat, rice, etc.), starchy vegetables, nuts, and legumes. The complex carbohydrates are good sources of fiber with the exception of refined grains and cereals. For a healthy diet, it is recommended to limit the amount of added sugar and when consuming grains or cereals choose whole over refined ones. In this way, we ensure a high fiber and low sugars intake, a low glycemic index, and therefore a low rise of blood glucose levels, reducing the risk for obesity and type-2 diabetes. This recommendation should be made to all chronic pain patients in order to prevent or manage body weight, diabetes, and other metabolic disorders which at the same time could promote chronic inflammation.

Generally, when the intake of carbohydrates exceeds the requirements our body transforms them in fats which are stored in adipocytes, favoring weight gain and therefore obesity. This is the reason why the amount of carbohydrates in diet must be adapted to individual characteristics and energy needs. Nevertheless, as they are a main energy source, it is recommended that around 50% of daily calories come from this macronutrient, even in overweight people. Diets that are high in protein and reduced in carbohydrate provide a common approach for achieving weight loss in obese humans, but some of them could not be completely a safe option. In the case that they are poor in fiber and rich in saturated fats, there is no benefit for health and even long-term effect on microbiota-derived metabolites that influence colonic health has not been established (Russell et al., 2011). In this sense, the total amount of carbohydrates may be less important than the type of carbohydrate we eat. Sugars and refined foods are associated with weight gain and metabolic disorders, especially type-2 diabetes, therefore to reduce them is critical. In line with current guidelines (from the American Diabetes Association and others), reducing total energy intake to promote weight loss should be the main strategy, because there still is not enough evidence to promote an ideal percentage of energy coming from carbohydrates, protein, and fat. Although some studies have shown that the Mediterranean, vegan and low-glycemic index diets appear to be promising, further research that controls for weight loss is needed (Emadian, Andrews, England, Wallace, & Thompson, 2015).

And, what about microbiota? Depending on diet gut bacteria composition will vary considerably. Soluble fibers, fermented foods, nondigestible carbohydrates, presence of antioxidant substances as flavonoids and reduced content on sugars, and saturated fatty acids are recognized as improving factors for gut microbiota.

While the "healthy" gut microbiota is seen to be a stable community, there are stages within the life cycle of humans during which there can be alterations in the structure and function of this population. The microbiota produces numerous compounds of a hormonal nature which are released into the blood stream and act at distal sites. Among the targets for these substances are many other organs including the brain. The microbiota releases its hormonal products into interstitial tissue, to be picked up by blood and lymph capillaries. These secretions are usually effective in low concentrations on target organs or tissues remote from the enteric milieu. Thus, considering the ability to influence the function of distal organs and systems, in many respects the gut microbiota resembles an endocrine organ. When dysregulation among these bacterial communities occurs (dysbiosis), it can lead to inflammatory disorders, including inflammatory bowel disease, obesity, diabetes, and autism. It has been also shown that the gut microbiota plays an important role in weight control, in addition to diet, lifestyle, genetics, and the environment. One postulated explanation for this is that the higher presence of Firmicutes in obese produce more complete metabolism of a given energy source than do Bacteroidetes (prevailing in normal weight individuals), thus promoting more efficient absorption of calories and subsequent weight gain. However, other possible mechanism by which the intestinal microbiome could affect host obesity state is the induction of a low-grade inflammation which would alter metabolism (Bermon et al., 2015). Moreover, it is proposed that proinflammatory dietary compounds, such as saturated fat, together with genetic predisposition may alter the gut microbiota and increase caloric load. Some data also show how the intake of some antiinflammatory foods could be beneficial, it is the case of eating almonds and pistachios which has been found to increase the number of beneficial butyrate producing bacteria and reduce the number of lactic acid producing bacteria (Ukhanova et al., 2014). Curiously, one study found that the viable count of lactic acid producing *Enterococcus* and *Streptococcus* spp. in the fecal samples from chronic fatigue syndrome patients were significantly higher than those for the control group, leading to a possible relationship with their symptoms (Sheedy et al., 2009). On the other hand, butyrate, but not lactic acid, is the major energy source for colonocytes and is involved in the maintenance of colonic mucosal health. Recently several intestinal (trans-epithelial ion transport, inflammatory and oxidative status, nonspecific intestinal defense mechanisms, intestinal motility) and extra-intestinal (cholesterol and body weight regulation) effects of butyrate have been demonstrated (Canani et al., 2011). Along with diet, it seems that exercise may exert a beneficial role in energy homeostasis, it might also modulate and help to restore the gut microbiota when altered by an inadequate diet (Bermon et al., 2015). Whether exercise is a potential external agent with the capacity to improve gut microbiota it would not be a benefit for those chronic pain and obese patients who have very reduced physical activity. These and more data show the relevance of microbiota and the concept of a microbiome–brain–gut axis relevant to homeostasis and possibly linked to complex stress-related CNS disorders (Moloney, Desbonnet, Clarke, Dinan, & Cryan, 2014).

Scientific data is emerging about the possible relationship between some chronic pain conditions, such as FM and food intolerances, such as celiac disease. Gluten is been pointed as the possible trigger of FM or at least of some cases, nevertheless this hypothesis needs to be confirmed with more studies. Several studies have demonstrated an elevated comorbidity of IBS among patients with FM. Other studies have investigated the frequency of presentation of gastrointestinal symptoms in FM in a nonspecific approach describing several gastrointestinal complaints frequently reported by these patients, such as abdominal pain, dyspepsia, and bowel changes, among others. Several underlying mechanisms that require further investigation could serve as potential explanatory hypotheses for the appearance of such manifestations. These include sensitivity to dietary constituents, such as gluten, lactose or FODMAPs, or alterations in the brain–gut axis as a result of small intestinal bacterial overgrowth or subclinical enteric infections, such as giardiasis (Slim et al., 2015). As it is known nontreated celiac disease has some similar symptoms to FM, as, for example, body pain, therefore it is obvious that within the dietary management of chronic pain patient food intolerances deserve special attention. In any case, it is needed to diagnose properly and afterward apply only the strictly necessary dietary restrictions. When patients complain about gastrointestinal disorders it is important to check whether current diet or habits may be the cause or not, and to find out whether there is a problem, such as IBS or a primary food intolerance to gluten or other dietary compounds, such as lactose, fructose, or even FODMAPs (a sort of carbohydrates which are fermentable oligo-, di- and monosaccharides). It's important to understand why some foods are not well tolerated by these patients to establish an adequate individual diet management. At the moment, there is a big amount of emerging science about this issue, trying to find out which is the role of food intolerances in chronic pain conditions and even in obesity, however, it is needed more research to know exactly whether gastrointestinal disorders are directly associated to obesity and pain or are independent factors which obviously may need dietary treatment.

CONCLUSIONS

Obesity is an increasingly prevalent problem characterized by weight gain through excess food and fat intake and a sedentary lifestyle. Adipose tissue is not only an energy store but also an active organ involved in the regulation of inflammation. Overweight and obese people are more prone to a proinflammatory state, manifested by metabolic syndrome but also by a higher prevalence of chronic pain comorbidities. Patients who have FM, OA, RA, LBP, or other chronic pain conditions have worse functional capacity and QoL when obesity coexists. Most studies of chronic pain conditions evaluating the effect of obesity or BMI on QoL have noted that physical function and general health perception are the most affected domains. Growing evidence suggests that chronic systemic inflammation may be involved in the onset and perpetuation of chronic pain conditions. Moreover, sedentary living is associated with systemic inflammation, depression, lack of sleep, and poor self-rated health, which are worsened by lack of exercise and an unhealthy diet. As a result, obesity and pain reduce functional capacity and QoL, creating a vicious circle that is difficult to interrupt.

For obese people with chronic pain conditions, changes in lifestyle, behavior, physical activity, and diet have demonstrated benefits in functional capacity and QoL. Therefore, more studies are needed to assess the relationship among high BMI, metabolic syndrome, and pain, including the impact of dietary changes, individualized exercise, and cognitive–behavioral therapy that reduces fear of movement, psychological and sleep disorders, and stress. This approach would lead to healthier lifestyles and, consequently, to better functional capacity and QoL in overweight or obese patients with chronic pain conditions.

Additional research is needed to provide more details about the relationship between the pathophysiologic mechanism of pain and excess body weight and their impact on functionality and QoL. Current studies have used various methodologic approaches in different populations. However, standardized protocols are needed to study and compare various populations with different social, racial, and other critical characteristics in different geographic settings. Available data suggest the benefits of multidimensional management of patients with chronic pain conditions and obesity, including analgesic drugs but also weight loss diets, exercise, and cognitive–behavioral therapy. Special attention should be paid to specific populations, such as children, women, and older individuals.

With all the information we have right now about possible nutritional treatment for chronic pain, we can have the general idea that diet is a relevant factor to include in a multidisciplinary management of patients. With an optimization of diet we may achieve a better nutrients intake, a healthier body weight, and also an improvement of metabolic disorders. At the moment, we can draw the basic characteristics of an ideal diet moving to an antiinflammatory nutrient profile which may be reached by these recommendations:

- increase polyunsaturated omega-3 fatty acids through oily fish, nuts, and seeds,
- increase antioxidants (vitamins, minerals, and flavonoids) with a real 5-a-day intake of fruits and vegetables,
- increase monounsaturated fatty acids basically with the use of olive oil,
- fit calories to individual needs to avoid excess of energy intake and fat accumulation,
- reduce the amount of saturated fats by lowering intake of meat, dairy, and processed foods,
- reduce salt content in food,
- reduce added sugar and sugar rich foods and soft-drinks,
- add fiber, prebiotics and probiotics to diet through legumes, whole grain cereals, vegetables, and fermented foods.

Following these recommendations the nutritional profile of diet would change completely, giving to our body a better macronutrients proportion and an optimal content of micronutrients, antioxidant substances, and antiinflammatory.

Regarding the role of diet and some food components, there are many studies considering how some nutrients are involved in physiological mechanisms and how they are needed for a proper functioning. Obviously, it has been pointed out how diet is critical to manage obesity, metabolic disorders, and even proinflammatory status in some patients. Moreover, some studies give a relevant role to microbiota disorders and food intolerances which must be treated by an adequate diet in each case. Nevertheless, although in the last years we have gained more knowledge of all these relationships, but require an intense research to find out exactly which dietary recommendations are the better and how they can help in obesity, pain relief, functionality, and QoL.

References

Ackerman, I. N., & Osborne, R. H. (2012). Obesity and increased burden of hip and knee joint disease in Australia: results from a national survey. *BMC Musculoskeletal Disorders, 13*, 254.

Amy Janke, E., & Kozak, A. T. (2012). "The more pain I have, the more I want to eat": obesity in the context of chronic pain. *Obesity, 20*(10), 2027–2034.

Anandacoomarasamy, A., Caterson, I., Sambrook, P., et al. (2008). The impact of obesity on the musculoskeletal system. *International Journal of Obesity, 32*(2), 211–222.

Anandacoomarasamy, A., Fransen, M., & March, L. (2009). Obesity and the musculoskeletal system. *Current Opinion in Rheumatology, 21*(1), 71–77.

Aparicio, V. A., Ortega, F. B., Carbonell-Baeza, A., et al. (2011a). Relationship of weight status with mental and physical health in female fibromyalgia patients. *Obesity Facts, 4*(6), 443–448.

Aparicio, V. A., Ortega, F. B., Heredia, J. M., et al. (2011b). Analysis of the body composition of Spanish women with fibromyalgia [in Spanish]. *Reumatology Clinical, 7*(1), 7–12.

Arranz, L. I., Canela, M. A., & Rafecas, M. (2010). Fibromyalgia and nutrition, what do we know? *Rheumatology International, 30*(11), 1417–1427.

Arranz, L., Canela, M. A., & Rafecas, M. (2012). Relationship between body mass index, fat mass and lean mass with SF-36 quality of life scores in a group of fibromyalgia patients. *Rheumatology International, 32*(11), 3605–3611.

Arranz, L. I., Rafecas, M., & Alegre, C. (2014 Jan). Effects of obesity on function and quality of life in chronic pain conditions. *Curr Rheumatol Rep., 16*(1), 390.

Beauchamp, C. K., Keast, R. S., Morel, D., Lin, J., Pika, J., Han, Q., et al. (2005). Phytochemistry: ibuprofen-like activity in extra-virgin olive oil. *Nature, 437*, 45–46.

Belluzi, A., Boschi, S., Brignola, C., Munarini, A., Cariani, G., & Miglio, F. (2000). Polyunsaturated fatty acids and inflammatory bowel disease. *American Journal of Clinical Nutrition, 71*(Suppl. 1), 339S–342S.

Bennett, R. M., Jones, J., Turk, D. C., et al. (2007). An internet survey of 2,596 people with fibromyalgia. *BMC Musculoskeletal Disorders, 8*, 27.

Bermon, S., Petriz, B., Kajėnienė, A., Prestes, J., Castell, L., & Franco, O. L. (2015). The microbiota: an exercise immunology perspective. *Exercise Immunology Review, 21*, 70–79.

Bliddal, H, Leeds, A. R., & Christensen, R. (2014). Osteoarthritis, obesity and weight loss: evidence, hypotheses and horizons—a scoping review. *Obesity Review, 15*(7), 578–586.

Bollinger, T., Bollinger, A., Oster, H., et al. (2010). Sleep, immunity, and circadian clocks: a mechanistic model. *Gerontology, 56*(6), 574–580.

Bultink, I. E., Vis, M., van der Horst-Bruinsma, I. E., et al. (2012). Inflammatory rheumatic disorders and bone. *Current Rheumatology Reports, 14*(3), 224–230.

Calder, P. C. (2013). Omega-3 polyunsaturated fatty acids and inflammatory processes: nutrition or pharmacology? *British Journal of Clinical Pharmacology, 75*, 645–662.

Caldwell, J., Hart-Johnson, T., & Green, C. R. (2009). Body mass index and quality of life: examining blacks and whites with chronic pain. *Journal of Pain, 10*(1), 60–67.

Canani, R. B., Costanzo, M. D., Leone, L., Pedata, M., Meli, R., & Calignano, A. (2011). Potential beneficial effects of butyrate in intestinal and extraintestinal diseases. *World Journal of Gastroenterology, 17*(12), 1519–1528.

Carville, S. F., Arendt-Nielsen, S., Bliddal, H., et al. (2008). EULAR evidence-based recommendations for the management of fibromyalgia syndrome. *Annals of the Rheumatic Diseases, 67*, 536–541.

Castres, I., Folope, V., Dechelotte, P., et al. (2010). Quality of life and obesity class relationships. *International Journal of Sports Medicine, 31*(11), 773–778.

Chakrabarty, S., & Zoorob, R. (2007). Fibromyalgia. *American Family Physician, 76*(2), 247–254.

Chaput, J. P., Klingenberg, L., & Sjödin, A. (2010). Do all sedentary activities lead to weight gain? Sleep does not. *Current Opinion in Clinical Nutrition and Metabolic Care, 13*(6), 601–607.

Christensen, R., Astrup, A., & Bliddal, H. (2005). Weight loss: the treatment of choice for knee osteoarthritis? A randomized trial. *Osteoarthritis Cartilage, 13*(1), 20–27.

Christensen, R., Bartels, E. M., Astrup, A., et al. (2007). Effect of weight reduction in obese patients diagnosed with knee osteoarthritis: a systematic review and meta-analysis. *Annals of the Rheumatic Diseases, 66*(4), 433–439.

Creamer, P., Lethbridge-Cejku, M., & Hochberg, M. C. (2000). Factors associated with functional impairment in symptomatic knee osteoarthritis. *Rheumatology, 39*(5), 490–496.

Cuesta-Vargas, A. I., & González-Sánchez, M. (2013). Obesity effect on a multimodal physiotherapy program for low back pain suffers: patient reported outcome. *Journal of Occupational Medicine and Toxicology*, *8*(1), 13.

D'Arcy, Y. (2011). Managing pain in obese patients. *Nurse Practitioner*, *36*(12), 28–32.

Dao, H. H., Do, Q. T., & Sakamoto, J. (2010). Increased frequency of metabolic syndrome among Vietnamese women with early rheumatoid arthritis: a cross-sectional study. *Arthritis Research and Therapy*, *12*(6), R218.

Dixon, J. B. (2010). The effect of obesity on health outcomes. *Molecular and Cellular Endocrinology*, *316*(2), 104–108.

Dixon, J. B., Schachter, L. M., & O'Brien, P. E. (2001). Sleep disturbance and obesity: changes following surgically induced weight loss. *Archives of Internal Medicine*, *161*(1), 102–106.

Duruöz, M. T., Turan, Y., Gürgan, A., et al. (2012). Evaluation of metabolic syndrome in patients with chronic low back pain. *Rheumatology International*, *32*(3), 663–667.

Elbaz, A., Debbi, E. M., Segal, G., et al. (2011). Sex and body mass index correlate with Western Ontario and McMaster Universities Osteoarthritis Index and quality of life scores in knee osteoarthritis. *Archives of Physical Medicine and Rehabilitation*, *92*(10), 1618–1623.

Emadian, A., Andrews, R. C., England, C. Y., Wallace, V., & Thompson, J. L. (2015). The effect of macronutrients on glycaemic control: a systematic review of dietary randomised controlled trials in overweight and obese adults with type 2 diabetes in which there was no difference in weight loss between treatment groups. *British Journal of Nutrition*, *114*(10), 1656–1666.

Escudero, G. E., Romañuk, C. B., Toledo, M. E., Olivera, M. E., Manzo, R. H., & Laino, C. H. (2015). Analgesia enhancement and prevention of tolerance to morphine: beneficial effects of combined therapy with omega-3 fatty acids. *Journal of Pharmacy and Pharmacology*, *67*(9), 1251–1262.

Fanuele, J. C., Abdu, W. A., Hanscom, B., et al. (2002). Association between obesity and functional status in patients with spine disease. *Spine*, *27*(3), 306–312.

Fontaine, K. R., & Barofsky, I. (2001). Obesity and health-related quality of life. *Obesity Review*, *2*(3), 173–182.

Fontaine, K. R., Conn, L., & Clauw, D. J. (2011). Effects of lifestyle physical activity in adults with fibromyalgia: results at follow-up. *Journal of Clinical Rheumatology*, *17*(2), 64–68.

Fontana, L, & Partridge, L (2015). Promoting health and longevity through diet: from model organisms to humans. *Cell*, *161*(1), 106–118.

Frilander, H, Solovieva, S, Mutanen, P, Pihlajamäki, H, Heliövaara, M, & Viikari-Juntura, E (2015). Role of overweight and obesity in low back disorders among men: a longitudinal study with a life course approach. *BMJ Open*, *5*(8), e007805.

Gandhi, R., Razak, F., Davey, I. R., et al. (2010). Metabolic syndrome and the functional outcomes of hip and knee arthroplasty. *Journal Rheumatology*, *37*(9), 1917–1922.

García-Poma, A., Segami, M. I., Mora, C. S., et al. (2007). Obesity is independently associated with impaired quality of life in patients with rheumatoid arthritis. *Clinical Rheumatology*, *26*(11), 1831–1835.

George, MD, & Baker, J. F. (2016). The obesity epidemic and consequences for rheumatoid arthritis care. *Current Rheumatology Reports*, *18*(1), 6.

Giles, J. T., Ling, S. M., Ferrucci, L., et al. (2008). Abnormal body composition phenotypes in older rheumatoid arthritis patients: association with disease characteristics and pharmacotherapies. *Arthritis Rheumatism*, *59*(6), 807–815.

Goldberg, R. J., & Katz, J. (2007). A meta-analysis of the analgesic effects of omega-3 polyunsaturated fatty acid supplementation for inflammatory joint pain. *Pain*, *129*, 210–223.

Gómez-Vaquero, C., Nolla, J. M., Fiter, J., et al. (2001). Nutritional status in patients with rheumatoid arthritis. *Joint Bone Spine*, *68*(5), 403–409.

Gota, C. E., Kaouk, S., & Wilke, W. S. (2015). Fibromyalgia and obesity: the association between body mass index and disability, depression, history of abuse, medications, and comorbidities. *Journal of Clinical Rheumatology*, *21*(6), 289–295.

Grandner, M. A., Sands-Lincoln, M. R., Pak, V. M., et al. (2013). Sleep duration, cardiovascular disease, and proinflammatory biomarkers. *Nature Science Sleep*, *5*, 93–107.

Greer, S. M., Goldstein, A. N., & Walker, M. P. (2013). The impact of sleep deprivation on food desire in the human brain. *Nature Communications*, *4*, 2259.

Guo, X., Tresserra-Rimbau, A., Estruch, R., Martínez-González, M. A., Medina-Remón, A., Castañer, O., Corella, D., Salas-Salvadó, J., & Lamuela-Raventós, R. M. (2016). Effects of polyphenol, measured by a biomarker of total polyphenols in urine, on cardiovascular risk factors after a long-term follow-up in the predimed study. *Oxidative Medicine and Cellular Longevity*, *2016*, 2572606.

Hainsworth, K. R., Davies, W. H., Khan, K. A., et al. (2009). Co-occurring chronic pain and obesity in children and adolescents: the impact on health-related quality of life. *Clinical Journal of Pain*, *25*(8), 715–721.

Heo, M., Allison, D. B., Faith, M. S., et al. (2003). Obesity and quality of life: mediating effects of pain and comorbidities. *Obesity Research*, *11*(2), 209–216.

Heuch, I., Hagen, K., Heuch, I., et al. (2010). The impact of body mass index on the prevalence of low back pain: the HUNT study. *Spine*, *35*(7), 764–768.

Heuch, I., Heuch, I., Hagen, K., et al. (2013). Body mass index as a risk factor for developing chronic low back pain: a follow-up in the Nord-Trøndelag Health Study. *Spine*, *38*(2), 133–139.

Humphreys, J. H., Verstappen, S. M., Mirjafari, H., et al. (2013). Association of morbid obesity with disability in early inflammatory polyarthritis: results from the Norfolk Arthritis Register. *Arthritis Care Research*, *65*(1), 122–126.

Ibn Yacoub, Y., Amine, B., Laatiris, A., et al. (2012). Prevalence of overweight in Moroccan patients with rheumatoid arthritis and its relationships with disease features. *Clinical Rheumatology*, *31*(3), 479–482.

Ide, M. R., Gonzalez-Gay, M. A., Yano, K. C., et al. (2011). Functional capacity in rheumatoid arthritis patients: comparison between Spanish and Brazilian sample. *Rheumatology International*, *31*(2), 221–226.

Janke, E. A., Collins, A., & Kozak, A. T. (2007). Overview of the relationship between pain and obesity: what do we know? Where do we go next? *Journal of Rehabilitation Research and Development*, *44*(2), 245–262.

JoEriksen, W., Sandvik, L., & Bruusgaard, D. (1996). Does dietary supplementation of cod liver oil mitigate musculoskeletal pain? *European Journal of Clinical Nutrition*, *50*, 689–693.

Johannes, C. B., Le, T. K., Zhou, X., et al. (2010). The prevalence of chronic pain in United States adults: results of an Internet-based survey. *Journal Pain*, *11*(11), 1230–1239.

John, S., Luben, R., Shrestha, S. S., Welch, A., Khaw, K. T., & Hart, A. R. (2010). Dietary n-3 polyunsaturated fatty acids and the aetiology of ulcerative colitis: a UK prospective cohort study. *European Journal of Gastroenterology and Hepatology*, *22*, 602–606.

Karvonen-Gutierrez, C. A., Harlow, S. D., Mancuso, P., et al. (2013). Association of leptin levels with radiographic knee osteoarthritis among a cohort of midlife women. *Arthritis Care Research*, *65*(6), 936–944.

Kilkens, T. O., Honig, A., van Nieuwenhoven, M. A., Riedel, W. J., & Brummer, R. J. (2004). Acute tryptophan depletion affects brain-gut responses in irritable bowel syndrome patients and controls. *Gut*, *53*(12), 1794–1800.

Kim, C. H., Luedtke, C. A., Vincent, A., et al. (2012). Association of body mass index with symptom severity and quality of life in patients with fibromyalgia. *Arthritis Care Research, 64*(2), 222–228.

Kroes, MC, van Wingen, G. A., Wittwer, J., Mohajeri, M. H., Kloek, J., & Fernández, G. (2014). Food can lift mood by affecting mood-regulating neurocircuits via a serotonergic mechanism. *Neuroimage, 84*, 825–832.

Krystal, A. D. (2012). Psychiatric disorders and sleep. *Neurologic Clinics, 30*(4), 1389–1413.

Lebovits, A., Hainline, B., Stone, L. S., et al. (2009). Struck from behind: maintaining quality of life with chronic low back pain. *Journal of Pain, 10*(9), 927–931.

Ledochowski, M, Widner, B., Murr, C., Sperner-Unterweger, B., & Fuchs, D. (2001). Fructose malabsorption is associated with decreased plasma tryptophan. *Scandinavian Journal of Gastroenterology, 36*(4), 367–371.

Levy, B. D. (2010). Resolvins and protectins: natural pharmacophores for resolution biology. *Prostaglandins Leukotrienes and Essential Fatty Acids, 82*, 327–332.

Lidar, Z., Behrbalk, E., Regev, G. J., et al. (2012). Intervertebral disc height changes after weight reduction in morbidly obese patients and its effect on quality of life and radicular and low back pain. *Spine, 37*(23), 1947–1952.

Lorente-Cebrián, S., Costa, A. G., Navas-Carretero, S., Zabala, M., Laiglesia, L. M., Martínez, J. A., & Moreno-Aliaga, M. J. (2015). An update on the role of omega-3 fatty acids on inflammatory and degenerative diseases. *Journal of Physiology and Biochemistry, 71*(2), 341–349.

Mangwani, J., Giles, C., Mullins, M., et al. (2010). Obesity and recovery from low back pain: a prospective study to investigate the effect of body mass index on recovery from low back pain. *Annals of the Royal College of Surgeons of England, 92*(1), 23–26.

Marcus, D. A. (2004). Obesity and the impact of chronic pain. *Clinical Journal of Pain, 20*(3), 186–191.

Marks, R. (2007). Obesity profiles with knee osteoarthritis: correlation with pain, disability, disease progression. *Obesity, 15*(7), 1867–1874.

Martínez-González, M. A., Salas-Salvadó, J., Estruch, R., Corella, D., Fitó, M., & Ros, E. PREDIMED Investigators. (2015). Benefits of the Mediterranean diet: insights from the PREDIMED study. *Progress in Cardiovascular Diseases, 58*(1), 50–60.

Maskrey, B. H., Megson, I. L., Rossi, A. G., & Whitfield, P. D. (2013). Emerging importance of omega-3 fatty acids in the innate immune response: molecular mechanisms and lipidomic strategies for their analysis. *Molecular Nutrition and Food Research, 57*, 1390–1400.

McBeth, J., Wilkie, R., Bedson, J., Chew-Graham, C., & Lacey, R. J. (2015). Sleep disturbance and chronic widespread pain. *Current Rheumatology Reports, 17*(1), 469.

McVinnie, D. S. (2013). Obesity and pain. *British Journal of Pain, 7*(4), 163–170.

Melissas, J., Kontakis, G., Volakakis, E., et al. (2005). The effect of surgical weight reduction on functional status in morbidly obese patients with low back pain. *Obesity Surgery, 15*(3), 378–381.

Melissas, J., Volakakis, E., & Hadjipavlou, A. (2003). Low-back pain in morbidly obese patients and the effect of weight loss following surgery. *Obesity Surgery, 13*(3), 389–393.

Messier, S. P., Loeser, R. F., Miller, G. D., et al. (2004). Exercise and dietary weight loss in overweight and obese older adults with knee osteoarthritis: the arthritis, diet, and activity promotion trial. *Arthritis and Rheumatism, 50*(5), 1501–1510.

Miller, G. D., Rejeski, W. J., Williamson, J. D., ADAPT Investigators. et al. (2003). The arthritis, diet and activity promotion trial (ADAPT): design, rationale, and baseline results. *Control Clinical Trials, 24*(4), 462–480.

Moloney, R. D., Desbonnet, L., Clarke, G., Dinan, T. G., & Cryan, J. F. (2014). The microbiome: stress, health and disease. *Mammalian Genome, 25*(1–2), 49–74.

Müller, H., de Toledo, F. W., & Resch, K. L. (2001). Fasting followed by vegetarian diet in patients with rheumatoid arthritis: a systematic review. *Scandinavian Journal of Rheumatology, 30*(1), 1–10.

Nakamoto, K., Nishinaka, T., Ambo, A., Mankura, M., Kasuya, F., & Tokuyama, S. (2011). Possible involvement of β-endorphin in docosahexaenoic acid-induced antinociception. *European Journal of Pharmacology, 666*, 100–104.

Namkung, J., Kim, H, & Park, S. (2015). Peripheral serotonin: a new player in systemic energy homeostasis. *Molecules and Cells, 38*(12), 1023–1028.

Neumann, L., Lerner, E., Glazer, Y., et al. (2008). A cross-sectional study of the relationship between body mass index and clinical characteristics, tenderness measures, quality of life, and physical functioning in fibromyalgia patients. *Clinical Rheumatology, 27*(12), 1543–1547.

Nijs, J., Roussel, N., Van Oosterwijck, J., et al. (2013). Fear of movement and avoidance behaviour toward physical activity in chronic-fatigue syndrome and fibromyalgia: state of the art and implications for clinical practice. *Clinical Rheumatology, 32*(8), 1121–1129.

Okifuji, A., Donaldson, G. W., Barck, L., et al. (2010). Relationship between fibromyalgia and obesity in pain, function, mood, and sleep. *Journal of Pain, 11*(12), 1329–1337.

Okifuji, A., & Hare, B. D. (2011). Do sleep disorders contribute to pain sensitivity? *Current Rheumatology Reports, 13*(6), 528–534.

Okifuji, A., & Hare, B. D. (2015). The association between chronic pain and obesity. *Journal of Pain Research, 8*, 399–408.

Okręglicka, K. (2015). Health effects of changes in the structure of dietary macronutrients intake in western societies. *Roczniki Panstwowego Zakladu Higieny, 66*(2), 97–105.

Oliva-Moreno, J., & Gil-Lacruz, A. (2013). Body weight and health-related quality of life in Catalonia, Spain. *European Journal Health Econ, 14*(1), 95–105.

O'Mahony SM, Clarke G, Borre YE, Dinan TG, & Cryan, J. F. (2015). Serotonin, tryptophan metabolism and the brain-gut-microbiome axis. *Behavioural Brain Research, 277*, 32–48.

Omodei, D., & Fontana, L. (2011). Calorie restriction and prevention of age-associated chronic disease. *FEBS letters, 585*(11), 1537–1542.

Paans, N., van den Akker-Scheek, I., van der Meer, K., et al. (2009). The effects of exercise and weight loss in overweight patients with hip osteoarthritis: design of a prospective cohort study. *BMC Musculoskeletal Disorders, 10*, 24.

Palego, L, Betti, L, Rossi, A, & Giannaccini, G. (2016). Tryptophan biochemistry: structural, nutritional, metabolic, and medical aspects in humans. *Journal of Amino Acids, 2016*, 8952520.

Peanpadungrat, P. (2015 Apr). Efficacy and safety of fish oil in treatment of knee osteoarthritis. *Journal of the Medical Association of Thailand, 98*(Suppl 3), S110–S114.

Pells, J. J., Shelby, R. A., Keefe, F. J., et al. (2008). Arthritis self-efficacy and self-efficacy for resisting eating: relationships to pain, disability, and eating behavior in overweight and obese individuals with osteoarthritic knee pain. *Pain, 136*(3), 340–347.

Perez, J., Ware, M. A., Chevalier, S., Gougeon, R., & Shir, Y. (2005). Dietary omega-3 fatty acids may be associated with increased neuropathic pain in nerve-injured rats. *Anesthesia and Analgesia, 101*, 444–448.

Peyrin-Biroulet, L., Beisner, J., Wang, G., Nuding, S., Oommen, S. T., Kelly, D., Parmentier-Decrucq, E., Dessein, R., Merour, E., Chavatte, P., Grandjean, T., Bressenot, A., Desreumaux, P., Colombel, J. F., Desvergne, B., Stange, E. F., Wehkamp, J., & Chamaillard, M. (2010). Peroxisome proliferator-activated receptor gamma activation is required for maintenance of innate antimicrobial immunity in the colon. *Proceedings of the National Academy of Sciences of the United States of America, 107*, 8772–8777.

Piechota, G., Małkiewicz, J., & Karwat, I. D. (2005). Obesity as a cause and result of disability. *Przeglad Epidemiologiczny, 59*(1), 155–161.

Poggiogalle, E, Lubrano, C, Gnessi, L, Marocco, C, Di Lazzaro, L, Polidoro, G, Luisi, F, Merola, G, Mariani, S, Migliaccio, S, Lenzi, A, &

Donini, L. M. (2016). Reduced sleep duration affects body composition, dietary intake and quality of life in obese subjects. *Eating and Weight Disorders, 21*(3), 501–505.

Possley, D., Budiman-Mak, E., O'Connell, S., et al. (2009). Relationship between depression and functional measures in overweight and obese persons with osteoarthritis of the knee. *Journal of Rehabilitation and Research Development, 46*(9), 1091–1098.

Richette, P., Poitou, C., Garnero, P., et al. (2011). Benefits of massive weight loss on symptoms, systemic inflammation and cartilage turnover in obese patients with knee osteoarthritis. *Annals of the Rheumatic Diseases, 70*(1), 139–144.

Riecke, B. F., Christensen, R., Christensen, P., et al. (2010). Comparing two low-energy diets for the treatment of knee osteoarthritis symptoms in obese patients: a pragmatic randomized clinical trial. *Osteoarthritis Cartilage, 18*(6), 746–754.

Russell, W. R., Gratz, S. W., Duncan, S. H., Holtrop, G., Ince, J., Scobbie, L., Duncan, G., Johnstone, A. M., Lobley, G. E., Wallace, R. J., Duthie, G. G., & Flint, H. J. (2011). High-protein, reduced-carbohydrate weight-loss diets promote metabolite profiles likely to be detrimental to colonic health. *American Journal of Clinical Nutrition, 93*(5), 1062–1072.

Sala-Vila, A., Guasch-Ferré, M., Hu, F. B., Sánchez-Tainta, A., Bulló, M., Serra-Mir, M., López-Sabater, C., Sorlí, J. V., Arós, F., Fiol, M., Muñoz, M. A., Serra-Majem, L., Martínez, J. A., Corella, D., Fitó, M., Salas-Salvadó, J., Martínez-González, M. A., Estruch, R., & Ros, E. PREDIMED investigators. (2016). Dietary α-linolenic acid, marine ω-3 fatty acids, and mortality in a population with high fish consumption: findings from the prevención con dieta mediterránea (PREDIMED) study. *Journal of American Heart Association, 5*(1), pii: e002543.

Sañudo, B., Carrasco, L., de Hoyo, M., et al. (2012). Effects of exercise training and detraining in patients with fibromyalgia syndrome: a 3-yr longitudinal study. *American Journal of Physical Medicine Rehabilitation, 91*(7), 561–569quiz 570–573.

Seaman, D. R. (2013). Body mass index and musculoskeletal pain: is there a connection? *Chiropractic Manual Therapies, 21*(1), 15.

Sellinger, J. J., Clark, E. A., Shulman, M., et al. (2010). The moderating effect of obesity on cognitive-behavioral pain treatment outcomes. *Pain Medicine, 11*(9), 1381–1390.

Sendi, P., Brunotte, R., Potoczna, N., et al. (2005). Health-related quality of life in patients with class II and class III obesity. *Obesity Surgery, 15*(7), 1070–1076.

Senna, M. K, Ahmad, H. S., & Fathi, W. (2013). Depression in obese patients with primary fibromyalgia: the mediating role of poor sleep and eating disorder features. *Clinical Rheumatology, 32*(3), 369–375.

Senna, M. K., Sallam, R. A., Ashour, H. S., et al. (2012). Effect of weight reduction on the quality of life in obese patients with fibromyalgia syndrome: a randomized controlled trial. *Clinical Rheumatology, 31*(11), 1591–1597.

Shapiro, J. R., Anderson, D. A., & Danoff-Burg, S. (2005). A pilot study of the effects of behavioral weight loss treatment on fibromyalgia symptoms. *Journal of Psychosomatic Research, 59*(5), 275–282.

Sheedy, J. R., Wettenhall, R. E., Scanlon, D., Gooley, P. R., Lewis, D. P., McGregor, N., Stapleton, D. I., Butt, H. L., & DE Meirleir, K. L. (2009). Increased d-lactic Acid intestinal bacteria in patients with chronic fatigue syndrome. *In Vivo, 23*(4), 621–628.

Shiri, R., Karppinen, J., Leino-Arjas, P., et al. (2010). The association between obesity and low back pain: a meta-analysis. *American Journal of Epidemiology, 171*(2), 135–154.

Simopoulos, A. P. (2002). The importance of the ratio of omega-6/omega-3 essential fatty acids. *Biomedicine and Pharmacotherapy, 56*(8), 365–379.

Simopoulos, A. P. (2006). Evolutionary aspects of diet, the omega-6/omega-3 ratio and genetic variation: nutritional implications for chronic diseases. *Biomedicine Pharmacotherapy, 60*(9), 502–507.

Simopoulos, A. P. (2008). The importance of the omega-6/omega-3 fatty acid ratio in cardiovascular disease and other chronic diseases. *Experimental Biology and Medicine, 233*(6), 674–688.

Sirtori, A., Brunani, A., Villa, V., et al. (2012). Obesity is a marker of reduction in QoL and disability. *Scientific World Journal, 2012*, 167520.

Smedslund, G., Byfuglien, M. G., Olsen, S. U., & Hagen, K. B. (2010). Effectiveness and safety of dietary interventions for rheumatoid arthritis: a systematic review of randomized controlled trials. *Journal of the American Dietetic Association, 110*(5), 727–735.

Solon-Biet, S. M., McMahon, A. C., Ballard, J. W., Ruohonen, K., Wu, L. E, Cogger, V. C., Warren, A., Huang, X., Pichaud, N., Melvin, R. G., Gokarn, R., Khalil, M., Turner, N., Cooney, G. J., Sinclair, D. A., Raubenheimer, D., Le Couteur, D. G., & Simpson, S. J. (2014). The ratio of macronutrients, not caloric intake, dictates cardiometabolic health, aging, and longevity in ad libitum-fed mice. *Cell Metabolism, 19*(3), 418–430.

Solon-Biet, S. M., Mitchell, S. J., de Cabo, R., Raubenheimer, D., Le Couteur, D. G., & Simpson, S. J. (2015). Macronutrients and caloric intake in health and longevity. *Journal of Endocrinology, 226*(1), R17–R28.

Somers, T. J., Keefe, F. J., Carson, J. W., et al. (2008). Pain catastrophizing in borderline morbidly obese and morbidly obese individuals with osteoarthritic knee pain. *Pain Research and Management, 13*(5), 401–406.

Souza, P. R., & Norling, L. V. (2016). Implications for eicosapentaenoic acid- and docosahexaenoic acid-derived resolvins as therapeutics for arthritis. *European Journal of Pharmacology, 785*, 165–173.

Stavropoulos-Kalinoglou, A., Metsios, G. S., Koutedakis, Y., et al. (2011). Obesity in rheumatoid arthritis. *Rheumatology, 50*(3), 450–462.

Stavropoulos-Kalinoglou, A., Metsios, G. S., Panoulas, V. F., et al. (2009). Underweight and obese states both associate with worse disease activity and physical function in patients with established rheumatoid arthritis. *Clinical Rheumatology, 28*(4), 439–444.

Stevens, M., Paans, N., Wagenmakers, R., et al. (2012). The influence of overweight/obesity on patient-perceived physical functioning and health-related quality of life after primary total hip arthroplasty. *Obesity Surgery, 22*(4), 523–529.

Symmons, D. P. (2002). Epidemiology of rheumatoid arthritis: determinants of onset, persistence and outcome. *Best Practice and Research Clinical Rheumatology, 16*(5), 707–722.

Tanamas, S. K., Wluka, A. E., Berry, P., et al. (2012). Relationship between obesity and foot pain and its association with fat mass, fat distribution, and muscle mass. *Arthritis Care Research, 64*(2), 262–268.

Thalacker-Mercer, A. E., & Drummond, M. J. (2014). The importance of dietary protein for muscle health in inactive, hospitalized older adults. *Annals of the New York Academy of Sciences, 1328*, 1–9.

Touma, C., & Pannain, S. (2011). Does lack of sleep cause diabetes? *Cleveland Clinic Journal of Medicine, 78*(8), 549–558.

Tukker, A., Visscher, T. L., & Picavet, H. S. (2009). Overweight and health problems of the lower extremities: osteoarthritis, pain and disability. *Public Health Nutrition, 12*(3), 359–368.

Ukhanova, M., Wang X., Baer D.J., Novotny J.A., Fredborg M., & Mai, V. (2014). Effects of almond and pistachio consumption on gut microbiota composition in a randomised cross-over human feeding study. *British Journal of Nutrition, 111*(12), 2146–2152.

Urquhart, D. M., Berry, P., Wluka, A. E., et al. (2011). 2011 Young Investigator Award winner: Increased fat mass is associated with high levels of low back pain intensity and disability. *Spine, 36*(16), 1320–1325.

van Gool, C. H., Penninx, B. W., Kempen, G. I., et al. (2005). Effects of exercise adherence on physical function among overweight older adults with knee osteoarthritis. *Arthritis and Rheumatism, 53*(1), 24–32.

Vincent, H. K., Heywood, K., Connelly, J., et al. (2012a). Weight loss and obesity in the treatment and prevention of osteoarthritis. *PM & R*, 4(Suppl. 5), S59–S67.

Vincent, H. K., Horodyski, M., Gearen, P., et al. (2012b). Obesity and long term functional outcomes following elective total hip replacement. *Journal of Orthopedics and Surgical Research*, *7*, 16.

Vincent, H. K., Lamb, K. M., Day, T. I., et al. (2010). Morbid obesity is associated with fear of movement and lower quality of life in patients with knee pain-related diagnoses. *PM & R*, *2*(8), 713–722.

Vincent, H. K., Omli, M. R., Day, T., et al. (2011). Fear of movement, quality of life, and self-reported disability in obese patients with chronic lumbar pain. *Pain Medicine*, *12*(1), 154–164.

Vincent, H. K., Seay, A. N., Montero, C., et al. (2013). Functional pain severity and mobility in overweight older men and women with chronic low-back pain—part I. *American Journal of Physical Medicine and Rehabilitation*, *92*(5), 430–438.

Vorona, R. D., Winn, M. P., Babineau, T. W., et al. (2005). Overweight and obese patients in a primary care population report less sleep than patients with a normal body mass index. *Archives of Internal Medicine*, *165*(1), 25–30.

Wang, J., Sereika, S. M., Styn, M. A., et al. (2013). Factors associated with health-related quality of life among overweight or obese adults. *Journal of Clinical Nursing*, *22*(15–16), 2172–2182.

Westhoff, G., Rau, R., & Znk, A. (2007). Radiographic joint damage in early rheumatoid arthritis is highly dependent on body mass index. *Arthritis and Rheumatism*, *56*(11), 3575–3582.

WHO, 2000. Obesity: preventing and managing the global epidemic. Report of a WHO Consultation. WHO Technical Report Series 894. Geneva: World Health Organization.

World Health Organization, 2007. "Protein and amino acid requirements in human nutrition. Report of a joint WHO/FAO expert consultation", WHO Technical Report Series 935, Word Health Organization (WHO), Geneva, Switzerland.

WHO, 2008. Scoping Document for WHO Treatment Guideline on Non-malignant Pain in Adults. Adopted in WHO Steering Group on Pain Guidelines, October 14, 2008.

World Health Organization (WHO). (2009). *Global Health Risks: Mortality and burden of disease attributable to selected major risks.* Geneva, Switzerland: World Health Organization.

Wolfe, F., & Michaud, K. (2012). Effect of body mass index on mortality and clinical status in rheumatoid arthritis. *Arthritis Care Research*, *64*(10), 1471–1479.

Wright, L. J., Schur, E., Noonan, C., et al. (2010). Chronic pain, overweight, and obesity: findings from a community-based twin registry. *Journal of Pain*, *11*(7), 628–635.

Yancy, W. S., Jr., Olsen, M. K., Westman, E. C., et al. (2002). Relationship between obesity and health-related quality of life in men. *Obesity Research*, *10*(10), 1057–1064.

Yunus, M. B., Arslan, S., & Aldag, J. C. (2002). Relationship between body mass index and fibromyalgia features. *Scandinavian Journal of Rheumatology*, *31*(1), 27–31.

CHAPTER

14

Postoperative Analgesia in Morbid Obesity: An Overview of Multimodal Analgesia and Complimentary Therapies

M.M. Aman, A. Mahmoud**, A.C. Sinha**

*Department of Anesthesiology, Drexel University College of Medicine, Philadelphia, PA, United States; **Department of Anesthesiology, John H. Stroger, Jr. Hospital of Cook County, Chicago, IL, United States

INTRODUCTION

The prevalence of obesity in the United States arguably presents one of the most concerning public health issues over the last 2 decades (Ogden, Carroll, Kit, & Flegal, 2014; Sturm & Hattori, 2013). Obesity is defined as having an elevated body mass index (BMI) >30 kg/m^2, which serves as a simplified surrogate of body fat content. Predetermined values defining various weight classifications are demonstrated in Table 14.1. There is ample data to suggest an exponential increase in the incidence of morbidly obese population relative to being overweight (Adams et al., 2006; Hensrud & Klein, 2006). With over a third of the nation suffering from obesity, we continue to see these patients presenting for various procedural and surgical interventions. After having failed conservative measures including diets, supplements, exercise, and often-medical therapy in effort to lose weight, patients look toward bariatric surgery. Understanding the core physiologic changes in morbid obesity as it relates to post operative pain control helps facilitate a safe and comfortable perioperative experience for our patients. This chapter will aim to highlight physiologic changes that modulate pain control, anatomic concerns, the role of multimodal techniques, and supplements for optimizing postoperative analgesia.

BURDEN OF MORBID OBESITY

There is a profound burden of excess adipose tissue on both a systemic and cellular level. The effect of obesity on body systems leads to an increase in all cause mortality from metabolic syndrome (Lakka et al., 2002), elevated risk of cardiovascular disease, diabetes, cancer, and premature death (Kopelman, 2007; Lau, Dhillon, Yan, Szmitko, & Verma, 2005; Lundgren, Brown, Nordt, Sobel, & Fujii, 1996; Neligan, 2010). Many of these changes are reversible with weight reduction. Owing to an increase in overall oxygen consumption, and reduced functional residual capacity morbidly obese patients have a propensity to quickly become hypoxemic in the setting of airway compromise. Oxygenation and ventilation are further complicated by the various anatomic changes including large necks, and redundant tissue that obstructs the airway. Patients that report fatigue, loud snoring, daytime sleepiness, and witnessed apneic episodes by family should be evaluated for obstructive sleep apnea (OSA) with polysomnography (Alam, Lewis, Stephens, & Baxter, 2007; Grunstein, Wilcox, Yang, Gould, & Hedner, 1993). For undiagnosed patients, an effective screening can be performed using common questionnaire, such as STOP–BANG (Chung et al., 2012; Chung et al., 2008). The clinical implication

Nutritional Modulators of Pain in the Aging Population. http://dx.doi.org/10.1016/B978-0-12-805186-3.00014-X
Copyright © 2017 Elsevier Inc. All rights reserved.

TABLE 14.1 Disease Risk for Type 2 Diabetes, Hypertension, and CVD

			Disease risk relative to normal weight and waist circumference	
	BMI (kg/m²)	Obesity class	Men 102 cm (40 in.) or less women 88 cm (35 in.) or less	Men > 102 cm (40 in.) women > 88 cm (35 in.)
Underweight	<18.5		—	—
Normal	18.5–24.9		—	—
Overweight	25.0–29.9		Increased	High
Obesity	30.0–34.9	I	High	Very high
	35.0–39.9	II	Very high	Very high
Morbid obesity	40.0[a]	III	Extremely high	Extremely high

[a]*Increased waist circumference also can be a marker for increased risk, even in persons of normal weight.*
Source: National Heart, Lung, and Blood Institute, National Institutes of Health.

of OSA on perioperative pain management relates to opioid induced somnolence, subsequent airway compromise and hypoxemia.

PAIN IN THE OBESE PATIENT

Morbid obesity and systemic pain have a complex relation. Morbidly obese individuals are more likely to suffer from chronic pain disorders of the musculoskeletal system when compared to those with a normal BMI (Hitt, McMillen, Thornton-Neaves, Koch, & Cosby, 2007; Janke, Collins, & Kozak, 2007). Consequently, much of this pain is improved postbariatric surgery weight loss (Hooper, Stellato, Hallowell, Seitz, & Moskowitz, 2007), as much of this pain is mechanical. The challenge lies in appreciating the balance of factors that result in excess chronic pain, and factors that potentially raise the threshold to acute pain. Obesity is thought of as a proinflammatory state with many immune and hormonal variables interacting in producing chronic pain (McVinnie, 2013). On the other hand, it is suggested that acute pain is modulated by excess endogenous opioids, and increase threshold to pain. We will discuss variables that affect acute perioperative pain.

OBESITY AND HORMONAL REGULATION OF ACUTE PAIN

The role of various endocrine and paracrine cytokines in inducing metabolic changes that lead to the comorbidities associated with obesity is well established (Hotamisligil, Arner, Caro, Atkinson, & Spiegelman, 1995; Kern et al., 1995; Kong, Chan, & Chan, 2006; Steppan et al., 2001). Our understanding of adipokines (leptin, resistin, adipsin, and adiponectin), endogenous opioids, and dopaminergic systems as it relates to the neuromodulation of pain in obesity shows varying results. While the desire to eat may be initiated by the dopaminergic system, endogenous opioids, such as beta-endorphins and endomorphins provide the pleasurable sensation when food is consumed (Berridge, Ho, Richard, & DiFeliceantonio, 2010). There are two important phenomenon that are postulated to interplay in regulating eating habits in obesity-elevation in the levels of endogenous opioids (Khawaja, Chattopadhyay, & Green, 1991), and reduction in mu-receptor (MOR) binding sites in the brain (Karlsson et al., 2015b). Randomized, double blind, placebo controlled human trials and animal data has suggested inhibition of opioid receptors in the brain leads to reduced food consumption (Greenway et al., 2010; Ikeda et al., 2015). As with systemic comorbidities, recent data examining human positron emission tomography pre- and postbariatric surgery suggests these biochemical changes are reversible after bariatric surgery (Karlsson et al., 2015c). Most data on endogenous opiates discusses their effects on diet. It is difficult to extrapolate whether a parallel exists between increased endogenous opioids, reduced MOR, and postoperative pain control. Given our current understanding of endogenous opioids in obesity, a study examined the sensitivity to pain by measuring electrical threshold to pain after significant weight loss (mean 32 kg). The threshold to pain remained higher in obese participants compared to normal weight lean individuals (Dodet et al., 2013). While this suggests a sensory impairment in the detection of pain that may be caused my numerous hormonal factors, the opioid requirement to treat the pain is not assessed. In effort to answer this question, a large retrospective analysis of 11,719 patients who underwent bariatric surgery was conducted. Eight percent (n = 933) were chronic opioid users, and it was found that postoperative opioid consumption increased 13% at year one and 18% by year three postoperatively (Raebel et al., 2013). This could be in part due to the reduction of endogenous opioids from weight loss. In summary, excess endogenous opiate, high threshold to induce pain, and decreased opioid receptors in the brain all support the reduction of dosage of narcotic pain medicine in obese patients.

SYSTEMIC OPIOIDS IN THE MORBIDLY OBESE

Opioid therapy has long been the cornerstone for providing analgesia in the acute postoperative setting ("Practice guidelines for acute pain management in the perioperative setting. A report by the American Society of Anesthesiologists Task Force on Pain Management, Acute Pain Section," Practice guidelines, 1995). Inadequate analgesia due to fear of opioid related complications in the morbidly obese can have numerous adverse consequences. Patients are unlikely to participate in postoperative respiratory physiotherapy (incentive spirometrey or coughing) thereby increasing the incidence of postoperative pulmonary atelectasis and pneumonia. Furthermore, with the change in healthcare paradigm that emphasizes patient satisfaction in reimbursement models, it is important to achieve adequate postoperative analgesia for that reason as well.

Opioid Pharmacology and Pharmacokinetics in the Morbidly Obese

The properties of specific opioids depend on the binding receptor, degree of affinity, and the drug/receptor interaction (agonists, antagonists, and partial agonists). Four major classes of opioid receptors have been identified: mu, kappa, delta, and sigma with the majority located throughout the central nervous system.

It is important to remain cognizant the multiple physiological effects of morbid obesity when considering opioid use for acute postoperative analgesia. Factors affecting altered pharmacokinetics include, increased adipose tissue, increased blood volume, higher cardiac output, decreased total body water, altered protein binding and increased renal blood flow and glomerular filtration rate (GFR) (Banicek & Butcher, 2011). These changes should be considered alongside the physical characteristics of individual opioids (ionization, protein binding, and lipid solubility) to help guide opioid selection.

Disparities regarding regional circulation have been described in the morbidly obese. While the percentage of fat is increased in obesity, the blood flow per gram of fat is less than in nonobese individuals (Cheymol, 1988). These alterations result in changes with drug distribution in tissue such that lipophilic opioids are more likely to accumulate in fat tissue raising concern for redistribution from the adipose tissue to the blood stream. For these reasons, opioid dosing is a particular challenge in the morbidly obese. Regardless of the agent employed, diligent monitoring and titration is encouraged. Loading doses should be based on ideal body weight for agents that are restricted to lean tissues, namely hydrophilic opioids (morphine). When considering lipophilic agents (fentanyl) loading doses should be based on total body weight.

Opioid Patient Controlled Analgesia

Utilization of patient-controlled analgesia (PCA) pumps in the acute postoperative period has been associated with increased patient satisfaction. Determining the appropriate agent, bolus dose, lockout interval and background infusion rate in the morbidly obese can help minimize the risks associated with opioid overdose.

Selection of a hydrophilic agent (morphine) offers a more predictable clinical effect and is less likely to accumulate in adipose tissue. Best practice recommendations when considering a PCA in morbidly obese population include; adjusting initial PCA dose settings on estimated lean body mass, avoidance of routine use of continuous opioid background infusion PCA mode and utilizing an opioid-based PCA with local anesthetic wound infiltration and adjunct (nonnarcotic) analgesic medications (unless contraindicated) (Schumann et al., 2005). Given the propensity for morbidly obese patients to experience respiratory complications with opioid therapy, significant consideration should be made for continuous monitoring during PCA therapy. The Anesthesia Patient Safety Foundation has published recommendations intended to facilitate detection for clinically significant drug-induced respiratory depression. Recommendations include continuous oxygenation monitoring by continuous pulse oximetry, continuous ventilation monitoring by capnography when supplemental oxygen is needed "Opioid-Induced Ventilatory Impairment (OIVI): Time for a change in the Monitoring Strategy for Postoperative PCA Patients," OIVI (2011).

Multimodal Strategies in the Acute Postoperative Phase

Obese patients are at increased risk for opioid induced over sedation and respiratory depression. Risk factors for over sedation include coexisting sleep apnea, snoring, older age, being opiate naïve, longer length of time receiving general anesthesia, receiving other sedating drugs, preexisting pulmonary, or cardiac disease, thoracic incisions and smoking (Commission, 2012). As most of these risk factors are more prevalent in the morbidly obese, a call for opioid sparing multimodal strategies in the acute postoperative phase has emerged. Current American Society of Anesthesiologist (ASA) guidelines recommend that unless contraindicated, all surgical patients should receive an around-the-clock regimen of a nonopioid agent, such as acetaminophen or a nonsteroidal antiinflammatory drug (NSAID) "Practice guidelines for acute pain management in the perioperative setting: an updated report by the American Society of Anesthesiologists Task Force on Acute Pain Management," Practice guidelines (2012). Multiple professional organizations including the American society for Pain Management Nursing (ASPMN) (Jarzyna et al., 2011), the Agency for Healthcare Research and Quality (AHEQ) (Hughes, 2008), and the Joint Commission (Commission, 2012) encourage a multimodal approach that utilizes two or more analgesics acting by different mechanism to provide perioperative analgesia. These opioid-sparing strategies can be divided into nonopioid analgesics, systemic adjuvants and regional anesthesia and analgesia.

Nonopioid Systemic Analgesics

Concerns regarding nonopioid analgesics include inadequate analgesia secondary to their "ceiling" effect and agent specific side effects. Knowledge about existing patient comorbidities and dosing guidelines can affectively minimize these occurrences. Complete intraoperative nonopioid analgesia has been compared to a fentanyl-based analgesia in the morbidly obese for open gastric bypass with results showing decreased postoperative opioid use and sedation (Feld, Laurito, Beckerman, Vincent, & Hoffman, 2003). NSAIDS inhibit the production of cyclooxygenase (COX)-1 and COX-2 enzymes preventing the sensitization of pain at the injury site receptors. They are also commonly utilized for their anti-inflammatory and antipyretic properties. Intravenous Ketorolac has been heavily studied in the morbidly obese population and the management of acute postoperative pain. Ketorolac administration during the first 24 h post operatively reduces narcotic requirements leading to improved patient satisfaction and enthusiastic participation in respiratory physical therapy in morbidly obese patients undergoing laparoscopic surgery (Govindarajan et al., 2005). Consideration must be given to underlying renal function as morbidly obese individuals are more likely to have associated comorbidities (diabetes, hypertension) that may compromise renal functional.

Intravenous acetaminophen is a centrally acting nonopioid analgesic approved for moderate to severe pain. Administration of a normal dose of acetaminophen to an obese patient should yield plasma levels in the same range as persons of normal weight (Lee, Kramer, & Granville, 1981). In abdominal laparoscopic surgery acetaminophen lead to both reduced pain intensity rating in the first 24 h and shorter time to meaningful pain relief (Wininger et al., 2010). In orthopedic surgery (total hip and total knee replacement), acetaminophen plus PCA morphine demonstrated superior pain control compared to PCA morphine alone in addition to reducing pain intensity ratings (Sinatra et al., 2005).

Furthermore, combinations of nonopioid analgesics have been shown to be beneficial. Multimodal-approach with intravenous Ketorolac and acetaminophen every 6 h for 24 h in bariatric surgery reduced opioid consumption by 41%. In addition the time with oxygen saturation below 90% reduced by 33.2% (Ziemann-Gimmel, Hensel, Koppman, & Marema, 2013).

Systemic Adjuvants

Alpha-2 agonist: Clonidine and Dexmedetomidine are alpha-2 agonists with known clinical analgesic and opioid sparing effects. Oral clonidine premedication in patients with sleep apnea has been shown to reduce the amount of intraoperative anesthetics and postoperative opioid consumption (Pawlik, Hansen, Waldhauser, Selig, & Kuehnel, 2005). In the postoperative setting, an infusion of clonidine (4 μg/kg) when combined with PCA morphine/clonidine (1 mg and 20 μg respectively) was shown to reduce both morphine consumption at 12 h and incidence of nausea and vomiting (Jeffs, Hall, & Morris, 2002). When compared to the intravenous route, epidural administration of clonidine has been shown to provide comparable postoperative analgesia while simultaneously providing lower sedation levels (Bernard, Kick, & Bonnet, 1995).

Dexmedetomidine exhibits many folds higher selectively for the alpha2 receptors than clonidine. Intraoperative Dexmedetomidine infusions in open bariatric surgery resulted in lower volatile anesthetic requirements, with improved pain scores and decrease morphine use in the postanesthesia care unit (Feld, Hoffman, Stechert, Hoffman, & Ananda, 2006). In patients undergoing laparoscopic bariatric surgery, intraoperative infusions have demonstrated similar results with better postoperative recovery profiles and reduced opioid requirements (Bakhamees, El-Halafawy, El-Kerdawy, Gouda, & Altemyatt, 2007).

Ketamine is an N-methyl-D-aspartate (NMDA) receptor antagonist with known analgesic properties. It possesses potent antiinflammatory properties through interaction with numerous other receptor systems (De Kock, Loix, & Lavand'homme, 2013). Its use in conjunction with opioids offers a synergistic analgesic effect (Gupta, Devi, & Gomes, 2011). In addition, the preoperative administration of low-dose ketamine and clonidine at induction has been shown to facilitate early extubation and lowers postoperative analgesic requirements in patients presenting for weight loss surgery (Sollazzi et al., 2009). A Cochrane database of systemic review demonstrated that the perioperative use of subanesthetic doses of ketamine were effective at reducing morphine requirements in the first 24 h (Bell, Dahl, Moore, & Kalso, 2006).

REGIONAL ANESTHESIA AND ANALGESIA

Regional anesthesia can be broadly divided into neuraxial anesthesia and peripheral nerve blocks. Regional techniques, whether used as sole anesthetics or in combination with general anesthesia, can offer many advantages in the obese population. These blocks allow for opioid-free local anesthetic solutions to be utilized in the multimodal approach to post operative pain control. In the acute postoperative setting, successful peripheral nerve blocks will reduce both opioid consumption and the incidence of PONV. As the surface landmarks that guide needle insertion can be obscured, ultrasound utilization can help identify key underlying structures improving block success rate (Chantzi, Saranteas, Zogogiannis, Alevizou, & Dimitriou, 2007; Schwemmer, Papenfuss, Greim, Brederlau, & Roewer, 2006).

To preform these blocks safely and successfully, familiarity with the attempted block and associated anatomical changes is necessary. Upper limb brachial plexus blocks are relatively easier to perform in morbidly obese patients due to a disproportionate increase lower limb and abdominal fat distribution. Various lumbo-sacral approaches are markedly difficult to visualize (Al-Nasser, 2012; Hayashi & Ueyama, 2010). Proper patient positioning and additional time should be allotted to allow accurate identification of nerve structures thereby improve success rates (Schwemmer et al., 2006). Independent risk factors contributing to block failure include a BMI of more than 25 kg/m^2 and an ASA physical status IV (Cotter et al., 2004).

THORACIC EPIDURAL CATHETERIZATION IN THE OBESE

The successful identification of anatomical landmarks that guide thoracic epidural placement can be challenging in the morbidly obese population. Ultrasonography can be used to overcome these challenges. In patients undergoing bariatric surgery, ultrasound scanning was useful in identifying anatomical landmarks and estimating epidural space depth during thoracic epidural catheterization (Nishiyama, 2014). In addition to superior postoperative analgesia and decreased opioid consumption, neuraxial blockade (epidural or spinal anesthesia) has been shown to reduce postoperative mortality and other serious complications (von Ungern-Sternberg, Regli, Reber, & Schneider, 2005; Rodgers et al., 2000).

Epidural solution selection must be tailored to every individual patient. Careful consideration of underlying comorbidities must be considered prior to selection. Available solutions include local anesthetic, opioid, or a combination of local anesthetic and opioid. The combination of local anesthetics and opioids provides superior analgesia when compared to either agent being used individually (Jorgensen, Wetterslev, Moiniche, & Dahl, 2000). However, in patients with OSA, epidural solution should be opioid free or contain the lowest efficacious dose to minimize the risk of respiratory depression (*Practice Guidelines for the Prevention, Detection, and Management of Respiratory Depression Associated with Neuraxial Opioid Administration: An Updated Report by the American Society of Anesthesiologists Task Force on Neuraxial Opioids and the American Society of Regional Anesthesia and Pain Medicine*, Practice Guidelines, 2016). In addition to solution selection, careful titration should be instituted, as obese patients require less local anesthetic in order to achieve a similar block level when compared with non-obese patients (Hodgkinson & Husain, 1980).

The benefits of thoracic epidural use on postoperative pain control have been studied extensively. Finally, when compared to patients who received conventional postoperative PCA's patients who received thoracic epidurals had significantly improved postoperative pain relief, decreased postoperative side effects and a decrease in hospital stay following laparoscopic gastric bypass surgery (Rudram Muppuri & Hong, 2015).

COMPLEMENTARY AND ALTERNATIVE MEDICINE THERAPIES

Interest in integrative or holistic approaches to various medical conditions has seen a drastic rise in developed countries (Leach, 2013). Traditionally, these therapies have been practiced for centuries across the Asian subcontinent. Broadly, complementary and alternative medicine (CAM) can be divided into nutraceutical and dietary therapies, manipulation, and procedural therapies, and mind-body energy therapies. A detailed review of all aspects of complementary therapy is beyond the scope of this chapter and we recommend (Woodbury, Soong, Fishman, & Garcia, 2016) for a comprehensive analysis. We will overview the nutraceutical and dietary aspects of CAM as it relates to postoperative pain management.

DIETS

Numerous dietary plans have been developed to aid in weight reduction and primarily focus on either restriction of total calories consumed daily, or alter the type of caloric intake. Alterations in the amount of protein, carbohydrate, or fat consumed affect the body in much beyond weight gain or loss.

LOW CARBOHYDRATE DIET

The low carbohydrate, high protein, and high fat diet surged in popularity as a method for relatively rapid weight reduction. However, randomized trials examining its utility for sustained weight loss when compared to low calorie diets consisting of high carbohydrate and low fat was not impressive (Foster et al., 2003). In the perioperative setting carbohydrate rich drinks prior to surgery have been shown to reduce postoperative nausea and vomiting, results in earlier mobilization and reduced length of stay

(Awad, Varadhan, Ljungqvist, & Lobo, 2013). Various enhanced recovery after surgery (ERAS) protocols often include carbohydrate nutrition preoperatively with these goals. A study examining postoperative pain in patients who presented for bariatric surgery on low carbohydrate diets preoperatively, did not show a difference amongst carbohydrate rich drink, protein rich drink, or tap water (Karlsson, Wendel, Polits, Gislason, & Hedenbro, 2015). More data is needed to assess the impact of the low carbohydrate state on postoperative pain in morbidly obese patients.

KETOGENIC DIET

High fat, very low carbohydrate, and moderate protein consumption limits available glucose, resulting in the use of ketone bodies for cellular energy. This diet has been thought to reduce seizures since the turn of the twentieth century, and recent data still supports its judicious use (Martin, Jackson, Levy, & Cooper, 2016). As with seizures, pain is thought to involve excitability of neurons hence the use of various epileptic medications for the management of neuropathic pain. Although data examining the role of ketogenic diets and their direct role in reducing pain is lacking, a parallel has been suggested by reduction in reactive oxygen species and inflammation (Kim do et al., 2007; Maalouf, Sullivan, Davis, Kim, & Rho, 2007; Masino & Ruskin, 2013). However, in the perioperative setting patients should be well advised to avoid drastic physiological changes that are caused by such diets. Optimization should focus of maintaining homeostasis and correcting nutritional deficiencies. The risks involved with undergoing anesthesia compounded by the surgical stress response, far outweigh any potential benefit of a ketotic state.

PERIOPERATIVE CONSIDERATIONS OF DIETARY SUPPLEMENTS

The use of dietary supplements including minerals, vitamins, amino acids, fatty acids, fiber, and other nutrients has seen a dramatic rise in the last 2 decades (Barnes, Bloom, & Nahin, 2008; Wu, Wang, & Kennedy, 2011). It is helpful to be familiar with commonly used supplements for pain, anxiety, depression, and other ailments as they have various adverse interactions in the perioperative setting. As with other medications, there is risk for drug–drug interaction. Inquiry about specific supplement use should be made during preanesthetic evaluations, as a large majority of patients will not volunteer this information (Kaye et al., 2000). The pharmacological effects of these medications are best examined into two broad categories: pharmacokinetics, and pharmacodynamics.

TABLE 14.2 Common Supplements Affecting CYP Isoenzymes

Enzyme	Inducers	Inhibitors	Common substrates
CYP3A4	*Gingko*, St. Johns wort	Kava	Fentanyl, Tramadol, Alfentanil, benzodiazapenes
CYP2D6	—	*Gingko*	Codeine, hydrocodone, beta blockers, Ondansetron
CYP2C9	St. Johns wort	*Gingko*, java	NSAIDS, ketamine, THC, sulfonylureas
CYP2C19	*Gingko*, St. Johns wort	Kava	Proton pump inhibitors, Clopidogrel, Coumadin

Modified from (Abe, Kaye, Gritsenko, Urman, & Kaye, 2014).

Pharmacokinetics examines all aspects of how the body processes medications and supplements. Drugs undergo absorption, distribution, metabolism, and excretion. When examining the role of supplements in the perioperative setting, metabolism is arguably the most relevant. The liver is responsible for biotransformation of drugs via Phase 1 and Phase 2 reactions. Phase 1 reactions include oxidation, hydroxylation, reduction, and hydrolysis by various cytochrome P450 (CYP) isoenzymes, while Phase 2 facilitates conjugation to increase water solubility and elimination. It is during the Phase 1 reactions that supplements can either induce or inhibit specific CYP isoenzymes leading to potentially dangerous side effects. Inducing of an isoenzyme will cause increased metabolism, and reduction of desired effect. Inhibition of an isoenzyme will result in build up of drug to potentially toxic effects. A brief, nonexhaustive list of common supplements affecting CYP isoenzymes is displayed in Table 14.2.

Pharmacodynamics assesses how a given drug affects the body. When supplements interact with medications used in the perioperative setting it will result in either a synergistic, or antagonistic pharmacological affect. We emphasize vigilance toward anticoagulant, central nervous system depressant, and myocardial depressant affects of various supplements when combined with anesthetic agents.

Melatonin

The anticipation of postoperative pain is a common cause of anxiety in the perioperative setting. As a result, the use of benzodiazepines has become the mainstay of anxiolysis. However, a recent large randomized controlled trial failed to demonstrate a correlation between the use of Lorazepam for anxiolysis in patients undergoing general anesthesia for elective surgery and self reported patient satisfaction that day after surgery. Its use resulted in modest prolongation to extubation and lower rate of early cognitive recovery

(Maurice-Szamburski et al., 2015). Melatonin is secreted by pineal gland in the brain and is well known for its role as a regulatory hormone of circadian rhythms. Based on data from animal models it was demonstrated that melatonin also has antinociceptive and antiinflammatory functions (Padhy & Kumar, 2005; Wang et al., 2009). Clinical trials demonstrate its utility as an anxiolytic (Naguib & Samarkandi, 1999, 2000) and analgesic (Caumo, Levandovski, & Hidalgo, 2009; Caumo et al., 2007). A dose of melatonin 5 mg the night before and morning of surgery is found to be adequate and reduce postoperative opioid consumption by as much as 30% (Caumo et al., 2009).

St. John's Wort (*Hypericum perforatum*)

Commonly used for mild to moderate depression and sleep disorders, many patients use St. John's wort for anxiety, and pain disorders. Proposed mechanisms of action involve multiple pathways including inhibition of monoamine oxidase, serotonin, norepinephrine, and potentiation of gamma-aminobutyric acid (Hodges & Kam, 2002). It has been shown that a short 2-week course of St. John's wort can induce the activity of CYP-3A4, which is responsible for the metabolism of close to half of all prescribed medications. A study ascertained normal metabolism of Alprazolam in healthy volunteers, and reassessed various parameters after a 2-week course of St. John's wort. A twofold reduction in plasma concentration and doubling in the rate of clearance was noted (Markowitz et al., 2003). Reports of transplant organ rejection from reduced cyclosporine levels, and serotonergic crisis in patients taking antidepressants has sparked interest in effects during the perioperative setting. This signifies an increase in dosage needed to achieve a desired affect of medications metabolized by the CYP3A4 isoenzyme. Cessation of this supplement 2 weeks prior to surgery is reasonable.

Gingko Biloba

G. biloba is used by patients for the treatment of cognitive deficits from dementia and Alzheimer's and pain from intermittent claudication (IC). While mild side effects are primarily gastrointestinal, multiple reports suggest elevated risk of spontaneous bleeding. Alveolar hemorrhages, anterior chamber of eye bleeds, significant subdural and subarachnoid hemorrhages are reported in otherwise healthy individuals (Kaye, Baluch, Kaye, Frass, & Hofbauer, 2007). In effort to shed light on the effects of *Gingko* on clot formation, a group of investigators measured various aspects of clotting by rotational thromboelastometer (ROTEM). With the exception of Omega-3 fish oil multiple naturopathic medications including Gingko, failed to demonstrate a decrease in platelet aggregation or delay in clot formation (Bagge, Schott, & Kander, 2016). Patients often ask for council on supplements in the perioperative setting, and while these questions are correctly deferred to primary care providers, it may be of benefit to be informed on recent opinion. A metaanalysis of patients taking *G. biloba* for IC did not find any clinically significant reduction in pain from peripheral arterial disease (Nicolai et al., 2013), while its use for dementia showed promise (Le Bars et al., 1997). Given the potential for significant risk, we advise caution and a conservative approach toward invasive pain management techniques given the risk of bleeding.

Kava Kava

Kava is used as an anxiolytic, and sedative sleep aid. Reports have suggested synergistic affects with benzodiazepine's causing profound depressed cognition and coma (Almeida & Grimsley, 1996). Long-term use can lead to toxicity consisting of dry, flaky skin and reddened eyes (Norton & Ruze, 1994). Interaction with multiple CYP450 enzymes is displayed in Table 14.2. If kava was consumption was maintained preceding surgery, it is advised to administer benzodiazepines with caution.

Omega 3 Fish Oil

Fish oil is one of the most extensively researched supplements and is being used for its efficacy in reducing the risk of heart disease, musculoskeletal degeneration, and in the treatment of inflammatory (Proudman et al., 2015) and neuropathic pain. It is sensible to advise patients to withhold consumption at least three days prior to surgical intervention. Data has shown increased risk of bleeding in patients taking fish oil. As cited previously, delayed clot formation was noted on ROTEM with the use of fish oil (Bagge et al., 2016).

Honokiol

Honokiol is extracted from Magnolia plants indigenous to Japan, and is commonly used in homeopathic medications across the Asian subcontinent. It's has broad application owing to its analgesic, anxiolytic, and neuroprotective properties to name a few (Woodbury, Yu, Wei, & Garcia, 2013). Animal models have highlighted the utility of Honokiol and its structural analog magnolol in the treatment of inflammatory pain (Lin, Chen, Ko, & Chan, 2007). Interestingly, Honokiol has a similar polyphenolic structure to Propofol, which has been hypothesized to account for its similar hypnotic pharmacologic affects. As with other herbals, Honokiol has been implicated in increased risk of bleeding, and has a potential for neurotoxicity at high doses (Hu, Zhang, Wang, & Chen, 2005).

THE FUTURE OF PAIN-PHARMACOGENETIC TESTING

When categorizing how we metabolize a given drug, four subsets of metabolism are defined: poor, intermediate, extensive, and ultrarapid. The extensive metabolizer subset of patients is considered "normal" and what current dosing models use. Traditionally, it has been a trial and error process finding the right balance of desired effect versus overdose. When a clinically appropriate dosage of drug is administered and causes a profound adverse reaction, it may be secondary to the patient's genetics. For example, an extensive gastrointestinal bleed with a Celecoxib 200 mg TID in a poor metabolizer will quickly lead to toxic levels of the drug causing the bleed. From Watson and Crick describing the DNA double helix in the 1950s to the completion of the Human Genome Project, we have come a long way in our understanding of how we process medication. Genetic testing using an oral swab collecting a small sample of saliva can identify how our body will metabolize a given drug. The sample is run against a specific pain medication, and the result will categorize the patient's metabolism for that given CYP isoenzyme. This genetic make up becomes a part of the permanent medical record. If the same patient from the example previously develops atrial fibrillation and requires Warfarin (which is metabolized by the same isoenzyme), the drug dosage will be reduced in effort to prevent excessive anticoagulation. While beneficial for all patients, pharmacogenetic testing is particularly interesting in morbidly obese patients where the balance of pain control and overdose is more difficult to achieve.

References

Abe, A., Kaye, A. D., Gritsenko, K., Urman, R. D., & Kaye, A. M. (2014). Perioperative analgesia and the effects of dietary supplements. *Best Practice Research and Clinical Anaesthesiology, 28*(2), 183–189.

Adams, K. F., Schatzkin, A., Harris, T. B., Kipnis, V., Mouw, T., Ballard-Barbash, R., …, Leitzmann, M. F. (2006). Overweight, obesity, and mortality in a large prospective cohort of persons 50 to 71 years old. *New England Journal of Medicine, 355*(8), 763–778.

Al-Nasser, B. (2012). Review of interscalene block for postoperative analgesia after shoulder surgery in obese patients. *Acta Anaesthesiol Taiwan, 50*(1), 29–34.

Alam, I., Lewis, K., Stephens, J. W., & Baxter, J. N. (2007). Obesity, metabolic syndrome and sleep apnoea: all pro-inflammatory states. *Obesity Reviews, 8*(2), 119–127.

Almeida, J. C., & Grimsley, E. W. (1996). Coma from the health food store: interaction between kava and alprazolam. *Annals of Internal Medicine, 125*(11), 940–941.

Awad, S., Varadhan, K. K., Ljungqvist, O., & Lobo, D. N. (2013). A meta-analysis of randomised controlled trials on preoperative oral carbohydrate treatment in elective surgery. *Clinical Nutrition, 32*(1), 34–44.

Bagge, A., Schott, U., & Kander, T. (2016). Effects of naturopathic medicines on Multiplate and ROTEM: a prospective experimental pilot study in healthy volunteers. *BMC Complement Alternate Medicine, 16*(1), 64.

Bakhamees, H. S., El-Halafawy, Y. M., El-Kerdawy, H. M., Gouda, N. M., & Altemyatt, S. (2007). Effects of dexmedetomidine in morbidly obese patients undergoing laparoscopic gastric bypass. *Middle East Journal of Anaesthesiology, 19*(3), 537–551.

Banicek, J., & Butcher, D. (2011). Acute pain management following Roux-en-Y gastric bypass surgery. *Nursing Standard, 25*(18), 35–40.

Barnes, P. M., Bloom, B., & Nahin, R. L. (2008). Complementary and alternative medicine use among adults and children: United States, 2007. *National Health Statistics Report*(12), 1–23.

Bell, R. F., Dahl, J. B., Moore, R. A., & Kalso, E. (2006). Perioperative ketamine for acute postoperative pain. *Cochrane Database Systems Review*(1), Cd004603.

Bernard, J. M., Kick, O., & Bonnet, F. (1995). Comparison of intravenous and epidural clonidine for postoperative patient-controlled analgesia. *Anesthesia and Analgesia, 81*(4), 706–712.

Berridge, K. C., Ho, C. Y., Richard, J. M., & DiFeliceantonio, A. G. (2010). The tempted brain eats: pleasure and desire circuits in obesity and eating disorders. *Brain Research, 1350*, 43–64.

Caumo, W., Levandovski, R., & Hidalgo, M. P. (2009). Preoperative anxiolytic effect of melatonin and clonidine on postoperative pain and morphine consumption in patients undergoing abdominal hysterectomy: a double-blind, randomized, placebo-controlled study. *Journal of Pain, 10*(1), 100–108.

Caumo, W., Torres, F., Moreira, N. L., Jr., Auzani, J. A., Monteiro, C. A., Londero, G., …, Hidalgo, M. P. (2007). The clinical impact of preoperative melatonin on postoperative outcomes in patients undergoing abdominal hysterectomy. *Anesthesia and Analgesia, 105*(5), 1263–1271.

Chantzi, C., Saranteas, T., Zogogiannis, J., Alevizou, N., & Dimitriou, V. (2007). Ultrasound examination of the sciatic nerve at the anterior thigh in obese patients. *Acta Anaesthesiologica Scandinavica, 51*(1), 132.

Cheymol, G. (1988). Drug pharmacokinetics in the obese. *Fundamental and Clinical Pharmacology, 2*(3), 239–256.

Chung, F., Subramanyam, R., Liao, P., Sasaki, E., Shapiro, C., & Sun, Y. (2012). High STOP-Bang score indicates a high probability of obstructive sleep apnoea. *British Journal of Anaesthesia, 108*(5), 768–775.

Chung, F., Yegneswaran, B., Liao, P., Chung, S. A., Vairavanathan, S., Islam, S., …, Shapiro, C. M. (2008). Validation of the Berlin questionnaire and American Society of Anesthesiologists checklist as screening tools for obstructive sleep apnea in surgical patients. *Anesthesiology, 108*(5), 822–830.

Commission, T. J. (2012). Sentinel Event Alert. Available from: http://www.jointcommission.org/assets/1/18/sea_49_opioids_8_2_12_final.pdf

Cotter, J. T., Nielsen, K. C., Guller, U., Steele, S. M., Klein, S. M., Greengrass, R. A., & Pietrobon, R. (2004). Increased body mass index and ASA physical status IV are risk factors for block failure in ambulatory surgery—an analysis of 9,342 blocks. *Canadian Journal of Anaesthesia, 51*(8), 810–816.

De Kock, M., Loix, S., & Lavand'homme, P. (2013). Ketamine and peripheral inflammation. *CNS Neuroscience and Therapeutics, 19*(6), 403–410.

Dodet, P., Perrot, S., Auvergne, L., Hajj, A., Simoneau, G., Decleves, X., …, Lloret-Linares, C. (2013). Sensory impairment in obese patients? Sensitivity and pain detection thresholds for electrical stimulation after surgery-induced weight loss, and comparison with a nonobese population. *Clinical Journal of Pain, 29*(1), 43–49.

Feld, J. M., Hoffman, W. E., Stechert, M. M., Hoffman, I. W., & Ananda, R. C. (2006). Fentanyl or dexmedetomidine combined with desflurane for bariatric surgery. *Journal of Clinical Anesthesia, 18*(1), 24–28.

Feld, J. M., Laurito, C. E., Beckerman, M., Vincent, J., & Hoffman, W. E. (2003). Non-opioid analgesia improves pain relief and decreases sedation after gastric bypass surgery. *Canadian Journal of Anaesthesia, 50*(4), 336–341.

Foster, G. D., Wyatt, H. R., Hill, J. O., McGuckin, B. G., Brill, C., Mohammed, B. S., …, Klein, S. (2003). A randomized trial of a low-carbohydrate diet for obesity. New England Journal of Medicine, 348(21), 2082–2090.

Govindarajan, R., Ghosh, B., Sathyamoorthy, M. K., Kodali, N. S., Raza, A., Aronsohn, J., ..., Abadir, A. (2005). Efficacy of ketorolac in lieu of narcotics in the operative management of laparoscopic surgery for morbid obesity. *Surgery for Obesity and Related Diseases, 1*(6), 530–535; discussion 535–536.

Greenway, F. L., Fujioka, K., Plodkowski, R. A., Mudaliar, S., Guttadauria, M., Erickson, J., ..., Dunayevich, E. (2010). Effect of naltrexone plus bupropion on weight loss in overweight and obese adults (COR-I): a multicentre, randomised, double-blind, placebo-controlled, phase 3 trial. *Lancet, 376*(9741), 595–605.

Grunstein, R., Wilcox, I., Yang, T. S., Gould, Y., & Hedner, J. (1993). Snoring and sleep apnoea in men: association with central obesity and hypertension. *International Journal of Obesity and Related Metabolic Disorders, 17*(9), 533–540.

Gupta, A., Devi, L. A., & Gomes, I. (2011). Potentiation of mu-opioid receptor-mediated signaling by ketamine. *Journal of Neurochemistry, 119*(2), 294–302.

Hayashi, H., & Ueyama, H. (2010). [Experience of ultrasound-guided popliteal sciatic nerve block and femoral nerve perineural catheter placement in a morbidly obese patient undergoing total knee arthroplasty]. *Masui, 59*(10), 1260–1262.

Hensrud, D. D., & Klein, S. (2006). Extreme obesity: a new medical crisis in the United States. *Mayo Clinic Proceedings, 81*(Suppl. 10), S5–S10.

Hitt, H. C., McMillen, R. C., Thornton-Neaves, T., Koch, K., & Cosby, A. G. (2007). Comorbidity of obesity and pain in a general population: results from the Southern Pain Prevalence Study. *Journal of Pain, 8*(5), 430–436.

Hodges, P. J., & Kam, P. C. (2002). The peri-operative implications of herbal medicines. *Anaesthesia, 57*(9), 889–899.

Hodgkinson, R., & Husain, F. J. (1980). Obesity and the cephalad spread of analgesia following epidural administration of bupivacaine for Cesarean section. *Anesthesia and Analgesia, 59*(2), 89–92.

Hooper, M. M., Stellato, T. A., Hallowell, P. T., Seitz, B. A., & Moskowitz, R. W. (2007). Musculoskeletal findings in obese subjects before and after weight loss following bariatric surgery. *International Journal of Obesity (London), 31*(1), 114–120.

Hotamisligil, G. S., Arner, P., Caro, J. F., Atkinson, R. L., & Spiegelman, B. M. (1995). Increased adipose tissue expression of tumor necrosis factor-alpha in human obesity and insulin resistance. *Journal of Clinical Investigation, 95*(5), 2409–2415.

Hu, H., Zhang, X. X., Wang, Y. Y., & Chen, S. Z. (2005). Honokiol inhibits arterial thrombosis through endothelial cell protection and stimulation of prostacyclin. *Acta Pharmacologica Sinica, 26*(9), 1063–1068.

Ikeda, H., Ardianto, C., Yonemochi, N., Yang, L., Ohashi, T., Ikegami, M., ..., Kamei, J. (2015). Inhibition of opioid systems in the hypothalamus as well as the mesolimbic area suppresses feeding behavior of mice. *Neuroscience, 311*, 9–21.

Janke, E. A., Collins, A., & Kozak, A. T. (2007). Overview of the relationship between pain and obesity: what do we know? Where do we go next? *Journal of Rehabilitation Research and Development, 44*(2), 245–262.

Jarzyna, D., Jungquist, C. R., Pasero, C., Willens, J. S., Nisbet, A., Oakes, L., ..., Polomano, R. C. (2011). American Society for Pain Management Nursing guidelines on monitoring for opioid-induced sedation and respiratory depression. *Pain Management Nursing, 12*(3), 118–145.e110.

Jeffs, S. A., Hall, J. E., & Morris, S. (2002). Comparison of morphine alone with morphine plus clonidine for postoperative patient-controlled analgesia. *British Journal of Anaesthesia, 89*(3), 424–427.

Jorgensen, H., Wetterslev, J., Moiniche, S., & Dahl, J. B. (2000). Epidural local anaesthetics versus opioid-based analgesic regimens on postoperative gastrointestinal paralysis. PONV and pain after abdominal surgery. *Cochrane Database System Review*(4), Cd001893.

Karlsson, A., Wendel, K., Polits, S., Gislason, H., & Hedenbro, J. L. (2015a). Preoperative nutrition and postoperative discomfort in an eras setting: a randomized study in gastric bypass surgery. *Obesity Surgery*.doi: 10.1007/s11695-015-1848-7.

Karlsson, H. K., Tuominen, L., Tuulari, J. J., Hirvonen, J., Parkkola, R., Helin, S., ..., Nummenmaa, L. (2015). Obesity is associated with decreased mu-opioid but unaltered dopamine D2 receptor availability in the brain. *Journal of Neuroscience, 35*(9), 3959–3965.

Karlsson, H. K., Tuulari, J. J., Tuominen, L., Hirvonen, J., Honka, H., Parkkola, R., ..., Nummenmaa, L. (2015). Weight loss after bariatric surgery normalizes brain opioid receptors in morbid obesity. *Molecular Psychiatry*.

Kaye, A. D., Baluch, A., Kaye, A. J., Frass, M., & Hofbauer, R. (2007). Pharmacology of herbals and their impact in anesthesia. *Current Opinion in Anaesthesiology, 20*(4), 294–299.

Kaye, A. D., Clarke, R. C., Sabar, R., Vig, S., Dhawan, K. P., Hofbauer, R., & Kaye, A. M. (2000). Herbal medicines: current trends in anesthesiology practice--a hospital survey. *Journal of Clinical Anesthesia, 12*(6), 468–471.

Kern, P. A., Saghizadeh, M., Ong, J. M., Bosch, R. J., Deem, R., & Simsolo, R. B. (1995). The expression of tumor necrosis factor in human adipose tissue. Regulation by obesity, weight loss, and relationship to lipoprotein lipase. *Journal of Clinical Investigation, 95*(5), 2111–2119.

Khawaja, X. Z., Chattopadhyay, A. K., & Green, I. C. (1991). Increased beta-endorphin and dynorphin concentrations in discrete hypothalamic regions of genetically obese (ob/ob) mice. *Brain Research, 555*(1), 164–168.

Kim do, Y., Davis, L. M., Sullivan, P. G., Maalouf, M., Simeone, T. A., van Brederode, J., & Rho, J. M. (2007). Ketone bodies are protective against oxidative stress in neocortical neurons. *Journal of Neurochemistry, 101*(5), 1316–1326.

Kong, A. P., Chan, N. N., & Chan, J. C. (2006). The role of adipocytokines and neurohormonal dysregulation in metabolic syndrome. *Current Diabetes Reviews, 2*(4), 397–407.

Kopelman, P. (2007). Health risks associated with overweight and obesity. *Obesity Reviews, 8*(Suppl. 1), 13–17.

Lakka, H. M., Laaksonen, D. E., Lakka, T. A., Niskanen, L. K., Kumpusalo, E., Tuomilehto, J., & Salonen, J. T. (2002). The metabolic syndrome and total and cardiovascular disease mortality in middle-aged men. *Jama, 288*(21), 2709–2716.

Lau, D. C., Dhillon, B., Yan, H., Szmitko, P. E., & Verma, S. (2005). Adipokines: molecular links between obesity and atheroslcerosis. *American Journal of Physiology—Heart and Circulatory Physiology, 288*(5), H2031–2041.

Le Bars, P. L., Katz, M. M., Berman, N., Itil, T. M., Freedman, A. M., & Schatzberg, A. F. (1997). A placebo-controlled, double-blind, randomized trial of an extract of Ginkgo biloba for dementia. North American EGb Study Group. *Jama, 278*(16), 1327–1332.

Leach, M. J. (2013). Profile of the complementary and alternative medicine workforce across Australia, New Zealand, Canada, United States and United Kingdom. *Complementary Therapies in Medicine, 21*(4), 364–378.

Lee, W. H., Kramer, W. G., & Granville, G. E. (1981). The effect of obesity on acetaminophen pharmacokinetics in man. *Journal of Clinical Pharmacology, 21*(7), 284–287.

Lin, Y. R., Chen, H. H., Ko, C. H., & Chan, M. H. (2007). Effects of honokiol and magnolol on acute and inflammatory pain models in mice. *Life Science, 81*(13), 1071–1078.

Lundgren, C. H., Brown, S. L., Nordt, T. K., Sobel, B. E., & Fujii, S. (1996). Elaboration of type-1 plasminogen activator inhibitor from adipocytes. A potential pathogenetic link between obesity and cardiovascular disease. *Circulation, 93*(1), 106–110.

Maalouf, M., Sullivan, P. G., Davis, L., Kim, D. Y., & Rho, J. M. (2007). Ketones inhibit mitochondrial production of reactive oxygen species production following glutamate excitotoxicity by increasing NADH oxidation. *Neuroscience, 145*(1), 256–264.

Markowitz, J. S., Donovan, J. L., DeVane, C. L., Taylor, R. M., Ruan, Y., Wang, J. S., & Chavin, K. D. (2003). Effect of St John's wort on drug metabolism by induction of cytochrome P450 3A4 enzyme. *Jama, 290*(11), 1500–1504.

Martin, K., Jackson, C. F., Levy, R. G., & Cooper, P. N. (2016). Ketogenic diet and other dietary treatments for epilepsy. *Cochrane Database Systematic Review, 2*, Cd001903.

Masino, S. A., & Ruskin, D. N. (2013). Ketogenic diets and pain. *Journal of Child Neurology, 28*(8), 993–1001.

Maurice-Szamburski, A., Auquier, P., Viarre-Oreal, V., Cuvillon, P., Carles, M., Ripart, J., …, Bruder, N. (2015). Effect of sedative premedication on patient experience after general anesthesia: a randomized clinical trial. *Jama, 313*(9), 916–925.

McVinnie, D. S. (2013). Obesity and pain. *Br Journal of Pain, 7*(4), 163–170.

Naguib, M., & Samarkandi, A. H. (1999). Premedication with melatonin: a double-blind, placebo-controlled comparison with midazolam. *British Journal of Anaesthesia, 82*(6), 875–880.

Naguib, M., & Samarkandi, A. H. (2000). The comparative dose-response effects of melatonin and midazolam for premedication of adult patients: a double-blinded, placebo-controlled study. *Anesthesia and Analgesia, 91*(2), 473–479.

Neligan, P. J. (2010). Metabolic syndrome: anesthesia for morbid obesity. *Current Opinion in Anesthesiology, 23*(3), 375–383.

Nicolai, S. P., Kruidenier, L. M., Bendermacher, B. L., Prins, M. H., Stokmans, R. A., Broos, P. P., & Teijink, J. A. (2013). *Ginkgo biloba* for intermittent claudication. *Cochrane Database Systematic Review, 6*, Cd006888.

Nishiyama, T. (2014). Thoracic epidural catheterization using ultrasound in obese patients for bariatric surgery. *Journal of Research in Obesity, 6*.

Norton, S. A., & Ruze, P. (1994). Kava dermopathy. *Journal of the American Academy of Dermatology, 31*(1), 89–97.

Ogden, C. L., Carroll, M. D., Kit, B. K., & Flegal, K. M. (2014). Prevalence of childhood and adult obesity in the United States, 2011–2012. *Jama, 311*(8), 806–814.

Opioid-Induced Ventilatory Impairment (OIVI): Time for a change in the Monitoring Strategy for Postoperative PCA Patients. (2011). Available from: http://www.apsf.org/resources/oivi/

Padhy, B. M., & Kumar, V. L. (2005). Inhibition of Calotropis procera latex-induced inflammatory hyperalgesia by oxytocin and melatonin. *Mediators of Inflammation, 2005*(6), 360–365.

Pawlik, M. T., Hansen, E., Waldhauser, D., Selig, C., & Kuehnel, T. S. (2005). Clonidine premedication in patients with sleep apnea syndrome: a randomized, double-blind, placebo-controlled study. *Anesthesia and Analgesia, 101*(5), 1374–1380.

Practice guidelines for acute pain management in the perioperative setting: an updated report by the American Society of Anesthesiologists Task Force on Acute Pain Management. (2012). *Anesthesiology, 116*(2), 248–273.

Practice guidelines for acute pain management in the perioperative setting. A report by the American Society of Anesthesiologists Task Force on Pain Management, Acute Pain Section. (1995). *Anesthesiology, 82*(4), 1071–1081.

Practice guidelines for the prevention, detection, and management of respiratory depression associated with neuraxial opioid administration: an updated report by the American Society of Anesthesiologists Task Force on Neuraxial Opioids and the American Society of Regional Anesthesia and Pain Medicine. (2016). *Anesthesiology, 124*(3), 535–552.

Proudman, S. M., James, M. J., Spargo, L. D., Metcalf, R. G., Sullivan, T. R., Rischmueller, M., …, Cleland, L. G. (2015). Fish oil in recent onset rheumatoid arthritis: a randomised, double-blind controlled trial within algorithm-based drug use. Ann Rheum Dis, 74(1), 89–95.

Raebel, M. A., Newcomer, S. R., Reifler, L. M., Boudreau, D., Elliott, T. E., DeBar, L., …, Bayliss, E. A. (2013). Chronic use of opioid medications before and after bariatric surgery. *Jama, 310*(13), 1369–1376.

Rodgers, A., Walker, N., Schug, S., McKee, A., Kehlet, H., van Zundert, A., …, MacMahon, S. (2000). Reduction of postoperative mortality and morbidity with epidural or spinal anaesthesia: results from overview of randomised trials. *British Medical Journal, 321*(7275), 1493.

Hughes, R. G. (Ed.) (2008). *Patient safety and quality: An evidence-based handbook for nurse*. Agency for Healthcare Research and Quality. Publication No. 08-0043.

Rudram Muppuri, G. M. M., Hong W. (2015). Comparison of Patient Controlled Analgesia to Epidural Analgesia for Postoperative Pain Management after Laparoscopic Gastric Bypass Surgery: A Retrospective Study. *J Anesth Perioper Med, 2*(5), 251–255. Available from: http://www.japmnet.com/content-8-85-1.html

Schumann, R., Jones, S. B., Ortiz, V. E., Connor, K., Pulai, I., Ozawa, E. T., …, Carr, D. B. (2005). Best practice recommendations for anesthetic perioperative care and pain management in weight loss surgery. *Obes Res, 13*(2), 254–266.

Schwemmer, U., Papenfuss, T., Greim, C., Brederlau, J., & Roewer, N. (2006). Ultrasound-guided interscalene brachial plexus anaesthesia: differences in success between patients of normal and excessive weight. *Ultraschall in der Medizin, 27*(3), 245–250.

Sinatra, R. S., Jahr, J. S., Reynolds, L. W., Viscusi, E. R., Groudine, S. B., & Payen-Champenois, C. (2005). Efficacy and safety of single and repeated administration of 1 gram intravenous acetaminophen injection (paracetamol) for pain management after major orthopedic surgery. *Anesthesiology, 102*(4), 822–831.

Sollazzi, L., Modesti, C., Vitale, F., Sacco, T., Ciocchetti, P., Idra, A. S., …, Perilli, V. (2009). Preinductive use of clonidine and ketamine improves recovery and reduces postoperative pain after bariatric surgery. *Surgery for Obesity and Related Diseases, 5*(1), 67–71.

Steppan, C. M., Bailey, S. T., Bhat, S., Brown, E. J., Banerjee, R. R., Wright, C. M., …, Lazar, M. A. (2001). The hormone resistin links obesity to diabetes. *Nature, 409*(6818), 307–312.

Sturm, R., & Hattori, A. (2013). Morbid obesity rates continue to rise rapidly in the United States. *International Journal of Obesity (London), 37*(6), 889–891.

von Ungern-Sternberg, B. S., Regli, A., Reber, A., & Schneider, M. C. (2005). Effect of obesity and thoracic epidural analgesia on perioperative spirometry. *British Journal of Anaesthesia, 94*(1), 121–127.

Wang, S., Zhang, L., Lim, G., Sung, B., Tian, Y., Chou, C. W., …, Mao, J. (2009). A combined effect of dextromethorphan and melatonin on neuropathic pain behavior in rats. *Brain Research, 1288*, 42–49.

Wininger, S. J., Miller, H., Minkowitz, H. S., Royal, M. A., Ang, R. Y., Breitmeyer, J. B., & Singla, N. K. (2010). A randomized, double-blind, placebo-controlled, multicenter, repeat-dose study of two intravenous acetaminophen dosing regimens for the treatment of pain after abdominal laparoscopic surgery. *Clinical Therapeutics, 32*(14), 2348–2369.

Woodbury, A., Soong, S. N., Fishman, D., & Garcia, P. S. (2016). Complementary and alternative medicine therapies for the anesthesiologist and pain practitioner: a narrative review. *Canadian Journal of Anaesthesia, 63*(1), 69–85.

Woodbury, A., Yu, S. P., Wei, L., & Garcia, P. (2013). Neuro-modulating effects of honokiol: a review. *Frontiers of Neurology, 4*, 130.

Wu, C. H., Wang, C. C., & Kennedy, J. (2011). Changes in herb and dietary supplement use in the US adult population: a comparison of the 2002 and 2007 National Health Interview Surveys. *Clinical Therapeutics, 33*(11), 1749–1758.

Ziemann-Gimmel, P., Hensel, P., Koppman, J., & Marema, R. (2013). Multimodal analgesia reduces narcotic requirements and antiemetic rescue medication in laparoscopic Roux-en-Y gastric bypass surgery. Surgery for Obesity and Related Diseases, 9(6), 975–980.

SECTION E

NUTRIENTS IN PAIN IN PREVENTION AND TREATMENT

CHAPTER

15

Vitamin D Deficiency in Joint Pain: Effects of Vitamin D Supplementation

*B. Antony**, *C. Ding**,**

*Menzies Institute for Medical Research, University of Tasmania, Hobart, TAS, Australia;
**Translational Research Centre, Academy of Orthopaedics, Southern Medical University, Guangzhou, Guangdong Province, China

INTRODUCTION

Vitamin D deficiency [defined as serum level of 25-hydroxyvitamin D (25-(OH)D) < 50 nmol/L] is the most common nutritional deficiency worldwide. It is the most underdiagnosed medical condition in children and adults. In the United States and Europe, >40% of the adult population >50 years of age is vitamin D deficient. More than a dozen different studies of serum 25-(OH)D concentrations in 55,000 adults and children from many countries within the European Union reported that 13% of individuals had 25-(OH)D concentrations of <30 nmol/L and 40% had concentrations of <50 nmol/L (Cashman et al., 2016). In Australia, 4% of the population had a 25-(OH)D level <25 nmol/L, 31% (22% men; 39% women) had a level of <50 nmol/L, and 73% had a level of <75 nmol/L (Daly et al., 2012).

The prevalence of vitamin D deficiency increases significantly with age, in women, in those of non-Europid origin, in the obese and those who are physically inactive, and in those with a higher level of education (Daly et al., 2012). The main role of vitamin D is the regulation of serum calcium levels and maintenance and remodeling of bone formation as well as muscle function. However, the emerging evidence suggests that the benefits of vitamin D extend beyond healthy bones and muscles and it plays crucial roles in optimizing neuromuscular functioning, reducing inflammation, and decreasing the risks of many chronic diseases.

Vitamin D deficiency is linked with the risks of many chronic diseases, including cancer, autoimmune diseases (e.g., rheumatoid arthritis), type 2 diabetes, heart diseases and hypertension, and infectious diseases (including upper respiratory tract infections and tuberculosis), as well as osteoarthritis (OA) and joint pain. Vitamin D can exert neurological and immunological influences on pain manifestation, thereby playing a role in the etiology and maintenance of chronic pain and associated comorbidity (Holick, 2007; Shipton & Shipton, 2015). The following sections will outline the evidence of vitamin D deficiency in joint pain, specifically in knee and hip joint pain, and the effects of supplements in managing these pain conditions.

VITAMIN D DEFICIENCY AND JOINT PAIN

Prevalence of Joint Pain

Musculoskeletal pain is one of the most common causes of morbidity and presentation to primary care (Hasselstrom, Liu-Palmgren, & Rasjo-Wraak, 2002). Musculoskeletal pain ranges from chronic nonspecific pain to disease-specific pain mainly affecting the joints. Persistent musculoskeletal pain and weakness can be the result of many conditions including rickets, osteomalacia, osteopenia, cystic fibrosis, back pain, knee and hip OA, and costochondritic chest pain. Most of these conditions are associated with vitamin D deficiency.

Mechanisms Underlying Link Between Vitamin D and Joint Pain

The wide range of biological effects of vitamin D (e.g., calcium homeostasis; antiinflammatory, antiapoptotic, and antifibrotic effects; blood pressure regulation; and innate and adaptive immune system regulation) highlights

Nutritional Modulators of Pain in the Aging Population. http://dx.doi.org/10.1016/B978-0-12-805186-3.00015-1
Copyright © 2017 Elsevier Inc. All rights reserved.

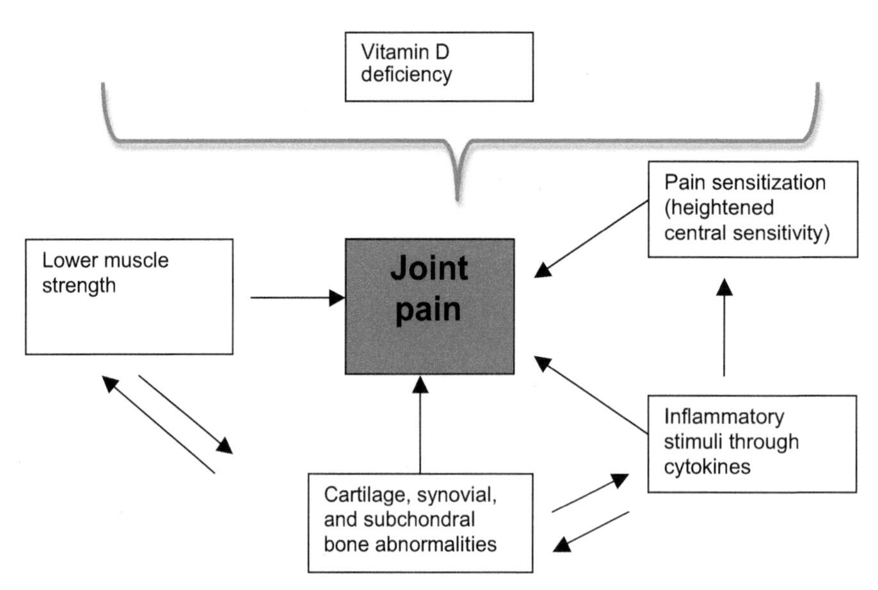

FIGURE 15.1 **Mechanisms underlying link between vitamin D and joint pain.**

the potential role of vitamin D deficiency in the development of symptoms that are associated with acute and chronic rheumatic diseases.

Epidemiological studies in patients with established inflammatory diseases identified associations between vitamin D deficiency and inflammatory conditions, including rheumatoid arthritis (Jeffery, Raza, & Hewison, 2016). Inflammatory pain may depend on the action of diverse cytokines and inflammatory stimuli, which can be triggered by vitamin D deficiency. This is supported by the finding that vitamin D supplementation for patients with musculoskeletal pain led to a faster decline of pain scores [assessed by visual analog scale (VAS)] and decreases in the levels of inflammatory and pain-related cytokines (Gendelman, Itzhaki, Makarov, Bennun, & Amital, 2015) (Fig. 15.1).

Low levels of vitamin D have been found to be associated with the presence of pain sensitization, which may mediate the association between vitamin D deficiency and musculoskeletal pain (Glover, Horgas, Fillingim, & Goodin, 2015). Low 25-(OH)D levels have been related to heightened central sensitivity (particularly augmented pain processing) on mechanical stimulation in chronic pain patients (von Kanel, Muller-Hartmannsgruber, Kokinogenis, & Egloff, 2014) (Fig. 15.1).

Low vitamin D intake and low 25-(OH)D levels have been associated with OA; similarly, loss of leg muscle strength is associated with knee OA. Studies have demonstrated a significant correlation of muscle strength with both serum vitamin D and knee pain, indicating a role for quadriceps muscle weakness in the association between serum vitamin D and osteoarthritic knee pain (Javadian et al., 2016) (Fig. 15.1).

Structural abnormalities of the diseases visualized using various imaging techniques such as magnetic resonance imaging (MRI) (e.g., subchondral bone marrow lesions, severe cartilage defects, effusion–synovitis) have been found to be modest predictors of the musculoskeletal complaints including knee osteoarthritic pain and disability. Vitamin D may have direct effects on the cartilage (chondrocytes) and presence of vitamin D receptors (VDRs) has been demonstrated in human articular chondrocytes (HACs) of osteoarthritic cartilage, especially the superficial zone (Tetlow & Woolley, 2001), and vitamin D deficiency may lead to joint pain through increasing cartilage damage. Similarly, vitamin D deficiency could impair the ability of bone to respond optimally to bone-specific pathophysiological processes (e.g., bone marrow lesions) in OA, thus leading to joint pain (Fig. 15.1).

Vitamin D synthesis requires longer periods of sun exposure for those with dark skin pigmentation. Therefore, vitamin D deficiency is common in black Americans. Studies indicate that 70% of white Americans and 95% of black Americans have insufficient levels of vitamin D (Ginde, Liu, & Camargo, 2009). Previous studies have found ethnic differences in response to experimental pain stimuli, with blacks reporting increased pain sensitivity (Campbell, Edwards, & Fillingim, 2005; Rahim-Williams et al., 2007). Therefore, we hypothesize that the race difference underlies the association between vitamin D deficiency and joint pain. However, recent studies examined whether variations in vitamin D levels contributed to race differences in knee osteoarthritic pain and reported that low levels of vitamin D mediated the relationship between race and experimental pain in older adults with symptomatic knee OA (Glover et al., 2012). Group differences in 25-(OH)D levels significantly predicted group differences in heat pain and pressure pain thresholds at the index knee and ipsilateral forearm (Glover et al., 2012).

Evidence of the Association Between Vitamin D and Joint Pain

Generalized Musculoskeletal Pain

Observational studies describing the association between vitamin D and musculoskeletal pain have shown inconsistent results with some studies reporting significant associations (Atherton et al., 2009; McBeth et al., 2010; McCabe et al., 2016) and others reporting no association between vitamin D and musculoskeletal pain (Al-Jarallah, Shehab, Abraham, Mojiminiyi, & Abdella, 2013). Hypovitaminosis D has been related with higher pain intensity and lower quality of life scores in patients with chronic widespread pain when compared with those in control group (Kuru, Akyuz, Yagci, & Giray, 2015). A meta-analysis of 12 observational studies in patients with chronic widespread pain reported that there was a positive association between hypovitaminosis D and chronic widespread pain (Hsiao, Hung, Chang, Han, & Wang, 2015). In a case–control study, mean vitamin D values were not statistically different in patients with generalized musculoskeletal pain [fibromyalgia, regional musculoskeletal pain (nonspecific low back pain and knee OA)] compared with those in controls (Al-Jarallah et al., 2013).

There is evidence to suggest that vitamin D deficiency modifies the risk of musculoskeletal symptoms experienced with statin use. A recent metaanalysis of seven studies provides evidence that low vitamin D levels are associated with myalgia in patients on statin therapy (Michalska-Kasiczak et al., 2015). Among adults ≥40 years old with 25-(OH)D <15 ng/mL (37.5 nmol/L), statin users had nearly two times greater odds of reporting musculoskeletal pain compared to nonstatin users (Morioka, Lee, Bertisch, & Buettner, 2015).

Osteoarthritic Pain

Observational studies of vitamin D in knee OA have reported consistent evidence with structural progression and incidence of radiographic knee OA. However, there were inconsistent results in the association between vitamin D deficiency and knee or hip pain resulting from OA.

In a case–control study, the mean serum 25-(OH)D in symptomatic knee OA patients was not significantly lower than that in controls, but in those aged <60 years the mean 25-(OH)D was significantly lower than in controls (Heidari, Heidari, & Hajian-Tilaki, 2011). Similarly, 93% of knee OA patients were vitamin D deficient, but there was no significant association between 25-(OH)D levels and severity of knee radiographic grading scores or different assessments including pain (Al-Jarallah et al., 2012).

A cross-sectional study explored the association of serum 25-(OH)D concentration and polymorphism in the VDR with knee pain and radiographic knee OA among men and women, and reported that 25-(OH)D level was not significantly associated with radiographic knee OA; however, low tertile of 25-(OH)D level tended to be associated with knee pain compared with high tertile of 25-(OH)D level. This study concluded that vitamin D might be associated with pain rather than radiographic change, but the evidence for an association between genetic variation in vitamin D–related genes and pain in knee OA was weak (Muraki et al., 2011). Another cross-sectional study reported that the knee OA patients with adequate 25-(OH)D levels had significantly less Western Ontario and McMaster Universities Osteoarthritis Index (WOMAC) knee pain compared with patients with deficient or insufficient 25-(OH)D levels, regardless of obesity status (Glover, Goodin, et al., 2015).

A longitudinal study in a population-based cohort of randomly selected older adults reported that the prevalence of moderate vitamin D deficiency (25-(OH)D 12.5–25 nmol/L) was 4.2% (Laslett et al., 2014). Moderate vitamin D deficiency predicted change in knee pain assessed using WOMAC score during 5 years with a similar effect size for hip pain during 2.4 years. No association was present when 25-(OH)D was analyzed as a continuous measure, suggesting that giving supplements to those with a higher 25-(OH)D level is unlikely to be effective for knee and hip pain (Laslett et al., 2014). Consistently, both sunlight exposure and serum 25-(OH)D levels were associated with decreased knee cartilage loss (assessed by radiograph or MRI), but this was best observed using the whole range of 25-(OH)D levels rather than predefined cut points (Ding et al., 2009).

A systematic review of 13 observational studies reported that there was insufficient or limited evidence for associations between 25-(OH)D and hand or hip OA, but low levels of 25-(OH)D were associated with increased progression of radiographic OA as assessed by the Kellgren and Lawrence (KL) score (Cao et al., 2013). Strong evidence for an association between 25-(OH)D and cartilage loss was reported when joint space narrowing and changes in cartilage volume were considered collectively as cartilage loss (Cao et al., 2013). However, there are inconsistent results in the association between vitamin D deficiency and knee or hip pain resulting from OA. In the systematic review mentioned earlier, authors found only limited evidence to support the association between 25-(OH)D levels and the prevalence or incidence of symptomatic OA (Cao et al., 2013).

Rheumatoid Arthritis Pain

In a case–control study, serum level of 25-(OH)D was markedly lower in the rheumatoid arthritis patient group than in the control group (Hong et al., 2014) and was inversely associated with pain VAS score, asthenia VAS, morning stiffness, number of tender joints, number of swollen joints, disease activity score (DAS), physical disability using Health Assessment Questionnaire (HAQ), and severity of the disease (Abourazzak et al., 2015; Hong et al., 2014). Recent meta-analyses demonstrated that serum vitamin D level was significantly lower in patients with rheumatoid arthritis than in controls, vitamin D deficiency was prevalent in patients with rheumatoid arthritis compared to in controls, and the 25-(OH)D level was correlated inversely with rheumatoid arthritis activity (Lee & Bae, 2016; Lin, Liu, Davies, & Chen, 2016).

SUPPLEMENTATION OF VITAMIN D FOR JOINT PAIN

The effects of vitamin D supplementation on joint pain have mainly been reported in patients with OA and rheumatoid arthritis. Randomized clinical trials (RCTs) have reported minimal effects of vitamin D supplementation on joint pain. In an RCT including immigrants from South Asia, the Middle East, and Africa living in Northern Europe (most prominent to vitamin D deficiency than native Western population), the musculoskeletal pain including joint pain and headache scores were improved at follow-up compared with baseline, but the use of vitamin D supplements (1000 or 400 IU/day), however, showed no significant effect on the occurrence, anatomical localization, and degree of pain compared to placebo during 16 weeks (Knutsen et al., 2014). Similarly, a post-hoc analysis from the Women's Health Initiative RCT to evaluate the influence of daily supplemental calcium (1000 mg) and vitamin D (400 IU) on joint symptoms for 2 years reported no statistically significant differences between supplement and placebo groups in joint pain frequency, joint swelling frequency, or severity scores for either outcome (Chlebowski et al., 2013). In an RCT with 3-month duration, adding 4000 IU of vitamin D for patients with musculoskeletal pain led to a faster decline of consecutive VAS scores and decreases in the levels of inflammatory and pain-related cytokines [tumor necrosis factor (TNF)-α levels decreased by 54.3% and prostaglandin (PG) E2 decreased by 39.2% in the treatment group] compared to placebo (Gendelman et al., 2015).

A Cochrane systematic review compared the efficacy and safety of vitamin D supplementation with placebo or active comparators for the treatment of chronic painful conditions and suggested that a large beneficial effect of vitamin D across different chronic painful conditions is unlikely (Straube, Derry, Straube, & Moore, 2015). Similarly, a recent meta-analysis of three clinical trials reported a moderate level of evidence showing a null effect of vitamin D supplementation on pain in patients with chronic nonspecific musculoskeletal pain (Gaikwad, Vanlint, Mittinity, Moseley, & Stocks, 2016).

Vitamin D Supplementation in Osteoarthritis

A nonrandomized and noncontrolled study in knee OA patients with vitamin D deficiency (<20 ng/mL or 50 nmol/L) reported that supplementation with 50,000 IU of oral cholecalciferol weekly was associated with significant increase in quadriceps muscle strength and decreases in WOMAC knee pain and VAS knee pain, compared to the baseline values (Heidari, Javadian, Babaei, & Yousef-Ghahari, 2015).

In an RCT on patients with symptomatic knee OA, supplementation with oral cholecalciferol, 2000 IU/day for 2 years, at a dose sufficient to elevate 25-(OH)D plasma levels to higher than 90 nmol/L, when compared with placebo, did not reduce knee pain or cartilage volume loss in patients with symptomatic knee OA (Table 15.1) (McAlindon et al., 2013). In a similar but larger RCT on participants with symptomatic knee OA and low vitamin D levels (12.5–60 nmol/L), supplementation with oral vitamin D (50,000 IU/month) for 2 years, compared with placebo, did not result in significant differences in change in MRI-measured tibial cartilage volume or WOMAC knee pain score (Jin et al., 2016). However, there was more reduction in knee pain assessed using VAS score and more improvement of knee function in vitamin D group (Jin et al., 2016). There were more Outcome Measures in Rheumatology Clinical trials–Osteoarthritis Research Society International (OMERACT-OARSI) responders in the vitamin D group than in the placebo group (35% vs. 25%, $P = 0.029$) (Table 15.1). A recent double-blind placebo-controlled RCT of 474 participants with knee OA reported that daily supplementation of 800 IU cholecalciferol for 3 years did not improve the rate of joint space narrowing (measured using X-ray) relative to the control group. Similarly, the secondary outcomes including WOMAC pain did not significantly differ between vitamin D and control group (Arden et al., 2016).

In a pilot placebo-controlled RCT of 107 patients with knee OA and vitamin D insufficiency (25-(OH) D ≤50nmol/L), supplementation with oral vitamin D (60,000 IU/day for 10 days followed by 60,000 IU/month for 6 months) for 1 year resulted in a small but statistically significant benefit on WOMAC and VAS knee pain (Table 15.1). However, the clinical importance of these results is unknown as the effect sizes observed for pain and function were statistically significant but small (Sanghi et al., 2013).

Vitamin D Supplementation in Rheumatoid Arthritis

Studies in rheumatoid arthritis did not show a consistent direction of effect of vitamin D on clinical outcomes including joint pain. Studies even suggest that multiple

TABLE 15.1 RCTs Examining the Effects of Vitamin D Supplementation on Osteoarthritic Pain

Authors	Patients	Control	Intervention Treatment	Outcomes	Conclusions
McAlindon et al. (2013)	Knee OA patients older than 45 years	Placebo (n = 73)	Vitamin D3, 2000 IU/day for 2 years (n = 73)	WOMAC pain; cartilage volume loss assessed using MRI	Vitamin D supplementation had no symptom or structure-modifying benefits for knee OA
Sanghi et al. (2013)	Knee OA patients older than 40 years with 25-(OH)D <50 nmol/L	Placebo (n = 51)	Calciferol (D2), 60,000 IU/day for 10 days followed by 60,000 IU/month for 6 months (n = 52)	WOMAC, VAS for pain; KL scoring for radiographic OA	Vitamin D intake had a small beneficial effect in improvement of knee pain and physical function in knee OA No significant difference in radiological features
Jin et al. (2016)	Knee OA patients aged 50–79 years with 25-(OH)D <60 nmol/L	Placebo (n = 204)	Vitamin D3, 50,000 IU/month for 24 months (n = 209)	Cartilage volume loss assessed using MRI; WOMAC for pain	Vitamin D supplementation had no significant effect on tibial cartilage volume or WOMAC knee pain. Secondary analyses showed vitamin D group had significant reduction in VAS knee pain, improvement in knee function, and more OMERACT-OARSI responders
Arden et al. (2016)	Knee OA patients older than 50 years	Placebo (n = 237)	Vitamin D3, 800 IU/day for 3 years (n = 237)	Rate of JSN during 3 years from X-ray; WOMAC for pain	Vitamin D supplementation did not improve the rate of joint space narrowing (measured using X-ray). Secondary outcomes including WOMAC pain, stiffness, and dysfunction did not significantly differ between vitamin D and control group

JSN, joint space narrowing; KL, Kellgren and Lawrence; MRI, magnetic resonance imaging; OA, osteoarthritis; 25-(OH)D, 25-hydroxyvitamin D; OMERACT-OARSI, Outcome Measures in Rheumatology Clinical Trials–Osteoarthritis Research Society International; RCT, randomized clinical trial; VAS, visual analog scale; WOMAC, Western Ontario and McMaster Universities Osteoarthritis Index.

high vitamin D exposures may increase the incidence of rheumatoid arthritis (Racovan et al., 2012). An open-labeled randomized trial comparing triple disease-modifying antirheumatic drug (DMARD) therapy and 500-IU 1,25-dihydroxy vitamin D3 + calcium combination versus triple DMARD and calcium alone was conducted with time to pain relief as the primary outcome. The prevalence of vitamin D deficiency in the study population was 68.1% (Gopinath & Danda, 2011). The study reported a significantly higher pain relief (50% vs. 30%) at the end of 3 months in vitamin D group (n = 59) compared to that in control group (n = 62), but there was no significant difference in the time taken for initial pain relief between the two groups (Gopinath & Danda, 2011).

Brohult and Jonson (1973) conducted a clinical trial of calciferol (vitamin D2) 100,000 IU daily during 12 months in patients with rheumatoid arthritis, and reported that the consumption of analgesics and antiinflammatory drugs decreased significantly in the calciferol group while there was no change in the placebo group (no direct pain relations were reported)). A recent study investigated the effects of ergocalciferol (vitamin D2) 50,000 IU plus calcium on disease activity in patients with rheumatoid arthritis (initially three times weekly and then twice monthly for a total duration of 12 months), and reported that vitamin D did not improve pain and physical function compared with placebo (just calcium) (Hansen, Bartels, Gangnon, Jones, & Gogineni, 2014); however, this study is limited by small sample size (n = 22).

In 117 patients with active rheumatoid arthritis receiving stable doses of methotrexate (MTX), vitamin D 50,000 IU treatment weekly for a duration of 12 weeks showed no improvement in DAS 28 and VAS pain scores compared to placebo (Salesi & Farajzadegan, 2012). Another trial reported that in 140 patients with rheumatoid arthritis treated with alfacalcidol (1-hydroxycholecalciferol, 1α-OH-D3) or placebo for 16 weeks, the percentage of patients with slight improvement was about 10% higher in 1α-OH-D3 than in placebo groups, but there was no significant difference with regard to duration of morning stiffness, number of joints with pain, number of joints with swelling, and Lansbury index (Yamauchi et al., 1989).

CONCLUSIONS

There are inconsistent findings from the observational studies that explored the association between vitamin D deficiency and joint pain relating to different musculoskeletal conditions. Some of these studies reported a weak, but statistically significant association with knee and hip joint pain, but others reported that vitamin D deficiency was not significantly associated with musculoskeletal pain.

There is evidence for and against the use of vitamin D supplementation for the treatment of joint pain. The non-RCTs have reported a small beneficial effect of vitamin D supplementation on chronic pain including joint pain. There are only a few randomized placebo-controlled clinical trials that have explored the effect of vitamin D supplementation on joint pain. The findings from these placebo-controlled RCTs suggest that there is no clinically significant benefit of vitamin D supplementation for knee pain. Future RCTs are required to address whether vitamin D supplementation is effective on musculoskeletal pain, particularly in those with vitamin D deficiency, and can act to increase the effectiveness of existing analgesics and/or reduce the dose and duration of their use.

Acknowledgment

The authors have no conflict of interest to declare.

Benny Antony would like to thank the fellowship support (as salary) from Arthritis Australia, Farrell Family and National Health and Medical Research Council of Australia. Changhai Ding would like to thank the fellowship support from Australian Research Council.

References

Abourazzak, F. E., Talbi, S., Aradoini, N., Berrada, K., Keita, S., & Hazry, T. (2015). 25-Hydroxy vitamin D and its relationship with clinical and laboratory parameters in patients with rheumatoid arthritis. *Clinical Rheumatology*, *34*(2), 353–357.

Al-Jarallah, K., Shehab, D., Abraham, M., Mojiminiyi, O. A., & Abdella, N. A. (2013). Musculoskeletal pain: should physicians test for vitamin D level? *International Journal of Rheumatic Diseases*, *16*(2), 193–197.

Al-Jarallah, K. F., Shehab, D., Al-Awadhi, A., Nahar, I., Haider, M. Z., & Moussa, M. A. (2012). Are 25(OH)D levels related to the severity of knee osteoarthritis and function? *Medical Principles and Practice*, *21*(1), 74–78.

Arden, N. K., Cro, S., Dore, C., Cooper, C., O'Neil, T., Birrell, F., . . ., Keen, R. (2016). Effect of vitamin D supplementation on radiographic knee osteoarthritis. *Osteoarthritis and Cartilage*, 24, 1858–1866.

Atherton, K., Berry, D. J., Parsons, T., Macfarlane, G. J., Power, C., & Hypponen, E. (2009). Vitamin D and chronic widespread pain in a white middle-aged British population: evidence from a cross-sectional population survey. *Annals of the Rheumatic Diseases*, *68*(6), 817–822.

Brohult, J., & Jonson, B. (1973). Effects of large doses of calciferol on patients with rheumatoid arthritis. A double-blind clinical trial. *Scandinavian Journal of Rheumatology*, *2*(4), 173–176.

Campbell, C. M., Edwards, R. R., & Fillingim, R. B. (2005). Ethnic differences in responses to multiple experimental pain stimuli. *Pain*, *113*(1–2), 20–26.

Cao, Y., Winzenberg, T., Nguo, K., Lin, J., Jones, G., & Ding, C. (2013). Association between serum levels of 25-hydroxyvitamin D and osteoarthritis: a systematic review. *Rheumatology*, *52*(7), 1323–1334.

Cashman, K. D., Dowling, K. G., Skrabakova, Z., Gonzalez-Gross, M., Valtuena, J., De Henauw, S., . . ., Kiely, M. (2016). Vitamin D deficiency in Europe: pandemic? *American Journal of Clinical Nutrition*, *103*(4), 1033–1044.

Chlebowski, R. T., Pettinger, M., Johnson, K. C., Wallace, R., Womack, C., Mossavar-Rahmani, Y., . . ., Kooperberg, C. L. (2013). Calcium plus vitamin D supplementation and joint symptoms in postmenopausal women in the women's health initiative randomized trial. *Journal of the Academy of Nutrition and Dietetics*, *113*(10), 1302–1310.

Daly, R. M., Gagnon, C., Lu, Z. X., Magliano, D. J., Dunstan, D. W., Sikaris, K. A., . . ., Shaw, J. E. (2012). Prevalence of vitamin D deficiency and its determinants in Australian adults aged 25 years and older: a national, population-based study. *Clinical Endocrinology*, *77*(1), 26–35.

Ding, C., Cicuttini, F., Parameswaran, V., Burgess, J., Quinn, S., & Jones, G. (2009). Serum levels of vitamin D, sunlight exposure, and knee cartilage loss in older adults: the Tasmanian older adult cohort study. *Arthritis and Rheumatism*, *60*(5), 1381–1389.

Gaikwad, M., Vanlint, S., Mittinity, M., Moseley, G. L., & Stocks, N. (2016). Does vitamin D supplementation alleviate chronic nonspecific musculoskeletal pain? A systematic review and meta-analysis. *Clinical Rheumatology*, Epub ahead of print.

Gendelman, O., Itzhaki, D., Makarov, S., Bennun, M., & Amital, H. (2015). A randomized double-blind placebo-controlled study adding high dose vitamin D to analgesic regimens in patients with musculoskeletal pain. *Lupus*, *24*(4–5), 483–489.

Ginde, A. A., Liu, M. C., & Camargo, C. A., Jr. (2009). Demographic differences and trends of vitamin D insufficiency in the US population, 1988–2004. *Archives of Internal Medicine*, *169*(6), 626–632.

Glover, T. L., Goodin, B. R., Horgas, A. L., Kindler, L. L., King, C. D., Sibille, K. T., . . ., Fillingim, R. B. (2012). Vitamin D, race, and experimental pain sensitivity in older adults with knee osteoarthritis. *Arthritis and Rheumatism*, *64*(12), 3926–3935.

Glover, T. L., Goodin, B. R., King, C. D., Sibille, K. T., Herbert, M. S., Sotolongo, A. S., . . ., Fillingim, R. B. (2015). A cross-sectional examination of vitamin D, obesity, and measures of pain and function in middle-aged and older adults with knee osteoarthritis. *The Clinical Journal of Pain*, *31*(12), 1060–1067.

Glover, T. L., Horgas, A. L., Fillingim, R. B., & Goodin, B. R. (2015b). Vitamin D status and pain sensitization in knee osteoarthritis: a critical review of the literature. *Pain Management*, *5*(6), 447–453.

Gopinath, K., & Danda, D. (2011). Supplementation of 1,25 dihydroxy vitamin D3 in patients with treatment naive early rheumatoid arthritis: a randomised controlled trial. *International Journal of Rheumatic Diseases*, *14*(4), 332–339.

Hansen, K. E., Bartels, C. M., Gangnon, R. E., Jones, A. N., & Gogineni, J. (2014). An evaluation of high-dose vitamin D for rheumatoid arthritis. *Journal of Clinical Rheumatology*, *20*(2), 112–114.

Hasselstrom, J., Liu-Palmgren, J., & Rasjo-Wraak, G. (2002). Prevalence of pain in general practice. *European Journal of Pain*, *6*(5), 375–385.

Heidari, B., Heidari, P., & Hajian-Tilaki, K. (2011). Association between serum vitamin D deficiency and knee osteoarthritis. *International Orthopaedics*, *35*(11), 1627–1631.

Heidari, B., Javadian, Y., Babaei, M., & Yousef-Ghahari, B. (2015). Restorative effect of vitamin D deficiency on knee pain and quadriceps muscle strength in knee osteoarthritis. *Acta Medica Iranica*, *53*(8), 466–470.

Holick, M. F. (2007). Vitamin D deficiency. *The New England Journal of Medicine*, *357*(3), 266–281.

Hong, Q., Xu, J., Xu, S., Lian, L., Zhang, M., & Ding, C. (2014). Associations between serum 25-hydroxyvitamin D and disease activity, inflammatory cytokines and bone loss in patients with rheumatoid arthritis. *Rheumatology*, *53*(11), 1994–2001.

Hsiao, M. Y., Hung, C. Y., Chang, K. V., Han, D. S., & Wang, T. G. (2015). Is serum hypovitaminosis D associated with chronic widespread pain including fibromyalgia? A meta-analysis of observational studies. *Pain Physician*, *18*(5), E877–E887.

Javadian, Y., Adabi, M., Heidari, B., Babaei, M., Firouzjahi, A., Ghahhari, B. Y., & Hajian-Tilaki, K. (2016). Quadriceps muscle strength correlates with serum vitamin D and knee pain in knee osteoarthritis. *The Clinical Journal of Pain*, Epub ahead of print.

Jeffery, L. E., Raza, K., & Hewison, M. (2016). Vitamin D in rheumatoid arthritis—towards clinical application. *Nature Reviews. Rheumatology, 12*(4), 201–210.

Jin, X., Jones, G., Cicuttini, F., Wluka, A., Zhu, Z., Han, W., . . ., Ding, C. (2016). Effect of vitamin D supplementation on tibial cartilage volume and knee pain among patients with symptomatic knee osteoarthritis: a randomized clinical trial. *JAMA: The Journal of the American Medical Association, 315*(10), 1005–1013.

Knutsen, K. V., Madar, A. A., Brekke, M., Meyer, H. E., Natvig, B., Mdala, I., & Lagerlov, P. (2014). Effect of vitamin D on musculoskeletal pain and headache: a randomized, double-blind, placebo-controlled trial among adult ethnic minorities in Norway. *Pain, 155*(12), 2591–2598.

Kuru, P., Akyuz, G., Yagci, I., & Giray, E. (2015). Hypovitaminosis D in widespread pain: its effect on pain perception, quality of life and nerve conduction studies. *Rheumatology International, 35*(2), 315–322.

Laslett, L. L., Quinn, S., Burgess, J. R., Parameswaran, V., Winzenberg, T. M., Jones, G., & Ding, C. (2014). Moderate vitamin D deficiency is associated with changes in knee and hip pain in older adults: a 5-year longitudinal study. *Annals of the Rheumatic Diseases, 73*(4), 697–703.

Lee, Y. H., & Bae, S. C. (2016). Vitamin D level in rheumatoid arthritis and its correlation with the disease activity: a meta-analysis. *Clinical and Experimental Rheumatology*, Epub ahead of print.

Lin, J., Liu, J., Davies, M. L., & Chen, W. (2016). Serum vitamin D level and rheumatoid arthritis disease activity: review and meta-analysis. *PLoS One, 11*(1), e0146351.

McAlindon, T., LaValley, M., Schneider, E., Nuite, M., Lee, J. Y., Price, L. L., . . ., Dawson-Hughes, B. (2013). Effect of vitamin D supplementation on progression of knee pain and cartilage volume loss in patients with symptomatic osteoarthritis: a randomized controlled trial. *JAMA: The Journal of the American Medical Association, 309*(2), 155–162.

McBeth, J., Pye, S. R., O'Neill, T. W., Macfarlane, G. J., Tajar, A., Bartfai, G., . . ., Group, E. (2010). Musculoskeletal pain is associated with very low levels of vitamin D in men: results from the European Male Ageing Study. *Annals of the Rheumatic Diseases, 69*(8), 1448–1452.

McCabe, P. S., Pye, S. R., McBeth, J., Lee, D. M., Tajar, A., Bartfai, G., . . ., Group, E. S. (2016). Low vitamin D and the risk of developing chronic widespread pain: results from the European male ageing study. *BMC Musculoskeletal Disorders, 17*(1), 32.

Michalska-Kasiczak, M., Sahebkar, A., Mikhailidis, D. P., Rysz, J., Muntner, P., Toth, P. P., . . ., Blood Pressure Meta-Analysis Collaboration, G. (2015). Analysis of vitamin D levels in patients with and without statin-associated myalgia—a systematic review and meta-analysis of 7 studies with 2420 patients. *International Journal of Cardiology, 178*, 111–116.

Morioka, T. Y., Lee, A. J., Bertisch, S., & Buettner, C. (2015). Vitamin D status modifies the association between statin use and musculoskeletal pain: a population based study. *Atherosclerosis, 238*(1), 77–82.

Muraki, S., Dennison, E., Jameson, K., Boucher, B. J., Akune, T., Yoshimura, N., . . ., Cooper, C. (2011). Association of vitamin D status with knee pain and radiographic knee osteoarthritis. *Osteoarthritis and Cartilage/OARS, Osteoarthritis Research Society, 19*(11), 1301–1306.

Racovan, M., Walitt, B., Collins, C. E., Pettinger, M., Parks, C. G., Shikany, J. M., . . ., Howard, B. V. (2012). Calcium and vitamin D supplementation and incident rheumatoid arthritis: The Women's Health Initiative calcium plus vitamin D trial. *Rheumatology International, 32*(12), 3823–3830.

Rahim-Williams, F. B., Riley, J. L., 3rd, Herrera, D., Campbell, C. M., Hastie, B. A., & Fillingim, R. B. (2007). Ethnic identity predicts experimental pain sensitivity in African Americans and Hispanics. *Pain, 129*(1–2), 177–184.

Salesi, M., & Farajzadegan, Z. (2012). Efficacy of vitamin D in patients with active rheumatoid arthritis receiving methotrexate therapy. *Rheumatology International, 32*(7), 2129–2133.

Sanghi, D., Mishra, A., Sharma, A. C., Singh, A., Natu, S. M., Agarwal, S., & Srivastava, R. N. (2013). Does vitamin D improve osteoarthritis of the knee: a randomized controlled pilot trial. *Clinical Orthopaedics and Related Research, 471*(11), 3556–3562.

Shipton, E. A., & Shipton, E. E. (2015). Vitamin D and pain: vitamin D and its role in the aetiology and maintenance of chronic pain states and associated comorbidities. *Pain Research and Treatment, 2015*, 904967.

Straube, S., Derry, S., Straube, C., & Moore, R. A. (2015). Vitamin D for the treatment of chronic painful conditions in adults. *Cochrane Database of Systematic Reviews, 5*, CD007771.

Tetlow, L. C., & Woolley, D. E. (2001). Expression of vitamin D receptors and matrix metalloproteinases in osteoarthritic cartilage and human articular chondrocytes in vitro. *Osteoarthritis and Cartilage/OARS, Osteoarthritis Research Society, 9*(5), 423–431.

von Kanel, R., Muller-Hartmannsgruber, V., Kokinogenis, G., & Egloff, N. (2014). Vitamin D and central hypersensitivity in patients with chronic pain. *Pain Medicine, 15*(9), 1609–1618.

Yamauchi, Y., Tsunematsu, T., Konda, S., Hoshino, T., Itokawa, Y., & Hoshizaki, H. (1989). A double blind trial of alfacalcidol on patients with rheumatoid arthritis (RA). *Ryumachi, 29*(1), 11–24.

C H A P T E R

16

Nutritional Modulators of Pain in the Aging Population

J. Smithson, K.A. Kellick, K. Mergenhagen

VA Western New York Healthcare System, Buffalo, NY, United States

BACKGROUND

Pain is a common condition for which many patients seek treatment. According to the International Association for the Study of Pain (IASP), pain is defined as a sensory or emotional experience that causes discomfort and is related to actual or potential tissue damage. It may also be labeled by the patient in terms of this damage (Loeser & Treede, 2008). Unfortunately, there is no objective measure of pain. Instead, it can be subjectively described using a pain scale. As expected, patient self-reported pain scores are highly variable and are non-comparable between patients. Classified as either acute or chronic, pain can be further distributed into the following categories: neuropathic, nociceptive, or psychogenic. These categories explain the effects and origin of the pain, which help providers tailor patient-specific treatment recommendations.

Acute pain is defined as the typical, anticipated physiological response to adverse thermal, chemical, or mechanical stimulus (Carr & Goudas, 1999). Referred to as a warning signal, acute pain usually resolves when the stimulus is removed. Acute pain is usually associated with surgery, trauma, or acute stimulus. However, if left untreated, acute pain can develop into chronic pain. Most patients describe acute pain as a sharp pain that begins suddenly (Loeser & Treede, 2008). Response to acute pain is based on patient-specific characteristics including attitudes, beliefs, and personalities. Common physiological responses include dilated pupils, anxiety, diaphoresis, tachycardia, increased blood pressure, and increased respiratory rate (Carr & Goudas, 1999).

Chronic pain is defined as a persistent pain that extends beyond typical healing time of the tissue (Loeser & Treede, 2008). It can also be described as acute pain that lasted longer than normal healing time, typically 3–6 months. About 20% of people are affected by chronic pain. Common types of chronic pain include cancer pain, posttraumatic/postsurgical pain, headache, visceral pain, and musculoskeletal pain (Treede et al., 2015). Unlike acute pain, common physiological responses include depressed mood, fatigue, loss of libido, and loss of appetite.

Neuropathic pain is defined as pain as a consequence of disease or abnormality impacting the somatosensory system (Loeser & Treede, 2008). It can be classified according to the pathology, including genetic, metabolic, traumatic, vascular, neoplastic, immunological, infectious, and toxic. This encompasses a wide variety of disease states including diabetic neuropathy, stroke, Guillain–Barré syndrome, HIV, chemotherapy, encephalitis, and multiple sclerosis (MS), to name a few. Symptoms can be divided into positive and negative. Negative symptoms include numbness, weakness, and loss of reflexes. It is estimated that neuropathic pain affects 8% of all people (Gilron, Baron, & Jensen, 2015).

Nociceptive pain refers to pain from an injury triggering nociceptors in peripheral tissues. Described as throbbing, sharp, or aching, nociceptive pain can be classified as either somatic or visceral in nature. Somatic pain refers to pain generated by damage to the body surface, deep tissues, and bone. Visceral pain is caused by pain generated in the chest or abdominal or pelvic areas. An example of nociceptive pain is the pain most patients feel after surgery (Loeser & Treede, 2008).

Nutritional Modulators of Pain in the Aging Population. http://dx.doi.org/10.1016/B978-0-12-805186-3.00016-3
Copyright © 2017 Elsevier Inc. All rights reserved.

Natural medicine is a topic of great debate. Today, complementary and alternative medicine is used by 40–60% of Americans. Of these patients, 30% cite pain as the primary condition being treated (Barnes, 2008). It has been proposed that pain is linked to nutritional modulators. Some of these modulators have more scientific evidence supporting their use. Nutritional modulators include probiotics, omega-3 fatty acids, magnesium, glucosamine/chondroitin, and vitamin D. Other proposed modulators have minimal or contradictory evidence to support their use, including turmeric, devil's claw, methylsulfonylmethane (MSM), *Boswellia*, white willow bark, and green tea (Bell, Borzan, Kalso, & Simonnet, 2012). The correlation between these modulators and pain provides natural treatment options for patients.

VITAMIN D DEFICIENCY

Vitamin D, calciferol, is a fat-soluble vitamin classified as a secosteroid. Calciferol collectively refers to the two main forms, vitamin D2 (ergocalciferol) and vitamin D3 (cholecalciferol). Vitamin D2 can be obtained from plant sources and vitamin D3 can be obtained from animal sources. While vitamin D can be obtained from the diet, the vast majority of vitamin D is synthesized in the human body. Excessive vitamin D can be stored in fat cells. Even though vitamin D deficiency is fairly common, vitamin D toxicity is rare (Holick, 2007).

Clinically, vitamin D status is determined by serum 25-hydroxyvitamin D. The preferred range of serum vitamin D is 30–60 ng/mL. A deficiency in vitamin D is classified as a serum vitamin D level below 20 ng/mL. As expected, many people are affected by vitamin D deficiency. Since a majority of vitamin D is synthesized in the skin through exposure to UVB radiation, the major cause of vitamin D deficiency is decreased exposure to the sun. This most commonly affects the elderly and women who have to remain covered due to religious or cultural reasons. Another common cause of vitamin D deficiency is dark skin pigmentation. According to one source, those with darker skin pigmentation require three to five times more exposure to sunlight than those with lighter skin tones. Additional causes of vitamin D deficiency can be divided into the following categories: reduced skin synthesis, decreased bioavailability, increased catabolism, breast-feeding, decreased synthesis of 25-hydroxyvitamin D, increased urinary loss of 25-hydroxyvitamin D, heritable disorders, and acquired disorders. A complete list of causes can be seen in Table 16.1 (Holick, 2007).

The most widely accepted function of vitamin D is the regulation of calcium and phosphorous homeostasis. Research has shown that vitamin D receptors are found in most tissues and cells in the body. This provides many possibilities for the increased function of vitamin D. Given the low cost of vitamin D, if an association is found, vitamin D may be a valid treatment option for pain. Of great interest is its use in chronic illnesses including autoimmune disorders, infectious diseases, cardiovascular diseases, and pain (Holick, 2007).

TABLE 16.1 Causes of Vitamin D Deficiency

Reduced skin synthesis:
• Sunscreen use • Darker skin pigmentation • Aging • Location (season, latitude, and time of day) • Skin grafting
Decreased bioavailability
• Malabsorption • Obesity
Increased catabolism
• Anticonvulsants, glucocorticoids, Highly Active Antiretroviral Therapy (HAART), antirejection medications • Breast-feeding
Decreased synthesis of 25-hydroxyvitamin D
• Liver failure
Increased urinary loss of 25-hydroxyvitamin D
• Nephrotic syndrome
Decreased synthesis of 1,25-dihydroxyvitamin D
• Chronic kidney disease
Heritable disorders
• Pseudovitamin D deficiency rickets • Vitamin D–resistant rickets • Vitamin D–dependent rickets • Autosomal dominant hypophosphatemic rickets • X-linked hypophosphatemic rickets
Acquired disorders
• Tumor-induced osteomalacia • Primary hyperparathyroidism • Granulomatous disorders, sarcoidosis, tuberculosis • Hyperthyroidism

Current studies have evaluated the correlation between vitamin D deficiency and chronic pain conditions such as polymyalgia rheumatica, fibromyalgia, osteoarthritis, nonspecific pain, and statin myopathies. A positive association was shown between calcium and vitamin D supplementation and pain associated with polymyalgia rheumatica (Di Munno et al., 1989). In patients with fibromyalgia, studies have shown that patients who received supplementation to maintain a serum calciferol level between 32 and 48 ng/mL reported a reduction in pain (Wepner et al., 2014). Elderly patients who received high-dose vitamin D supplementation had increased quality of life, decreased pain, and improved functional mobility (Sakalli, Arslan, & Yucel, 2012). Patients who received high-dose statins were more likely to develop myalgias if they were vitamin D deficient (Mergenhagen, Ott, Heckman, Rubin, & Kellick, 2014).

The cited studies are only several of the studies regarding the association between vitamin D and pain. As expected the methods as well as vitamin D dose varies based on patient characteristics. In general, vitamin D supplementation is well tolerated. Although rare, symptoms of vitamin D toxicity include hypercalcemia, azotemia, and anemia (Koutkia, Chen, & Holick, 2001). While some studies have failed to show favorable results, this still is a topic that is being widely investigated.

OMEGA-3 POLYUNSATURATED FATTY ACIDS

Omega-3 polyunsaturated fatty acids (PUFAs) are composed of linoleic acid (LA), α-linolenic acid (ALA), and long-chain derivatives. Most commonly found in high abundance in fish and fish oil, these are essential components of the human diet. Specifically, eicosapentaenoic acid (EPA) and docosahexaenoic acid (DHA) are the two active components responsible for the medicinal usefulness of PUFAs. The ideal ratio of omega-6/omega-3 is 1:1. Recommended dosing of PUFAs is 2.7 g of EPA and DHA daily (Simopoulos, 1999).

While the exact mechanism through which PUFAs work is unknown, ingestion of PUFAs is known to decrease production of prostaglandin (PG) E2 metabolites, decrease concentrations of thromboxane A2, decrease formation of leukotriene B4, increase concentration of prostacyclin PG13, and increase concentration of leukotriene B5. Thromboxane A2 is responsible for vasoconstriction and plate aggregation. Leukotriene B4 induces leukocyte chemotaxis and adherence as well as inflammation. Prostacyclin PG13 and prostacyclin PG12 are responsible for vasodilation and inhibition of platelet aggregation. PUFAs specifically increase only PG13. Leukotriene B5 is a chemotactic agent that is a weak inducer of inflammation (Simopoulos, 1999). In general, PUFAs reduce cytokine secretion as well as competitively inhibit cyclooxygenase and lipoxygenase, which is proposed to relieve pain (Goldberg & Katz, 2007).

Current studies have evaluated the association between PUFA supplementation and pain. Pain states including joint pain, rheumatoid arthritis, inflammatory bowel, and dysmenorrhea have been studied. In patients with rheumatoid arthritis, those who received PUFA supplementation reported decreased nonsteroidal antiinflammatory drug (NSAID) consumption (Lau, Morley, & Belch, 1993; Geusens, Wouters, Nijs, Jiang, & Dequeker, 1994; Adam et al., 2003). As expected, methods as well as PUFA doses varied based on patient characteristics. Orally PUFAs are well tolerated. When consumed in excess, they can lead to weight gain and increase the patient's cardiac risk. In general, doses of 2.7 g of EPA and DHA daily have been effective in reducing pain. While there are unfavorable studies in the literature, the majority of literature concurs that PUFA supplementation may help decrease the patient's pain.

MAGNESIUM

Clinical pain is caused by overactivation of excitatory glutamate/*N*-methyl-D-aspartate receptor (NMDA-R). The receptor is involved in activity-dependent central sensitization. Medications that inhibit NMDA-R are typically not recommended or used due to side effects. A way to decrease NMDA-R activity is reducing dietary polyamine intake or through magnesium supplementation (Treede et al., 2015).

Magnesium, which is commonly found in the diet, can be obtained through dietary sources including chocolate, green leafy vegetables, almonds, avocados, pumpkin, and bananas (U.S. Department of Agriculture, 2011). As with vitamin D deficiency, it is proposed that a magnesium deficiency can lead to overactivation of NMDA-R leading to hypersensitivity to pain. Magnesium also mediates neurogenic inflammation and is a smooth muscle relaxant.

Oral magnesium supplementation in patients with neuropathic pain resulted in reduced pain (Pickering et al., 2011). Magnesium supplementation in relation to menstrual pain was also studied. While magnesium did reduce PG concentrations, there was no significant difference in pain scores. The number of ibuprofen tablets consumed did not significantly differ between magnesium and placebo groups (Lloyd & Hornsby, 2009). The dosages used in studies have ranged from 300 to 600 mg daily.

The effect of topical magnesium application has also been studied in patients with fibromyalgia. It has been proposed that the pain associated with fibromyalgia is due to a decreased concentration of intracellular magnesium. Studies have shown that when magnesium, in the form of magnesium chloride, is applied transdermally to limbs, patients report a decreased amount of pain (Engen et al., 2015).

In general, magnesium supplementation can cause gastrointestinal problems including nausea, vomiting, and diarrhea. Although rare, hypermagnesemia can cause increased thirst, hypotension, muscle weakness, respiratory depression, and cardiac arrhythmias (Wang et al., 2003). As expected, results vary between studies. While there are unfavorable studies in the literature, both oral and topical magnesium have been shown to be effective in reducing pain in patients.

WILLOW BARK

Willow bark has been used for many years for antiinflammatory, antipyretic, and analgesic effects. Efficacy of willow bark is believed to be due to salicin content. When willow bark is ingested, 80% of salicin content is absorbed. Once absorbed, the salicin is metabolized by the intestinal flora to saligenin. This is further metabolized by the liver to salicylic acid (Shara & Stohs, 2015). It is believed that white willow bark acts as a nonselective inhibitor of cyclooxygenase (COX-1 and COX-2). This blocks inflammatory PGs (Chrubasik et al., 2000). Typical doses range from 120 to 240 mg of salicin daily. Willow bark has been studied in patients with joint/knee pain, acute back pain, osteoarthritis, headache, menstrual cramps, tendonitis, and generalized pain.

Willow bark's effectiveness in reduction of pain was studied in patients who suffered from rheumatic pain as a result of osteoarthritis or back conditions. While 33% of the patients withdrew from the study due to lack of efficacy, results showed a positive correlation between willow bark use and reduction of pain. Based on this study, willow bark can be used to treat musculoskeletal pain disorders with or without combination with other pain medications (Uehleke, Muller, Stange, Kelber, & Melzer, 2013).

Another study examined the use of willow bark in osteoarthritis. In general, pain was reduced from baseline by 14% after 2 weeks. However, this study did use the upper limit of the recommended dose (Schmid et al., 2001).

Willow bark's efficacy in reduction of pain is highly variable. Most studies that examine clinical efficacy of willow bark are studies with a small treatment population. While there have been positive correlations established between willow bark and pain, some studies find only that willow bark is effective at higher doses or when combined with other pain relievers. When taken orally, willow bark can cause gastrointestinal symptoms or itching and rash. In general, willow bark could potential be used to reduce pain in patients with a variety of conditions.

PROBIOTICS

Probiotics may restore or maintain gut microbiota. While the gut microbiota have many purposes, the most well-known purposes are metabolism of nutrients and protection from pathogens. The most common bacteria are *Lactobacillus acidophilus*, *Lactobacillus salivarius*, *Lactobacillus paracasei*, and *Bifidobacterium lactis* (Rousseaux et al., 2007).

The exact mechanism of probiotics association and pain is unknown. Many hypotheses exist. One hypothesis is that intestinal bacteria secrete cytokines that are known to affect visceral pain response (Maroon, Bost, & Maroon, 2010). Specifically, probiotics are responsible for induction of expression of receptors that are located on epithelial cells. These receptors control transmission of nociceptive information to intestinal nervous system. It is believed that these receptors include opioid and cannabinoid receptors. These receptors are known to have many functions including analgesic and antiinflammatory functions (Rousseaux et al., 2007).

Some studies have shown that probiotic supplementation can decrease visceral pain. As expected, this is specific to abdominal pain that can be experienced by many patients including those with irritable bowel syndrome (Maroon et al., 2010). There is, however, insufficient evidence to make a positive correlation between reduction of pain and probiotic use.

GLUCOSAMINE AND CHONDROITIN

Glucosamine and chondroitin are well-known natural supplements that many people consume for joint health. Both supplements have conflicting evidence regarding their clinical efficacy in reducing pain. Derived from exoskeletons of marine animals, glucosamine is a component of cartilage proteoglycans. Once cleaved and ionized in the stomach, it stimulates metabolism of chondrocytes in synovial tissues and articular cartilage (Pavelka et al., 2002). Made from shark and bovine cartilage, chondroitin is a substrate for formation of joint matrix structure. Some evidence even suggests that chondroitin prevents degradation of cartilage (Gallagher et al., 2015).

In patients with osteoarthritis, some studies show no significant decrease in pain reduction (Gallagher et al., 2015). Other studies demonstrated 42% less pain as compared to placebo (Uebelhart et al., 2004). In the well-known GAIT trial, patients with osteoarthritis were given glucosamine, chondroitin, a combination of glucosamine and chondroitin, celecoxib, or placebo. The results showed insignificant trends for improvement in joint pain with celecoxib and glucosamine. There was no effect with chondroitin or glucosamine–chondroitin when used as monotherapy (Sawitzke et al., 2010).

Dosages may be responsible for disparate results. The recommended dose of glucosamine, available as glucosamine hydrochloride, is 500 mg three times daily. When taken orally, glucosamine can cause mild gastrointestinal symptoms including gas, abdominal bloating, and pain. For diabetic patients, it can also cause elevated blood glucose levels. The recommended dose of chondroitin, available as chondroitin sulfate, is 400 mg three times daily. When taken orally, chondroitin is well tolerated. Despite inconclusive evidence, patients continue to take glucosamine and chondroitin supplementation.

TURMERIC

Curcumin, a derivative of turmeric, is a naturally occurring substance obtained from a flowering plant. While many people use curcumin for its color and spice, it also has medicinal properties including antiinflammatory, digestive, antineoplastic, and antioxidant properties. Researchers propose that turmeric works by inhibiting COX-1 and COX-2. Alternatively, it has been proposed that curcumin inhibits NF-κB, PGE2, leukotrienes, and nitric oxide that provide turmeric its medicinal properties. Effective dosages range from 400 to 600 mg usually taken up to three times a day (Maroon et al., 2010). Lower doses can be used in combination with NSAIDs. Dosages are based on percentage of curcumin provided. The standard recommended dose is 1200 mg of curcumin daily in divided doses. When taken orally, turmeric is well tolerated. The most commonly reported symptoms are gastrointestinal problems.

Turmeric has been studied in patients with conditions including colitis, neurodegenerative diseases, arthritis, and cancer. It has been proven effective in patients with osteoarthritis when 500 mg is taken twice daily. A reduction in pain, improved functionality, and decreased NSAID consumption were reported (Belcaro et al., 2010).

In comparison with NSAID use, evidence is mixed depending on which type of NSAID is used. In patients taking ibuprofen, a dose of 500 mg three to four times a day was effective in reducing osteoarthritic knee pain. In patients on 500-mg turmeric twice daily and diclofenac 25 mg daily, there was no significant reduction in pain (Kuptniratsaikul, Thanakhumtorn, Chinswangwatanakul, Wattanamongkonsil, & Thamlikitkul, 2009). Other studies have indicated that turmeric in combination with other natural medicines can help reduce pain in patients. However, there remains insufficient evidence to demonstrate that taking turmeric can help reduce joint pain.

DEVIL'S CLAW

Devil's claw contains iridoid glycoside that appears to have an antiinflammatory effect. It is proposed that through inhibition of COX-2 and nitric oxide synthase, devil's claw reduces pain. It specifically affects PGE2, thromboxane B2 (TXB2), interleukin (IL)-1, B2, and tumor necrosis factor (TNF)-α. However, there is no effect on the arachidonic acid pathway (Jang et al., 2003). Dosages are standardized to 2% harpagosides and 3% iridoid glycosides. Typical dose is 600 mg four times daily (Chantre et al., 2000). Generally well tolerated, the most commonly reported symptom is diarrhea and other gastrointestinal problems.

When taken orally, devil's claw may be effective when utilized for back pain and osteoarthritis. Devil's claw exhibited a decreased low back pain when compared to other NSAIDs (Chrubasik et al., 2002). When taken for osteoarthritis either alone or in combination with NSAIDs, there was a decrease in osteoarthritis pain. Some patients even report a decrease in NSAID use (Chantre et al., 2000). There remains insufficient evidence for use of devil's claw for rheumatoid arthritis pain (Grahame & Robinson, 1981).

METHYLSULFONYLMETHANE

MSM is used both orally and topically for a wide variety of pain etiologies and exhibits antiinflammatory properties. A naturally occurring substance, it is found in green plants, algae, fruits, vegetables, adrenal glands, milk, and urine (Barrager, Veltmann, Schauss, & Schiller, 2002).

MSM is obtained from about 15% of ingested dimethylsulfoxide (DMSO). It is used as a source of sulfur for amino acid formation. It is suggested that MSM inhibits changes in joints and could inhibit inflammation through a variety of mechanisms (Murav'ev Iu, Venikova, Pleskovskaia, Riazantseva, & Sigidin Ia, 1991). Generally well tolerated, effective doses typically range from 3 to 6 g daily.

When used both topically and orally, MSM has been shown to be effective in reducing osteoarthritic pain. It was shown to significantly reduce symptoms of osteoarthritis including pain and swelling but not stiffness (Usha & Naidu, 2004).

BOSWELLIA

Boswellia is known in the Western world as frankincense. This substance has antiinflammatory, antiarthritic, and analgesic properties. It has been used for osteoarthritis, rheumatoid arthritis, bursitis, and tendonitis. Other uses include ulcerative colitis, painful menstruation, and abdominal pain. It is proposed to inhibit leukotriene biosynthesis. This leads to reduction in white blood cells (WBCs). The reduction in WBC and leukocyte esterase makes *Boswellia* useful in rheumatoid arthritis (Maroon et al., 2010).

Boswellia consumption resulted in significant improvement in knee arthritis pain after 8 weeks of treatment (Keplinger, Laus, Wurm, Dierich, & Teppner, 1999). Other studies have shown that when combined with curcumin, the combination was superior to diclofenac when treating osteoarthritis (Maroon et al., 2010).

The dosage of *Boswellia* is based on the percentage of boswellic acids. Standard dosages contain 30–40% boswellic acid. This is equivalent to a dose of 300–500 mg two to three times a day (Maroon et al., 2010). There is sufficient evidence to prove the clinical efficacy of *Boswellia* in patients with osteoarthritis. However, there is insufficient evidence to prove the clinically efficacy of *Boswellia* in patients with rheumatoid arthritis.

GREEN TEA

Green tea, while commonly used for cardiovascular and cancer preventative purposes, has recently been recognized for antiinflammatory properties. It contains catechins that are polyphenolic compounds. In green tea, the most abundant compound is epigallocatechin-3-galate. This compound leads to inhibition of IL-1–stimulated proteoglycan release and collagen degradation. Effective dosages are 300–400 mg daily (Maroon et al., 2010). When taken orally, green tea can cause gastrointestinal symptoms as well as central nervous stimulation. This is most commonly seen with higher doses of green tea.

SUMMARY

In summary, pain is a common condition that is treated by less than 50% of Americans by complementary and alternative medicine. Nutritional modulators studied include vitamin D, PUFAs, polyamines, magnesium, flavonoids, α-lipoic acid, and vitamin E. These provide options to patients that are cheap. While the data are inclusive, these nutritional modulators are not 100% effective. However, studies have shown that they reduce pain in specific patient populations. Future research is ongoing and the place of these nutritional modulators in clinical practice is based on provider's discretion (Table 16.2).

TABLE 16.2 Summary of Nutritional Modulators of Pain

Name	Proposed mechanism	Dosage	Types of pain
Green tea	• Antiinflammatory properties	• 300–400 mg daily	
Omega-3 polyunsaturated fatty acids	• Reduce cytokine secretion • Competitively inhibit cyclooxygenase and lipoxygenase	• 2.7 g of EPA and DHA daily	• Rheumatoid arthritis • Inflammatory bowel disease • Dysmenorrhea
Magnesium	• Mediates neurogenic inflammation • Smooth muscle relaxant	• 300–600 mg daily • Maintain serum levels of 1.7–2.4 mg/dL	• Fibromyalgia • Menstrual pain • Neuropathic pain
Vitamin D	• Calcium and phosphorous homeostasis • Found in most tissue and muscle cells	• Maintains serum levels above 20 ng/mL	• Polymyalgia rheumatica • Fibromyalgia • Osteoarthritis • Elderly • Nonspecific pain • Statin myopathies
Willow bark	• Nonselective inhibitor of cyclooxygenase	• 120–240 mg salicin daily	• Joint/knee pain • Acute back pain • Osteoarthritis • Headache • Menstrual cramps • Tendonitis • Generalized pain
Lactobacillus	• Secretes cytokines that affect visceral pain	• 1–10 billion organisms daily	• Abdominal pain
Turmeric (curcumin)	• Nonselective inhibitor of cyclooxygenase	• 1200 mg daily	• Osteoarthritis • Joint pain
Glucosamine and chondroitin	• Glucosamine: component of cartilage proteoglycans • Chondroitin: joint matrix substrate	• Glucosamine 500 mg three times daily • Chondroitin 400 mg three times daily	• Osteoarthritis • Joint pain
Boswellia	• Inhibits leukotriene biosynthesis	• 300–500 mg two to three times daily	• Rheumatoid arthritis • Osteoarthritis
Devil's claw	• COX-2 inhibition	• 600 mg four times daily	• Osteoarthritis • Rheumatoid arthritis • Back pain
MSM	• Inhibits oxidative damage	• 3–6 g daily	• Osteoarthritis
Green tea	• Inhibits IL-1	• 300–400 mg daily	• Osteoarthritis

DHA, Docosahexaenoic acid; EPA, eicosapentaenoic acid; IL, interleukin; MSM, methylsulfonylmethane.

References

Adam, O., Beringer, C., Kless, T., Lemmen, C., Adam, A., Wiseman, M., Adam, P., Klimmek, R., & Forth, W. (2003). Anti-inflammatory effects of a low arachidonic acid diet and fish oil in patients with rheumatoid arthritis. *Rheumatology International, 23*(1), 27–36.

Barnes, P. (2008). *Complementary and alternative medicine use among adults and children: United States, 2007* (pp. 1–24).

Barrager, E., Veltmann, J. R., Jr., Schauss, A. G., & Schiller, R. N. (2002). A multicentered, open-label trial on the safety and efficacy of methylsulfonylmethane in the treatment of seasonal allergic rhinitis. *Journal of Alternative and Complementary Medicine (New York, N.Y.), 8*(2), 167–173.

Belcaro, G., Cesarone, M. R., Dugall, M., Pellegrini, L., Ledda, A., Grossi, M. G., Togni, S., & Appendino, G. (2010). Efficacy and safety of Meriva(R), a curcumin–phosphatidylcholine complex, during extended administration in osteoarthritis patients. *Alternative Medicine Review, 15*(4), 337–344.

Bell, R. F., Borzan, J., Kalso, E., & Simonnet, G. (2012). Food, pain, and drugs: does it matter what pain patients eat? *Pain, 153*(10), 1993–1996.

Carr, D. B., & Goudas, L. C. (1999). Acute pain. *Lancet, 353*(9169), 2051–2058.

Chantre, P., Cappelaere, A., Leblan, D., Guedon, D., Vandermander, J., & Fournie, B. (2000). Efficacy and tolerance of *Harpagophytum procumbens* versus diacerhein in treatment of osteoarthritis. *Phytomedicine, 7*(3), 177–183.

Chrubasik, S., Eisenberg, E., Balan, E., Weinberger, T., Luzzati, R., & Conradt, C. (2000). Treatment of low back pain exacerbations with willow bark extract: a randomized double-blind study. *The American Journal of Medicine, 109*(1), 9–14.

Chrubasik, S., Thanner, J., Kunzel, O., Conradt, C., Black, A., & Pollak, S. (2002). Comparison of outcome measures during treatment with the proprietary *Harpagophytum* extract doloteffin in patients with pain in the lower back, knee or hip. *Phytomedicine, 9*(3), 181–194.

Di Munno, O., Beghe, F., Favini, P., Di Giuseppe, P., Pontrandolfo, A., Occhipinti, G., & Pasero, G. (1989). Prevention of glucocorticoid-induced osteopenia: effect of oral 25-hydroxyvitamin D and calcium. *Clinical Rheumatology, 8*(2), 202–207.

Engen, D. J., McAllister, S. J., Whipple, M. O., Cha, S. S., Dion, L. J., Vincent, A., Bauer, B. A., & Wahner-Roedler, D. L. (2015). Effects of transdermal magnesium chloride on quality of life for patients with fibromyalgia: a feasibility study. *Journal of Integrative Medicine, 13*(5), 306–313.

Gallagher, B., Tjoumakaris, F. P., Harwood, M. I., Good, R. P., Ciccotti, M. G., & Freedman, K. B. (2015). Chondroprotection and the prevention of osteoarthritis progression of the knee: a systematic review of treatment agents. *The American Journal of Sports Medicine, 43*(3), 734–744.

Geusens, P., Wouters, C., Nijs, J., Jiang, Y., & Dequeker, J. (1994). Long-term effect of omega-3 fatty acid supplementation in active rheumatoid arthritis. A 12-month, double-blind, controlled study. *Arthritis and Rheumatism, 37*(6), 824–829.

Gilron, I., Baron, R., & Jensen, T. (2015). Neuropathic pain: principles of diagnosis and treatment. *Mayo Clinic Proceedings, 90*(4), 532–545.

Goldberg, R. J., & Katz, J. (2007). A meta-analysis of the analgesic effects of omega-3 polyunsaturated fatty acid supplementation for inflammatory joint pain. *Pain, 129*(1–2), 210–223.

Grahame, R., & Robinson, B. V. (1981). Devils's claw (*Harpagophytum procumbens*): pharmacological and clinical studies. *Annals of the Rheumatic Diseases, 40*(6), 632.

Holick, M. F. (2007). Vitamin D deficiency. *The New England Journal of Medicine, 357*(3), 266–281.

Jang, M. H., Lim, S., Han, S. M., Park, H. J., Shin, I., Kim, J. W., Kim, N. J., Lee, J. S., Kim, K. A., & Kim, C. J. (2003). *Harpagophytum procumbens* suppresses lipopolysaccharide-stimulated expressions of cyclooxygenase-2 and inducible nitric oxide synthase in fibroblast cell line L929. *Journal of Pharmacological Sciences, 93*(3), 367–371.

Keplinger, K., Laus, G., Wurm, M., Dierich, M. P., & Teppner, H. (1999). *Uncaria tomentosa* (Willd.) DC.—ethnomedicinal use and new pharmacological, toxicological and botanical results. *Journal of Ethnopharmacology, 64*(1), 23–34.

Koutkia, P., Chen, T. C., & Holick, M. F. (2001). Vitamin D intoxication associated with an over-the-counter supplement. *The New England Journal of Medicine, 345*(1), 66–67.

Kuptniratsaikul, V., Thanakhumtorn, S., Chinswangwatanakul, P., Wattanamongkonsil, L., & Thamlikitkul, V. (2009). Efficacy and safety of *Curcuma domestica* extracts in patients with knee osteoarthritis. *Journal of Alternative and Complementary Medicine (New York, N.Y.), 15*(8), 891–897.

Lau, C. S., Morley, K. D., & Belch, J. J. (1993). Effects of fish oil supplementation on non-steroidal anti-inflammatory drug requirement in patients with mild rheumatoid arthritis—A double-blind placebo controlled study. *British Journal of Rheumatology, 32*(11), 982–989.

Lloyd, K. B., & Hornsby, L. B. (2009). Complementary and alternative medications for women's health issues. *Nutrition in Clinical Practice, 24*(5), 589–608.

Loeser, J. D., & Treede, R. D. (2008). The Kyoto protocol of IASP basic pain terminology. *Pain, 137*(3), 473–477.

Maroon, J. C., Bost, J. W., & Maroon, A. (2010). Natural anti-inflammatory agents for pain relief. *Surgical Neurology International, 1*, 80.

Mergenhagen, K., Ott, M., Heckman, K., Rubin, L. M., & Kellick, K. (2014). Low vitamin D as a risk factor for the development of myalgia in patients taking high-dose simvastatin: a retrospective review. *Clinical Therapeutics, 36*(5), 770–777.

Murav'ev Iu, V., Venikova, M. S., Pleskovskaia, G. N., Riazantseva, T. A., & Sigidin Ia, A. (1991). Effect of dimethyl sulfoxide and dimethyl sulfone on a destructive process in the joints of mice with spontaneous arthritis. *Patologicheskaia Fiziologiia i Eksperimental'naia Terapiia*(2), 37–39.

Pavelka, K., Gatterova, J., Olejarova, M., Machacek, S., Giacovelli, G., & Rovati, L. C. (2002). Glucosamine sulfate use and delay of progression of knee osteoarthritis: a 3-year, randomized, placebo-controlled, double-blind study. *Archives of Internal Medicine, 162*(18), 2113–2123.

Pickering, G., Morel, V., Simen, E., Cardot, J. M., Moustafa, F., Delage, N., Picard, P., Eschalier, S., Boulliau, S., & Dubray, C. (2011). Oral magnesium treatment in patients with neuropathic pain: a randomized clinical trial. *Magnesium Research: Official Organ of the International Society for the Development of Research on Magnesium, 24*(2), 28–35.

Rousseaux, C., Thuru, X., Gelot, A., Barnich, N., Neut, C., Dubuquoy, L., Dubuquoy, C., Merour, E., Geboes, K., Chamaillard, M., Ouwehand, A., Leyer, G., Carcano, D., Colombel, J. F., Ardid, D., & Desreumaux, P. (2007). *Lactobacillus acidophilus* modulates intestinal pain and induces opioid and cannabinoid receptors. *Nature Medicine, 13*(1), 35–37.

Sakalli, H., Arslan, D., & Yucel, A. E. (2012). The effect of oral and parenteral vitamin D supplementation in the elderly: a prospective, double-blinded, randomized, placebo-controlled study. *Rheumatology International, 32*(8), 2279–2283.

Sawitzke, A. D., Shi, H., Finco, M. F., Dunlop, D. D., Harris, C. L., Singer, N. G., Bradley, J. D., Silver, D., Jackson, C. G., Lane, N. E., Oddis, C. V., Wolfe, F., Lisse, J., Furst, D. E., Bingham, C. O., Reda, D. J., Moskowitz, R. W., Williams, H. J., & Clegg, D. O. (2010). Clinical efficacy and safety of glucosamine, chondroitin sulphate, their combination, celecoxib or placebo taken to treat osteoarthritis of the knee: 2-year results from GAIT. *Annals of the Rheumatic Diseases, 69*(8), 1459–1464.

Schmid, B., Ludtke, R., Selbmann, H. K., Kotter, I., Tschirdewahn, B., Schaffner, W., & Heide, L. (2001). Efficacy and tolerability of a standardized willow bark extract in patients with osteoarthritis: randomized placebo-controlled, double blind clinical trial. *Phytotherapy Research: PTR, 15*(4), 344–350.

Shara, M., & Stohs, S. J. (2015). Efficacy and safety of white willow bark (*Salix alba*) extracts. *Phytotherapy Research: PTR*, *29*(8), 1112–1116.

Simopoulos, A. P. (1999). Essential fatty acids in health and chronic disease. *The American Journal of Clinical Nutrition*, *70*(3 suppl.), 560S–569S.

Treede, R. D., Rief, W., Barke, A., Aziz, Q., Bennett, M. I., Benoliel, R., Cohen, M., Evers, S., Finnerup, N. B., First, M. B., Giamberardino, M. A., Kaasa, S., Kosek, E., Lavand'homme, P., Nicholas, M., Perrot, S., Scholz, J., Schug, S., Smith, B. H., Svensson, P., Vlaeyen, J. W., & Wang, S. J. (2015). A classification of chronic pain for ICD-11. *Pain*, *156*(6), 1003–1007.

U.S. Department of Agriculture, A.R.S. (2011). *USDA national nutrient database for standard reference* (p. 24). Available at http://www.ars.usda.gov/ba/bhnrc/ndl.

Uebelhart, D., Malaise, M., Marcolongo, R., de Vathaire, F., Piperno, M., Mailleux, E., Fioravanti, A., Matoso, L., & Vignon, E. (2004). Intermittent treatment of knee osteoarthritis with oral chondroitin sulfate: a one-year, randomized, double-blind, multicenter study versus placebo. *Osteoarthritis and Cartilage/OARS, Osteoarthritis Research Society*, *12*(4), 269–276.

Uehleke, B., Muller, J., Stange, R., Kelber, O., & Melzer, J. (2013). Willow bark extract STW 33-I in the long-term treatment of outpatients with rheumatic pain mainly osteoarthritis or back pain. *Phytomedicine*, *20*(11), 980–984.

Usha, P. R., & Naidu, M. U. (2004). Randomised, double-blind, parallel, placebo-controlled study of oral glucosamine, methylsulfonylmethane and their combination in osteoarthritis. *Clinical Drug Investigation*, *24*(6), 353–363.

Wang, F., Van Den Eeden, S. K., Ackerson, L. M., Salk, S. E., Reince, R. H., & Elin, R. J. (2003). Oral magnesium oxide prophylaxis of frequent migrainous headache in children: a randomized, double-blind, placebo-controlled trial. *Headache*, *43*(6), 601–610.

Wepner, F., Scheuer, R., Schuetz-Wieser, B., Machacek, P., Pieler-Bruha, E., Cross, H. S., Hahne, J., & Friedrich, M. (2014). Effects of vitamin D on patients with fibromyalgia syndrome: a randomized placebo-controlled trial. *Pain*, *155*(2), 261–268.

CHAPTER

17

Trace Elements Alleviate Pain in Mice and Humans

B.I. Tamba, T. Alexa-Stratulat

Centre for the Study and Therapy of Pain, Grigore T. Popa University of Medicine and Pharmacy, Iasi, Romania

INTRODUCTION

Chronic pain has become one of the most pressing public health issues; current estimates show a prevalence of 40% in adults (Tsang et al., 2008) and a prevalence of 4–40% in children (King et al., 2011). Individuals affected by chronic pain have a decreased quality of life and impaired social functioning, and experience sleep, mood, and anxiety disorders. Pain complicates preexisting medical conditions and significantly hinders work productivity. From an economical point of view, costs related to chronic pain are greater than the annual costs of heart disease, cancer, or diabetes, ranging from $560 to 635 billion per year in the United States (Gaskin & Richard, 2012).

Current options for chronic pain management are diverse, and mostly focus on pharmacological treatment with drugs pertaining to opioid or nonopioid classes, which have not significantly changed in the past decade. Most recently developed compounds are just improved versions of classic drugs with similar side effects and addiction issues. As such, we need to explore new analgesic compounds that target different pain mechanisms and have a better safety profile and better treatment adherence. In recent years, more and more studies have focused on the potential benefits of dietary supplements. The theoretical rationale behind this shift in focus includes their effect on inflammation, oxidative stress, mitochondrial dysfunction, and nerve health, as well as the increase of unbalanced diets that lead to different chronic deficiencies (which dietary supplements might reverse). As such, mineral supplements were shown to reduce symptoms in patients with chronic lower back pain (Vormann, Worlitschek, Goedecke, & Silver, 2001), chronic pelvic pain syndrome (Lombardo et al., 2012), chronic pancreatitis (Cai et al., 2013), tendon injuries (Curtis, 2015), and migraine (Dhillon, Singh, & Lyall, 2011).

However, available data are scarce and often contradictory (Siriwardena, Mason, Sheen, Makin, & Shah, 2012); furthermore, the heterogeneity of current studies makes it difficult to identify which compound of the dietary supplement is truly beneficial. The aim of this chapter is to individually review the main trace elements and minerals most often encountered in dietary supplements and to discuss their potential role as analgesics or coanalgesics in acute and chronic pain syndromes.

ZINC

Theoretical Background

The second most prevalent trace element in the body, zinc (Zn) is essential to several metalloproteins and transcription factors and is crucial to the body's antioxidant defense (Nozaki et al., 2011). Zn is found in high concentrations in the epidermis, where nociceptive nerve endings begin the complex processing and transmission of pain (Nelson et al., 2007). One other site that contains high quantities of Zn is the nervous system, where Zn can be found either free or protein bound (90% of CNS Zn) or sequestered in the synaptic vesicles (10% of CNS Zn) of certain neuronal subtypes (Larson & Kitto, 1997) that are most often GABAergic or glutamatergic. Zn-containing neurons are highly expressed in laminas I and II of the spine and in the central nervous system and are involved in both motor control and sensory transmission—they

Nutritional Modulators of Pain in the Aging Population. http://dx.doi.org/10.1016/B978-0-12-805186-3.00017-5
Copyright © 2017 Elsevier Inc. All rights reserved.

act on several types of ion channels and modulate the excitability of peripheral and central neurons (Jo, Danscher, Schrøder, & Suh, 2008). After being released, Zn ions inhibit the *N*-methyl-D-aspartate (NMDA) receptor and the presynaptic release of glutamate, both of which are associatedv with hyperalgesia and neuropathic pain. Also, Zn appears to modulate Transient receptor potential A (TRPA1) channels used as polymodal receptors for noxious stimuli in nociceptive neurons (Hu, Bandell, Petrus, Zhu, & Patapoutian, 2009). Zn is also a key modulator of pain through the matrix metalloproteinases that are Zn-dependent and are essential to the physiological functioning of the central nervous system.

In the medical practice, Zn is currently used in peptic ulcer treatment, age-related macular degeneration, reducing the duration of cold symptoms, sickle cell disease, attention deficit hyperactivity disorder, and Wilson disease. Topical Zn is used in several types of dermatologic lesions (minor cuts, scrapes, burns, poison ivy, and poison oak rashes). Not all uses are FDA-approved, but Zn-based compounds are readily available as over-the-counter drugs or dietary supplements.

Fundamental Studies

Single Agent

Zn was shown to significantly activate a population of neurons from mouse dorsal root ganglia by increasing calcium influx, most likely through TRPA1 (Hu et al., 2009). One other study suggested that Zn has antinociceptive effects through modulating the NMDA receptor, as shown by the increased hyperalgesic response of knock-in NMDA receptor mutant mice in which Zn cannot bind to the NR2A channel-like N-terminal domain (Nozaki et al., 2011).

In murine models, intrathecal Zn administration led to a significant decrease of pain behavior in the writhing test, whereas Zn chelators induced a significant hyperalgesic effect in the tail-flick test, results that suggest a direct role of spinal Zn in pain modulation (Larson & Kitto, 1997). Liu, Walker, and Tracey (1999) reported that Zn chloride has dose-dependent analgesic effects no matter the form of administration (intrathecal, intraplantar, or systemic) in a rat model of sciatic nerve injury. Similarly, research performed in our department indicates a 17% increase in tail-flick and hot-plate latency and a 25% decrease in pain-related behavior in the writhing test in mice treated with intraperitoneal Zn chloride (Tamba, Leon, & Petreus, 2013). Somewhat in opposition to these results, an older study observed that Zn concentration increases in a murine model of trigeminal neuralgia and Zn supplementation worsens this condition's symptoms (Megdiatov, Vorobeĭchik, Dolgikh, & Reshetniak, 1995).

Regarding the effect of Zn on inflammation, fundamental studies report contradictory results. Systemic Zn administration significantly reduced inflammatory hyperalgesia secondary to the intraplantar administration of Freund's adjuvant and decreased IL-1 and nerve growth factor (NGF) levels (Safieh-Garabedian et al., 1996). Similarly, one other study concluded that oral (25 mg/kg) or subcutaneous (15 mg/kg) Zn administration significantly reduced carrageenan-induced paw edema (Abou-Mohamed, el-Kashef, Salem, & Elmazar, 1995). However, another group reported that administering 30-nM Zn acetate in the mouse's hind paw led to increased pain-like behavior, an effect that was absent when administering the same quantity of calcium acetate (Hu et al., 2009).

In an animal model of interstitial cystitis, polaprezinc (a Zn-based drug used in the clinical setting for the treatment of peptic ulcer) 30, 100, 200, or 400 mg/kg was administered orally 1 h before or 3 h after i.p. administration of cyclophosphamide (300 mg/kg). Results indicated that mice treated with polaprezinc experienced a decrease in both inflammatory symptoms and pain intensity for both localized and referred pain and hyperalgesia (Murakami-Nakayama et al., 2015).

Other arguments that support Zn's involvement in pain modulation include the symptoms of Zn deficiency and the hyperalgesic (Matsunami, Kirishi, Okui, & Kawabata, 2011) and neuropathic effect of Zn chelators (Jo et al., 2008) in pain animal models. Agents that decrease Zn availability or Zn chelators have been shown to promote central sensitization and lower the threshold for nociceptor excitability, most likely through depleting Zn off the histidine residues in Ca^{2+} channels (Nelson et al., 2007). Both nanosized and conventional-sized Zn oxide were shown to increase hot-plate latency in an opioid-independent manner (Kesmati & Torabi, 2014), thus suggesting a potential benefit for Zn and opioid combinations in pain management.

Coadministration With Analgesics

A recent study assessed the effect of trace elements on the release of diclofenac sodium from tablets and capsules and found that Zn coadministration enhances enteric release of coated diclofenac, leading to a higher absorption in the GI tract (Biernat, Musiał, Gosławska, & Pluta, 2014).

In our department, coadministration of tramadol and Zn (0.6, 1.2, or 2.4 mg/kg b.w.) leads to a significant enhancement of tramadol's effect, with an added analgesic effect of approximately 20% in both tail-flick and hot-plate tests. The smallest dose (0.6 mg/kg b.w.) was determined to be the most efficient, possibly due to Zn's neurotoxic effect in high concentrations (Alexa, Aurelia, Tudor, & Bogdan, 2015). Similarly, subcutaneous coadministration of Zn (15 mg/kg) and indometacin (5 mg/kg) or diclofenac (10 mg/kg) led to a more important decrease in paw edema than that of either agent alone (Abou-Mohamed et al., 1995). More recently, coadministration of Zn and tenoxicam was found to have a good antiinflammatory profile, inhibiting carrageenan-induced paw edema and decreasing pain behavior in the writhing test, and significantly reducing tenoxicam's gastric toxicity (Nascimento et al., 2003). A combination between nanosized Zn oxide and morphine was shown to be more effective than morphine alone as assessed by the hot-plate test (Kesmati & Torabi, 2014).

Clinical Studies

In the clinical setting, there is an increasing body of evidence that indicates a beneficial effect of Zn supplementation in primary dysmenorrhea. Although the information first came from retrospective case series and clinical observations, it was shortly followed by results from randomized clinical trials. Zekavat, Karimi, Amanat, and Alipour (2015) enrolled 120 females and randomized them to receive either oral Zn supplementation (50 mg/day from the first day of menses to 3 days prior to the end of menses) or placebo and concluded that Zn decreases both pain duration and pain severity in the study population. Similarly, Kashefi, Khajehei, Tabatabaeichehr, Alavinia, and Asili (2014) assessed both Zn and ginger in young girls with this condition (150 participants) and found that both supplements were efficient in reducing pain severity.

Cancer patients undergoing certain chemotherapy regimens are more prone to developing mucositis, a condition characterized by inflammation, pain, and an increased analgesic requirement. Zn supplementation (220 mg/day) throughout *chemotherapy* decreased the intensity of mucositis and xerostomia, together with providing pain alleviation (an average of two points as assessed by a visual analog scale) in a clinical trial (Arbabi-kalati, Arbabi-kalati, Deghatipour, & Ansari Moghadam, 2012). Similar results were reported in cancer patients with *radiotherapy*-induced mucositis—each of the two small clinical trials that enrolled approximately 30 patients found that Zn supplementation delays the development of severe mucositis and decreases oral discomfort in head and neck cancer patients (Lin, Que, Lin, & Lin, 2006; Ertekin, Koç, Karslioglu, & Sezen, 2004). In contrast to these findings, however, the results of a larger trial (144 patients) were published in 2013 and showed that Zn supplementation (50 mg three times per day) has no significant benefit in decreasing the incidence of mucositis (Sangthawan, Phungrassami, & Sinkitjarurnchai, 2013). However, this study did not report any pain measurement and serum Zn levels were not assessed prior to treatment. Also, it was carried out in an Asian population and the supplementation was done with 150-mg Zn, a dose that might be insufficient in these patients, especially since Thailand has an estimated Zn deficiency incidence of 15–25% (Wessells & Brown, 2012). Zn supplementation was also found to be inefficient in patients receiving chemotherapy for bone marrow transplant (Mansouri et al., 2012), although another study performed on the same type of patients found that Zn-based mouthwash is effective (Mehdipour, Taghavi Zenoz, Asvadi Kermani, & Hosseinpour, 2011). As a rinsing solution, polaprezinc was assessed for preventing mucositis in 2 clinical trials (approximately 30 patients each) with patients undergoing chemoradiotherapy and was found superior to azulene gargle in terms of incidence and severity of mucositis and pain intensity (Hayashi et al., 2014; Watanabe, Ishihara, Matsuura, Mizuta, & Itoh, 2010). Because data are somewhat in contradiction and high-quality evidence is lacking, no definitive recommendation has yet been issued regarding the efficacy of Zn supplementation in mucositis.

A small study in cirrhotic patients assessed the effect of oral Zn sulfate supplementation (220 mg 2 times per day, 3 times per week, 12 weeks) on the frequency and severity of muscle cramps and found a significant improvement in 10 of the 12 enrolled patients (Kugelmas, 2000). This potential analgesic effect of Zn was not related to Zn deficiency/toxicity, taking into account the fact that no relationship between serum Zn levels and the incidence of cramps was found in this population (Baskol et al., 2004).

In trigeminal neuralgia patients, a small study concluded that treatment with a Zn chelator (xydiphone) led to a significant improvement in pain in 15 of 25 carbamazepine-treated patients (Megdiatov et al., 1995). One other intriguing hypothesis states that Zn might be useful in preventing and treating angina in patients without Zn deficiency. Zn sulfate was reported as beneficial in angina patient case series in the 1970s and 1980s and professional exposure to Zn was associated with a decreased incidence of effort angina in a large cohort study in the 1990s (Eby & Halcomb, 2006). Although the exact mechanism by which Zn may influence angina is unknown, it is most likely an antioxidant and antiinflammatory mechanism that acts both in the coronary vessels and in the general circulation.

Cutaneous Zn administration has also shown benefits in several types of conditions. It has been shown to stimulate reepithelialization and decrease inflammation, together with having a local antibacterial effect (Arbabi-kalati et al., 2012). Leg ulcers showed improved healing and decreased pain after using either the Unna boot (a Zn oxide delivery system to the wound bed) (Stebbins, Hanke, & Petersen, 2011) or a compression system with Zn paste bandages (Mosti, Crespi, & Mattaliano, 2011). In neonates, a skin care product containing Zn oxide as a skin protector was ranked as better than or similar to other products in terms of reducing the baby's discomfort by the nurses working in the department (Young, Chakravarthy, Drower, & Reyna, 2014). Coadministration of a Zn chloride spray and a magnesium hydroxide ointment contributed to faster healing, lower infection rate, and decreased pain in a randomized double-blind placebo-controlled clinical study that enrolled 85 patients with incisional wounds after obstetric and gynecological surgery (Pastorfide, Gorgonio, Ganzon, & Alberto, 1989). Also, the antiinflammatory effects of Zn were used to create a topical ointment (Theraflex-TMJ) that also contains copper pyrocarboxylate. In a clinical study, 52 patients with masseter muscle and temporomandibular joint pain were instructed to apply the cream twice daily for 2 weeks. The authors observed that the treatment significantly decreased pain levels throughout the 2 weeks and in the follow-up period, suggesting its efficacy in this population (Lobo et al., 2004).

TAKE-HOME MESSAGES: ZINC AND PAIN

- Zn is one of the most promising minerals potentially beneficial in the treatment of pain.
- There is an increasingly strong body of evidence that suggests coadministration of Zn and opioid analgesics increases the effect of both morphine and tramadol.
- Because it is already used in the clinical setting, trials assessing Zn's effects as an analgesic or as a coanalgesic should be encouraged.

MAGNESIUM

Theoretical Background

Magnesium (Mg) is an essential trace element required for the adequate functioning of more than 200 proteins and enzymes. The mineral is known for its vasodilator and antiinflammatory effects, stimulating endothelial-dependent NO release (Brousseau, Scott, Hillery, & Panepinto, 2004) and protecting the endothelium from ischemia and secondary dysfunction. Clinical studies have shown that Mg deficiency leads to increased levels of interleukin-6 and tumor necrosis factor-α (inflammatory cytokines) and increased expression of endothelial vascular cell adhesion molecule 1 (Brousseau et al., 2015). Mg inhibits inositol triphosphate calcium channel and modulates several other types of voltage-gated calcium channels, being considered an intracellular calcium antagonist (Singh, Jindal, & Singh, 2011), a mechanism that explains its involvement in pain modulation. Also, Mg is a noncompetitive antagonist of the NMDA receptor ion channel (Galgon et al., 2015), another analgesic mechanism of this trace element.

Mg has been the focus of intense preclinical and clinical research in several fields of medical science. The International Society for the Development of Research on Magnesium publishes a quarterly journal focused solely on original articles, reviews, and updates in Mg-related research. Due to limited space, we could not include all the studies involving pain and Mg and focused mainly on recent clinical research with practice-altering potential.

Fundamental Studies

In an animal study, Mg and ketamine were found to similarly reduce spinal c-Fos expression, a marker for neuronal activation in pain, which suggested they had similar analgesic effects (Lee, Jee, Kim, Kim, & Lee, 2006). On acute pain, three different doses of Mg chloride were assessed (37.5, 75, 150 mg/kg), exhibiting direct antinociceptive effects as assessed by tail-flick and hot-plate tests (Tamba et al., 2013). Regarding inflammatory pain, subcutaneous magnesium sulfate ($MgSO_4$) significantly decreased pain behavior after hind paw carrageenan administration (Srebro, Vučković, Vujović, & Prostran, 2014).

In neuropathic animals, Mg administration was associated with good outcomes. In a rat model of diabetes, oral Mg supplementation in drinking water for 3 weeks did not influence the parameters of diabetes, but it abolished thermal and tactile allodynia and delayed the development of mechanical hypersensitivity, together with decreasing the phosphorylation of the NMDA receptor NR1 subunit (correlated with the development of neuropathic pain) (Rondón et al., 2010). In another study, neuropathic rats (after spinal cord injury) received 300 or 600 mg $MgSO_4$ or saline via the intraperitoneal route. The authors reported an increase in tail-flick and hot-plate latency and lower scores in the acetone test for both Mg-treated groups when compared with saline (Farsi, Afshari, et al., 2015).

Coadministration of morphine (0.1 mg/kg) and $MgSO_4$ (125 mg/kg) was significantly more efficient than either of the drugs alone in alleviating neuropathic pain induced by sciatic nerve ligation in rats (Ulugol et al., 2002). Similar results were reported for Mg pretreatment and morphine, fentanyl, and buprenorphine administration in rats with vincristine-induced neuropathy (Bujalska, Makulska-Nowak, & Gumułka, 2009) and for methylprednisolone–Mg combination in rats with neuropathic pain after spinal cord injury (Farsi, Naghib Zadeh, et al., 2015). In our department, coadministration of tramadol and Mg led to a significant enhancement of tramadol's analgesic effect as assessed by the tail-flick and hot-plate tests (Alexa et al., 2015). Similar results on acute pain were reported for $MgSO_4$ and ketamine coadministration by another research group (Savic Vujovic et al., 2015). One interesting study reported that Mg and diclofenac coadministration enhances enteric-coated diclofenac's release, leading to a higher absorption from the GI tract (Biernat et al., 2014).

Clinical Studies

Propofol injections are used in anesthesiology and are considered in most cases a painful and unpleasant experience. Several clinical trials that assess the role of Mg in alleviating this type of pain have been published to date. In 2002, the results of a randomized trial that enrolled 100 patients showed that i.v. pretreatment with $MgSO_4$ (2.48 mmol) decreased the pain score rated after propofol injection—64% of the patients in the $MgSO_4$ group reported no pain when compared with 16% in the placebo group (Memiş, Turan, Karamanlioğlu, Süt, & Pamukçu, 2002). A subsequent study compared the efficacy of i.v. Mg (1 g) and lidocaine (40 mg) pretreatment in this setting and found that although they are similar in terms of pain alleviation (68% of patients reported no pain in the Mg group and 58% in the lidocaine group), Mg injection by itself causes pain, which is why lidocaine administration should be preferred (Agarwal et al., 2004). One study compared Mg with other analgesics and with placebo and found that the most effective drug in this setting is i.v. granisetron; i.v. Mg, however, was associated with less pain than the placebo (an approximate decrease of 10–20% in pain incidence) (Singh et al., 2011). These results are similar to those of another study that randomized patients in six groups [control, granisetron, lidocaine, acetaminophen, $MgSO_4$ (2 mmol), and ondansetron] and found that lidocaine and granisetron were the most effective drugs in reducing propofol-related pain frequency. However, although $MgSO_4$ was found to be less effective than the aforementioned drugs, it was superior to the control and more efficient than paracetamol or ondansetron (51.78% of the patients in the Mg group reported no pain) (Alipour, Tabari, & Alipour, 2014). As a coanalgesic, Mg pretreatment had contradicting results. A large clinical trial (158 patients) reported that adding $MgSO_4$ (0.25 mg) to lidocaine (50 mg) pretreatment did not enhance lidocaine's analgesic effects (Galgon et al., 2015), whereas another trial (300 patients) reached the opposite conclusion—$MgSO_4$ (300 mg) + lidocaine (40 mg) is significantly more efficient than lidocaine alone, with lower pain scores and no complications (Sun, Zhou, Lin, Zhou, & Wang, 2016). The marked differences between these two trials are probably due to the $MGSO_4$ dose—it is more than 10 times higher in the study performed by Sun et al. To date, there are no firm recommendations issued regarding the benefits of Mg in propofol injections. However, since there are already-established treatments associated with better outcomes and less pain at the injection site, Mg should be explored as a therapeutic option only in selected cases, such as lidocaine allergy.

Mg was assessed as a novel pain therapy in pediatric patients with sickle cell disease, an inherited hematologic disease characterized by recurrent intensely painful episodes secondary to vasoocclusion (Goldman, Mounstephen, Kirby-Allen, & Friedman, 2013). Chronic Mg supplementation was found to significantly decrease the number of days with painful episodes in this population in a small clinical trial (17 patients)—with an average of 15 days in 6 months in the control group and 1 day in the Mg supplementation group (De Franceschi et al., 2000). In another small clinical trial, 19 children with acute pain crisis secondary to sickle cell disease received $MgSO_4$ after being admitted together with standardized therapy and the length of stay was compared with the department's previous experience. The authors concluded that $MgSO_4$ was beneficial in decreasing the amount of time the child spent in the hospital (Brousseau et al., 2004). Subsequently, larger trials were designed to assess these findings—104 children with sickle cell disease were randomized to receive either $MgSO_4$ or placebo after admission, alongside standard therapy in a trial published in 2013. The authors found that Mg was well tolerated, but did not benefit the patients in terms of duration of hospital stay, pain scores, or analgesic requirements (Goldman et al., 2013). Similar results were reported from a National Institute of Health (NIH)-registered trial in 2015—a total of 204 children from 8 pediatric centers were randomized to receive placebo or Mg (40 mg/kg) 6 doses every 8 h; the investigators found no significant difference between the two groups (Brousseau et al., 2015).

Mg has been investigated in several clinical trials, together with calcium, as an agent for the prevention of chemotherapy-induced neuropathy. Currently, due to the results of a large trial (NCCTG N08CB), the American Society of Clinical Oncology guidelines do not endorse this treatment (Hershman et al., 2014). However, Mg has been investigated in other neuropathic pain states as well. A small clinical study published in 1998 reported that $MgSO_4$ treatment has analgesic effects in six of eight patients with refractory neuropathic pain (Tanaka et al., 1998).

In patients with postherpetic chronic neuralgia refractory to treatment, 3-day consecutive administration of i.v. $MgSO_4$ 30 mg/kg was as efficient as ketamine in decreasing pain intensity as assessed by a visual analog scale 2 weeks after the first infusion (Kim, Lee, & Oh, 2015). Another small study assessed the effects of two $MgSO_4$ doses (500 mg and 1 g) in neuropathic pain secondary to malignant infiltration of the brachial or lumbosacral plexus and found that both doses alleviated pain in 10 of the 12 enrolled patients (Crosby, Wilcock, & Corcoran, 2000). Good outcomes were also reported from a combination of i.v. lidocaine (100 mg) and $MgSO_4$ (1.2 g) in patients suffering from intractable trigeminal neuralgia—a retrospective analysis from a pain center reported that treatment with this combination once a week for 3 weeks reduced pain intensity in all patients due to their different mechanisms that have a synergic effect on pain modulation and transmission (Arai et al., 2013). Also, a 2-week intravenous Mg infusion followed by 4 weeks of oral Mg supplementation decreased pain intensity in patients with chronic low back pain with a neuropathic component as reported by a prospective study that enrolled 80 patients (Yousef & Al-deeb, 2013). However, not all studies reported neuropathic pain alleviation following Mg supplementation—in a clinical research involving 50 patients with surgical, traumatic, or postherpetic neuropathic pain, the authors assessed the effect of oral Mg chloride administration (419 mg two times per day) and found that pain intensity and quality of life were similar in the Mg and in the placebo groups. Nonetheless, the authors did observe that Mg-treated patients reported a decrease in paroxysmal pain attacks and an improved emotional component as assessed by one of the questionnaires (Pickering et al., 2011).

Administering Mg alone or in combination with other analgesics has been intensely studied in patients undergoing surgery—either for alleviating postoperative pain, as an adjuvant to regional anesthesia, or for preventing different painful postoperative conditions. For instance, the results of a clinical study that enrolled 75 patents reported that $MgSO_4$ coadministered with lidocaine leads to an earlier onset of sensory block and increases postoperative analgesia in patients requiring regional anesthesia when compared to lidocaine alone (Bansal, Baduni, Bhalla, & Mahawar, 2015). Similar results were reported in another clinical study (90 patients), where lidocaine–$MgSO_4$ proved to be superior to lidocaine–paracetamol and lidocaine–placebo (Mirkheshti, Aryani, Shojaei, & Dabbagh, 2012).

Regarding its effects on postoperative pain, intraarticular Mg treatment significantly reduced pain scores when compared with control in a clinical study that enrolled 67 patients undergoing arthroscopy (Saritas, Borazan, Okesli, Yel, & Otelcioglu, 2015). In patients undergoing elective colorectal surgery, however, $MgSO_4$ administration (30 mg/kg followed by 10 mg/kg/h for 20 h) had no effect on morphine consumption after surgery (Zarauza et al., 2000). The effect of continuous Mg i.v. administration during surgery was also assessed in patients undergoing lower limb orthopedic surgery in one study that enrolled 60 patients and randomized them to receive Mg or placebo; the results showed that patients in the Mg group reported less pain and required less morphine in the early postoperative setting (the first 24 h) (Dabbagh, Elyasi, Razavi, Fathi, & Rajaei, 2009). In contradiction with these results, postoperative Mg (bolus 50 mg/kg followed by 10 mg/kg/h infusion) administration did not decrease analgesic requirements when compared with placebo and was inferior to ketamine treatment in a clinical trial that enrolled 120 patients undergoing total abdominal hysterectomy (Arıkan, Aslan, Arıkan, Horasanlı, & But, 2016). Similar contradictory results are reported from other types of surgery as well—one study reported that coadministration of Mg and metamizol significantly enhanced metamizol's effect in terms of analgesic efficacy in posttonsillectomy patients (Tugrul et al., 2014), whereas another study reported that Mg has no influence on ropivacaine's efficacy in the same surgical procedure (Sun, Wu, Zhao, Chen, & Wang, 2015). A recently published review analyzed 18 trials involving neuraxial administration of $MgSO_4$ as a perioperative analgesic adjuvant and concluded that the time to first analgesic request increases by 72.2% after epidural Mg administration (Albrecht, Kirkham, Liu, & Brull, 2013). Another systematic review assessed intravenous Mg administration as an adjuvant to morphine for alleviating postoperative pain and concluded that coadministration of the two drugs has synergistic effects that decrease morphine requirements (Murphy et al., 2013).

Mg administration has also been investigated as a potential treatment in migraine. $MgSO_4$ was more effective and had a more rapid analgesic onset when compared with dexamethasone/metoclopramide in 70 patients referred to the emergency department for migraine headaches (Shahrami et al., 2015). Also, in a large pediatric study, 160 children diagnosed with migraine received acetaminophen and ibuprofen with or without Mg pretreatment. Results showed that pain intensity and frequency were significantly reduced in the Mg–ibuprofen and Mg–acetaminophen groups (Gallelli et al., 2014). In 2014, a metaanalysis assessed the effect of i.v. $MgSO_4$ in acute migraine and concluded that this treatment had no effect and that side effects/adverse events were more likely in Mg-treated patients (Choi & Parmar, 2014). However, 2 years later, another metaanalysis included articles that assessed the effect of oral and intravenous Mg administration on migraine. The authors included 21 high-quality studies and reported that intravenous Mg reduces pain in migraine attacks within 15–45 min, whereas oral Mg supplementation reduces both the frequency and the intensity of migraine (Chiu, Yeh, Huang, & Chen, 2016).

TAKE-HOME MESSAGES: MAGNESIUM AND PAIN

- Mg exerts its effects on pain through NMDA modulation and by blocking different types of calcium channels.
- As an analgesic, Mg has been shown to have some effect, largely dependent on dose, route of administration, and type of pain assessed.
- Mg is a very promising coanalgesic, although determining the best associations and the optimal dose still requires additional research.

MANGANESE

Theoretical Background

Manganese (Mn) is an essential cofactor for ATP due to its role in gluconeogenesis and has antioxidant effects through mitochondrial superoxide dismutase (Mn-SOD). In the central nervous system, Mn is mostly encountered in the basal ganglia, especially in regions that are also rich in iron (Preedy, Watson, & Martin, 2011). Mn toxicity clinically manifests similarly to Parkinson disease, which is why dopaminergic neurons have been considered as Mn's target. However, currently, the mechanisms underlying Mn's neurotoxicity also involve the metal's effect on GABA projections and on the extracellular levels of glutamate (Fitsanakis, Au, Erikson, & Aschner, 2006). Because it is an essential component of Mn-SOD, which converts superoxide into hydrogen peroxide, which is further metabolized to water and molecular oxygen, Mn deficiency may increase oxidative stress and contribute to mitochondrial dysfunction, both of which are mechanisms highly involved in pain modulation (Schwartz et al., 2009). Also, Mn blocks voltage-dependent Ca^{2+} channels and nerve-evoked neurotransmitter release, showcasing the two mechanisms through which it might influence pain transmission (Takeda, 2003).

Fundamental Studies

An animal study in the 1980s reported that the hyperalgesic effects of intracerebroventricular acetylcholine on the tail-flick test were reduced by Mn administration (Widman, Rosin, & Dewey, 1978). More recently, coadministration of Mn (3.6, 7.2, or 14.4 mg/kg) and tramadol was shown to significantly enhance tramadol's analgesic effect. These results were seen in all Mn doses but more intensely in the 7.2-mg schedule of administration. The added analgesic effect was greater than 20% when compared with tramadol alone (Alexa et al., 2015) and was mostly expressed in the tail-flick test, which suggests a spinal effect of Mn coadministration.

One other fundamental study assessed the effect of an Mn complex, MnL4, known to mimic SOD activity, in different fundamental pain models and compared it with standard analgesic drugs. Results indicated that i.p. administration of 15 mg/kg MnL4 3 h after subcutaneous carrageenan significantly increased mechanical thresholds, whereas ibuprofen and diclofenac (same dose as MnL4) had no effect. Similarly, 7 days after complete Freund's adjuvant intraarticular administration (fundamental model of inflammatory arthritis), MnL4 significantly increased the withdrawal threshold starting 15 min after i.p. administration, whereas ibuprofen and diclofenac (same dose as MnL4) had no effect. The authors also tested MnL4 in another osteoarthritis model where neuropathic pain is prevalent and found the substance to be as efficient as gabapentin (Di Cesare Mannelli et al., 2013).

Clinical Studies

Currently, to our knowledge, there are no clinical studies assessing the potential analgesic role of Mn in pain. On the contrary, available clinical data suggest that Mn has a pronociceptive effect in the clinical setting. Mn is well known to have neurotoxic effects and acute high-level exposure induces a condition called manganism, similar to Parkinson disease, that includes muscular pain and cephalalgia (Michalke & Fernsebner, 2014). In the past years, however, most available data have been derived from studies assessing the effect of chronic Mn exposure. For instance, Bouchard, Mergler, Baldwin, and Panisset (2008) assessed long-term exposure to Mn through inhalation and found that workers from an Mn-alloy production plant reported more often fatigue, musculoskeletal pain, and muscular weakness than matched controls 14 years after the plant had closed.

However, there are also some observations that indicate a potential role for Mn in analgesia. For instance, a small study involving women and their menstrual cycle symptoms found that decreased Mn levels are associated with increased pain intensity (Penland & Johnson, 1993). A more recent study found that a complex calcium polyuronate dressing supplemented with Zn and Mn significantly decreased pain in patients with necrotizing dermohypodermitis when compared with the reference therapeutic combination (Danino, Guberman, Mondié, Jebrane, & Servant, 2010).

TAKE-HOME MESSAGES: MANGANESE AND PAIN

- An optimal level of Mn is important in pain modulation: by influencing dopaminergic, glutamate, and GABA systems, Mn can be neurotoxic in high doses, while Mn deficiency promotes oxidation and mitochondrial dysfunction.
- Coadministration of Mn and tramadol is analgesic in animal studies and should be assessed in the clinical setting.

SELENIUM

Theoretical Background

Selenium (Se) is an essential trace element required for the optimal functioning of more than 25 proteins that mostly play a part in antioxidant defense. It competes with sulfur and can be incorporated in sulfur-containing amino acids such as cystine and methionine or in the structure of different enzymes from the glutathione/thioredoxin reductase family (Bujalska, Winecka, & Gumułka, 2008). In the central nervous system, Se is involved in neuronal signal transduction and in brain development, most likely due to its ability to inhibit apoptosis and mitochondrial stress and to modulate transient receptor potential (TRP) channels (Nazıroğlu, Çelik, Uğuz, & Bütün, 2015). Se modulates both cannabinoid and serotoninergic systems, thus exerting analgesic and antineuropathic activity (Del Fabbro et al., 2012). In its elemental form, Se is very rare and is acquired in humans mainly through diet, with various concentrations that depend on the local Se concentration in the water and soil. Organoselenium compounds are the form in which Se is most often used in medicine and research; these substances have glutathione peroxidase–like activity and have become very popular in the past years due to their important antioxidant effects (Savegnago et al., 2006); currently a large number of Se-based drugs are under development. Se is available as an over-the-counter dietary supplement, either alone or in combination with other trace elements and minerals; in large quantities it can be toxic, leading to a condition called selenosis characterized by nausea and vomiting, hair and nail anomalies, and headache (MacFarquhar et al., 2010).

Fundamental Studies

Oral administration of different doses of organoselenium compounds (1, 5, 10, 25, and 50 mg/kg, p.o.) was found to significantly decrease pain behavior in both phases of the paw formalin test and in capsaicin-induced and carrageenan-induced hyperalgesia. The compound exhibited analgesic effects in several other pain tests where nociception was induced by means of a chemical irritant (Donato et al., 2015). Diphenyl diselenide, one of the more promising organoselenium compounds, was assessed in two studies by either oral or subcutaneous route with favorable results—the substance significantly inhibited pain behavior in the formalin, capsaicin, glutamate, bradykinin, and writhing test (Savegnago et al., 2007; Nogueira, Quinhones, Jung, Zeni, & Rocha, 2003) with little to no associated toxicity.

Subcutaneous pretreatment with bis-selenide alkene derivatives was found to be effective in decreasing the number of writhes after acetic acid administration, and increased tail-flick latency and exerted antiinflammatory effects in capsaicin-induced pain, with an estimated potency two to four times higher than aspirin and acetaminophen. The effect was not reversed by naloxone, as it would have been for morphine treatment, suggesting an opioid-independent analgesic effect of the substances (Savegnago et al., 2006). Selol, another organoselenium compound, was assessed as a coanalgesic in rats with diabetic neuropathy after streptozocin administration. The authors found that pretreatment with selol significantly and persistently enhanced the effects of morphine, fentanyl, and buprenorphine; the cumulative effect was significantly higher than that of any of the substances in monotherapy (Bujalska et al., 2008).

Selol has also been investigated as an analgesic and coanalgesic of morphine in chemotherapy-induced neuropathy, with promising results from a study on mice with vincristine-induced neuropathy (Bujalska & Gumułka, 2008). In another model of induced neuropathy by brachial plexus avulsion, thermal and mechanical hyperalgesia were significantly alleviated by an oral organoselenic compound (25 mg/kg) administration. Its analgesic effects were prevented by selective cannabinoid receptor antagonists, suggesting that modulation of the cannabinoid system is a key mechanism by which Se exerts its effects (Del Fabbro et al., 2012). Another study assessed the effects of Se and riboflavin coadministration on a rat model testing cephalalgia and found that this drug combination had a protective effect on glutathione peroxidase (GSH), GSH-peroxidase, and antioxidant vitamin concentration and on the activity of brain microsomal Ca-ATPase (Nazıroğlu et al., 2015).

Clinical Studies

Clinical studies involving organoselenium compounds have so far focused on cancer and critically ill patients. In these populations, there is an increase in oxidative stress with augmented reactive oxygen and nitrogen species generation and decreased antioxidant defense, which promotes cell death, mitochondrial dysfunction, and systemic inflammation. In critically ill patients, plasma Se levels are significantly decreased when compared to those in the general population, an observation that has provided the theoretical rationale for assessing the benefit of Se supplementation in these patients. A metaanalysis published in 2014 included nine high-quality randomized clinical trials and concluded that Se supplementation is safe and may have a beneficial effect on 28-day mortality (Landucci, Mancinelli, De Gaudio, & Virgili, 2014). In cancer patients, Se supplementation (200 μg/day) was beneficial in decreasing abdominal pain in a small study that included women with ovarian cancer (Sieja & Talerczyk, 2004) and was associated with a lower incidence of radiation-associated lymphedema after radiotherapy (Micke et al., 2003). However, a Cochrane review from 2006 stated that there is insufficient evidence for recommending Se supplementation for alleviating side effects of cancer treatment or for increasing the quality of life in cancer patients (Dennert & Horneber, 2006). Furthermore, a more recent clinical trial reported that Se had only limited effects in preventing radiotherapy-associated toxicities in 39 head and neck cancer patients (Büntzel et al., 2010). To date, there are no formal recommendations indicating Se supplementation in critically ill or cancer patients.

Other areas of clinical research in which Se has been investigated include administering the substance as an analgesic in chronic pancreatitis, but available data are currently insufficient to draw any conclusions (Cai et al., 2013). Se, in coadministration with lycopene and *Serenoa repens*, was evaluated in chronic pelvic pain syndrome/chronic prostatitis and was found to be beneficial in terms of symptomatic improvement (Morgia et al., 2010). Also, patients with erosive-ulcerative lesions of oral lichen planus reported a significant decrease in pain intensity and had a superior trend toward healing when adding topical Se, vitamin A, and vitamin C to the standard treatment (topical corticosteroids and antifungals) (Belal, 2015).

TAKE-HOME MESSAGES: SELENIUM AND PAIN

- Organoselenium compounds are powerful antioxidants with potent antiinflammatory and analgesic effects as assessed by several animal studies.
- Their analgesic mechanism is opioid-independent and relies on Ca^{2+}, TRP, and mitochondrial modulation.
- Clinical studies assessing the effects of Se supplementation on pain are inconclusive, although Se seems to improve symptoms in conditions associated with increased oxidation.

COPPER

Theoretical Background

Copper (Cu) is essential to various metalloproteins and is involved in oxidation and electron transfer, which is why it has been hypothesized that it has analgesic and antiinflammatory effects (Gumilar et al., 2012). However, the metal can also behave as a prooxidant and proinflammatory agent (Turgut et al., 2013), depending on the available Cu quantity and the status of the patient. Cu is required for both ceruloplasmin and cytochrome *c* oxidase activity, proteins highly involved in the antioxidative and antiinflammatory defenses (Spain, Leist, & De Sousa, 2009). The metal's levels increase during inflammatory states and an adequate Cu intake has been suggested to modulate rheumatoid arthritis. In the central nervous system, Cu is involved in the synthesis of catecholamines, opioid peptides, and neuropeptides (Tamba et al., 2013) and through a high-affinity Cu-binding protein it can modulate NMDA and α-amino-3-hydroxy-5-methyl-4-isoxazolepropionic acid (AMPA) receptors, together with blocking T-type Ca^{2+} channels in a manner somewhat similar to Zn's (Preedy et al., 2011). Complexes of Cu and nonsteroidal antiinflammatory drugs (NSAIDs) seem to have special added effects on SOD (Agotegaray, Boeris, & Quinzani, 2010) and catechol oxidase, which leads to an enhanced protective role in chronic conditions such as cardiovascular disease, cancer, or diabetes.

Currently, in the clinical setting, Cu is mostly used as part of some intrauterine contraceptive devices (IUDs), due to Cu's toxicity to sperm. Also, Cu bracelets are available as over-the-counter remedies for arthritic pain.

Fundamental Studies

In one study, Cu salts [Cu chloride (0.5, 1.0, 2.0 mg/kg) and Cu sulfate (0.5, 1.0 mg/kg)] exhibited antinociceptive and antiinflammatory effects in mice assessed by means of the tail-flick, hot-plate, and writhing tests (Tamba et al., 2013).

Due to its aforementioned antiinflammatory effects, Cu has been most often assessed in coadministration with NSAIDs in different models of pain. Oral Cu salicylate was shown to decrease sensitivity to mechanical stimuli, in both arthritic and nonarthritic rats, with a more pronounced effect in arthritic animals, suggesting two synergistic mechanisms of action—inflammation-dependent and inflammation-independent (Jacka, Bernard, & Singer, 1983). A Cu(II)–fenoprofenate complex was compared with a calcium salt of fenoprofenate in mice undergoing carrageenan administration and was found to have more robust and longer-lasting antiinflammatory effects on paw edema (Agotegaray et al., 2010). Two years later, another study using fenoprofen–Cu complexes was published with similar results: adding Cu significantly enhanced fenoprofen's activity in both the writhing test and the second phase of the formalin inflammatory pain test—percentage inhibition was increased with almost 100% for both (Gumilar et al., 2012).

Clinical Studies

There is a limited amount of information regarding Cu's effect on pain. An excess of systemic Cu leads to digestive symptoms that include intense abdominal pain. An inappropriately high quantity of Cu in drinking water induced severe vomiting and abdominal pain in 12 people from rural Cheshire (Hoveyda, Yates, Bond, & Hunter, 2003). A case–control study assessed Cu levels in women with endometriosis, a well-known painful condition, and found that they were significantly increased when compared with Cu levels in age-matched controls (Turgut et al., 2013). On the other hand, clinical experience mostly acquired through isolated case reports (Spain et al., 2009) suggests that Cu deficiency leads to painful states secondary to neurological disorders—myeloneuropathy, distal paresthesias, and sensory ataxia.

As an analgesic, Cu has been assessed together with salicylate in topical gel application for pain relief in osteoarthritis. The Cu-salicylate gel (1.5 g twice daily) was more often associated with skin rashes when compared with the placebo and had no analgesic effect as assessed by the pain score and additional analgesic requirements in 116 patients with hip or knee osteoarthritis (Shackel, Day, Kellett, & Brooks, 1997). Cu has also been used in the treatment of osteoarthritis as a medical bracelet, available in several pharmacies, based on some nonrandomized clinical data from the 1980s (Walker & Keats, 1976) and on the 100-year-old concept of metallotherapy. However, subsequent studies did not support the efficacy of Cu bracelets and reported that 4 or 5 weeks of use did not influence pain as assessed by visual analog scales, nor did it decrease analgesic requirements, inflammation, or physical limitations secondary to the condition (Richmond et al., 2009; Richmond, Gunadasa, Bland, & Macpherson, 2013).

In 2012, a topical formulation containing Cu sulfate and hypericum perforatum was assessed in patients with herpes skin lesions. Almost 150 participants with active lesions were randomized in 2 groups—one that received the aforementioned gel (topical applications) and the other that received standard 5% acyclovir cream. Results indicated a superior effect of the new formula, with a significant decrease of both burning/stinging sensations and symptoms of acute pain (Clewell, Barnes, Endres, Ahmed, & Ghambeer, 2012).

Numerous studies have been performed assessing the risk/benefit ratio of Cu-IUDs and the incidence of local pain due to growing concern regarding Cu's toxicity. One clinical trial assessed the differences between Cu-IUD users and women who did not use contraception and found that Cu-IUD is associated with a higher incidence of localized pain (Sakinci et al., 2016), but most available data indicate that there is no significant difference between IUDs, oral contraceptives, and progestogen injections (Li et al., 2004), although levonorgestrel-releasing IUDs seem to be better tolerated than Cu-IUDs (Skrzypulec & Drosdzol, 2008) and to decrease the incidence of dysmenorrhea (Kelekci, Kelekci, & Yilmaz, 2012).

TAKE-HOME MESSAGES: COPPER AND PAIN

- Cu can either promote or alleviate pain and inflammation depending on dose and preexisting plasma Cu levels.
- Cu significantly enhances the effect of NSAIDs on pain and inflammation and clinical studies should focus on developing and testing topical and oral Cu–NSAID combinations.
- Cu bracelets are not efficient in osteoarthritis.

STRONTIUM

Introduction

Strontium (Sr) is a nonessential trace element currently used in the ceramic and glass industry. In its natural state, it is nonradioactive (stable Sr) and human exposure occurs most often through inhalation and water ingestion (Gad, 2014). Because it is a chemical analogue of Ca^{2+}, Sr will replace Ca^{2+} in the bones and in all other tissues with high Ca^{2+} concentration. The relationship between Sr and pain is not completely understood and is mainly based on its similarity to Ca^{2+}. In the clinical setting, current therapeutic uses of Sr in painful conditions include using Sr salts such as Sr ranelate (SR) in preventing osteoporotic fractures (Meunier et al., 2004) and radioactive Sr (Sr 89) is frequently used to treat painful bone metastases (Furubayashi, Negishi, Ura, Hirai, & Nakamura, 2015). Since the mechanisms and roles of radioactive Sr in oncology are well determined, we will focus only on presenting the data available for stable Sr and Sr salts and their effect on pain.

Fundamental Studies

Intracerebroventricular administration of Sr has an antinociceptive effect in mice as assessed by the tail-flick test (Welch, Vocci, & Dewey, 1983). In dogs, SR administration was associated with a decrease in the progression of articular osteoarthritis as assessed by both functional and structural tests (Pelletier et al., 2013) and similar results were obtained after administering SR in a rat model of osteoarthritic pain (Yu et al., 2013). Due to its antiinflammatory effects, SR was also assessed in a rat model of ulcerative collitis and the authors reported a significant improvement in the expression of inflammatory cytokines and in histological colitis-induced changes in rats treated with SR—the outcomes of SR-treated groups were similar to those of prednisolone-treated groups (Topal et al., 2014).

Clinical Studies

Besides its effects on osteoporosis, an increasing body of evidence from fundamental studies indicated that SR has antiinflammatory effects and might be beneficial in painful conditions of the bone. As such, the SEKOIA trial aimed to assess the effects of SR in the treatment of knee osteoarthritis and found that 58% of the patients who received SR 2 g/day experienced a statistically significant decrease in pain intensity, especially after 6 months of treatment (Bruyere et al., 2008). Subsequently, SR was assessed in rheumatoid arthritis in one case report and the authors concluded that it has similar beneficial outcomes (Liu, Shen, & Chen, 2013).

In the clinical setting, stable Sr was investigated as a topical agent in the treatment of dermatologic disorders. One small clinical study found that using a lactic acid and Sr cream is associated with less pain, burning, and stinging than an ammonium lactate lotion 12% (Haddican, Gagliotti, & Lebwohl, 2013).

As a desensitizing agent, Sr-containing toothpaste was shown to alleviate painful local symptoms in hypersensitive patients, according to data published after a small clinical trial (Liu & Hu, 2012). Two years after, the results of a larger trial became available, where the authors had reached a similar conclusion: 10% Sr chloride gel significantly lowered the pain score in patients with dentin hypersensitivity (Antoniazzi, Machado, Grellmann, Santos, & Zanatta, 2014). One other study pointed out the benefits of using an Sr acetate/silica toothpaste for pain reduction in dentine hypersensitivity (West et al., 2013).

TAKE-HOME MESSAGES: STRONTIUM AND PAIN

- Sr most likely modulates bone pain due to its antiinflammatory effects.
- Because it is already used in medical practice, further clinical trials of SR in osteoarthritis should be performed as soon as possible in order to consolidate the findings of the SEKOIA trial.
- Sr is a promising ingredient for oral gels and toothpastes used for dentin hypersensitivity.

OTHER ESSENTIAL AND NONESSENTIAL TRACE ELEMENTS

Aluminum is a light ductile metal intensely used in industry. Routes of exposure include inhalation and ingestion, although the rate of absorption is quite low—2.4% through inhalation and a maximum of 10% through ingestion (Nordberg, Koji, & Nordberg, 2015). The metal has several uses in medical practice, such as: (1) it is used as an adjuvant in several types of vaccines; (2) aluminum hydroxide, aluminum phosphate, and sucralfate are used in dyspepsia and gastroesophageal reflux disease; (3) aluminum salts are used in dialysis as phosphate binders (to decrease plasma phosphate levels); and (4) aluminum chloride, aluminum–zirconium–glycine complex, and aluminum chlorohydrate are used in antiperspirants and in the management of hyperhidrosis (Yokel, 2014). Current fundamental research indicates that high aluminum doses are toxic for most organs, although the metal is particularly recognized for its neurotoxicity—several studies have linked increased aluminum exposure with the development of Alzheimer disease (Krewski et al., 2007; Walton, 2014) and Parkinson disease (Altschuler, 1999) due to aluminum's age-related increase in the brain, activation of the glia, and cytokine production (Campbell, Becaria, Lahiri, Sharman, & Bondy, 2004) and its prooxidant effects (Exley, 2004). Aluminum is also toxic to the mitochondria by inhibiting mitochondrial monoamine oxidase; the metal depletes glutathione and impairs the activity of cytochrome *c* (Bosetti et al., 2001).

Animal studies frequently use aluminum administration to test neuroprotective agents and antiinflammatory substances—a prostate extract with aluminum hydroxide injection was reported to be a valid animal model of chronic pelvic pain syndrome (Qi et al., 2012) and oral aluminum chloride administration was used as a model of oxidative stress, procarcinogenicity, and neurotoxicity (Abdel Moneim, 2012). A recently published study found that pretreatment with aluminum chloride intensified cold allodynia induced by oxaliplatin and increased the expression of TRPA1 in dorsal root ganglia (DRGs) exposed to platinum-based drugs, suggesting that the metal worsens this type of chemotherapy-induced neuropathy (Park et al., 2015). In humans, chronic aluminum exposure is associated with airway inflammation and administration of aluminum-containing vaccines is believed to be responsible for macrophagic myofasciitis, a local lesion that appears due to the long-term persistence of aluminum at the site of vaccination (Israeli, Agmon-Levin, Blank, & Shoenfeld, 2011) and leads to arthromyalgias, muscle weakness, marked asthenia, hemisensory or sensorimotor symptoms, bilateral pyramidal signs, and chronic fatigue (Ragunathan-Thangarajah et al., 2013).

Cadmium is a highly toxic heavy metal considered to be an environmental contaminant and a human carcinogen with a very long half-life (Wang & Du, 2013). Exposure is most often related to occupational hazard or tobacco use. In animal studies, intraperitoneal cadmium administration was associated with systemic inflammation and an increase in oxidative stress that, in turn, led to thromboembolic events (Fahim et al., 2012), changes associated with hyperalgesia, and pain processing anomalies. Another potential mechanism for cadmium's effect on pain is elevating intracellular Ca^{2+} concentrations and activating TRPA1—in vitro cadmium administration significantly stimulated mouse sensory neurons and intraplantar cadmium injection induced a formalin-like local effect (Miura et al., 2013). In humans, acute cadmium inhalation determines metal fume fever, characterized by several painful symptoms such as headache and chest pain (Beton, Andrews, Davies, Howells, & Smith, 1966), and acute ingestion leads to abdominal pain, diarrhea, nausea, and vomiting that occur within minutes (Nordberg et al., 2015). Chronic cadmium exposure is associated with severe pain in the joints and spine, secondary to either cadmium's toxic effect on the kidneys or cadmium's effect on bone metabolism (Kazantzis, 2004; Nordberg et al., 2015).

Nickel is a heavy and malleable transition metal intensely used in different industries, from jewelry to aeronautics. It enters the body through inhalation or ingestion and it is currently considered a human carcinogen (Yalçın Tepe, 2014). There are little data regarding the relationship between nickel and pain. In 1988, three different concentrations of intrathecal nickel (2.5, 5.0, and 10.0 μmol/mouse) were found to have no effect on the writhing test (Doğrul & Yeşilyurt, 1998). More recently, another group of researchers found that intrathecal pretreatment with nickel chloride (1–10 μg) dose dependently decreased pain behavior after formalin administration, most likely due to the metal's blocking effect on spinal T-type Ca^{2+} channels (Cheng, Lin, Chen, Yang, & Chiou, 2007). Similar results were reported in 2015 in mice with chronic pain after nerve ligation—a 7-day nickel chloride administration schedule was associated with a decrease in both mechanical allodynia and thermal hyperalgesia (Chen et al., 2015).

To our knowledge, nickel has not yet been assessed as an analgesic/coanalgesic in the clinical setting. Most data available involve reports of pain secondary to nickel allergy after orthopedic or orthodontic implants (Dezulovic, Baur, Stangl, Baur, & Lenz, 2012) or painful complaints (headache, back pain, chest pain) of people with chronic Ni inhalation (Ekosse, 2011).

Bromine has been recently established as an essential trace element, necessary for the collagen IV scaffold involved in the functionality of the basement membranes of all animal phyla (McCall et al., 2014). Historically, bromine has been used as a sedative and as an anticonvulsant (most likely due to its indirect modulation of the GABA-A receptor), but the FDA has discouraged the use of Br salts since 1975, when Bromo-Seltzer (a well-known sedative) was removed from the market (Garnier, Rambourg-Schepens, Müller, & Hallier, 1996). Although some countries still allow bromide salts as anticonvulsants, they are currently mostly limited to veterinary use (Steinmetz, Tipold, Bilzer, & Schenk, 2012). Animal studies indicate that adding bromine to propofol (4-bromopropofol) is associated with lower rates of discharge in ventral horn neurons, most likely through a glycine-mediated mechanism, an effect that could lead to muscle relaxation and have potential clinical benefits in chronic low back pain (Eckle et al., 2014). Unfortunately, data from fundamental studies of bromine are limited and most studies are outdated.

In clinical practice, exposure to methyl bromide is well documented due to the compound's use as an insecticidal fumigant for crops. Acute poisoning is associated with headache, dizziness, abdominal pain, nausea, vomiting, and visual disturbances (Suwanlaong & Phanthumchinda, 2008). Long-term side effects include muscle cramps, convulsions, peripheral neuropathy, demyelination, degeneration of neurons, and gliosis, together with significant changes in EEG patterns (Verberk, Rooyakkers-Beemster, de Vlieger, & van Vliet, 1979). In countries that still allow their use, studies indicate that bromine salts are a good choice as drugs of tertiary choice in the treatment of children with epilepsy (Korinthenberg, Burkart, Woelfle, Moenting, & Ernst, 2007), although they have a narrow therapeutic index and their overdose is associated with lethargy, drowsiness, and headache. Cutaneous bromine exposure is most often reported to be toxic; however, small doses seem to be beneficial in dermatologic conditions such as psoriasis as indicated by a clinical study published in 2014 where highly mineralized bromine–iodine brine was shown to be highly effective in inhibiting lipid peroxidation and inducing clinical remission of psoriasis (El'kin, Koriukina, Datskovskiĭ, & Plotnikova, 2014).

TAKE-HOME MESSAGES: OTHER TRACE ELEMENTS AND PAIN

- Aluminum is neurotoxic, proinflammatory, and prooxidant. Animal and human studies indicate that it is hyperalgesic due to both local and systemic effects.
- Cadmium is a proinflammatory metal with hyperalgesic and allodynic affects.
- Nickel blocks spinal T-type Ca^{2+} channels, thus blocking pain transmission.
- The relationship between bromine and pain is insufficiently investigated, but bromine-containing combinations (e.g., bromine–propofol) may have clinical benefit.

CONCLUSIONS

Trace elements influence pain transmission and perception by modulating several key peripheral or central elements of the pain pathway. Most trace elements have more than one analgesic mechanism, acting on inflammation, oxidative stress, mitochondrial dysfunction, and ion channels or receptors involved in pain pathways. More and more preclinical and clinical studies have focused in recent years on exploring the potential use of trace elements as cheaper and safer alternatives to analgesics. A promising new direction in the field of pain research has emerged—the use of trace elements as co-analgesics that enhance the drug's effect and thus lead to better pain control or lower analgesic requirements. However, these studies need to enter the daily practice with caution due to the risk of overdose, toxicity, and hyperalgesia associated with chronic supplementation of some of these minerals and metals.

References

Abdel Moneim, A. E. (2012). Evaluating the potential role of pomegranate peel in aluminum-induced oxidative stress and histopathological alterations in brain of female eats. *Biological Trace Element Research*, *150*(1–3), 328–336.

Abou-Mohamed, G., el-Kashef, H. A., Salem, H. A., & Elmazar, M. M. (1995). Effect of zinc on the anti-inflammatory and ulcerogenic activities of indometacin and diclofenac. *Pharmacology*, *50*(4), 266–272.

Agarwal, A., Dhiraj, S., Raza, M., Pandey, R., Pandey, C. K., Singh, P. K., Singh, U., & Gupta, D. (2004). Vein pretreatment with magnesium sulfate to prevent pain on injection of propofol is not justified. *Canadian Journal of Anaesthesia = Journal Canadien D'anesthésie*, *51*(2), 130–133.

Agotegaray, M., Boeris, M., & Quinzani, O. (2010). Significant anti-inflammatory properties of a copper(II) fenoprofenate complex compared with its parent drug. Physical and chemical characterization of the complex. *Journal of the Brazilian Chemical Society*, *21*(12), 2294–2301.

Albrecht, E., Kirkham, K. R., Liu, S. S., & Brull, R. (2013). The analgesic efficacy and safety of neuraxial magnesium sulphate: a quantitative review. *Anaesthesia*, *68*(2), 190–202.

Alexa, T., Aurelia, M., Tudor, V., & Bogdan, T. (2015). Enhanced analgesic effects of tramadol and common trace element coadministration in mice. *Journal of Neuroscience Research*, *93*(10), 1534–1541.

Alipour, M., Tabari, M., & Alipour, M. (2014). Paracetamol, ondansetron, granisetron, magnesium sulfate and lidocaine and reduced propofol injection pain. *Iranian Red Crescent Medical Journal*, *16*(3), e16086.

Altschuler, E. (1999). Aluminum-containing antacids as a cause of idiopathic Parkinson's disease. *Medical Hypotheses*, *53*(1), 22–23.

Antoniazzi, R. P., Machado, M. E., Grellmann, A. P., Santos, R. C. V., & Zanatta, F. B. (2014). Effectiveness of a desensitizing agent for topical and home use for dentin hypersensitivity: a randomized clinical trial. *American Journal of Dentistry*, *27*(5), 251–257.

Arai, Y. -C. P., Hatakeyama, N., Nishihara, M., Ikeuchi, M., Kurisuno, M., & Ikemoto, T. (2013). Intravenous lidocaine and magnesium for management of intractable trigeminal neuralgia: a case series of nine patients. *Journal of Anesthesia*, *27*(6), 960–962.

Arbabi-kalati, F., Arbabi-kalati, F., Deghatipour, M., & Ansari Moghadam, A. (2012). Evaluation of the efficacy of zinc sulfate in the prevention of chemotherapy-induced mucositis: a double-blind randomized clinical trial. *Archives of Iranian Medicine*, *15*(7), 413–417.

Arıkan, M., Aslan, B., Arıkan, O., Horasanlı, E., & But, A. (2016). Comparison of the effects of magnesium and ketamine on postoperative pain and morphine consumption. A double-blind randomized controlled clinical study. *Acta Cirúrgica Brasileira/Sociedade Brasileira Para Desenvolvimento Pesquisa Em Cirurgia*, *31*(1), 67–73.

Bansal, P., Baduni, N., Bhalla, J., & Mahawar, B. (2015). A comparative evaluation of magnesium sulphate and nitroglycerine as potential adjuncts to lidocaine in intravenous regional anaesthesia. *International Journal of Critical Illness and Injury Science*, *5*(1), 27–31.

Baskol, M., Ozbakir, O., Coşkun, R., Baskol, G., Saraymen, R., & Yucesoy, M. (2004). The role of serum zinc and other factors on the prevalence of muscle cramps in non-alcoholic cirrhotic patients. *Journal of Clinical Gastroenterology*, *38*(6), 524–529.

Belal, M. H. (2015). Management of symptomatic erosive-ulcerative lesions of oral lichen planus in an adult Egyptian population using selenium-ACE combined with topical corticosteroids plus antifungal agent. *Contemporary Clinical Dentistry*, *6*(4), 454–460.

Beton, D. C., Andrews, G. S., Davies, H. J., Howells, L., & Smith, G. F. (1966). Acute cadmium fume poisoning. Five cases with one death from renal necrosis. *British Journal of Industrial Medicine*, *23*(4), 292–301.

Biernat, P., Musiał, W., Gosławska, D., & Pluta, J. (2014). The impact of selected preparations of trace elements—magnesium, potassium, calcium, and zinc on the release of diclofenac sodium from enteric coated tablets and from sustained release capsules. *Advances in Clinical and Experimental Medicine: Official Organ Wroclaw Medical University*, *23*(2), 205–213.

Bosetti, F., Solaini, G., Tendi, E. A., Chikhale, E. G., Chandrasekaran, K., & Rapoport, S. I. (2001). Mitochondrial cytochrome *c* oxidase subunit III is selectively down-regulated by aluminum exposure in PC12S cells. *Neuroreport*, *12*(4), 721–724.

Bouchard, M., Mergler, D., Baldwin, M. E., & Panisset, M. (2008). Manganese cumulative exposure and symptoms: a follow-up study of alloy workers. *Neurotoxicology*, *29*(4), 577–583.

Brousseau, D. C., Scott, J. P., Badaki-Makun, O., Darbari, D. S., Chumpitazi, C. E., Airewele, G. E., Ellison, A. M., et al. (2015). A multicenter randomized controlled trial of intravenous magnesium for sickle cell pain crisis in children. *Blood*, *126*(14), 1651–1657.

Brousseau, D. C., Scott, J. P., Hillery, C. A., & Panepinto, J. A. (2004). The effect of magnesium on length of stay for pediatric sickle cell pain crisis. *Academic Emergency Medicine: Official Journal of the Society for Academic Emergency Medicine*, *11*(9), 968–972.

Bruyere, O., Delferriere, D., Roux, C., Wark, J. D., Spector, T., Devogelaer, J. -P., Brixen, K., et al. (2008). Effects of strontium ranelate on spinal osteoarthritis progression. *Annals of the Rheumatic Diseases*, *67*(3), 335–339.

Bujalska, M., & Gumułka, S. W. (2008). Effect of selenium compound (selol) on the opioid activity in vincristine induced hyperalgesia. *Neuroendocrinology Letters*, *29*(4), 552–557.

Bujalska, M., Makulska-Nowak, H., & Gumułka, S. W. (2009). Magnesium ions and opioid agonists in vincristine-induced neuropathy. *Pharmacological Reports: PR*, *61*(6), 1096–1104.

Bujalska, M., Winecka, R., & Gumułka, S. W. (2008). Effect of selol on the opioids activity in streptozotocin induced hyperalgesia. *Acta Poloniae Pharmaceutica*, *65*(6), 691–696.

Büntzel, J., Riesenbeck, D., Glatzel, M., Berndt-Skorka, R., Riedel, T., Mücke, R., Kisters, K., et al. (2010). Limited effects of selenium substitution in the prevention of radiation-associated toxicities. Results of a randomized study in head and neck cancer patients. *Anticancer Research*, *30*(5), 1829–1832.

Cai, G. -H., Huang, J., Zhao, Y., Chen, J., Wu, H. -H., Dong, Y. -L., Smith, H. S., Li, Y. -Q., Wang, W., & Wu, S. -X. (2013). Antioxidant therapy for pain relief in patients with chronic pancreatitis: systematic review and meta-analysis. *Pain Physician*, *16*(6), 521–532.

Campbell, A., Becaria, A., Lahiri, D. K., Sharman, K., & Bondy, S. C. (2004). Chronic exposure to aluminum in drinking water increases inflammatory parameters selectively in the brain. *Journal of Neuroscience Research, 75*(4), 565–572.

Chen, Y. L., Tsaur, M. L., Wang, S. W., Wang, T. Y., Hung, Y. C., Lin, C. S., Chang, Y. F., Wang, Y. C., Shiue, S. J., & Cheng, J. K. (2015). Chronic intrathecal infusion of mibefradil, ethosuximide and nickel attenuates nerve ligation-induced pain in rats. *British Journal of Anaesthesia, 115*(1), 105–111.

Cheng, J. -K., Lin, C. -S., Chen, C. -C., Yang, J. -R., & Chiou, L. -C. (2007). Effects of intrathecal injection of T-type calcium channel blockers in the rat formalin test. *Behavioural Pharmacology, 18*(1), 1–8.

Chiu, H. -Y., Yeh, T. -H., Huang, Y. -C., & Chen, P. -Y. (2016). Effects of intravenous and oral magnesium on reducing migraine: a meta-analysis of randomized controlled trials. *Pain Physician, 19*(1), E97–E112.

Choi, H., & Parmar, N. (2014). The use of intravenous magnesium sulphate for acute migraine: meta-analysis of randomized controlled trials. *European Journal of Emergency Medicine: Official Journal of the European Society for Emergency Medicine, 21*(1), 2–9.

Clewell, A., Barnes, M., Endres, J. R., Ahmed, M., & Ghambeer, D. K. S. (2012). Efficacy and tolerability assessment of a topical formulation containing copper sulfate and hypericum perforatum on patients with herpes skin lesions: a comparative, randomized controlled trial. *Journal of Drugs in Dermatology: JDD, 11*(2), 209–215.

Crosby, V., Wilcock, A., & Corcoran, R. (2000). The safety and efficacy of a single dose (500 mg or 1 g) of intravenous magnesium sulfate in neuropathic pain poorly responsive to strong opioid analgesics in patients with cancer. *Journal of Pain and Symptom Management, 19*(1), 35–39.

Curtis, L. (2016). Nutritional research may be useful in treating tendon injuries. *Nutrition, 32*(6), 617–619.

Dabbagh, A., Elyasi, H., Razavi, S. S., Fathi, M., & Rajaei, S. (2009). Intravenous magnesium sulfate for post-operative pain in patients undergoing lower limb orthopedic surgery. *Acta Anaesthesiologica Scandinavica, 53*(8), 1088–1091.

Danino, A. M., Guberman, S., Mondié, J. -M., Jebrane, A., & Servant, J. -M. (2010). Calcium polyuronate dressing supplemented with zinc and manganese (Trionic®) in necrotizing dermohypodermitis of the extremities: a randomized multicentre study. *Annals of Burns and Fire Disasters, 23*(2), 95–101.

De Franceschi, L., Bachir, D., Galacteros, F., Tchernia, G., Cynober, T., Neuberg, D., Beuzard, Y., & Brugnara, C. (2000). Oral magnesium pidolate: effects of long-term administration in patients with sickle cell disease. *British Journal of Haematology, 108*(2), 284–289.

Del Fabbro, L., Borges Filho, C., Cattelan Souza, L., Savegnago, L., Alves, D., Henrique Schneider, P., de Salles, H. D., & Jesse, C. R. (2012). Effects of Se-phenyl thiazolidine-4-carboselenoate on mechanical and thermal hyperalgesia in brachial plexus avulsion in mice: mediation by cannabinoid CB1 and CB2 receptors. *Brain Research, 1475*(October), 31–36.

Dennert, G., & Horneber, M. (2006). Selenium for alleviating the side effects of chemotherapy, radiotherapy and surgery in cancer patients. *The Cochrane Database of Systematic Reviews*(3), CD005037.

Dezulovic, M., Baur, U., Stangl, R., Baur, W., & Lenz, E. (2012). Nickel allergy and painful unicondylar knee arthroplasty. *Zeitschrift Für Orthopädie Und Unfallchirurgie, 150*(3), 269–271.

Dhillon, K. S., Singh, J., & Lyall, J. S. (2011). A new horizon into the pathobiology, etiology and treatment of migraine. *Medical Hypotheses, 77*(1), 147–151.

Di Cesare Mannelli, L., Bani, D., Bencini, A., Brandi, M. L., Calosi, L., Cantore, M., Carossino, A. M., Ghelardini, C., Valtancoli, B., & Failli, P. (2013). Therapeutic effects of the superoxide dismutase mimetic compound MnIIMe2DO2A on experimental articular pain in rats. *Mediators of Inflammation, 2013*(January), 905360.

Doğrul, A., & Yeşilyurt, O. (1998). Effects of intrathecally administered aminoglycoside antibiotics, calcium-channel blockers, nickel and calcium on acetic acid-induced writhing test in mice. *General Pharmacology, 30*(4), 613–616.

Donato, F., Pavin, N. F., Goes, A. T. R., Souza, L. C., Soares, L. C., Rodrigues, O. E. D., Jesse, C. R., & Savegnago, L. (2015). Antinociceptive and anti-hyperalgesic effects of bis(4-methylbenzoyl) diselenide in mice: evidence for the mechanism of action. *Pharmaceutical Biology, 53*(3), 395–403.

Eby, G. A., & Halcomb, W. W. (2006). High-dose zinc to terminate angina pectoris: a review and hypothesis for action by ICAM inhibition. *Medical Hypotheses, 66*(1), 169–172.

Eckle, V. S., Grasshoff, C., Mirakaj, V., O'Neill, P. M., Berry, N. G., Leuwer, M., & Antkowiak, B. (2014). 4-Bromopropofol decreases action potential generation in spinal neurons by inducing a glycine receptor-mediated tonic conductance. *British Journal of Pharmacology, 171*(24), 5790–5801.

Ekosse, G-I. E. (2011). Health status within the precincts of a nickel–copper mining and smelting environment. *African Health Sciences, 11*(1), 90–96.

El'kin, V. D., Koriukina, I. P., Datskovskiĭ, I. A. S., & Plotnikova, E. V. (2014). The clinical results and lipid peroxidation dynamics in the patients presenting with psoriasis treated by the applications of a natural highly mineralized bromine–iodine brine. *Voprosy Kurortologii, Fizioterapii, I Lechebnoĭ Fizicheskoĭ Kultury*(2), 38–42.

Ertekin, M. V., Koç, M., Karslioglu, I., & Sezen, O. (2004). Zinc sulfate in the prevention of radiation-induced oropharyngeal mucositis: a prospective, placebo-controlled, randomized study. *International Journal of Radiation Oncology, Biology, Physics, 58*(1), 167–174.

Exley, C. (2004). The pro-oxidant activity of aluminum. *Free Radical Biology & Medicine, 36*(3), 380–387.

Fahim, M. A., Nemmar, A., Dhanasekaran, S., Singh, S., Shafiullah, M., Yasin, J., Zia, S., & Hasan, M. Y. (2012). Acute cadmium exposure causes systemic and thromboembolic events in mice. *Physiological Research/Academia Scientiarum Bohemoslovaca, 61*(1), 73–80.

Farsi, L., Afshari, K., Keshavarz, M., Naghib Zadeh, M., Memari, F., & Norouzi-Javidan, A. (2015a). Postinjury treatment with magnesium sulfate attenuates neuropathic pains following spinal cord injury in male rats. *Behavioural Pharmacology, 26*(3), 315–320.

Farsi, L., Naghib Zadeh, M., Afshari, K., Norouzi-Javidan, A., Ghajarzadeh, M., Naghshband, Z., & Keshavarz, M. (2015b). Effects of combining methylprednisolone with magnesium sulfate on neuropathic pain and functional recovery following spinal cord injury in male rats. *Acta Medica Iranica, 53*(3), 149–157.

Fitsanakis, V. A., Au, C., Erikson, K. M., & Aschner, M. (2006). The effects of manganese on glutamate, dopamine and γ-aminobutyric acid regulation. *Neurochemistry International, 48*(6–7), 426–433.

Furubayashi, N., Negishi, T., Ura, S., Hirai, Y., & Nakamura, Mo. (2015). Palliative effects and adverse events of strontium-89 for prostate cancer patients with bone metastasis. *Molecular and Clinical Oncology, 3*(1), 257–263.

Gad, S. C. (2014). *Encyclopedia of toxicology*. San Diego, CA: Elsevier.

Galgon, R. E., Strube, P., Heier, J., Groth, J., Wang, S., & Schroeder, K. M. (2015). Magnesium sulfate with lidocaine for preventing propofol injection pain: a randomized, double-blind, placebo-controlled trial. *Journal of Anesthesia, 29*(2), 206–211.

Gallelli, L., Avenoso, T., Falcone, D., Palleria, C., Peltrone, F., Esposito, M., De Sarro, G., Carotenuto, M., & Guidetti, V. (2014). Effects of acetaminophen and ibuprofen in children with migraine receiving preventive treatment with magnesium. *Headache, 54*(2), 313–324.

Garnier, R., Rambourg-Schepens, M. O., Müller, A., & Hallier, E. (1996). Glutathione transferase activity and formation of macromolecular adducts in two cases of acute methyl bromide poisoning. *Occupational and Environmental Medicine, 53*(3), 211–215.

Gaskin, D. J., & Patrick, R. (2012). The economic costs of pain in the United States. *The Journal of Pain: Official Journal of the American Pain Society*, *13*(8), 715–724.

Goldman, R. D., Mounstephen, W., Kirby-Allen, M., & Friedman, J. N. (2013). Intravenous magnesium sulfate for vaso-occlusive episodes in sickle cell disease. *Pediatrics*, *132*(6), e1634–e1641.

Gumilar, F., Agotegaray, M., Bras, C., Gandini, N. A., Minetti, A., & Quinzani, O. (2012). Anti-nociceptive activity and toxicity evaluation of Cu(II)–fenoprofenate complexes in mice. *European Journal of Pharmacology*, *675*(1–3), 32–39.

Haddican, M., Gagliotti, M., & Lebwohl, M. (2013). Reduced burning and stinging associated with topical application of lactic acid 10% with strontium versus ammonium lactate 12%. *Cutis*, *91*(5), 260–262.

Hayashi, H., Kobayashi, R., Suzuki, A., Ishihara, M., Nakamura, N., Kitagawa, J., Kanemura, N., et al. (2014). Polaprezinc prevents oral mucositis in patients treated with high-dose chemotherapy followed by hematopoietic stem cell transplantation. *Anticancer Research*, *34*(12), 7271–7277.

Hershman, D. L., Lacchetti, C., Dworkin, R. H., Lavoie Smith, E. M., Bleeker, J., Cavaletti, G., Chauhan, C., et al. (2014). Prevention and management of chemotherapy-induced peripheral neuropathy in survivors of adult cancers: American Society of Clinical Oncology clinical practice guideline. *Journal of Clinical Oncology: Official Journal of the American Society of Clinical Oncology*, *32*(18), 1941–1967.

Hoveyda, N., Yates, B., Bond, C. R., & Hunter, P. R. (2003). A cluster of cases of abdominal pain possibly associated with high copper levels in a private water supply. *Journal of Environmental Health*, *66*(2), 29–32.

Hu, H., Bandell, M., Petrus, M. J., Zhu, M. X., & Patapoutian, A. (2009). Zinc activates damage-sensing TRPA1 ion channels. *Nature Chemical Biology*, *5*(3), 183–190.

Israeli, E., Agmon-Levin, N., Blank, M., & Shoenfeld, Y. (2011). Macrophagic myofaciitis a vaccine (alum) autoimmune-related disease. *Clinical Reviews in Allergy & Immunology*, *41*(2), 163–168.

Jacka, T., Bernard, C. C., & Singer, G. (1983). Copper salicylate as an anti-inflammatory and analgesic agent in arthritic rats. *Life Sciences*, *32*(9), 1023–1030.

Jo, S. M., Danscher, G., Schrøder, H. D., & Suh, S. W. (2008). Depletion of vesicular zinc in dorsal horn of spinal cord causes increased neuropathic pain in mice. *Biometals: An International Journal on the Role of Metal Ions in Biology, Biochemistry, and Medicine*, *21*(2), 151–158.

Kashefi, F., Khajehei, M., Tabatabaeichehr, M., Alavinia, M., & Asili, J. (2014). Comparison of the effect of ginger and zinc sulfate on primary dysmenorrhea: a placebo-controlled randomized trial. *Pain Management Nursing: Official Journal of the American Society of Pain Management Nurses*, *15*(4), 826–833.

Kazantzis, G. (2004). Cadmium, osteoporosis and calcium metabolism. *Biometals: An International Journal on the Role of Metal Ions in Biology, Biochemistry, and Medicine*, *17*(5), 493–498.

Kelekci, S., Kelekci, K. H., & Yilmaz, B. (2012). Effects of levonorgestrel-releasing intrauterine system and T380A intrauterine copper device on dysmenorrhea and days of bleeding in women with and without adenomyosis. *Contraception*, *86*(5), 458–463.

Kesmati, M., & Torabi, M. (2014). Interaction between analgesic effect of nano and conventional size of zinc oxide and opioidergic system activity in animal model of acute pain. *Basic and Clinical Neuroscience*, *5*(1), 80–87.

Kim, Y. H., Lee, P. B., & Oh, T. K. (2015). Is magnesium sulfate effective for pain in chronic postherpetic neuralgia patients comparing with ketamine infusion therapy? *Journal of Clinical Anesthesia*, *27*(4), 296–300.

King, S., Chambers, C. T., Huguet, A., MacNevin, R. C., McGrath, P. J., Parker, L., & MacDonald, A. J. (2011). The epidemiology of chronic pain in children and adolescents revisited: a systematic review. *Pain*, *152*(12), 2729–2738.

Korinthenberg, R., Burkart, P., Woelfle, C., Moenting, J. S., & Ernst, J. P. (2007). Pharmacology, efficacy, and tolerability of potassium bromide in childhood epilepsy. *Journal of Child Neurology*, *22*(4), 414–418.

Krewski, D., Yokel, R. A., Nieboer, E., Borchelt, D., Cohen, J., Harry, J., Kacew, S., Lindsay, J., Mahfouz, A. M., & Rondeau, V. (2007). Human health risk assessment for aluminium, aluminium oxide, and aluminium hydroxide, Journal of Toxicology and Environmental Health. Part B. *Critical Reviews*, *10*(suppl. 1), 1–269.

Kugelmas, M. (2000). Preliminary observation: oral zinc sulfate replacement is effective in treating muscle cramps in cirrhotic patients. *Journal of the American College of Nutrition*, *19*(1), 13–15.

Landucci, F., Mancinelli, P., De Gaudio, A. R., & Virgili, G. (2014). Selenium supplementation in critically ill patients: a systematic review and meta-analysis. *Journal of Critical Care*, *29*(1), 150–156.

Larson, A. A., & Kitto, K. F. (1997). Manipulations of zinc in the spinal cord, by intrathecal injection of zinc chloride, disodium-calcium-EDTA, or dipicolinic acid, alter nociceptive activity in mice. *The Journal of Pharmacology and Experimental Therapeutics*, *282*(3), 1319–1325.

Lee, D. H., Jee, D. L., Kim, S. Y., Kim, J. M., & Lee, H. M. (2006). Magnesium sulphate attenuates tourniquet-induced hypertension and spinal c-Fos mRNA expression: a comparison with ketamine. *The Journal of International Medical Research*, *34*(6), 573–584.

Li, R. H. W., Lo, S. S. T., Teh, D. K. G., Tong, N. -C., Tsui, M. H. Y., Cheung, K. -B., & Chung, T. K. H. (2004). Impact of common contraceptive methods on quality of life and sexual function in Hong Kong Chinese women. *Contraception*, *70*(6), 474–482.

Lin, L. -C., Que, J., Lin, L. -K., & Lin, F. -C. (2006). Zinc supplementation to improve mucositis and dermatitis in patients after radiotherapy for head-and-neck cancers: a double-blind, randomized study. *International Journal of Radiation Oncology, Biology, Physics*, *65*(3), 745–750.

Liu, A. L. -J., Shen, P. -W., & Chen, P. -J. (2013). Strontium ranelate in fracture healing and joint pain improvement in a rheumatoid arthritis patient. *Clinical Cases in Mineral and Bone Metabolism: The Official Journal of the Italian Society of Osteoporosis, Mineral Metabolism, and Skeletal Diseases*, *10*(3), 206–209.

Liu, H., & Hu, D. (2012). Efficacy of a commercial dentifrice containing 2% strontium chloride and 5% potassium nitrate for dentin hypersensitivity: a 3-day clinical study in adults in China. *Clinical Therapeutics*, *34*(3), 614–622.

Liu, T., Walker, J. S., & Tracey, D. J. (1999). Zinc alleviates thermal hyperalgesia due to partial nerve injury. *Neuroreport*, *10*(7), 1619–1623.

Lobo, S. L., Mehta, N., Forgione, A. G., Melis, M., Al-Badawi, E., Ceneviz, C., & Zawawi, K. H. (2004). Use of Theraflex-TMJ topical cream for the treatment of temporomandibular joint and muscle pain. *Cranio: The Journal of Craniomandibular Practice*, *22*(2), 137–144.

Lombardo, F., Fiducia, M., Lunghi, R., Marchetti, L., Palumbo, A., Rizzo, F., Koverech, A., Lenzi, A., & Gandini, L. (2012). Effects of a dietary supplement on chronic pelvic pain syndrome (category IIIA), leucocytospermia and semen parameters. *Andrologia*, *44*(suppl. 1), 672–678.

MacFarquhar, J. K., Broussard, D. L., Melstrom, P., Hutchinson, R., Wolkin, A., Martin, C., Burk, R. F., et al. (2010). Acute selenium toxicity associated with a dietary supplement. *Archives of Internal Medicine*, *170*(3), 256–261.

Mansouri, A., Hadjibabaie, M., Iravani, M., Shamshiri, A. R., Hayatshahi, A., Javadi, M. R., Khoee, S. H., Alimoghaddam, K., & Ghavamzadeh, A. (2012). The effect of zinc sulfate in the prevention of high-dose chemotherapy-induced mucositis: a double-blind, randomized, placebo-controlled study. *Hematological Oncology*, *30*(1), 22–26.

Matsunami, M., Kirishi, S., Okui, T., & Kawabata, A. (2011). Chelating luminal zinc mimics hydrogen sulfide-evoked colonic pain in mice: possible involvement of T-type calcium channels. *Neuroscience*, *181*(May), 257–264.

McCall, A. S., Cummings, C. F., Bhave, G., Vanacore, R., Page-McCaw, A., & Hudson, B. G. (2014). Bromine is an essential trace element for assembly of collagen IV scaffolds in tissue development and architecture. *Cell*, *157*(6), 1380–1392.

Megdiatov, R. S., Vorobeĭchik, I. M., Dolgikh, V. G., & Reshetniak, V. K. (1995). The role of zinc ions in the pathogenesis of trigeminal neuralgia (experimental and clinical research). *Zhurnal Nevrologii I Psikhiatrii Imeni S.S. Korsakova/Ministerstvo Zdravookhraneniia I Meditsinskoĭ Promyshlennosti Rossiĭskoĭ Federatsii, Vserossiĭskoe Obshchestvo Nevrologov [i] Vserossiĭskoe Obshchestvo Psikhiatrov*, *95*(5), 14–18.

Mehdipour, M., Taghavi Zenoz, A., Asvadi Kermani, I., & Hosseinpour, A. (2011). A comparison between zinc sulfate and chlorhexidine gluconate mouthwashes in the prevention of chemotherapy-induced oral mucositis. *Daru: Journal of Faculty of Pharmacy, Tehran University of Medical Sciences*, *19*(1), 71–73.

Memiş, D., Turan, A., Karamanlioğlu, B., Süt, N., & Pamukçu, Z. (2002). The use of magnesium sulfate to prevent pain on injection of propofol. *Anesthesia and Analgesia*, *95*(3), 606–608table of contents.

Meunier, P. J., Roux, C., Seeman, E., Ortolani, S., Badurski, J. E., Spector, T. D., Cannata, J., et al. (2004). The effects of strontium ranelate on the risk of vertebral fracture in women with postmenopausal osteoporosis. *The New England Journal of Medicine*, *350*(5), 459–468.

Michalke, B., & Fernsebner, K. (2014). New insights into manganese toxicity and speciation. *Journal of Trace Elements in Medicine and Biology: Organ of the Society for Minerals and Trace Elements (GMS)*, *28*(2), 106–116.

Micke, O., Bruns, F., Mücke, R., Schäfer, U., Glatzel, M., DeVries, A. F., Schönekaes, K., Kisters, K., & Büntzel, J. (2003). Selenium in the treatment of radiation-associated secondary lymphedema. *International Journal of Radiation Oncology, Biology, Physics*, *56*(1), 40–49.

Mirkheshti, A., Aryani, M. R., Shojaei, P., & Dabbagh, A. (2012). The effect of adding magnesium sulfate to lidocaine compared with paracetamol in prevention of acute pain in hand surgery patients under intravenous regional anesthesia (IVRA). *International Journal of Preventive Medicine*, *3*(9), 616–621.

Miura, S., Takahashi, K., Imagawa, T., Uchida, K., Saito, S., Tominaga, M., & Ohta, T. (2013). Involvement of TRPA1 activation in acute pain induced by cadmium in mice. *Molecular Pain*, *9*(January), 7.

Morgia, G., Mucciardi, G., Galì, A., Madonia, M., Marchese, F., Di Benedetto, A., Romano, G., et al. (2010). Treatment of chronic prostatitis/chronic pelvic pain syndrome category IIIA with *Serenoa repens* plus selenium and lycopene (Profluss) versus *S. repens* alone: an Italian randomized multicenter-controlled study. *Urologia Internationalis*, *84*(4), 400–406.

Mosti, G., Crespi, A., & Mattaliano, V. (2011). Comparison between a new, two-component compression system with zinc paste bandages for leg ulcer healing: a prospective, multicenter, randomized. controlled trial monitoring sub-bandage pressures. *Wounds: A Compendium of Clinical Research and Practice*, *23*(5), 126–134.

Murakami-Nakayama, M., Tsubota, M., Hiruma, S., Sekiguchi, F., Matsuyama, K., Kimura, T., Moriyama, M., & Kawabata, A. (2015). Polaprezinc attenuates cyclophosphamide-induced cystitis and related bladder pain in mice. *Journal of Pharmacological Sciences*, *127*(2), 223–228.

Murphy, J. D., Paskaradevan, J., Eisler, L. L., Ouanes, J. -P. P., Garcia Tomas, V. A., Freck, E. A., & Wu, C. L. (2013). Analgesic efficacy of continuous intravenous magnesium infusion as an adjuvant to morphine for postoperative analgesia: a systematic review and meta-analysis. *Middle East Journal of Anesthesiology*, *22*(1), 11–20.

Nascimento, J. W. L., Santos, L. H., Nothenberg, M. S., Coelho, M. M., Oga, S., & Tagliati, C. A. (2003). Anti-inflammatory activity and gastric lesions induced by zinc-tenoxicam. *Pharmacology*, *68*(2), 64–69.

Nazıroğlu, M., Çelik, Ö., Uğuz, A. C., & Bütün, A. (2015). Protective effects of riboflavin and selenium on brain microsomal Ca2+-ATPase and oxidative damage caused by glyceryl trinitrate in a rat headache model. *Biological Trace Element Research*, *164*(1), 72–79.

Nelson, M. T., Woo, J., Kang, H. -W., Vitko, I., Barrett, P. Q., Perez-Reyes, E., Lee, J. -H., Shin, H. -S., & Todorovic, S. M. (2007). Reducing agents sensitize C-type nociceptors by relieving high-affinity zinc inhibition of T-type calcium channels. *The Journal of Neuroscience: The Official Journal of the Society for Neuroscience*, *27*(31), 8250–8260.

Nogueira, C. W., Quinhones, E. B., Jung, E. A. C., Zeni, G., & Rocha, J. B. T. (2003). Anti-inflammatory and antinociceptive activity of diphenyl diselenide. *Inflammation Research: Official Journal of the European Histamine Research Society . . . [et al.]*, *52*(2), 56–63.

Nordberg, G., Koji, N., & Nordberg, M. (2015). *Handbook on the toxicology of metals* (4th ed.). Amsterdam: Elsevier B.V.

Nozaki, C., Vergnano, A. M., Filliol, D., Ouagazzal, A. -M., Le Goff, A., Carvalho, S., Reiss, D., et al. (2011). Zinc alleviates pain through high-affinity binding to the NMDA receptor NR2A subunit. *Nature Neuroscience*, *14*(8), 1017–1022.

Park, J. -H., Chae, J., Roh, K., Kil, E. -J., Lee, M., Auh, C. -K., Lee, M. -A., Yeom, C. -H., & Lee, S. (2015). Oxaliplatin-induced peripheral neuropathy via TRPA1 stimulation in mice dorsal root ganglion is correlated with aluminum accumulation. *PLoS One*, *10*(4), e0124875.

Pastorfide, G. B., Gorgonio, N. M., Ganzon, A. R., & Alberto, R. M. (1989). Zinc chloride spray—magnesium hydroxide ointment dual topical regimen in the treatment of obstetric and gynecologic incisional wounds. *Clinical Therapeutics*, *11*(2), 258–263.

Pelletier, J. -P., Kapoor, M., Fahmi, H., Lajeunesse, D., Blesius, A., Maillet, J., & Martel-Pelletier, J. (2013). Strontium ranelate reduces the progression of experimental dog osteoarthritis by inhibiting the expression of key proteases in cartilage and of IL-1β in the synovium. *Annals of the Rheumatic Diseases*, *72*(2), 250–257.

Penland, J. G., & Johnson, P. E. (1993). Dietary calcium and manganese effects on menstrual cycle symptoms. *American Journal of Obstetrics and Gynecology*, *168*(5), 1417–1423.

Pickering, G., Morel, V., Simen, E., Cardot, J. -M., Moustafa, F., Delage, N., Picard, P., Eschalier, S., Boulliau, S., & Dubray, C. (2011). Oral magnesium treatment in patients with neuropathic pain: a randomized clinical trial. *Magnesium Research*, *24*(2), 28–35.

Preedy, V. R., Watson, R. R., & Martin, C. R. (Eds.). (2011). *Handbook of behavior, food and nutrition*. New York, NY: Springer.

Qi, X., Han, L., Liu, X., Zhi, J., Zhao, B., Chen, D., Yu, F., & Zhou, X. (2012). Prostate extract with aluminum hydroxide injection as a novel animal model for chronic prostatitis/chronic pelvic pain syndrome. *Urology*, *80*(6), 1389e9–1389e15.

Ragunathan-Thangarajah, N., Le Beller, C., Boutouyrie, P., Bassez, G., Gherardi, R. K., Laurent, S., & Authier, F. -J. (2013). Distinctive clinical features in arthro-myalgic patients with and without aluminum hydroxyde-induced macrophagic myofasciitis: an exploratory study. *Journal of Inorganic Biochemistry*, *128*(November), 262–266.

Richmond, S. J., Brown, S. R., Campion, P. D., Porter, A. J. L., Klaber Moffett, J. A., Jackson, D. A., Featherstone, V. A., & Taylor, A. J. (2009). Therapeutic effects of magnetic and copper bracelets in osteoarthritis: a randomised placebo-controlled crossover trial. *Complementary Therapies in Medicine*, *17*(5–6), 249–256.

Richmond, S. J., Gunadasa, S., Bland, M., & Macpherson, H. (2013). Copper bracelets and magnetic wrist straps for rheumatoid arthritis--analgesic and anti-inflammatory effects: a randomised double-blind placebo controlled crossover trial. *PLoS One*, *8*(9), e71529.

Rondón, L. J., Privat, A. M., Daulhac, L., Davin, N., Mazur, A., Fialip, J., Eschalier, A., & Courteix, C. (2010). Magnesium attenuates chronic hypersensitivity and spinal cord NMDA receptor phosphorylation in a rat model of diabetic neuropathic pain. *The Journal of Physiology*, *588*(pt 21), 4205–4215.

Safieh-Garabedian, B., Poole, S., Allchorne, A., Kanaan, S., Saade, N., & Woolf, C. J. (1996). Zinc reduces the hyperalgesia and upregulation of NGF and IL-1 beta produced by peripheral inflammation in the rat. *Neuropharmacology*, *35*(5), 599–603.

Sakinci, M., Ercan, C. M., Olgan, S., Coksuer, H., Karasahin, K. E., & Kuru, O. (2016). Comparative analysis of copper intrauterine device impact on female sexual dysfunction subtypes. *Taiwanese Journal of Obstetrics & Gynecology, 55*(1), 30–34.

Sangthawan, D., Phungrassami, T., & Sinkitjarurnchai, W. (2013). A randomized double-blind, placebo-controlled trial of zinc sulfate supplementation for alleviation of radiation-induced oral mucositis and pharyngitis in head and neck cancer patients. *Journal of the Medical Association of Thailand = Chotmaihet Thangphaet, 96*(1), 69–76.

Saritas, T. B., Borazan, H., Okesli, S., Yel, M., & Otelcioglu, Ş. (2015). Is intra-articular magnesium effective for postoperative analgesia in arthroscopic shoulder surgery? *Pain Research & Management: The Journal of the Canadian Pain Society = Journal de La Société Canadienne Pour Le Traitement de La Douleur, 20*(1), 35–38.

Savegnago, L., Jesse, C. R., Moro, A. V., Borges, V. C., Santos, F. W., Rocha, J. B. T., & Nogueira, C. W. (2006). Bis selenide alkene derivatives: a class of potential antioxidant and antinociceptive agents. *Pharmacology, Biochemistry, and Behavior., 83*(2), 221–229.

Savegnago, L., Pinto, L. G., Jesse, C. R., Alves, D., Rocha, J. B. T., Nogueira, C. W., & Zeni, G. (2007). Antinociceptive properties of diphenyl diselenide: evidences for the mechanism of action. *European Journal of Pharmacology, 555*(2–3), 129–138.

Savic Vujovic, K. R., Vuckovic, S., Srebro, D., Medic, B., Stojanovic, R., Vucetic, C., & Prostran, M. (2015). A synergistic interaction between magnesium sulphate and ketamine on the inhibition of acute nociception in rats. *European Review for Medical and Pharmacological Sciences, 19*(13), 2503–2509.

Schwartz, E. S., Kim, H. Y., Wang, J., Lee, I., Klann, E., Chung, J. M., & Chung, K. (2009). Persistent pain is dependent on spinal mitochondrial antioxidant levels. *Journal of Neuroscience, 29*(1), 159–168.

Shackel, N. A., Day, R. O., Kellett, B., & Brooks, P. M. (1997). Copper-salicylate gel for pain relief in osteoarthritis: a randomised controlled trial. *The Medical Journal of Australia, 167*(3), 134–136.

Shahrami, A., Assarzadegan, F., Hatamabadi, H. R., Asgarzadeh, M., Sarehbandi, B., & Asgarzadeh, S. (2015). Comparison of therapeutic effects of magnesium sulfate vs. dexamethasone/metoclopramide on alleviating acute migraine headache. *The Journal of Emergency Medicine, 48*(1), 69–76.

Sieja, K., & Talerczyk, M. (2004). Selenium as an element in the treatment of ovarian cancer in women receiving chemotherapy. *Gynecologic Oncology, 93*(2), 320–327.

Singh, D. K., Jindal, P., & Singh, G. (2011). Comparative study of attenuation of the pain caused by propofol intravenous injection, by granisetron, magnesium sulfate and nitroglycerine. *Saudi Journal of Anaesthesia, 5*(1), 50–54.

Siriwardena, A. K., Mason, J. M., Sheen, A. J., Makin, A. J., & Shah, N. S. (2012). Antioxidant therapy does not reduce pain in patients with chronic pancreatitis: the ANTICIPATE study. *Gastroenterology, 143*(3), 655–63.e1.

Skrzypulec, V., & Drosdzol, A. (2008). Evaluation of quality of life and sexual functioning of women using levonorgestrel-releasing intrauterine contraceptive system—Mirena. *Collegium Antropologicum, 32*(4), 1059–1068.

Spain, R. I., Leist, T. P., & De Sousa, E. A. (2009). When metals compete: a case of copper-deficiency myeloneuropathy and anemia. *Nature Clinical Practice. Neurology, 5*(2), 106–111.

Srebro, D. P., Vučković, S., Vujović, K. S., & Prostran, M. (2014). Anti-hyperalgesic effect of systemic magnesium sulfate in carrageenan-induced inflammatory pain in rats: influence of the nitric oxide pathway. *Magnesium Research, 27*(2), 77–85.

Stebbins, W. G., Hanke, C. W., & Petersen, J. (2011). Enhanced healing of surgical wounds of the lower leg using weekly zinc oxide compression dressings. *Dermatologic Surgery: Official Publication for American Society for Dermatologic Surgery [et al.], 37*(2), 158–165.

Steinmetz, S., Tipold, A., Bilzer, T., & Schenk, H. C. (2012). Transient neuromyopathy after bromide intoxication in a dog with idiopathic epilepsy. *Irish Veterinary Journal, 65*(1), 19.

Sun, J., Wu, X., Zhao, X., Chen, F., & Wang, W. (2015). Pre-emptive peritonsillar infiltration of magnesium sulphate and ropivacaine vs. ropivacaine or magnesium alone for relief of post-adenotonsillectomy pain in children. *International Journal of Pediatric Otorhinolaryngology, 79*(4), 499–503.

Sun, J., Zhou, R., Lin, W., Zhou, J., & Wang, W. (2016). Magnesium sulfate plus lidocaine reduces propofol injection pain: a double-blind, randomized study. *Clinical Therapeutics, 38*(1), 31–38.

Suwanlaong, K., & Kammant, P. (2008). Neurological manifestation of methyl bromide intoxication. *Journal of the Medical Association of Thailand = Chotmaihet Thangphaet, 91*(3), 421–426.

Takeda, A. (2003). Manganese action in brain function. *Brain Research. Brain Research Reviews, 41*(1), 79–87.

Tamba, B. I., Leon, M. -M., & Petreus, T. (2013). Common trace elements alleviate pain in an experimental mouse model. *Journal of Neuroscience Research, 91*(4), 554–561.

Tanaka, M., Shimizu, S., Nishimura, W., Mine, O., Akatsuka, M., Inamori, K., & Mori, H. (1998). Relief of neuropathic pain with intravenous magnesium. *Masui. The Japanese Journal of Anesthesiology, 47*(9), 1109–1113.

Topal, F., Yonem, O., Tuzcu, N., Tuzcu, M., Ataseven, H., & Akyol, M. (2014). Strontium chloride: can it be a new treatment option for ulcerative colitis? *BioMed Research International, 2014*(January), 530687.

Tsang, A., Von Korff, M., Lee, S., Alonso, J., Karam, E., Angermeyer, M. C., Borges, G. L. G., et al. (2008). Common chronic pain conditions in developed and developing countries: gender and age differences and comorbidity with depression-anxiety disorders. *The Journal of Pain: Official Journal of the American Pain Society, 9*(10), 883–891.

Tugrul, S., Degirmenci, N., Eren, S. B., Dogan, R., Veyseller, B., & Ozturan, O. (2015). Analgesic effect of magnesium in post-tonsillectomy patients: a prospective randomised clinical trial. *European Archives of Oto-Rhino-Laryngology: Official Journal of the European Federation of Oto-Rhino-Laryngological Societies (EUFOS): Affiliated with the German Society for Oto-Rhino-Laryngology—Head and Neck Surgery, 272*(9), 2483–2487.

Turgut, A., Özler, A., Görük, N. Y., Tunc, S. Y., Evliyaoglu, O., & Gül, T. (2013). Copper, ceruloplasmin and oxidative stress in patients with advanced-stage endometriosis. *European Review for Medical and Pharmacological Sciences, 17*(11), 1472–1478.

Ulugol, A., Aslantas, A., Ipci, Y., Tuncer, A., Karadag, C. H., & Dokmeci, I. (2002). Combined systemic administration of morphine and magnesium sulfate attenuates pain-related behavior in mononeuropathic rats. *Brain Research, 943*(1), 101–104.

Verberk, M. M., Rooyakkers-Beemster, T., de Vlieger, M., & van Vliet, A. G. (1979). Bromine in blood, EEG and transaminases in methyl bromide workers. *British Journal of Industrial Medicine, 36*(1), 59–62.

Vormann, J., Worlitschek, M., Goedecke, T., & Silver, B. (2001). Supplementation with alkaline minerals reduces symptoms in patients with chronic low back pain. *Journal of Trace Elements in Medicine and Biology: Organ of the Society for Minerals and Trace Elements (GMS), 15*(2–3), 179–183.

Walker, W. R., & Keats, D. M. (1976). An investigation of the therapeutic value of the 'copper bracelet'—dermal assimilation of copper in arthritic/rheumatoid conditions. *Agents and Actions, 6*(4), 454–459.

Walton, J. R. (2014). Chronic aluminum intake causes Alzheimer's disease: applying Sir Austin Bradford Hill's causality criteria. *Journal of Alzheimer's Disease: JAD, 40*(4), 765–838.

Wang, B., & Du, Y. (2013). Cadmium and its neurotoxic effects. *Oxidative Medicine and Cellular Longevity, 2013*(January), 898034.

Watanabe, T., Ishihara, M., Matsuura, K., Mizuta, K., & Itoh, Y. (2010). Polaprezinc prevents oral mucositis associated with radiochemotherapy in patients with head and neck cancer. *International Journal of Cancer*, *127*(8), 1984–1990.

Welch, S. P., Vocci, F. J., & Dewey, W. L. (1983). Antinociceptive and lethal effects of intraventricularly administered barium and strontium: antagonism by atropine sulfate or naloxone hydrochlorine. *Life Sciences*, *33*(4), 359–364.

Wessells, K. R., & Brown, K. H. (2012). Estimating the global prevalence of zinc deficiency: results based on zinc availability in national food supplies and the prevalence of stunting. *PLoS One*, *7*(11), e50568.

West, N., Newcombe, R. G., Hughes, N., Mason, S., Maggio, B., Sufi, F., & Claydon, N. (2013). A 3-day randomised clinical study investigating the efficacy of two toothpastes, designed to occlude dentine tubules, for the treatment of dentine hypersensitivity. *Journal of Dentistry*, *41*(2), 187–194.

Widman, M., Rosin, D., & Dewey, W. L. (1978). Effects of divalent cations, lanthanum, cation chelators and an ionophore on acetylcholine antinociception. *Journal of Pharmacology and Experimental Therapy*, *205*(2), 311–318.

Yalçın Tepe, A. (2014). *Encyclopedia of food safety*. Amsterdam: Elsevier.

Yokel, R. A. (2014). *Encyclopedia of the neurological sciences*. Amsterdam: Elsevier.

Young, D. L., Chakravarthy, D., Drower, E., & Reyna S R. (2014). Skin care product evaluation in a group of critically ill, premature neonates: a descriptive study. *Journal of Wound, Ostomy, and Continence Nursing: Official Publication of the Wound, Ostomy and Continence Nurses Society/WOCN*, *41*(6), 519–527.

Yousef, A. A., & Al-deeb, A. E. (2013). A double-blinded randomised controlled study of the value of sequential intravenous and oral magnesium therapy in patients with chronic low back pain with a neuropathic component. *Anaesthesia*, *68*(3), 260–266.

Yu, D. -G., Ding, H. -F., Mao, Y. -Q., Liu, M., Yu, B., Zhao, X., Wang, X. -Q., et al. (2013). Strontium ranelate reduces cartilage degeneration and subchondral bone remodeling in rat osteoarthritis model. *Acta Pharmacologica Sinica*, *34*(3), 393–402.

Zarauza, R., Sáez-Fernández, A. N., Iribarren, M. J., Carrascosa, F., Adame, M., Fidalgo, I., & Monedero, P. (2000). A comparative study with oral nifedipine, intravenous nimodipine, and magnesium sulfate in postoperative analgesia. *Anesthesia and Analgesia*, *91*(4), 938–943.

Zekavat, O. R., Karimi, M. Y., Amanat, A., & Alipour, F. (2015). A randomised controlled trial of oral zinc sulphate for primary dysmenorrhoea in adolescent females. *The Australian & New Zealand Journal of Obstetrics & Gynaecology*, *55*(4), 369–373.

CHAPTER

18

Vitamin B_{12} for Relieving Pain in Aphthous Ulcers

H.-L. Liu

Department of Nursing, Central Taiwan University of Science and Technology, Beitun District, Taichung City, Taiwan

INTRODUCTION

Aphthous ulcers are painful oral mucosal inflammatory ulcers that can occur inside the mouth anywhere, and frequently impact daily life activities, such as eating, swallowing, and speaking. The term "aphthous" is derived from a Greek word "aphtha," which means ulceration (Preeti, Magesh, Rajkumar, & Karthik, 2011). Aphthous stomatitis was also known as canker sores or mouth ulcer, and this condition is a very common oral mucosal inflammatory ulcerative disease worldwide. However, most of the people who experience "canker sore" have sharply painful sores that can occur anywhere inside the oral cavity including the skin covering the inside of the lips and cheeks, the floor of the mouth, the tip or underside of the tongue, the soft palate, and the tonsillar area (Field & Longman, 2003). The aphthous ulcer condition is characterized by localized, shallow, rounded, painful, small, clean borders, a peripheral erythematous halo, and a yellow or grayish base, present first in childhood or adolescence (Jurge, Kuffer, Scully, & Porter, 2006).

Aphthous ulcers usually occur in recurrent bouts at intervals of a few days to a few months (Porter, Hegarty, Kaliakatsou, Hodgson, & Scully, 2000; Porter, Scully, & Pedersen, 1998; Ship, Chavez, Doerr, Henson, & Sarmadi, 2000). An aphthous ulcer usually heals within 7–14 days without scarring; however, in some people, it may often recur. If an ulcer persists for more than 3 weeks or if there is recurrent formation of new aphthous ulcers, the patient may also be suffering from other clinical abnormalities.

EPIDEMIOLOGY OF APHTHOUS ULCER

According to epidemiological studies, recurrent aphthous ulcer is prevalent worldwide and may affect between 2% and 50% of people within a general population, with most estimates falling between 5% and 25%, and with 3-month recurrence rates as high as 50% (Miller & Ship, 1977; Rees & Binnie, 1996; Scully & Porter, 2008; Ship, 1972); the exact cause of recurrent aphthous stomatitis is still unknown. There tends to be female predominance in some adult and child patient groups (Porter et al., 1998, 2000; Tabolli et al., 2009; Ship et al., 2000).

The onset of mouth aphthous ulcers typically occurs in childhood (Shulman, 2004), but 40% of children can have a history of recurrent aphthous stomatitis, with ulceration beginning at 5 years of age and the frequency of affected patients rising with age (Hakemer, Piatowska, & Zabinska, 1971; Miller, Garfunkel, Ram, & Ship, 1980; Peretz, 1994).

Several studies showed that children of higher socioeconomic status may be more commonly affected than those from low socioeconomic status (Crivelli, Aguas, Adler, Quarracino, & Bazerque, 1988; Hakemer et al., 1971; Miller et al., 1980; Peretz, 1994). According to a study from the United States, 39,206 school-year children, whose ages ranged from 5 to 17, went through examination, and approximately 37% of these children were reported to have recurrent aphthous stomatitis (Kleinman, Swango, & Pindborg, 1994). Spanish epidemiological studies have shown oral mucosal lesions most often in children, and the level of recurrent aphthous stomatitis reported ranges from 0.9% to 10.8%

Nutritional Modulators of Pain in the Aging Population. http://dx.doi.org/10.1016/B978-0-12-805186-3.00018-7
Copyright © 2017 Elsevier Inc. All rights reserved.

(Rioboo-Crespo Mdel, Planells-del Pozo, & Rioboo-García, 2005). In an epidemiological study conducted in Italy from 1997 to 2007, Majorana et al. (2010) surveyed 10,128 children between the ages 0 and 12 years, and found that the prevalence in children presenting with recurrent aphthous stomatitis was 14.8% and this condition is relatively common.

TYPES OF MOUTH ULCER

The symptoms of aphthous ulcers can present in three main forms, which have been described under three different clinical variants as classified by Stanley (1972): minor, major, or herpetiform ulcers.

Minor aphthous ulcers are the most common form, which vary from 8- to 10-mm size, round, clearly defined, painful ulcers. Healing occurs in 10–14 days without scarring (Field, Brookes, & Tyldesley, 1992). Major aphthous ulcer lesions are larger (greater than 1 cm in diameter). Healing of this form of ulcer may take 20–30 days or longer than that of minor aphthous ulcers, and frequently results in scarring (Wray, Ferguson, Mason, Hutcheon, & Dagg, 1975). Herpetiform ulceration is characterized by recurrent crops of multiple ulcers, which present with multiple small and painful ulcers, together with clusters of pinpoint lesions that often occur in multiples of 1–100, each being 2–3 mm. The ulcers tend to fuse, producing large irregular ulcers. These are more common in women and have a later age of onset than other clinical variants of recurrent aphthous stomatitis (Scully & Porter, 1989).

CAUSE OF CANKER SORES

The exact cause of most canker sores is still unknown; stress, tissue injury, or citrus or acidic fruits and vegetables (e.g., lemons, oranges, pineapples, strawberries, apples, and tomatoes) can trigger a mouth ulcer. Sometimes a food with sharp edges or dental appliance, such as braces or ill-fitting dentures, might also trigger mouth ulcers. Some cases of complex mouth ulcers are caused by an idiopathic condition in most patients (Porter et al., 2000), which may arise in multisystemic disease (Porter et al., 2000), including Sweet syndrome (Driban & Alvarez, 1984; von den Driesch, Gomez, Kiesewetter, & Hornstein, 1989), mouth and genital ulcers with inflamed cartilage (MAGIC) syndrome (Lê Thi Huong et al., 1993; Orme, Nordlund, Barich, & Brown, 1990), Behçet disease (Krause et al., 1998, 1999; Lee, 1997; Rogers, 1997), cyclic neutropenia (Lange & Jones, 1981; Scully, MacFadyen, & Campbell, 1982), benign familial neutropenia (Hastürk et al., 1998; Porter, Scully, & Standen, 1994), a periodic syndrome with fever and pharyngitis (Marshall, Edwards, Butler, & Lawton, 1987), various nutritional deficiencies with or without underlying gastrointestinal tract disorders (Eversole, 1994; Grattan & Scully, 1986; Weusten & van de Wiel, 1998), some other primary immunodeficiencies (Porter & Scully, 1993a, 1993b, 1993c, 1993d), and infection with human immunodeficiency virus (MacPhail & Greenspan, 1997; Zakrzewska, Robinson, & Williams, 1997). Nonsteroidal antiinflammatory drugs (NSAIDs) (Healy & Thornhill, 1995) or nicorandil (Shotts, Scully, Avery, & Porter, 1999), which are rarely seen, can give rise to oral ulcers. Nutritional deficiencies or hematologic diseases have been reported in 20% of patients with recurrent aphthous stomatitis (Casiglia, Morwski, & Nebesio, 2010; Nolan, McIntosh, Allam, & Lamey, 1991). The cause of aphthous ulcers remains unknown; in other words, an aphthous ulcer can occur due to a variety of reasons including systemic diseases, nutritional deficiencies, food allergies, genetic predisposition, immune disorders, medications, human immunodeficiency virus infection, and environmental factors (Porter et al., 1998, 2000).

APHTHOUS ULCER TREATMENT

The etiopathogenesis of this disease is yet unclear. Several studies recorded specific replacement therapy preparations from *Myrtus communis* (myrtle) herbs (Babaee, Mansourian, Momen-Heravi, Moghadamnia, & Momen-Beitollahi, 2010), licorice herbs (Brogden, Speight, & Avery, 1974; Das, Das, Gulati, & Singh, 1989; Moghadamnia et al., 2009), multivitamins (Lalla et al., 2012; Pedersen, Hougen, Klausen, & Winther, 1990), and adhesive pastes (Reznik & O'Daniels, 2001). Several topical agents are available for symptomatic relief such as local and systemic antibiotics (Kerr, Drexel, & Spielman, 2003), local antiseptics (Meiller et al., 1991), topical NSAIDs (Murray, McGuinness, Biagioni, Hyland, & Lamey, 2005), and topical corticosteroids (Gonzalez-Moles, Morales, Rodriguez-Archilla, Isabel, & Gonzalez-Moles, 2002), and even topical and systemic immunomodulators, immunosuppressants, and corticosteroids (Femiano, Gombos, & Scully, 2003; Hutchinson, Angenend, Mok, Cummins, & Richards, 1990; Katz, Langevitz, Shemer, Barak, & Livneh, 1994) were among the treatments given to patients with recurrent aphthous stomatitis.

VITAMIN B_{12} TREATMENT FOR MOUTH ULCER

The lack of clarity regarding the etiology of aphthous ulcers has resulted in treatments that are ad hoc (Porter et al., 2000). Aphthous ulcer treatment strategies must be directed toward providing symptomatic relief by reducing pain, increasing the duration of ulcer-free periods, and accelerating ulcer healing (Preeti et al., 2011).

Several vitamin B_{12} (cobalamin) treatments for recurrent aphthous ulcers aim to decrease the pain, healing time, and ulcer number and size, and increase the frequency and duration of disease-free periods. Vitamin B_{12} may play an important role in the treatment of aphthous ulcers. The most common etiology of vitamin B_{12} deficiency is food-cobalamin malabsorption resulting from gastric dysfunction (Dholakia et al., 2005). The prevalence of vitamin B_{12} deficiency increases with age and in the elderly (>65 years of age) (Dali-Youcef & Andrès, 2009). Studies of the impact of age suggest a high prevalence of subnormal cobalamin concentrations (Dali-Youcef & Andrès, 2009; Porter et al., 1998) and, in some reports, an inverse relationship between age and serum cobalamin concentration has been shown (Allen, 2009).

Burgess and Haley (2008) investigated 143 patients experiencing recurrent aphthous stomatitis and found that 26.6% of patients with recurrent aphthous stomatitis had a vitamin B_{12} deficiency, compared to 12.6% of the control patients. Piskin, Sayan, Durukan, and Senol (2002) reported that 35 patients with recurrent aphthous ulcers had vitamin B_{12} levels significantly lower than those of the 26 healthy control patients, while no significant differences were reported in the other hematologic factors measured. Volkov et al. (2009) used a randomized, double-blind, placebo-controlled trial to confirm the effectiveness of vitamin B_{12} in the treatment of recurrent aphthous ulcers. The study suggested that a 1000-μg daily dose of vitamin B_{12} dissolved under the tongue might prevent aphthous ulcers after 5–6 months of use. Such rapid relief has been termed the master key effect (Volkov, Press, & Rudoy, 2006). It is therefore suggested that high levels of vitamin B_{12} reduce the incidence of mouth ulcers (Volkov, Rudoy, Abu-Rabia, Masalha, & Masalha, 2005).

Vitamin B_{12} may play an important role for aphthous ulcers. Nutritional deficiencies or hematologic diseases have been documented in 20% of patients with recurrent aphthous ulcers (Nolan et al., 1991). Studies have found that recurrent aphthous stomatitis patients who present to physicians for treatment for deficiencies of iron, folate, and vitamin B_{12} record a 71% improvement in aphthous ulcer following replacement therapy for these deficiencies (Olson, Feinberg, Silverman, Abrams, & Greenspan, 1982). Several vitamin B_{12} (cobalamin) treatments for recurrent aphthous stomatitis have addressed the goals of decreasing pain, healing time, and number and size of the ulcer, and increasing the number and length of disease-free periods.

Brachmann (1954) first suggested that vitamin B_{12} deficiency could be associated with aphthous ulcers. The most common etiology of vitamin B_{12} deficiency is food-cobalamin malabsorption resulting from gastric dysfunction (Dholakia et al., 2005). Studies that have examined the impact of age suggest a high prevalence of subnormal cobalamin concentrations (Dali-Youcef & Andrès, 2009; Porter et al., 1998) and, in some reports, an inverse relationship between age and serum cobalamin concentrations (Allen, 2009; Davis, Lawton, Prouty, & Chow, 1965) has been shown.

Burgess and Haley (2008) conducted a trial where patients were treated with 30 (each disc is 500 μg) vitamin B_{12} discs with instructions to use 2 initially and then 1 each succeeding day, placing the discs on the sores on the buccal side of a tooth and allowing to dissolve over 20–40 min. The control group were given the same treatment with placebo/nonactive discs. All seven subjects who received the active discs, and eight who received the placebo nonactive discs, were instructed to make careful observations of their ulcers and report their observations at least once each week over a 30-day period. All of the participants in the intervention group reported a benefit from the vitamin B_{12} treatment. Six of seven participants reported a reduced duration of each ulcer, four of the seven reported less peak pain from each ulcer, and four of seven reported lower frequencies of ulcers. These initial data suggest that treatment with dissolvable vitamin B_{12} discs might reduce frequency of minor recurrent aphthous stomatitis and reduce duration and peak pain levels of ulcers (Burgess & Haley, 2008). Treatment with vitamin B_{12} by oral supplementation may be an effective therapy for recurrent aphthous stomatitis (Burgess & Haley, 2008; Volkov et al., 2005, 2009). Zhong, Mao, and Li (2010) investigated issues related to supplementing vitamin B_{12} for the treatment of recurrent aphthous stomatitis.

TREATMENT FOR PAIN IN APTHTHOUS ULCERS

Liu and Chiu (2015), Volkov et al. (2009), Burgess and Haley (2008), and Zhong et al. (2010) have been investigating issues related to supplementing vitamin B_{12} for treatment of aphthous ulcer to relieve pain. Burgess and Haley (2008) conducted a trial in which patients were treated with 30 discs (each disc is 500 μg) before sleep, placing into saliva via discs adhered to the buccal side of a tooth (with the disc dissolving over 20–40 min near an ulcer place when present) for 30 days, and reported significant improvement (4.55, $P < 0.03$) and pain reduction (4.82, $P < 0.02$) in the intervention group. Volkov et al. (2009) conducted a study on the effect of 1000 μg of vitamin B_{12} tablets orally each day before sleep for 6 months. The results showed that the average level of pain also showed statistically significant differences after 5 and 6 months in the vitamin B_{12} treatment group compared to in the control group. Zhong et al. (2010) conducted a study to observe the effect of inhalation of nebulized vitamin B_{12} solution to treat patients with surface-corticosteroid-inhalation-induced oral ulcers four times per day for 5 days (no record of daily dose was given), and reported level of pain and ulcer size with the vitamin B_{12} treatment compared to the placebo. Liu and Chiu (2015) conducted a randomized, double-blind, placebo-controlled trial, in which 22 patients were assigned to the intervention group and 20 to the control group undergoing aphthous ulcer treatment for 2 days, to confirm the analgesic benefit of treatment of mouth ulcers with vitamin B_{12} as adjunctive therapy. They used 500-μg vitamin B_{12} into 2 g triamcinolone ointment for 2 days of treatment. They found statistically significant differences in pain levels after 2 days of treatment between the intervention group and the control group ($P < 0.001$) (Liu & Chiu, 2015).

Burgess and Haley (2008) measured self-reported perception of improvement and found that vitamin B_{12} treatment led to an improvement in the treatment group (76.92%, $n = 26$) versus the control group (45.00%, $n = 20$) with an odds ratio (OR) of 0.25 and 95% confidence interval (CI) (0.07, 0.87). Burgess and Haley (2008) used 500-μg vitamin B_{12}—two doses initially and then one each succeeding day for 30 days, placing into saliva via discs adhered to the buccal side of a tooth, with discs dissolving over 20–40 min near an ulcer when present. The study was conducted over 30 days and reported significant perceived improvement ($P < 0.03$) and pain reduction ($P < 0.02$) in the intervention group (Burgess & Haley, 2008). Burgess and Haley (2008) reported that in a separate trial with 16 nonblinded participants, 100% of participants reported a benefit from vitamin B_{12} disc use. Seventy-three percent of the treatment group also reported reduced frequency of ulcers and no adverse reactions or complications were reported (Burgess & Haley, 2008).

Volkov et al. (2009) examined the number of days to recovery from a recurrent aphthous stomatitis and self-reported pain levels. This study also reported a statistically significant [OR = 0.16; 95% CI (0.05, 0.55)] protective effect of vitamin B_{12} in the treatment group (74.07%, $n = 31$) versus the control group (32%, $n = 27$). Volkov et al. (2009) used 1000 μg of vitamin B_{12} tablets taken orally each day before sleep for 6 months. The results showed that reported average number of recurrent aphthous stomatitis ulcers decreased significantly after 5 and 6 months [OR = −8.74, 95% CI (−16.62, −0.86); and OR =−9.51, 95% CI (−12.64, −6.40); $P = 0.03$ and <0.01, respectively], average duration of recurrent aphthous stomatitis episode decrease was significant after 5 and 6 months [OR = −2.38, 95% CI (−4.51, −0.25); and OR = −2.86, 95% CI (−5.39, −0.33); $P = 0.03$ and 0.03, respectively], and average level of pain also showed statistically significant difference after 5 and 6 months [OR = −1.42, 95% CI (−2.35, −0.49); and OR = −1.72, 95% CI (−2.70, −0.74); $P < 0.0001$ and <0.0001, respectively] for the vitamin B_{12} treatment group, compared with the control group (Liu, Chiu, & Chen, 2013).

Zhong et al. (2010) examined ulcer size and pain level in response to nebulized vitamin B_{12}. The delivered dosage of vitamin B_{12} was not reported and the intervention was delivered over 5 days. Liu et al. (2013) reviewed and analyzed the results that found a protective effect [OR = 0.04; 95% CI (0.00, 0.83), 100% vs. 65%] of vitamin B_{12} in the treatment group ($n = 20$), as compared with that in the control group ($n = 20$). Zhong et al. (2010) used vitamin B_{12} nebulizer solution inhalation to treat patients with surface-corticosteroid-inhalation-induced oral ulcer four times a day for 5 days (no record of daily dose was given). Zhong et al. (2010) showed an improvement in both reported level of pain and ulcer size with vitamin B_{12} treatment compared with a placebo (containing 2.5% sodium bicarbonate solution to gargle).

Liu and Chiu (2015) conducted a randomized, double-blind, placebo-controlled trial, in which 22 patients were assigned to the intervention group and 20 to the control group undergoing aphthous ulcer treatment for 2 days, to confirm the analgesic benefit of treatment of mouth ulcers with vitamin B_{12} as adjunctive therapy. They used 500-μg vitamin B_{12} into 2 g triamcinolone ointment for 2 days of treatment. They found statistically significant differences in pain levels after 2 days of treatment between the intervention group and the control group ($P < 0.001$). Liu and Chiu (2015) found that vitamin B_{12} treatment relieves the painful feeling in the treatment group (81.82%, $n = 22$) versus the control group (30.00%, $n = 20$). Liu and Chiu (2015) made the subjects feel the level of pain themselves, using a visual analog scale (VAS) device to measure pain. This research found differences in pain levels after 2 days of treatment between the intervention group and the control group [mean VAS 0.36 (95% CI, 0.01–0.71) vs. 1.80 (1.16–2.44), $P < 0.001$].

The studies by Burgess and Haley (2008), Liu and Chiu (2015), and Zhong et al. (2010) recorded their patients' pain relief, which is presented in Fig. 18.1. This meta-analysis showed significant improvement in pain relief among patients with aphthous stomatitis in the intervention group [OR = 0.13; 95% CI (0.05, 0.32); $P < 0.001$], and the homogeneity hypothesis was not rejected ($P = 0.59$). For details, please refer to Fig. 18.1. The trials in this review, evidence from three randomized controlled trials involving 95 participants showed that daily use of the vitamin B_{12} treatment as adjunctive care is associated with a decreased level of pain caused by an aphthous ulcer. Overall, our meta-analysis suggests that vitamin B_{12} may significantly reduce the intensity of pain during healing and should to provide relieves the painful feeling in the aphthous ulcers.

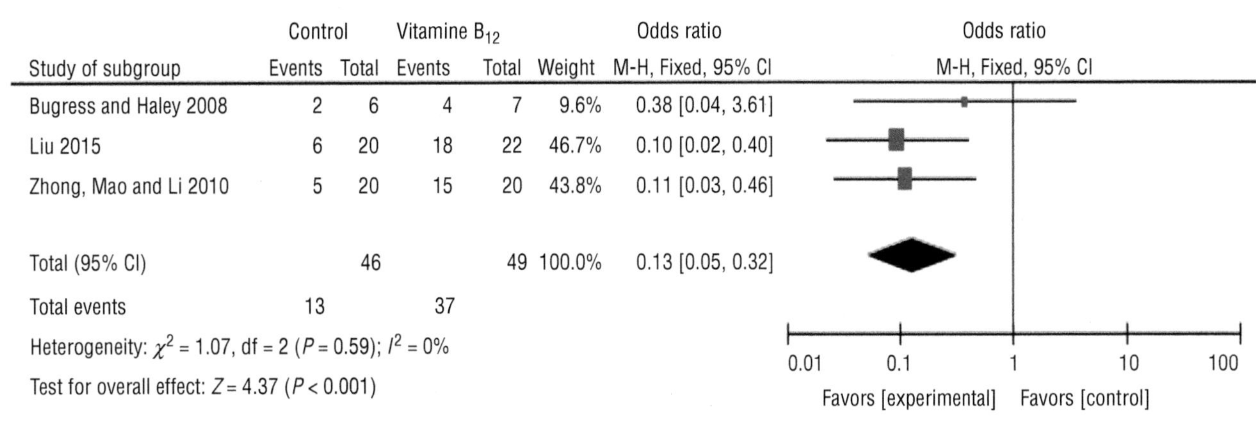

FIGURE 18.1 **Meta-analysis showing that vitamin B_{12} provides relief from pain in aphthous ulcers.** *CI*, Confidence interval.

In conclusion, vitamin B_{12} treatment may be beneficial to patients with mouth ulcers. According to our study, vitamin B_{12} is only for adjuvant therapy to relieve ulcer pain, which means that vitamin B_{12} not only is able to promote ulcer healing but also has good analgesic effect. Although the meta-analysis was statistically significant, we must interpret the results carefully because of the small size and the fact that the studies were very different with respect to vitamin B_{12} dosage, mode of delivery, and participant's length of the treatment. The meta-analysis demonstrates that vitamin B_{12} is an effective analgesic treatment for aphthous ulcers. Pain reduction is essential not only for providing comfort to aphthous ulcers patients but also because it can affect oral intake, swallowing, and speaking. Therefore, vitamin B_{12} is an effective method and beneficial as a simple, inexpensive therapy for aphthous stomatitis patients to reduce pain levels in patients with mouth ulcers.

Regarding the effectiveness of vitamin B_{12} in the treatment of aphthous ulcers, no solid conclusions can be drawn because of the limitation given earlier. This would suggest that further research is required to examine the relief of pain in the treatment of aphthous ulcers and to compare daily orally taken vitamin B_{12} alone versus daily orally taken vitamin B_{12} in addition to oral cavity mucous membrane absorption near site of a mouth ulcer.

References

Allen, L. H. (2009). How common is vitamin B-12 deficiency? *American Journal of Clinical Nutrition, 89*, 693S–696S.

Babaee, N., Mansourian, A., Momen-Heravi, F., Moghadamnia, A., & Momen-Beitollahi, J. (2010). The efficacy of a paste containing *Myrtus communis* (myrtle) in the management of recurrent aphthous stomatitis: a randomized controlled trial. *Clinical Oral Investigations, 14*, 65–70.

Brachmann, F. (1954). Treatment of chronically recurrent aphthae with vitamin B12. *Zohnarztl Welt, 9*, 58–59.

Brogden, R. N., Speight, T. M., & Avery, G. S. (1974). Deglycyrrhizinated liquorice: a report of its pharmacological properties and therapeutic efficacy in peptic ulcer. *Drugs, 8*, 330–339.

Burgess, J. A., & Haley, J. T. (2008). Effect of bioactive B12 in adhering discs on aphthous ulcers. *Inside Dentistry, 10*, 60–63.

Casiglia, J. M., Morwski, G. W., & Nebesio, C. L. (2010). Aphthous stomatitis. Emedicine dermatology. Available at: http://emedicine.medscape.com/article/1075570-overview (accessed February 3, 2010).

Crivelli, M. R., Aguas, S., Adler, I., Quarracino, C., & Bazerque, P. (1988). Influence of socioeconomic status on oral mucosa lesion prevalence in schoolchildren. *Community Dentistry and Oral Epidemiology, 16*, 58–60.

Dali-Youcef, N., & Andrès, E. (2009). An update on cobalamin deficiency in adults. *Oxford Journals Medicine: Monthly Journal of the Association of Physicians, 102*, 17–28.

Das, S. K., Das, V., Gulati, A. K., & Singh, V. P. (1989). Deglycyrrhizinated liquorice in aphthous ulcers. *Journal of Association of Physicians of India, 37*, 647.

Davis, R. L., Lawton, A. H., Prouty, R., & Chow, B. F. (1965). The absorption of oral vitamin B-12 in an aged population. *Journal of Gerontology, 20*, 169–172.

Dholakia, K. R., Dharmarajan, T. S., Yadav, D., Oiseth, S., Norkus, E. P., & Pitchumoni, C. S. (2005). Vitamin B12 deficiency and gastric histopathology in older patients. *World Journal of Gastroenterology, 11*, 7078–7083.

Driban, N. E., & Alvarez, M. A. (1984). Oral manifestations of Sweet's syndrome. *Dermatológica, 169*, 102–103.

Eversole, L. R. (1994). Immunopathology of oral mucosal ulcerative desquamative, and bullous diseases. *Oral Surgery, Oral Medicine, Oral Pathology, Oral Radiology, and Endodontology, 77*, 555–571.

Femiano, F., Gombos, F., & Scully, C. (2003). Recurrent aphthous stomatitis unresponsive to topical corticosteroids: a study of the comparative therapeutic effects of systemic prednisone and systemic sulodexide. *International Journal of Dermatology, 42*, 394–397.

Field, E. A., & Longman, L. P. (2003). *Tyldesley's oral medicine* (5th ed.). Oxford: Oxford University Press.

Field, E. A., Brookes, V., & Tyldesley, W. R. (1992). Recurrent aphthous ulceration in children—a review. *International Journal of Paediatric Dentistry, 2*, 1–10.

Gonzalez-Moles, M. A., Morales, P., Rodriguez-Archilla, A., Isabel, I. R., & Gonzalez-Moles, S. (2002). Treatment of severe chronic oral erosive lesions with clobetasol propionate in aqueous solution. *Oral Surgery, Oral Medicine, Oral Pathology, Oral Radiology, and Endodontology, 93*, 264–270.

Grattan, C. E., & Scully, C. (1986). Oral ulceration: a diagnostic problem. *British Medical Journal, 26*, 1093–1094.

Hakemer, D., Piatowska, D., & Zabinska, O. (1971). Chronic diseases of the oral mucosa in children in light of own observations. *Czas Stomatol, 24*, 871–875.

Hastürk, H., Tezcan, I., Yel, L., Ersoy, F., Sanal, O., Yamalik, N., & Berker, E. (1998). A case of chronic severe neutropenia: oral findings and consequences of short term granulocyte colony-stimulating factor treatment. *Australian Dental Journal, 43*, 9–13.

Healy, C. M., & Thornhill, M. H. (1995). An association between recurrent oro-genital ulceration and nonsteroidal anti-inflammatory drugs. *Journal of Oral Pathology & Medicine, 24*, 46–48.

Hutchinson, V. A., Angenend, J. L., Mok, W. L., Cummins, J. M., & Richards, A. B. (1990). Chronic recurrent aphthous stomatitis: oral treatment with low-dose interferon alpha. *Molecular Biotherapy, 2*, 160–164.

Jurge, S., Kuffer, R., Scully, C., & Porter, S. R. (2006). Recurrent aphthous stomatitis. *Oral Disease, 12*, 1–21.

Katz, J., Langevitz, P., Shemer, J., Barak, S., & Livneh, A. (1994). Prevention of recurrent aphthous stomatitis with colchicine: an open trial. *Journal of the American Academy of Dermatology, 31*, 459–461.

Kerr, A. R., Drexel, C. A., & Spielman, A. I. (2003). The efficacy and safety of 50 mg penicillin G potassium troches for recurrent aphthous ulcers. *Oral Surgery, Oral Medicine, Oral Pathology, Oral Radiology, and Endodontology, 96*, 685–694.

Kleinman, D. V., Swango, P. A., & Pindborg, J. J. (1994). Epidemiology of oral mucosal lesions in United States schoolchildren: 1986–87. *Community Dentistry and Oral Epidemiology, 22*(4), 243–253.

Krause, I., Uziel, Y., Guedj, D., Mukamel, M., Molad, Y., Amit, M., & Weinberger, A. (1998). Mode of presentation and multisystem involvement in Behcet's disease: the influence of sex and age of disease onset. *The Journal of Rheumatology, 25*, 1566–1569.

Krause, I., Rosen, Y., Kaplan, I., Milo, G., Guedj, D., Molad, Y., & Weinberger, A. (1999). Recurrent aphthous stomatitis in Behcet's disease: clinical features and correlation with systemic disease expression and severity. *Journal of Oral Pathology & Medicine, 28*, 193–196.

Lalla, R. V., Choquette, L. E., Feinn, R. S., Zawistowski, H., Latortue, M. C., Kelly, E. T., & Baccaglini, L. (2012). Multivitamin therapy for recurrent aphthous stomatitis: a randomized, double-masked, placebo-controlled trial. *The Journal of the American Dental Association, 143*(4), 370–376.

Lange, R. D., & Jones, J. B. (1981). Cyclic neutropenia: a review of clinical manifestations and management. *American Journal of Pediatric Hematology/Oncology, 3*, 363–367.

Lê Thi Huong, D., Wechsler, B., Piette, J. C., Papo, T., Jaccard, A., Jault, F., Gandjbakhch, I., & Godeau, P. (1993). Aortic insufficiency and recurrent valve prosthesis dehiscence in MAGIC syndrome. *The Journal of Rheumatology, 20*, 397–398.

Lee, S. (1997). Diagnostic criteria of Behcet's disease: problems and suggestions. *Yonsei Medical Journal, 38*, 365–369.

Liu, H. L., & Chiu, S. C. (2015). The effectiveness of vitamin B12 for relieving pain in aphthous ulcers: a randomized, double-blind, placebo-controlled trial. *Pain Management Nursing, 16*(3), 182–187.

Liu, H. L., Chiu, S. C., & Chen, K. H. (2013). Effectiveness of vitamin B12 on recurrent aphthous stomatitis in long term care: a systematic review. *JBI Database of Systematic Reviews & Implementation Reports, 11*(2), 281–307.

MacPhail, L. A., & Greenspan, J. S. (1997). Oral ulceration in HIV infection: investigation and pathogenesis. *Oral Diseases, 3*, S190–S194.

Majorana, A., Bardellini, E., Flocchini, P., Amadori, F., Conti, G., & Campus, G. (2010). Oral mucosal lesions in children from 0 to 12 years old: ten years' experience. *Oral Surgery, Oral Medicine, Oral Pathology, Oral Radiology, and Endodontics, 110*(1), e13–e18.

Marshall, G. S., Edwards, K. M., Butler, J., & Lawton, A. R. (1987). Syndrome of periodic fever, pharyngitis and aphthous stomatitis. *Journal of Pediatrics, 110*, 43–46.

Meiller, T. F., Kutcher, M. J., Overholser, C. D., Niehaus, C., DePaola, L. G., & Siegel, M. A. (1991). Effect of an antimicrobial mouthrinse on recurrent aphthous ulcerations. *Oral Surgery, Oral Medicine, Oral Pathology, Oral Radiology, and Endodontology, 72*, 425–429.

Miller, M. F., & Ship, I. I. (1977). A retrospective study of the prevalence and incidence of recurrent aphthous ulcers in a professional population, 1958–1971. *Oral Surgery, Oral Medicine, Oral Pathology, Oral Radiology, and Endodontology, 43*, 532–537.

Miller, M. F., Garfunkel, A. A., Ram, C. A., & Ship, I. I. (1980). The inheritance of recurrent aphthous stomatitis. Observations on susceptibility. *Oral Surgery, Oral Medicine, Oral Pathology, Oral Radiology, and Endodontology, 49*, 12.

Moghadamnia, A. A., Motallebnejad, M., Khanian, M., Moghadamnia, A. A., Motallebnejad, M., & Khanian, M. (2009). The efficacy of the bioadhesive patches containing licorice extract in the management of recurrent aphthous stomatitis. *Phytotherapy Research, 23*, 246–250.

Murray, B., McGuinness, N., Biagioni, P., Hyland, P., & Lamey, P. J. (2005). A comparative study of the efficacy of aphthae in the management of recurrent minor aphthous ulceration. *Journal of Oral Pathology & Medicine, 34*, 413–419.

Nolan, A., McIntosh, W. B., Allam, B. F., & Lamey, P. J. (1991). Recurrent aphthous ulceration: vitamin B1, B2 and B6 status and response to replacement therapy. *Journal of Oral Pathology & Medicine, 20*, 389–391.

Olson, J. A., Feinberg, I., Silverman, S., Jr., Abrams, D., & Greenspan, J. S. (1982). Serum vitamin B12 folate, and iron levels in recurrent oral ulceration. *Oral Surgery, Oral Medicine, Oral Pathology, Oral Radiology, and Endodontology, 54*, 517–520.

Orme, R. L., Nordlund, J. J., Barich, L., & Brown, T. (1990). The MAGIC syndrome (mouth and genital ulcers with inflamed cartilage). *Archives of Dermatology, 126*, 940–944.

Pedersen, A., Hougen, H. P., Klausen, B., & Winther, K. (1990). LongoVital in the prevention of recurrent aphthous ulceration. *Journal of Oral Pathology & Medicine, 19*, 371–375.

Peretz, B. (1994). Major recurrent aphthous stomatitis in an 11-year-old girl: case report. *The Journal of Clinical Pediatric Dentistry, 18*(4), 309–312.

Piskin, S., Sayan, C., Durukan, N., & Senol, M. (2002). Serum iron, ferritin, folic acid, and vitamin B12 levels in recurrent aphthous stomatitis. *Journal of the European Academy of Dermatology and Venereology, 16*, 66–67.

Porter, S. R., & Scully, C. (1993a). Orofacial manifestations in primary immunodeficiencies involving IgA deficiency. *Journal of Oral Pathology & Medicine, 22*, 117–119.

Porter, S. R., & Scully, C. (1993b). Orofacial manifestations in primary immunodeficiencies: common variable immunodeficiency. *Journal of Oral Pathology & Medicine, 22*, 157–158.

Porter, S. R., & Scully, C. (1993c). Orofacial manifestations in primary immunodeficiencies: T-lymphocyte defects. *Journal of Oral Pathology & Medicine, 22*, 308–309.

Porter, S. R., & Scully, C. (1993d). Orofacial manifestations in primary immunodeficiencies: polymorphonuclear leukocyte defects. *Journal of Oral Pathology & Medicine, 22*, 310–311.

Porter, S. R., Scully, C., & Standen, G. R. (1994). Oral ulceration as a manifestation of autoimmune neutropenia. *Oral Surgery, Oral Medicine, Oral Pathology, Oral Radiology, and Endodontology, 78*, 179–180.

Porter, S. R., Scully, C., & Pedersen, A. (1998). Recurrent aphthous stomatitis. *Critical Reviews in Oral Biology & Medicine, 9*, 306–321.

Porter, S. R., Hegarty, A., Kaliakatsou, F., Hodgson, T. A., & Scully, C. (2000). Recurrent aphthous stomatitis. *Clinics in Dermatology, 18*, 569–578.

Preeti, L., Magesh, K., Rajkumar, K., & Karthik, R. (2011). Recurrent aphthous stomatitis. *Journal of Oral and Maxillofacial Pathology, 15*(3), 252–256.

Rees, T. D., & Binnie, W. H. (1996). Recurrent aphthous stomatitis. *Dermatologic Clinics, 14*, 243–256.

Reznik, D., & O'Daniels, C. M. (2001). Clinical treatment evaluations of a new topical oral medication. *Compendium of Continuing Education in Dentistry, 32*, 17–21.

Rioboo-Crespo Mdel, R., Planells-del Pozo, P., & Rioboo-García, R. (2005). Epidemiology of the most common oral mucosal diseases in children. *Medicina Oral, Patología Oral y Cirugía Bucal, 10*(5), 376–387.

Rogers, R. (1997). Recurrent aphthous stomatitis in the diagnosis of Behcet's disease. *Yonsei Medical Journal*, *38*, 370–379.

Scully, C., & Porter, S. (1989). Recurrent aphthous stomatitis: current concepts of etiology, pathogenesis and management. *Journal of Oral Pathology & Medicine*, *18*, 21–27.

Scully, C., & Porter, S. (2008). Oral mucosal disease: recurrent aphthous stomatitis. *British Journal of Oral and Maxillofacial Surgery*, *46*, 198–206.

Scully, C., MacFadyen, E. E., & Campbell, A. (1982). Orofacial manifestations in cyclic neutropenia. *British Journal of Oral Surgery*, *20*, 96–101.

Ship, I. I. (1972). Epidemiologic aspects of recurrent aphthous ulcerations. *Oral Surgery, Oral Medicine, Oral Pathology, Oral Radiology, and Endodontology*, *33*, 400–406.

Ship, J. A., Chavez, E. M., Doerr, P. A., Henson, B. S., & Sarmadi, M. (2000). Recurrent aphthous stomatitis. *Quintessence International*, *31*, 95–112.

Shotts, R. H., Scully, C., Avery, C. M., & Porter, S. R. (1999). Nicorandil-induced severe oral ulceration: a newly recognized drug reaction. *Oral Surgery, Oral Medicine, Oral Pathology, Oral Radiology, and Endodontology*, *87*, 706–707.

Shulman, J. D. (2004). An exploration of point, annual, and lifetime prevalence in characterizing recurrent aphthous stomatitis in USA children and youths. *Journal of Oral Pathology & Medicine*, *33*, 558–566.

Stanley, H. R. (1972). Aphthous lesions. *Oral Surgery, Oral Medicine, Oral Pathology, Oral Radiology, and Endodontics*, *30*, 407–416.

Tabolli, S., Bergamo, F., Alessandroni, L., Di Pietro, C., Sampogna, F., & Abeni, D. (2009). Quality of life and psychological problems of patients with oral mucosal disease in dermatological practice. *Dermatology (Basel, Switzerland)*, *218*, 314–320.

Volkov, I., Rudoy, I., Abu-Rabia, U., Masalha, T., & Masalha, R. (2005). Case report: recurrent aphthous stomatitis responds to vitamin B12 treatment. *Canadian Family Physician*, *51*(6), 844–845.

Volkov, I., Press, Y., & Rudoy, I. (2006). Vitamin B12 could be a "master key" in the regulation of multiple pathological processes. *Journal of Nippon Medical School*, *73*(2), 65–69.

Volkov, I., Rudoy, I., Freud, T., Sardal, G., Naimer, S., Peleg, R., & Press, Y. (2009). Effectiveness of vitamin B12 in treating recurrent aphthous stomatitis: a randomized, double-blind, placebo-controlled trial. *Journal of the American Board of Family Medicine*, *22*, 9–16.

von den Driesch, P., Gomez, R. S., Kiesewetter, F., & Hornstein, O. P. (1989). Sweet's syndrome: clinical spectrum and associated conditions. *Cutis*, *44*, 193–200.

Weusten, B. L., & van de Wiel, A. (1998). Aphthous ulcers and vitamin B12 deficiency. *Netherlands Journal of Medicine*, *53*, 172–175.

Wray, D., Ferguson, M. M., Mason, D. K., Hutcheon, A. W., & Dagg, J. H. (1975). Recurrent aphthae: treatment with vitamin B12, folic acid, and iron. *British Medical Journal*, *2*, 490–493.

Zakrzewska, J. M., Robinson, P., & Williams, I. G. (1997). Severe oral ulceration in patients with HIV infection: a case series. *Oral Diseases*, *3*(suppl. 1), S194–S196.

Zhong, D., Mao, X., & Li, A. (2010). Observation on effect of compound vitamin B12 solution to treat patients with oral ulcers induced by nebulizating inhalation of surface corticosteroid. *Chinese General Nursing*, *8*, 1988–1989 (in Chinese).

CHAPTER

19

Vitamin K, Osteoarthritis, and Joint Pain

M.K. Shea, S.L. Booth

Jean Mayer Human Nutrition Research Center on Aging, Tufts University, Boston, MA, United States

Osteoarthritis is a debilitating disease that can develop in any joint, but in particular the knee and hand (Prieto-Alhambra et al., 2014). This disease is characterized by articular cartilage degradation, subarticular bone remodeling and hypertrophy, synovial inflammation, and pathological changes in other joint tissues (Fig. 19.1), leading to joint pain and impaired movement. Knee osteoarthritis is the leading cause of lower extremity pain and disability in older age (Duncan et al., 2007; Sharma et al., 2003), whereas hand osteoarthritis causes reduced grip strength and loss of function, thereby limiting ability to perform everyday tasks, such as opening containers and doors, writing, dressing, and eating (Lee, Paik, Lim, Kim, & Gong, 2012; Kwok et al., 2011; Zhang et al., 2002). There is currently no known cure for any form of osteoarthritis. In a joint report, the Centers for Disease Control and the Arthritis Foundation highlighted "the role of specific dietary components and nutritional supplements in the prevention and management of osteoarthritis" as a key research priority (Giles & Klippel, 2010). Vitamin K and vitamin K–dependent proteins have recently been linked to osteoarthritis in mechanistic and population-based studies, as summarized in this review.

VITAMIN K SOURCES

There is more than one naturally occurring form of vitamin K (Fig. 19.2). The primary dietary form is phylloquinone (vitamin K_1), which is plant-based. Phylloquinone is also the predominant form of vitamin K in circulation. The current recommended intakes (90–120 μg/day) are assumed to maintain normal coagulation, which is vitamin K's established function (Food and Nutrition Board, 2001). Yet even when vitamin K intakes are sufficient to maintain coagulation, subclinical vitamin K insufficiency can be apparent in extrahepatic tissues and associated with several chronic diseases, including osteoarthritis (McCann & Ames, 2009). Older adults generally consume less than the current recommended amounts of vitamin K and are at an increased risk for chronic diseases related to vitamin K insufficiency (Food and Nutrition Board, 2001; McCann & Ames, 2009). Menaquinones are a second form of vitamin K (known collectively as vitamin K_2) that differ from phylloquinone in the length and saturation of their side chain (Fig. 19.2). Menaquinone-4 (MK-4) is found in meat and dairy products because some animal feed contains its precursor, menadione. All other menaquinones are synthesized by bacteria and are present in fermented and/or animal-based foods (Beulens et al., 2013). Based on our current knowledge of vitamin K metabolism, bacterially synthesized menaquinones do not appear to contribute substantially to vitamin K nutritional status (Beulens et al., 2013). None of the menaquinone forms are detected in circulation, unless taken in high amounts in the form of supplements (Shea & Booth, 2016).

Vitamin K intakes are estimated using dietary surveys, most commonly using the food frequency questionnaire (FFQ) instrument. However, vitamin K intake measures carry limitations that are inherent to survey methods and unique to vitamin K that need to be considered when results are interpreted, as reviewed elsewhere (Shea & Booth, 2016). Specifically, it is important to consider the dietary sources of phylloquinone (green leafy vegetables and vegetable oils) that are characteristic of generally healthy diets. In US cohorts, higher phylloquinone intake reflected generally healthy lifestyles, so studies utilizing phylloquinone intake as an indicator of vitamin K status are prone to confounding by indication, which may not be completely eliminated by statistical adjustment (Erkkila & Booth, 2008; Braam et al., 2004; Shea & Booth, 2016). While this limitation may not pertain to menaquinone intake because menaquinone-rich

Nutritional Modulators of Pain in the Aging Population. http://dx.doi.org/10.1016/B978-0-12-805186-3.00019-9
Copyright © 2017 Elsevier Inc. All rights reserved.

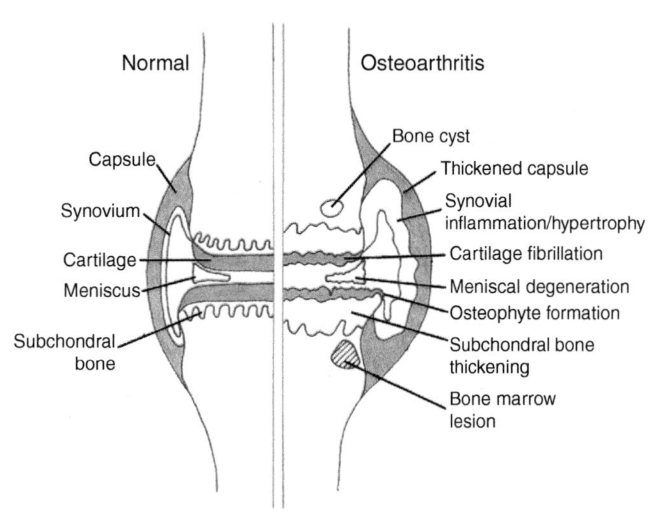

FIGURE 19.1 **Osteoarthritis is characterized by degradation and loss of articular cartilage, subchondral bone thickening, bone marrow lesions and cysts, osteophytes at the joint margins, meniscal degeneration (knee), and joint capsule swelling (Loeser, 2010).** *Source: From Loeser, R. F. (2010). Age-related changes in the musculoskeletal system and the development of osteoarthritis.* Clinics in Geriatric Medicine, *26(3), 371–386.*

foods are not necessarily characteristic of a healthy diet, there are other components of menaquinone-rich foods, such as individual fatty acids, that may have independent protective effect against risk of chronic diseases. In addition, food composition databases for menaquinones are not as complete as they are for phylloquinone, which places an additional limitation on analyses that rely on these databases (Shea & Booth, 2016).

VITAMIN K AND OSTEOARTHRITIS: UNDERLYING MECHANISMS

The only established function of vitamin K is as an enzymatic cofactor in the γ-carboxylation of vitamin K–dependent proteins, as summarized in Fig. 19.3. Carboxylation confers function to all vitamin K–dependent proteins. Warfarin, which is a coumarin-based oral anticoagulant, inhibits the VKOR enzyme, thereby limiting the carboxylation of vitamin K–dependent coagulation proteins. Phylloquinone and all of the menaquinone forms of vitamin K are capable of functioning as an enzymatic cofactor in this capacity.

In addition to clotting proteins, several vitamin K–dependent proteins are present in various extrahepatic tissues, including cartilage and bone, which is the proposed mechanism underlying vitamin K's potential role in osteoarthritis (Fig. 19.4). Currently the most studied vitamin K–dependent protein with respect to osteoarthritis is the calcification inhibitor matrix gla protein (MGP). Articular cartilage and meniscal calcification (chondrocalcinosis) and calcium crystal deposition contribute to osteoarthritis (Terkeltaub, 2002; Abhishek et al., 2013, 2014; Sanmarti et al., 1996; Rutsch & Terkeltaub, 2005; Felson, Anderson, Naimark, Kannel, & Meenan, 1989; Fuerst et al., 2009; Derfus et al., 2002; Abhishek, 2015; Hawellek et al., 2016). Mice lacking MGP develop severe cartilage and vascular calcification (Luo et al., 1997). Chondrocytes, the cells that secrete the cartilage matrix, synthesize MGP as well as the enzymes required for the carboxylation of vitamin K–dependent proteins (Wallin, Schurgers, & Loeser, 2010). MGP is synthesized as undercarboxylated MGP (ucMGP), and, without sufficient posttranslational availability of vitamin K, remains in the undercarboxylated form. The ucMGP is thought to have impaired capacity to inhibit calcification. This observation is supported by the observation that the ucMGP is abundant in human osteoarthritic articular cartilage, while the carboxylated MGP (cMGP) form is more abundant in healthy articular cartilage (Wallin et al., 2010). Furthermore, the γ-carboxylase enzyme is more active in healthy articular cartilage compared to in osteoarthritic cartilage, suggesting a reduced capability to carboxylate MGP and

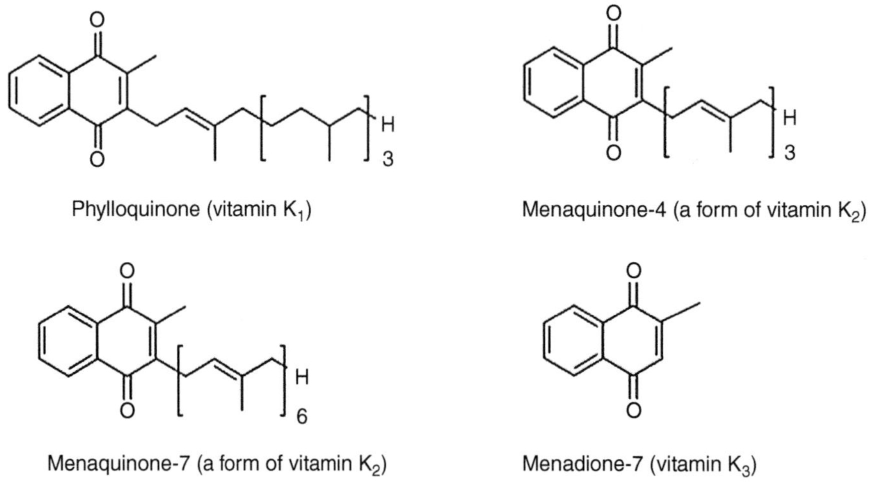

Phylloquinone (vitamin K_1)

Menaquinone-4 (a form of vitamin K_2)

Menaquinone-7 (a form of vitamin K_2)

Menadione-7 (vitamin K_3)

FIGURE 19.2 Forms of vitamin K.

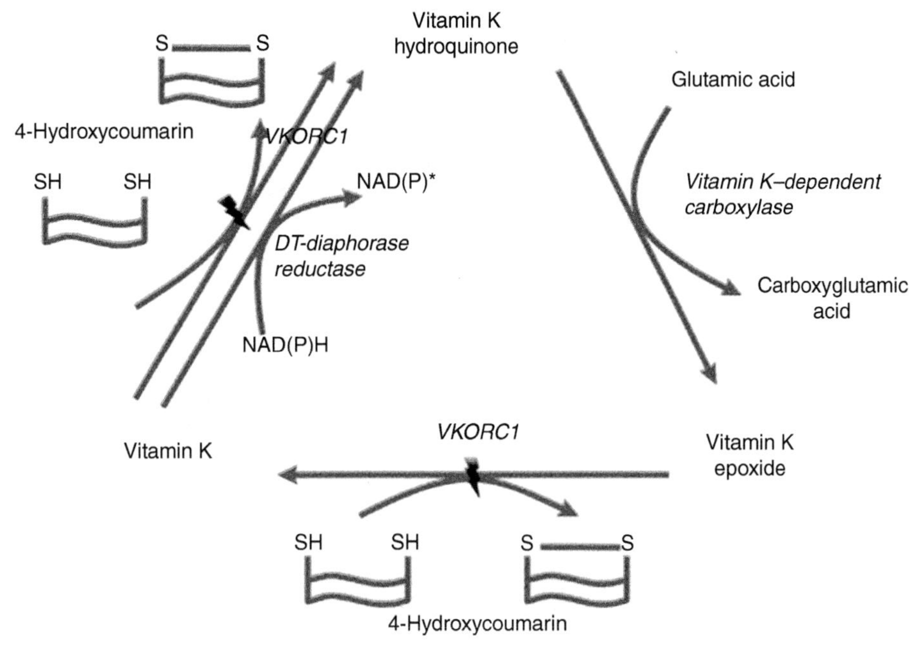

FIGURE 19.3 **Vitamin K, obtained from the diet, is reduced to vitamin K hydroquinone by the vitamin K epoxide reductase enzyme (VKORC1).** Vitamin K hydroquinone is a cofactor for the γ-carboxylase enzyme, which carboxylates glutamic acid (glu) residues [to γ-carboxyglutamic acid (gla) residues]. Vitamin K epoxide is generated, which is reduced back to vitamin K by VKORC1 (Garcia & Reitsma, 2008). *Source: From Garcia, A. A., & Reitsma, P. H. (2008). VKORC1 and the vitamin K cycle.* Vitamins and Hormones, *78, 23–33.*

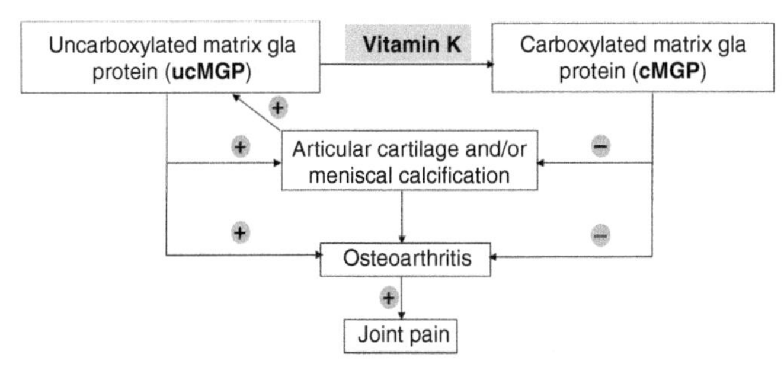

FIGURE 19.4 **Working model showing how vitamin K is implicated in osteoarthritis.**

other vitamin K–dependent proteins in osteoarthritis (Wallin et al., 2010).

Gla-rich protein (GRP) is another vitamin K–dependent protein identified in articular cartilage that has been implicated in cartilage mineralization. Similar to MGP, undercarboxylated GRP (ucGRP) was more abundant than carboxylated GRP in osteoarthritic articular cartilage. This pattern was reflected by an increased calcium deposition in osteoarthritic cartilage compared to that in healthy cartilage (Rafael et al., 2014; Cavaco et al., 2016).

In addition to articular cartilage damage, osteoarthritis is characterized by pathological changes in subarticular bone. Osteocalcin (OC), the most abundant noncartilaginous protein in bone, is a vitamin K–dependent protein synthesized by osteoblasts and increases during bone formation (Gundberg, Lian, & Booth, 2012). However, it is not known whether the carboxylation status of OC in joint tissues is implicated in osteoarthritis. Nonetheless, the presence of multiple vitamin K–dependent proteins in joint tissue (Wallin et al., 2010; Rafael et al., 2014; Cavaco et al., 2016; Loeser et al., 1997; Ohno et al., 2005) suggests that a role for vitamin K in joint health is plausible.

Independent of its role as an enzyme cofactor, vitamin K may also affect osteoarthritis and related outcomes through inflammatory pathways. Phylloquinone and MK-4 treatment in animal and in vitro experiments suppressed production of interleukin-6 and other inflammatory mediators (Hara, Akiyama, Tajima, & Shiraki, 1993; Ohsaki et al., 2006, 2010; Reddi et al., 1995). This anti-inflammatory effect appears to be mediated through the nuclear factor kappa B (NF-κB) pathway (Ohsaki et al., 2010). The NF-κB signaling pathways (Marcu, Otero, Olivotto, Borzi, & Goldring, 2010; Rigoglou & Papavassiliou, 2013) and proinflammatory mechanisms are well established in osteoarthritis (Greene & Loeser, 2015; Goldring, Otero, Tsuchimochi, Ijiri, & Li, 2008; Rahmati, Mobasheri, & Mozafari, 2016), pain (Felson, 2005), and poor function (Brinkley et al., 2009). However, the role of vitamin K on inflammatory cytokine production in joint tissues specifically needs to be evaluated.

BIOMARKERS OF VITAMIN K STATUS USED IN OSTEOARTHRITIS STUDIES

Nutritional biomarkers, which reflect nutrient intake and metabolism, are not limited by incomplete food composition database or other biases inherent to dietary questionnaires (Potischman, 2003). However, estimating vitamin K status using biomarkers is not straightforward because there is no single biomarker that is considered a robust measure of vitamin K status (Shea & Booth, 2016). Circulating phylloquinone is the only biomarker of vitamin K status for which there is an international quality assurance scheme to ensure the highest quality of control standards (Card, Shearer, Schurgers, & Harrington, 2009). Because phylloquinone is transported on triglyceride-rich lipoproteins, serum/plasma samples must be obtained in a fasted state and/or corrected for triglycerides in order for circulating phylloquinone to reflect vitamin K nutritional status. In contrast to other nutrients, there is not an established concentration of phylloquinone that is considered "sufficient." When the Institute of Medicine's adequate intakes are met, circulating concentrations generally approximate 1.0 nmol/L (Food and Nutrition Board, 2001; Booth et al., 2003). However, whether 1.0 nmol/L is indeed sufficient to meet all physiological needs of vitamin K has not been established.

The undercarboxylated fractions of some vitamin K–dependent proteins are detectable in circulation. Higher concentrations of these functional biomarkers reflect lower vitamin K status in tissues that utilize that vitamin K–dependent protein (Shea & Booth, 2016). For example, MGP functions as a calcification inhibitor in tissues that should not mineralize/calcify, such as cartilage and vascular tissue (Price, Faus, & Williamson, 1998; Schurgers et al., 2007; Yagami et al., 1999; Luo et al., 1997). Circulating (dephosphorylated) ucMGP [(dp)ucMGP] is thought to reflect vitamin K status in these tissues. In a similar manner, serum undercarboxylated osteocalcin (ucOC) reflects vitamin K status of bone and protein induced in vitamin K antagonism—factor II (PIVKA-II, a measure of undercarboxylated prothrombin) reflects vitamin K stores in the liver.

Growth arrest-specific 6 protein, which promotes chondrocyte survival, (Loeser et al., 1997), and transforming growth factor-β-inducible protein, which regulates chondrocyte differentiation (Ohno et al., 2005), are additional vitamin K–dependent proteins detected in cartilage. Because antibodies specific to the carboxylated and/or undercarboxylated forms of these proteins have not yet been developed, and hence no biomarkers are available, the role of carboxylation status of these specific proteins in osteoarthritis is unknown.

VITAMIN K AND OSTEOARTHRITIS: EVIDENCE FROM HUMAN STUDIES

The association of vitamin K nutritional status with joint health has been evaluated primarily in observational studies (Table 19.1), which requires estimating vitamin K status in community-dwelling or clinical groups. This can be done using dietary intakes and/or biomarkers (Shea & Booth, 2016).

In a cross-sectional analysis of the Research on Arthritis and Disability (ROAD) study, a cohort of older men and women from rural areas of Japan, a 1 standard deviation (SD) increase in vitamin K intake was associated with a 25% lower odds of having radiographic knee osteoarthritis (defined as a Kellgren and Lawrence grade ≥2) (Kellgren & Lawrence, 1957; Oka et al., 2009). In this same cohort, higher vitamin K intake was associated with less joint space narrowing and osteophytes (radiographic characteristics of knee osteoarthritis) in women, but not in men (Muraki et al., 2014). The overall mean ± SD vitamin K intake in this cohort was 244 ± 148 μg/day in men and 222 ± 117 μg/day in women (Oka et al., 2009), so the incremental benefit of increased vitamin K intake was roughly comparable to an intake 30% greater than the current US recommendation (120 and 90 μg/day for men and women, respectively). The higher intakes reported in Japan may reflect regional differences in food preferences. While phylloquinone is the primary dietary form in Western diets, menaquinone-7 is abundant in *natto*, a fermented soybean-based food commonly eaten in some regions of Japan (Kamao et al., 2007). Menaquinone-7 was also found to be the primary circulating form of vitamin K in postmenopausal women from Nagano, Japan (Tsugawa et al., 2006). The ROAD studies (Oka et al., 2009; Muraki et al., 2014) did not specify what dietary forms of vitamin K were evaluated. To the best of our knowledge, there are no other studies that report on the association between vitamin K intake and knee osteoarthritis or related outcomes.

In contrast, the association between vitamin K status biomarkers and osteoarthritis has been evaluated in three US cohorts (Table 19.1) (Neogi et al., 2006; Misra et al., 2013; Shea et al., 2015a). In the Framingham Offspring Study, plasma phylloquinone, categorized according to distribution quartiles, was inversely associated with knee and hand osteoarthritis prevalence (Neogi et al., 2006). These researchers proposed a plasma phylloquinone threshold of 1.0 nmol/L as potentially beneficial to joint health because there did not appear to be any additional reduction in odds for osteoarthritis above 1.0 nmol/L in this cohort (Neogi et al., 2006). In the Multisite Osteoarthritis (MOST) Study, participants with plasma phylloquinone ≤0.5 nmol/L were 1.5–2.0 times more likely to develop radiographic knee osteoarthritis and cartilage damage over 30 months [risk ratio (95% CI) 1.56 (1.08–2.25) and 2.39 (1.05–5.40), respectively], compared to those with plasma phylloquinone ≥0.5 nmol/L (Misra et al., 2013). In the Health Aging and Body Composition (Health ABC) Study, a cohort of generally well-functioning older adults (mean ± SD age = 74 ± 3 years), those with plasma phylloquinone <0.2 nmol/L (below the assay limit of detection) had a 1.7- and 2.6-fold higher odds of worsening cartilage damage and meniscal damage over 3 years. This analysis also suggested that

TABLE 19.1 Observational and Intervention Studies of Vitamin K and Osteoarthritis

Participants	Design	Exposure	Outcome(s)	Results	References
719 community-dwelling men and women; ≥60 years	Cross-sectional	Vitamin K intake (self-report)	Radiographic knee OA	Lower vitamin K intake associated with more knee OA	Oka et al. (2009)
25 patients (22 females) with radiographic knee OA; mean ± SD age 76 ± 8 years	Cross-sectional	Serum ucOC	Serum hyaluronan	Positive association, suggesting low vitamin K status associated with more knee synovitis	Naito et al. (2012)
672 community-dwelling men and women; mean ± SD age 66 ± 9 years	Cross-sectional	Plasma phylloquinone	Radiographic knee and hand OA	Plasma phylloquinone <1.0 nmol/L associated with more knee and hand OA	Neogi et al. (2006)
1180 community-dwelling men and women; mean ± SD age 62 ± 8 years	Longitudinal observational	Plasma phylloquinone	Radiographic knee OA	Plasma phylloquinone <0.5 nmol/L associated with 1.56-fold higher risk of developing knee OA over 30 months	Misra et al. (2013)
791 older community-dwelling men and women; mean ± SD age 74 ± 3 years	Cross-sectional and longitudinal observational	Plasma phylloquinone and (dp)ucMGP	Knee OA structural features measured with MRI	Cross-sectional: higher plasma (dp) ucMGP associated with higher odds of OA features (osteophytes, cartilage damage, bone marrow lesions, subarticular cysts) Longitudinal: very low plasma phylloquinone (<0.2 nmol/L) associated with a 1.7- and 2.6-fold higher odds of articular and meniscus and articular cartilage damage progression over 3 years	Shea et al. (2015a)
376 community-dwelling men and women; mean ± SD age 71 ± 6 years	Randomized controlled trial	Phylloquinone supplementation (500 μg/day; 3 years)	Radiographic hand OA	No association between phylloquinone supplementation and hand OA prevalence	Neogi et al. (2008)

(dp)ucMGP, (Dephosphorylated) undercarboxylated matrix gla protein; OA, osteoarthritis; SD, standard deviation; ucOC, undercarboxylated osteocalcin.

participants with plasma phylloquinone <0.2 nmol/L were more likely to have bone attrition, subarticular cyst, and osteophyte progression, but statistical significance was not reached [odds ratio (95% confidence interval): 1.9 (0.9–3.6), 1.5 (0.8–2.7), 1.5 (0.8–2.8), respectively] (Shea et al., 2015a). In this study, there were no differences in structural knee osteoarthritis progression detected at the 1.0-nmol/L plasma phylloquinone threshold.

The relevance of the circulating concentrations of undercarboxylated vitamin K–dependent proteins to osteoarthritis is still uncertain. In a small cross-sectional analysis of patients with radiographic knee osteoarthritis, elevated serum ucOC was associated with elevated serum hyaluronan, a marker of synovial inflammation (Naito et al., 2012). Synovial inflammation can occur in knee osteoarthritis. Serum OC is a biomarker of bone formation, so it increases during bone remodeling (Gundberg, Nieman, Abrams, & Rosen, 1998; Szulc & Delmas, 2008). The ucOC concentration depends on the amount of OC synthesized by bone as well as the availability of vitamin K because OC carboxylation occurs posttranslationally (Gundberg et al., 1998, 2012). Typically ucOC is expressed as a percent of total (%ucOC) or as a ratio to total OC or carboxylated OC (Gundberg et al., 1998, 2012). Unfortunately, this study did not report ucOC as a ratio and given that ucOC was positively correlated to several biomarkers of bone turnover, it is more likely that the elevated ucOC was influenced by bone turnover, and not necessarily reflective of low vitamin K status (Naito et al., 2012). Of note, bone turnover biomarkers have been associated with more knee osteoarthritis and articular cartilage loss in some (Berry et al., 2010; Bettica, Cline, Hart, Meyer, & Spector, 2002; Kumm, Tamm, Lintrop, & Tamm, 2013; Wang, Ebeling, Hanna, O'Sullivan, & Cicuttini, 2005), but not all (Hunter et al., 2008), studies.

In the Health ABC Study, participants with elevated (dp)ucMGP (defined as the highest quartile) were more likely to have knee osteophytes, bone marrow lesions, subarticular cysts, and meniscus damage cross-sectionally (Shea et al., 2015a). However, (dp)ucMGP was not associated with progression of any structural abnormalities in the longitudinal analysis, which could be explained by reverse causation because osteoarthritis appears to affect MGP carboxylation (Wallin et al., 2010). It may also suggest that the role of vitamin K in these pathologies is through modulation of proinflammatory cytokines. However, if vitamin K status were associated with inflammatory components of osteoarthritis, one would expect lower vitamin K status to be associated with synovitis (synovial inflammation), which was not the case in Health ABC (Shea et al., 2015a, 2016). In other community-based cohorts, higher phylloquinone intake and circulating phylloquinone were associated with a lower inflammatory burden (Juanola-Falgarona et al., 2013; Shea et al., 2008, 2014), but none of these studies evaluated osteoarthritis-related outcomes. Therefore, more translational studies are needed to clarify the pathways through which vitamin K may affect joint health.

The results of the only known randomized controlled vitamin K supplementation trial that evaluated osteoarthritis as an outcome found no difference in prevalent hand osteoarthritis in community-dwelling older adults randomized to receive phylloquinone supplementation (500 μg/day) for 3 years compared to those randomized to placebo (total n = 378) (Neogi, Felson, Sarno, & Booth, 2008). Unfortunately this trial was not designed to evaluate hand osteoarthritis and baseline osteoarthritis measures were not available, so hand osteoarthritis prevalence was evaluated at follow-up only. In a hypothesis-generating subgroup analysis, these same authors reported that participants with <1.0 nmol/L plasma phylloquinone at baseline and whose plasma phylloquinone increased to ≥1.0 nmol/L following supplementation were 47% less likely to have radiographic joint space narrowing [odds ratio (95% confidence interval): 0.53 (0.32–0.89)]. In these same participants, there was a nonsignificant trend toward less radiographic hand osteoarthritis [odds ratio (95% confidence interval): 0.78 (0.56–1.07)] but no association with osteophytes [odds ratio (95% confidence interval): 0.88 (0.56–1.40)]. This suggests that persons with low vitamin K status are more likely to benefit from vitamin K supplementation, but this finding needs to be confirmed in trials designed specifically to test the effect of vitamin K supplementation on osteoarthritis development and progression.

Since better vitamin K status appears to be associated with less osteoarthritis (Neogi et al., 2006; Misra et al., 2013; Shea et al., 2015a), it would follow that better vitamin K status would also be associated with better physical function because functional impairment is a primary consequence of osteoarthritis. To the best of our knowledge, there is only one study that has addressed this question. In a subcohort of Health ABC, those with ≥1.0 nmol/L plasma phylloquinone had better short physical performance battery (SPPB) scores and faster 20-m gait speed at baseline and after 4–5 years of follow-up. The rate of decline did not differ according to plasma phylloquinone, however. This may suggest that vitamin K has a role in maintaining function but not in altering the rate of functional decline. Participants in the lowest plasma (dp)ucMGP tertile also had better SPPB scores at baseline and but the association over follow-up was not consistent (Shea et al., 2016). In Health ABC, vitamin K status was measured in participants in the knee osteoarthritis substudy only. These participants were selected based on having qualifying knee pain [defined as having "knee pain, aching, or stiffness on most days for at least one month" at some point over the previous year or reporting moderate or worse knee pain during the previous month in association with at least one activity on the Western Ontario and McMaster Universities Arthritis Index (WOMAC) knee pain scale or for being a control (without knee pain)]. The association between vitamin K status and function did not appear to differ by knee pain status, but this subgroup analysis was underpowered (Shea et al., 2015a, 2016). Neither plasma phylloquinone nor (dp)ucMGP differed between participants with and without knee pain. Of interest, in this same cohort, participants with <0.2 nmol/L plasma phylloquinone were less likely to have structural knee osteoarthritis progression, while a threshold of 1.0 nmol/L was relevant to lower extremity function. Although the concentration of circulating phylloquinone considered sufficient has not been established, it is plausible that a lower threshold may apply to structural outcomes than to functional outcomes of joint health. This needs to be clarified in future studies.

CONCLUSIONS AND FUTURE DIRECTIONS

There is accumulating evidence to support a protective role for vitamin K in osteoarthritis. However, given the inconsistencies in results across the studies conducted to date, it is premature to make recommendations regarding vitamin K's efficacy in reducing osteoarthritis development and/or progression. Clinical trials designed to test the effect of vitamin K on osteoarthritis and its associated pain are needed to fill this gap, particularly given the uncertainty that current biomarkers are capturing the putative mechanisms by which vitamin K may have a protective role in joint health.

Acknowledgments

All authors have read and approved the final manuscript. This study was supported by the National Institute of Arthritis Musculoskeletal and Skin Diseases (K01AR063167) and US Department of Agriculture, Agricultural Research Service under Cooperative Agreement No. 58-1950-7-707. Any opinions, findings, conclusions, or recommendations expressed in this publication are those of the authors and do not necessarily reflect the view of the US Department of Agriculture. The authors have no conflicts of interest to disclose.

References

Abhishek, A. (2016). Calcium pyrophosphate deposition disease: a review of epidemiologic findings. *Current Opinion in Rheumatology, 28*, 133–139.

Abhishek, A., Doherty, S., Maciewicz, R., Muir, K., Zhang, W., & Doherty, M. (2013). Evidence of a systemic predisposition to chondrocalcinosis and association between chondrocalcinosis and osteoarthritis at distant joints: a cross-sectional study. *Arthritis Care & Research, 65*, 1052–1058.

Abhishek, A., Doherty, S., Maciewicz, R., Muir, K., Zhang, W., & Doherty, M. (2014). Association between low cortical bone mineral density, soft-tissue calcification, vascular calcification and chondrocalcinosis: a case–control study. *Annals of the Rheumatic Diseases., 73*, 1997–2002.

Berry, P. A., Maciewicz, R. A., Cicuttini, F. M., Jones, M. D., Hellawell, C. J., & Wluka, A. E. (2010). Markers of bone formation and resorption identify subgroups of patients with clinical knee osteoarthritis who have reduced rates of cartilage loss. *The Journal of Rheumatology, 37*, 1252–1259.

Bettica, P., Cline, G., Hart, D. J., Meyer, J., & Spector, T. D. (2002). Evidence for increased bone resorption in patients with progressive knee osteoarthritis: longitudinal results from the Chingford study. *Arthritis and Rheumatism, 46*, 3178–3184.

Beulens, J. W., Booth, S. L., van den Heuvel, E. G., Stoecklin, E., Baka, A., & Vermeer, C. (2013). The role of menaquinones (vitamin K2) in human health. *The British Journal of Nutrition, 110*, 1357–1368.

Booth, S. L., Martini, L., Peterson, J. W., Saltzman, E., Dallal, G. E., & Wood, R. J. (2003). Dietary phylloquinone depletion and repletion in older women. *The Journal of Nutrition, 133*, 2565–2569.

Braam, L., McKeown, N., Jacques, P., Lichtenstein, A., Vermeer, C., Wilson, P., & Booth, S. (2004). Dietary phylloquinone intake as a potential marker for a heart-healthy dietary pattern in the Framingham Offspring cohort. *Journal of the American Dietetic Association, 104*, 1410–1414.

Brinkley, T. E., Leng, X., Miller, M. E., Kitzman, D. W., Pahor, M., Berry, M. J., Marsh, A. P., Kritchevsky, S. B., & Nicklas, B. J. (2009). Chronic inflammation is associated with low physical function in older adults across multiple comorbidities. *The Journals of Gerontology. Series A, Biological Sciences and Medical Sciences, 64*, 455–461.

Card, D. J., Shearer, M. J., Schurgers, L. J., & Harrington, D. J. (2009). The external quality assurance of phylloquinone (vitamin K(1)) analysis in human serum. *Biomedical Chromatography: BMC, 23*, 1276–1282.

Cavaco, S., Viegas, C. S., Rafael, M. S., Ramos, A., Magalhaes, J., Blanco, F. J., Vermeer, C., & Simes, D. C. (2016). Gla-rich protein is involved in the cross-talk between calcification and inflammation in osteoarthritis. *Cellular and Molecular Life Sciences: CMLS, 73*, 1051–1065.

Derfus, B. A., Kurian, J. B., Butler, J. J., Daft, L. J., Carrera, G. F., Ryan, L. M., & Rosenthal, A. K. (2002). The high prevalence of pathologic calcium crystals in pre-operative knees. *The Journal of Rheumatology, 29*, 570–574.

Duncan, R., Peat, G., Thomas, E., Hay, E., McCall, I., & Croft, P. (2007). Symptoms and radiographic osteoarthritis: not as discordant as they are made out to be? *Annals of the Rheumatic Diseases, 66*, 86–91.

Erkkila, A. T., & Booth, S. L. (2008). Vitamin K intake and atherosclerosis. *Current Opinion in Lipidology, 19*, 39–42.

Felson, D. T. (2005). The sources of pain in knee osteoarthritis. *Current Opinion in Rheumatology, 17*, 624–628.

Felson, D. T., Anderson, J. J., Naimark, A., Kannel, W., & Meenan, R. F. (1989). The prevalence of chondrocalcinosis in the elderly and its association with knee osteoarthritis: the Framingham Study. *The Journal of Rheumatology, 16*, 1241–1245.

Food and Nutrition Board, Institute of Medicine. (2001). *Dietary reference intakes for vitamin A, vitamin K, arsenic, boron, chromium, copper, iodine, iron, manganese, molybdenum, nickel, silicon, vanadium, and Zinc*. Washington, D.C.: National Academy Press.

Fuerst, M., Bertrand, J., Lammers, L., Dreier, R., Echtermeyer, F., Nitschke, Y., Rutsch, F., Schafer, F. K., Niggemeyer, O., Steinhagen, J., Lohmann, C. H., Pap, T., & Ruther, W. (2009). Calcification of articular cartilage in human osteoarthritis. *Arthritis and Rheumatism, 60*, 2694–2703.

Garcia, A. A., & Reitsma, P. H. (2008). VKORC1 and the vitamin K cycle. *Vitamins and Hormones, 78*, 23–33.

Giles, W., & Klippel, J. H. (2010). *A national public health agenda for osteoarthritis 2010*. Atlanta, GA: Centers for Disease Control and Prevention, The Arthritis Foundation.

Goldring, M. B., Otero, M., Tsuchimochi, K., Ijiri, K., & Li, Y. (2008). Defining the roles of inflammatory and anabolic cytokines in cartilage metabolism. *Annals of the Rheumatic Diseases., 67*(suppl. 3), iii75–iii82.

Greene, M. A., & Loeser, R. F. (2015). Aging-related inflammation in osteoarthritis. *Osteoarthritis and Cartilage/OARS, Osteoarthritis Research Society, 23*, 1966–1971.

Gundberg, C. M., Lian, J. B., & Booth, S. L. (2012). Vitamin K-dependent carboxylation of osteocalcin: friend or foe? *Advances in Nutrition, 3*, 149–157.

Gundberg, C. M., Nieman, S. D., Abrams, S., & Rosen, H. (1998). Vitamin K status and bone health: an analysis of methods for determination of undercarboxylated osteocalcin. *The Journal of Clinical Endocrinology and Metabolism, 83*, 3258–3266.

Hara, K., Akiyama, Y., Tajima, T., & Shiraki, M. (1993). Menatetrenone inhibits bone resorption partly through inhibition of PGE2 synthesis in vitro. *Journal of Bone and Mineral Research, 8*, 535–542.

Hawellek, T., Hubert, J., Hischke, S., Vettorazzi, E., Wegscheider, K., Bertrand, J., Pap, T., Krause, M., Puschel, K., Ruther, W., & Niemeier, A. (2016). Articular cartilage calcification of the humeral head is highly prevalent and associated with osteoarthritis in the general population. *Journal of Orthopaedic Research*, Epub ahead of print.

Hunter, D. J., LaValley, M., Li, J., Bauer, D. C., Nevitt, M., DeGroot, J., Poole, R., Eyre, D., Guermazi, A., Gale, D., Totterman, S., & Felson, D. T. (2008). Biochemical markers of bone turnover and their association with bone marrow lesions. *Arthritis Research & Therapy, 10*, R102.

Juanola-Falgarona, M., Salas-Salvado, J., Estruch, R., Portillo, M. P., Casas, R., Miranda, J., Martinez-Gonzalez, M. A., & Bullo, M. (2013). Association between dietary phylloquinone intake and peripheral metabolic risk markers related to insulin resistance and diabetes in elderly subjects at high cardiovascular risk. *Cardiovascular Diabetology, 12*, 7.

Kamao, M., Suhara, Y., Tsugawa, N., Uwano, M., Yamaguchi, N., Uenishi, K., Ishida, H., Sasaki, S., & Okano, T. (2007). Vitamin K content of foods and dietary vitamin K intake in Japanese young women. *Journal of Nutritional Science and Vitaminology, 53*, 464–470.

Kellgren, J. H., & Lawrence, J. S. (1957). Radiological assessment of osteo-arthrosis. *Annals of the Rheumatic Diseases., 16*, 494–502.

Kumm, J., Tamm, A., Lintrop, M., & Tamm, A. (2013). Diagnostic and prognostic value of bone biomarkers in progressive knee osteoarthritis: a 6-year follow-up study in middle-aged subjects. *Osteoarthritis and Cartilage/OARS, Osteoarthritis Research Society, 21*, 815–822.

Kwok, W. Y., Kloppenburg, M., Rosendaal, F. R., van Meurs, J. B., Hofman, A., & Bierma-Zeinstra, S. M. (2011). Erosive hand osteoarthritis: its prevalence and clinical impact in the general population and symptomatic hand osteoarthritis. *Annals of the Rheumatic Diseases, 70*, 1238–1242.

Lee, H. J., Paik, N. J., Lim, J. Y., Kim, K. W., & Gong, H. S. (2012). The impact of digit-related radiographic osteoarthritis of the hand on grip-strength and upper extremity disability. *Clinical Orthopaedics and Related Research, 470*, 2202–2208.

Loeser, R. F. (2010). Age-related changes in the musculoskeletal system and the development of osteoarthritis. *Clinics in Geriatric Medicine, 26*, 371–386.

Loeser, R. F., Varnum, B. C., Carlson, C. S., Goldring, M. B., Liu, E. T., Sadiev, S., Kute, T. E., & Wallin, R. (1997). Human chondrocyte expression of growth-arrest-specific gene 6 and the tyrosine kinase receptor axl: potential role in autocrine signaling in cartilage. *Arthritis and Rheumatism*, *40*, 1455–1465.

Luo, G., Ducy, P., McKee, M. D., Pinero, G. J., Loyer, E., Behringer, R. R., & Karsenty, G. (1997). Spontaneous calcification of arteries and cartilage in mice lacking matrix GLA protein. *Nature*, *386*, 78–81.

Marcu, K. B., Otero, M., Olivotto, E., Borzi, R. M., & Goldring, M. B. (2010). NF-kappaB signaling: multiple angles to target OA. *Current Drug Targets*, *11*, 599–613.

McCann, J. C., & Ames, B. N. (2009). Vitamin K, an example of triage theory: is micronutrient inadequacy linked to diseases of aging? *The American Journal of Clinical Nutrition*, *90*, 889–907.

Misra, D., Booth, S. L., Tolstykh, I., Felson, D. T., Nevitt, M. C., Lewis, C. E., Torner, J., & Neogi, T. (2013). Vitamin K deficiency is associated with incident knee osteoarthritis. *The American Journal of Medicine*, *126*, 243–248.

Muraki, S., Akune, T., En-yo, Y., Yoshida, M., Tanaka, S., Kawaguchi, H., Nakamura, K., Oka, H., & Yoshimura, N. (2014). Association of dietary intake with joint space narrowing and osteophytosis at the knee in Japanese men and women: the ROAD study. *Modern Rheumatology*, *24*, 236–242.

Naito, K., Watari, T., Obayashi, O., Katsube, S., Nagaoka, I., & Kaneko, K. (2012). Relationship between serum undercarboxylated osteocalcin and hyaluronan levels in patients with bilateral knee osteoarthritis. *International Journal of Molecular Medicine*, *29*, 756–760.

Neogi, T., Booth, S. L., Zhang, Y. Q., Jacques, P. F., Terkeltaub, R., Aliabadi, P., & Felson, D. T. (2006). Low vitamin K status is associated with osteoarthritis in the hand and knee. *Arthritis and Rheumatism*, *54*, 1255–1261.

Neogi, T., Felson, D. T., Sarno, R., & Booth, S. L. (2008). Vitamin K in hand osteoarthritis: results from a randomised clinical trial. *Annals of the Rheumatic Diseases*, *67*, 1570–1573.

Ohno, S., Tanaka, N., Ueki, M., Honda, K., Tanimoto, K., Yoneno, K., Ohno-Nakahara, M., Fujimoto, K., Kato, Y., & Tanne, K. (2005). Mechanical regulation of terminal chondrocyte differentiation via RGD-CAP/beta ig-h3 induced by TGF-beta. *Connective Tissue Research*, *46*, 227–234.

Ohsaki, Y., Shirakawa, H., Hiwatashi, K., Furukawa, Y., Mizutani, T., & Komai, M. (2006). Vitamin K suppresses lipopolysaccharide-induced inflammation in the rat. *Bioscience, Biotechnology, and Biochemistry*, *70*, 926–932.

Ohsaki, Y., Shirakawa, H., Miura, A., Giriwono, P. E., Sato, S., Ohashi, A., Iribe, M., Goto, T., & Komai, M. (2010). Vitamin K suppresses the lipopolysaccharide-induced expression of inflammatory cytokines in cultured macrophage-like cells via the inhibition of the activation of nuclear factor kappaB through the repression of IKKalpha/beta phosphorylation. *The Journal of Nutritional Biochemistry*, *21*, 1120–1126.

Oka, H., Akune, T., Muraki, S., En-yo, Y., Yoshida, M., Saika, A., Sasaki, S., Nakamura, K., Kawaguchi, H., & Yoshimura, N. (2009). Association of low dietary vitamin K intake with radiographic knee osteoarthritis in the Japanese elderly population: dietary survey in a population-based cohort of the ROAD study. *Journal of Orthopaedic Science*, *14*, 687–692.

Potischman, N. (2003). Biologic and methodologic issues for nutritional biomarkers. *The Journal of Nutrition*, *133*(suppl. 3), 875S–880S.

Price, P. A., Faus, S. A., & Williamson, M. K. (1998). Warfarin causes rapid calcification of the elastic lamellae in rat arteries and heart valves. *Arteriosclerosis, Thrombosis, and Vascular Biology*, *18*, 1400–1407.

Prieto-Alhambra, D., Judge, A., Javaid, M. K., Cooper, C., Diez-Perez, A., & Arden, N. K. (2014). Incidence and risk factors for clinically diagnosed knee, hip and hand osteoarthritis: influences of age, gender and osteoarthritis affecting other joints. *Annals of the Rheumatic Diseases*, *73*, 1659–1664.

Rafael, M. S., Cavaco, S., Viegas, C. S., Santos, S., Ramos, A., Willems, B. A., Herfs, M., Theuwissen, E., Vermeer, C., & Simes, D. C. (2014). Insights into the association of Gla-rich protein and osteoarthritis, novel splice variants and gamma-carboxylation status. *Molecular Nutrition & Food Research*, *98*, 1636–1646.

Rahmati, M., Mobasheri, A., & Mozafari, M. (2016). Inflammatory mediators in osteoarthritis: a critical review of the state-of-the-art, current prospects, and future challenges. *Bone*, *85*, 81–90.

Reddi, K., Henderson, B., Meghji, S., Wilson, M., Poole, S., Hopper, C., Harris, M., & Hodges, S. J. (1995). Interleukin 6 production by lipopolysaccharide-stimulated human fibroblasts is potently inhibited by naphthoquinone (vitamin K) compounds. *Cytokine*, *7*, 287–290.

Rigoglou, S., & Papavassiliou, A. G. (2013). The NF-kappaB signalling pathway in osteoarthritis. *The International Journal of Biochemistry & Cell Biology*, *45*, 2580–2584.

Rutsch, F., & Terkeltaub, R. (2005). Deficiencies of physiologic calcification inhibitors and low-grade inflammation in arterial calcification: lessons for cartilage calcification. *Joint Bone Spine: Revue du Rhumatisme*, *72*, 110–118.

Sanmarti, R., Kanterewicz, E., Pladevall, M., Panella, D., Tarradellas, J. B., & Gomez, J. M. (1996). Analysis of the association between chondrocalcinosis and osteoarthritis: a community based study. *Annals of the Rheumatic Diseases.*, *55*, 30–33.

Schurgers, L. J., Spronk, H. M., Soute, B. A., Schiffers, P. M., DeMey, J. G., & Vermeer, C. (2007). Regression of warfarin-induced medial elastocalcinosis by high intake of vitamin K in rats. *Blood*, *109*, 2823–2831.

Sharma, L., Cahue, S., Song, J., Hayes, K., Pai, Y. C., & Dunlop, D. (2003). Physical functioning over three years in knee osteoarthritis: role of psychosocial, local mechanical, and neuromuscular factors. *Arthritis and Rheumatism*, *48*, 3359–3370.

Shea, M. K., & Booth, S. L. (2016). Concepts and controversies in evaluating vitamin K status in population-based studies. *Nutrients*, *8*.

Shea, M. K., Booth, S. L., Massaro, J. M., Jacques, P. F., D'Agostino, R. B., Sr., Dawson-Hughes, B., Ordovas, J. M., O'Donnell, C. J., Kathiresan, S., Keaney, J. F., Jr., Vasan, R. S., & Benjamin, E. J. (2008). Vitamin K and vitamin D status: associations with inflammatory markers in the Framingham Offspring Study. *American Journal of Epidemiology*, *167*, 313–320.

Shea, M. K., Cushman, M., Booth, S. L., Burke, G. L., Chen, H., & Kritchevsky, S. B. (2014). Associations between vitamin K status and haemostatic and inflammatory biomarkers in community-dwelling adults. The Multi-Ethnic Study of Atherosclerosis. *Thrombosis and Haemostasis*, *112*, 438–444.

Shea, M. K., Kritchevsky, S. B., Hsu, F. C., Nevitt, M., Booth, S. L., Kwoh, C. K., McAlindon, T. E., Vermeer, C., Drummen, N., Harris, T. B., Womack, C., & Loeser, R. F. (2015a). The association between vitamin K status and knee osteoarthritis features in older adults: the Health, Aging and Body Composition Study. *Osteoarthritis and Cartilage/OARS, Osteoarthritis Research Society*, *23*, 370–378.

Shea, M. K., Loeser, R. F., Hsu, F. C., Booth, S. L., Nevitt, M., Simonsick, E. M., Strotmeyer, E. S., Vermeer, C., & Kritchevsky, S. B. (2016). Vitamin K status and lower extremity function in older adults: the Health Aging and Body Composition Study. *The Journals of Gerontology. Series A, Biological Sciences and Medical Sciences*, *71*, 1348–1355.

Szulc, P., & Delmas, P. D. (2008). Biochemical markers of bone turnover: potential use in the investigation and management of postmenopausal osteoporosis. *Osteoporosis International*, *19*, 1683–1704.

Terkeltaub, R. A. (2002). What does cartilage calcification tell us about osteoarthritis? *The Journal of Rheumatology*, *29*, 411–415.

Tsugawa, N., Shiraki, M., Suhara, Y., Kamao, M., Tanaka, K., & Okano, T. (2006). Vitamin K status of healthy Japanese women: age-related vitamin K requirement for gamma-carboxylation of osteocalcin. *The American Journal of Clinical Nutrition*, *83*, 380–386.

Wallin, R., Schurgers, L. J., & Loeser, R. F. (2010). Biosynthesis of the vitamin K-dependent matrix Gla protein (MGP) in chondrocytes: a fetuin–MGP protein complex is assembled in vesicles shed from normal but not from osteoarthritic chondrocytes. *Osteoarthritis and Cartilage/OARS, Osteoarthritis Research Society*, *18*, 1096–1103.

Wang, Y., Ebeling, P. R., Hanna, F., O'Sullivan, R., & Cicuttini, F. M. (2005). Relationship between bone markers and knee cartilage volume in healthy men. *The Journal of Rheumatology*, *32*, 2200–2204.

Yagami, K., Suh, J. Y., Enomoto-Iwamoto, M., Koyama, E., Abrams, W. R., Shapiro, I. M., Pacifici, M., & Iwamoto, M. (1999). Matrix GLA protein is a developmental regulator of chondrocyte mineralization and, when constitutively expressed, blocks endochondral and intramembranous ossification in the limb. *The Journal of Cell Biology*, *147*, 1097–1108.

Zhang, Y., Niu, J., Kelly-Hayes, M., Chaisson, C. E., Aliabadi, P., & Felson, D. T. (2002). Prevalence of symptomatic hand osteoarthritis and its impact on functional status among the elderly: the Framingham Study. *American Journal of Epidemiology*, *156*, 1021–1027.

CHAPTER

20

Conservative and Postoperative Coanalgesic Therapy for Upper Limb Tendinopathy Using Dietary Supplements

*Giovanni Merolla**,**, *S. Cerciello*†,‡

*Shoulder and Elbow Surgery Unit, "D. Cervesi" Hospital, Cattolica, AUSL della Romagna Ambito Territoriale di Rimini, Cattolica, Rimini, Italy; **"Marco Simoncelli" Biomechanics Laboratory, "D. Cervesi" Hospital, Cattolica, AUSL della Romagna AmbitoTerritoriale di Rimini, Cattolica, Rimini, Italy; †Casa di cura Villa Betania, Rome, Italy; ‡Marrelli Hospital, Crotone, Italy

INTRODUCTION

Injuries to the shoulder tendons are highly common in orthopedic practice. Rotator cuff (RC) tendon rupture was first described by Smith in 1834 (Burkhead, 2011; Smith, 2010) and subsequently characterized by Duplay (Farrell, Sperling, & Cofield, n.d.; Meyer, 1924), Codman (1934), and Neer (2005). Tendon degeneration and its end stage, rupture, are a source of significant functional impairment and pain. According to Picavet and Schouten (2003), 30–40% of patients visit their general practitioner due to musculoskeletal pain; the shoulder accounts for more than 30% of complaints, ranking second after low back pain. The prevalence of shoulder conditions increases with age, peaking after 50 years (Hasvold & Johnsen, 1993). The supraspinatus tendon is the most susceptible to full-thickness RC tears (RCTs) (Millett & Warth, 2014). Conservative treatment, specifically prolonged rest and drug therapy, is indicated in the majority of cases; however, at 18-month follow-up, 61% of patients may still be symptomatic and 26% rate their symptoms as severe, despite appropriate conservative treatment. This is due to the fact that most RCTs are progressive and initially asymptomatic (Yamaguchi et al., 2006; Keener, Steger-May, Stobbs, & Yamaguchi, 2010), they do not heal spontaneously, and they tend to grow larger over time (Yamaguchi et al., 2006, n.d.). Acting on risk factors is critical. Manual workers are very prone to shoulder problems. The prevalence of RC tendinopathy among workers performing heavy manual tasks is as high as 18% (Silverstein et al., 2006; Kaergaard & Andersen, 2000). According to Webster and Snook, the mean cost of compensation per case of upper extremity work-related musculoskeletal disorders in 1993 was $8070, amounting to a total compensable cost of $563 million in the US workforce. Whereas the compensable cost includes only medical expenses and lost wages, when all other expenses (e.g., full lost wages, lost production, cost of recruiting and training replacements, and rehabilitation) are considered, the overall cost to the national economy is much steeper (Webster & Snook, 1994). Effective pain medications and successful rehabilitation programs would help reduce symptoms and recover function, allowing patients to go back to work. Pain control is also crucial after surgical repair, to enhance rehabilitation compliance and reduce stiffness (Kim, Kim, & Kim, 2014).

Nutritional Modulators of Pain in the Aging Population. http://dx.doi.org/10.1016/B978-0-12-805186-3.00020-5
Copyright © 2017 Elsevier Inc. All rights reserved.

TENDON DEGENERATION, INFLAMMATION, AND PAIN

Tendons are complex structures formed by soft, fibrous connective bands and an abundant, cell-rich extracellular matrix (Calve et al., n.d.; Andarawis-Puri, Flatow, & Soslowsky, 2015; James, Kesturu, Balian, & Chhabra, 2008). Tenoblasts and tenocytes account for 90–95% of tendon cellular elements (Andarawis-Puri et al., 2015), whereas the main elements of the matrix include collagen type I fibrils (95% of total tendon collagen), other collagen types (III and V), proteoglycans, elastin, and fibronectin (Andarawis-Puri et al., 2015; James et al., 2008; Bernard-Beaubois, Hecquet, Houcine, Hayem, & Adolphe, 1997; Rees et al., 2000). Such cell composition provides limited tissue healing properties (Butler, Juncosa, & Dressler, 2004). Tendon damage may be the consequence of strenuous exercise as well as aging. Repetitive, exhausting physical exercise involves an increased oxygen demand, which may elevate the rate of production of reactive oxygen species (ROS) and free radicals (Morillas-Ruiz et al., 2005). After intense physical activity, production of free radicals exceeds their degradation ability by the antioxidant defense system, resulting in accumulation of ROS and free radicals (Fisher-Wellman & Bloomer, 2009), cell damage, and, often, tendinopathy (Sharma & Maffulli, n.d.). RCTs have been demonstrated to result from primary intrinsic RC degeneration (Hashimoto, Nobuhara, & Hamada, 2003) due to a variety of factors that include natural aging, limited vascularity, altered biology, poor mechanical properties, and genetic factors (Lake, Miller, Elliott, & Soslowsky, 2010; Seitz, McClure, Finucane, Boardman, & Michener, 2011; Harvie et al., 2004). Anatomical damage may also result from the infiltration of macrophages and monocytes, which produce inflammatory cytokines such as interleukin (IL)-1β (Tsuzaki, Guyton, et al., 2003). Significantly increased levels of IL-1β, a potent proinflammatory cytokine, have been described in the synovium, where they enhance inflammatory reactions in injured joints (Gotoh et al., 2000, 2002). IL-1β induces activation of nuclear factor-kappa B (NF-κB), a central transcription factor and key gene expression regulator (Barnes & Karin, 1997; Largo et al., 2003). NF-κB is found in the cytoplasm in its resting stage as a heterotrimer complex consisting of two subunits and an additional inhibitory subunit, Iκ Bα (Kumar, Takada, Boriek, & Aggarwal, 2004). NF-κB activation is crucial in the regulation and expression of more than 500 inflammation-related gene products as well as in tumor cell transformation, survival, proliferation, invasion, angiogenesis, metastasis, and chemoresistance (Sung et al., 2008). IL-1β can also induce expression of inflammatory mediators such as COX-2, prostaglandin E2, and matrix metalloproteinases, which are involved in tendon matrix degradation (Archambault, Tsuzaki, Herzog, & Banes, 2002; Tsuzaki, Bynum, et al., 2003). Prostaglandins and leukotrienes are derivatives of oxidized arachidonic acid due to the action of arachidonate 5-lipoxygenase (5-LO) (Aley, Messing, Mochly-Rosen, & Levine, 2000). Leukotrienes, especially LTB, increase polymorphonuclear cell vascular permeability and chemotaxis, inducing their degranulation (Boden et al., 2001), activation of inflammation pathways, and hyperalgesia.

RATIONALE FOR THE USE OF STANDARD ANTIINFLAMMATORY DRUGS

The treatment of inflammation and tendon degeneration should aim at reducing COX-2 activity and the production of oxidized arachidonic acid derivatives.

Nonsteroidal antiinflammatory drugs (NSAIDs) are the medications most commonly prescribed for tendinopathy (Wang, Iosifidis, & Fu, 2006). They act principally by inhibiting the production of proinflammatory cytokines, prostaglandin, and thromboxane (Talalay, 2001; Rehman & Sack, 1999), but are associated with significant side effects (Fitzgerald, 2004; Harris & Von Schacky, 2004) such as delayed muscle regeneration and impaired ligament, tendon, and cartilage healing (Almekinders, 1999; Miller, Ahmed, Bobrowski, & Haqqi, 2006). These problems have prompted research into natural compounds, such as herbal remedies, capable of reducing inflammation and postoperative pain (Maroon, Bost, Borden, Lorenz, & Ross, 2006; Maroon, Bost, & Maroon, 2010).

ANTIINFLAMMATORY AND ANALGESIC ACTIVITY OF DIETARY SUPPLEMENTS

The mechanisms of action of antiinflammatory herbs and dietary supplements (DSs) have extensively been investigated. Some have a similar action to NSAIDs, that is, they inhibit inflammatory pathways (Maroon et al., 2006; Hostanska, Daum, & Saller, n.d.), whereas others mainly enhance the antiinflammatory and antinociceptive effects of NSAIDs. The most widely explored supplements are those containing *Boswellia serrata* and *Curcuma longa* (Fig. 20.1). *B. serrata* (Salai/Salai guggul) is a medium-sized tree of the Burseraceae family (genus *Boswellia*) growing in dry mountain areas in India, Northern Africa, and the Middle East, where its resin has been burnt as incense in religious and cultural ceremonies (frankincense) and used to treat a variety of inflammatory diseases since time immemorial (Khan & Abourashed, n.d.). It contains monoterpenes, diterpenes, triterpenes, tetracyclic triterpenic acid, and four major pentacyclic triterpenic acids—β-boswellic acid,

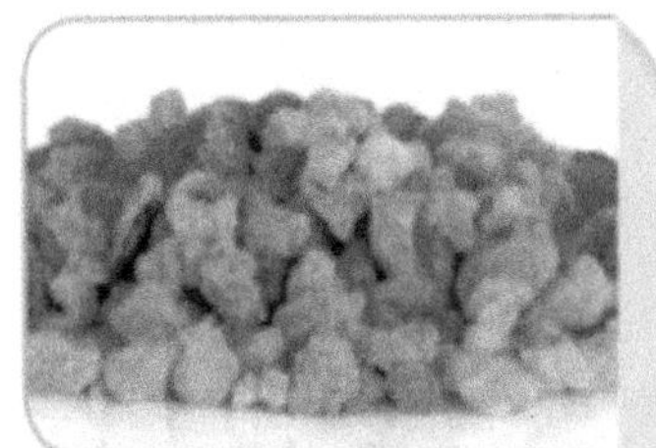

Boswellia •Analgesic and antiinflammatory activity

AKBA (acetyl-11-keto-β-boswellic acid) plays a role in the inhibition of the 5-LOX activity

Acetyl-11-a-keto-boswellic acid (AKBA): structure for binding and 5-lipoxygenase inibitory activity; British Journal of Pharmacology (1996) 117, 615–618.

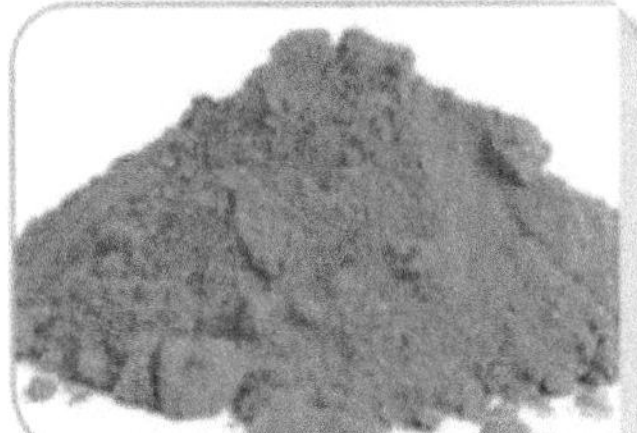

Curcumin •Antiinflammatory and antiapoptotic activity

Titrated in curcuminoids at 95%, has an inhibitory activity on the inflammatory processes IL-1β and NF-κB mediated

Curcumin modulates nuclear factor B (NF-B)-mediated inflammation in human tenocytes in vitro; The journal of Biological Chemistry vol. (2011) 286(32), pp. 28556–28566, August 12, 2011.

FIGURE 20.1 **Curcumin powder and *Boswellia serrata* extract.**

acetyl-β-boswellic acid, 11-keto-β-boswellic acid, and acetyl-11-keto-β-boswellic acid (AKBA)—which participate in proinflammatory enzyme regulation. AKBA has the stronger antiinflammatory action and inhibits 5-LO activity through a dual mechanism, where direct interaction with the enzyme is combined with regulation of the proteins that activate it (Ammon, Safayhi, Mack, & Sabieraj, 1993) (Fig. 20.2). 5-LO also generates inflammatory leukotrienes, which cause inflammation by promoting free radical damage, calcium dislocation, cell adhesion, and migration of inflammation-producing cells to the inflamed body area. AKBA reduces 5-LO activity and its proinflammatory and hyperalgesic effects. Singh and Atal (1986) have reported that it induced 25–46% inhibition of paw edema in rats and mice. Pure AKBA from *B. serrata* extract has demonstrated antiinflammatory properties in human peripheral blood mononuclear cells and mouse macrophages via inhibition of tumor necrosis factor (TNF)-α, IL-1β, nitric oxide, and mitogen-activated protein kinase production (Gayathri, Manjula, Vinaykumar, Lakshmi, & Balakrishnan, 2007). In addition, incensole acetate, a novel compound isolated from *Boswellia* resin, inhibits NF-κB activation (Moussaieff et al., 2007). Bishnoi, Patil, Kumar, and Kulkarni (2006) have found that AKBA and NSAIDs exert a synergistic effect. The finding is interesting, since this action would allow reducing the therapeutic doses of NSAIDs, hence their adverse effects. In a recent study of patients with knee arthritis, Vishal, Mishra, and Raychaudhuri (2011) showed that AKBA reduces pain and improves knee function. AKBA may thus provide an interesting alternative for patients with poor tolerance to NSAIDs. In addition, whereas NSAIDs severely impair glycosaminoglycan (GAG) synthesis, accelerating joint damage in arthritis patients, AKBA significantly reduces their degradation (Brandt & Palmoski, 1984).

B. serrata is generally sold as tablets or capsules, but different manufacturing processes have prevented an ideal dosage from being determined. However, standard treatments involve a total daily dose of 300–500 mg of

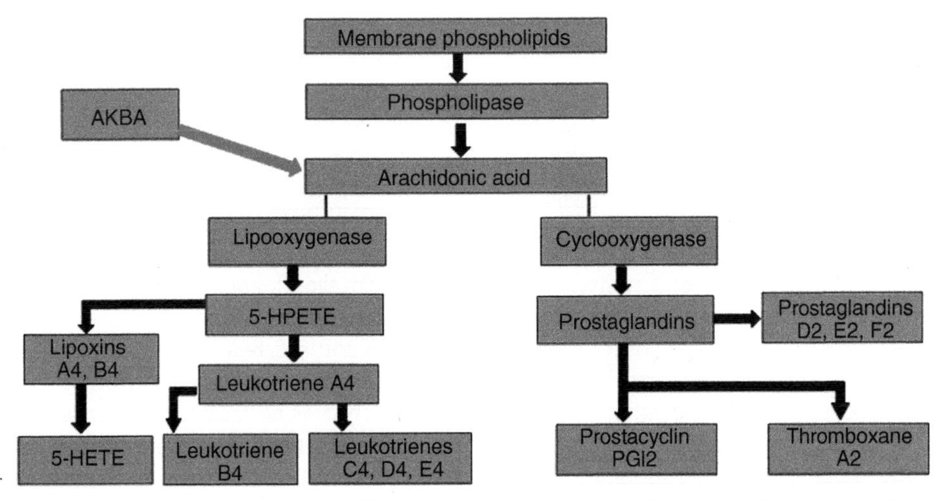

FIGURE 20.2 **Cascade of events and inflammatory mediators.** Acetyl-11-keto-β-boswellic acid (AKBA) inhibits 5-lipoxygenase activity.

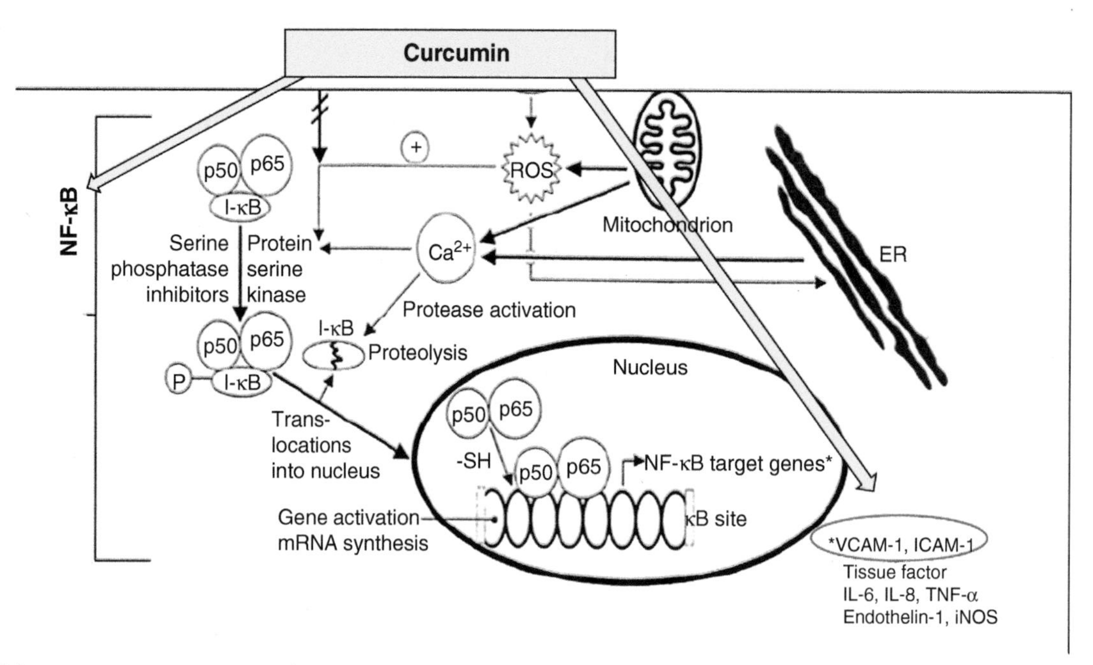

FIGURE 20.3 **Curcumin suppresses IL-β1–induced activation and nuclear translocation of NF-κB.** *IL*, Interleukin; *NF-κB*, nuclear factor-kappa B; *TNF*, tumor necrosis factor.

an extract standardized to contain 30–40% boswellic acids, divided into two or three daily administrations. *C. longa* (turmeric) is a curry spice and a traditional medicinal herb that has long been used in China and Southeast Asia to treat inflammatory conditions. It exerts an antioxidant and antiinflammatory action by inhibiting NF-κB, an activator of several pathways involved in inflammation (Bharti, Donato, Singh, & Aggarwal, 2003; Aggarwal, Kumar, & Bharti, n.d.). It also modulates other relevant molecular targets, including transcription factors (AP-1, β-catenin, and peroxisome proliferator–activated receptor-c), enzymes (COX-2, 5-LOX, and inducible nitric oxide synthase), proinflammatory cytokines (TNF-α, IL-1β, and IL-6), and cell surface adhesion molecules. The effect of curcumin has been investigated in several conditions, including inflammatory diseases (Aggarwal et al., n.d.; Shakibaei, John, Schulze-Tanzil, Lehmann, & Mobasheri, 2007). An in vitro study of human tenocytes has found that it suppresses IL-β1–induced activation and nuclear translocation of NF-κB in a concentration- and time-dependent manner (Buhrmann, 2011) (Fig. 20.3). Moreover, curcumin can either stimulate or inhibit apoptotic signaling, with an effect on different target cells that is closely dependent on treatment time and concentration (Chan, Wu, & Chang, 2006). Overall, nearly 100 companies in the world sell a wide range of curcumin products including beverages, tablets, capsules, creams, gels, nasal sprays, extracts, and coloring agents for both dietary and therapeutic purposes (Allison & Ditor, 2015). Such preparations contain three major components: curcumin (77%), demethoxycurcumin (17%), and bis-demethoxycurcumin (3%), which are collectively called "curcuminoids" (Buhrmann, Mobasheri, Matis, & Shakibaei, 2010; (Hatcher, Planalp, Cho, Torti, & Torti, 2008).

Also in this case, the optimal dosage is still debated; however, clinical trials have shown that a daily dose of 8–12 g is well tolerated and involves no adverse side effects (Sharma et al., 2001).

CLINICAL APPLICATIONS OF DIETARY SUPPLEMENTS TO TREAT TENDINOPATHY AND REDUCE PAIN AFTER TENDON REPAIR SURGERY

DSs have been suggested to enhance tendon healing and reduce pain due to inflammatory conditions of muscles and tendons (Notarnicola et al., 2012). Since DSs containing ascorbic acid raise growth hormone levels, they have been postulated to help healing of chronic tendon injuries (Allampallam, Chakraborty, & Robinson, 2000), whereas those containing amino acids such as glycine, lysine, and proline are held to enhance tendon and ligament repair. Nevertheless, administration of substances containing collagen is unlikely to affect the production of abnormal collagen by tenocytes. Indeed, the major scientific databases (Ovid, Cochrane Reviews, and Google Scholar) contain few papers reporting beneficial effects of DSs on tendon injuries.

Two studies describe the effects of DSs on postoperative pain and tendon healing. A prospective randomized controlled trial of 90 patients with posterosuperior RCTs (Gumina, Passaretti, Gurzì, & Candela, 2012) treated by arthroscopy assessed the effect of a compound containing arginine L-α-ketoglutarate, methylsulfonylmethane (MSM), hydrolyzed type I collagen, and bromelain administered daily for 30 months after surgery. Primary outcome measures were the difference between pre- and postoperative Constant scores and repair integrity assessed by MRI according to Sugaya's classification (Sugaya, Maeda, Matsuki, & Moriishi, 2007). The secondary outcome measure was the Simple Shoulder Test (SST) score. At 6 months, the treated group reported less shoulder pain and exhibited better repair integrity.

Very recently, Merolla, Dellabiancia, Ingardia, Paladini, and Porcellini (2015) assessed the effects of DS administration in an exhaustive study, where 100 patients with full-thickness supraspinatus tears treated by arthroscopic tendon reinsertion (Figs. 20.4a and b and 20.5a and b) were prospectively randomized to receive a preparation containing Tendisulfur (two daily sachets for 15 days and one sachet for the next 45 days) or a placebo since the first postoperative day. Both groups were also administered a conventional analgesic therapy with tramadol and/or paracetamol (maximum daily dosage 400 mg and 4 g, respectively). Tendisulfur is a commercially available DS containing a high dose of MSM, types I and II collagen, GAGs, the amino acids L-arginine and L-lysine, dry extract of *B. serrata* titrated to 30% in AKBA, and dry extract of *C. longa* titrated to 95% in curcuminoids. The ingredients of this nutraceutical preparation have documented analgesic and trophic effects on tendon, muscle, ligament, and cartilage (Maroon et al., 2006, 2010; Gumina et al., 2012; Merolla et al., 2015; Arafa, Hamuda, Melek, & Darwish, 2013; Kim, Axelrod, Howard, Buratovich, & Waters, 2006). The placebo contained the following natural constituents: sorbitol,

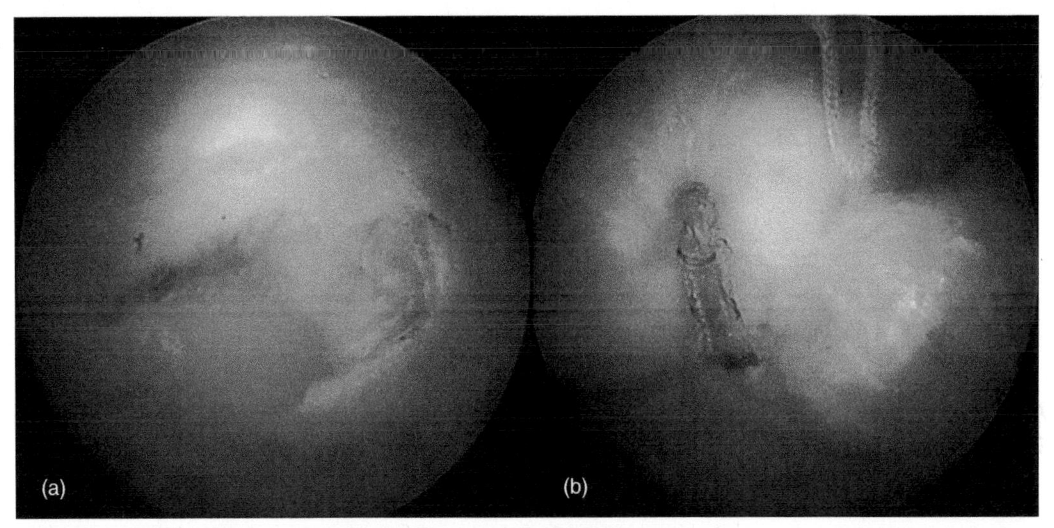

FIGURE 20.4 (a) Small insertional tear of the supraspinatus tendon, which exhibits good tissue quality and appropriate thickness; (b) the tendon is reattached to bone using a double-loaded suture anchor and simple stitches.

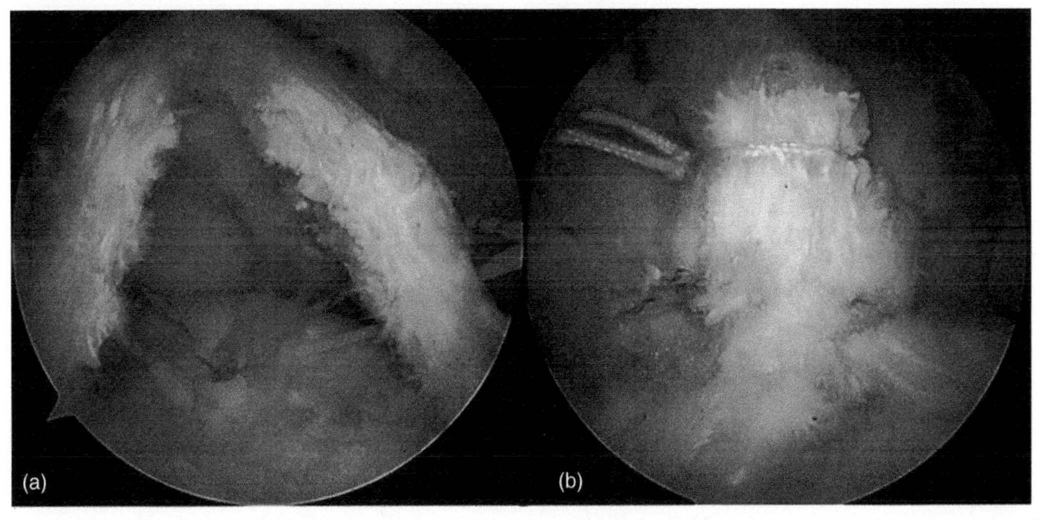

FIGURE 20.5 (a) Full-thickness (V-shaped) supraspinatus tear: thinning, degeneration, and fatty infiltration can be noted; (b) the tendon is reattached to the supraspinatus footprint using a triple-loaded suture anchor and side-to-side sutures.

acesulfame K, sucralose, silicon dioxide, xanthan gum, orange aroma, passion fruit flavor, β-carotene 1%, E 120, and anhydrous citric acid. Outcomes were evaluated using a pain visual analog scale (VAS) as the sole primary outcome measure; secondary outcome measures were as follows: (1) the Constant–Murley score (CMS); (2) the SST score; (3) the patient global assessment (PGA) score; and (4) preparation tolerability, including any adverse events after each administration. Special tests for RC assessment were also performed (Park, Yokota, Gill, El Rassi, & McFarland, 2005) (Fig. 20.6). Patients were assessed at baseline and then at 1, 2, 4, 6, 8, 12, and 24 weeks. At 1 week, the patients receiving Tendisulfur showed significantly lower pain scores ($P = 0.0477$), including pain at night; at 2 weeks their pain scores were still lower than those of the control group, but the difference was no longer significant ($P = 0.0988$). From the third week onward, there were no differences between the groups. The CMS and the SST score were comparable both at 12 weeks ($P = 0.884$ and 0.352, respectively) and at 24 weeks ($P = 0.523$ and 0.292, respectively). PGA scores were good in all participants. Compliance was high and no adverse events were recorded. The authors concluded that the significantly lower pain scores found at 1 week and the lower pain scores found at 2 weeks in the patients receiving Tendisulfur enhanced compliance with the rehabilitation protocol and minimized the risk of complications.

Another research group is exploring the efficacy of 90-day administration of a preparation containing Tendisulfur in professional baseball players with shoulder pain due to supraspinatus tendinopathy. The primary end point is tendon ultrastructure changes as assessed by elastography; the secondary end point is the analgesic effect of the treatment during and after sport activities. Clinical assessment includes the Hawkins, Yocum, and Neer tests for impingement syndrome (Park et al., 2005). The preliminary results in half of the patients are

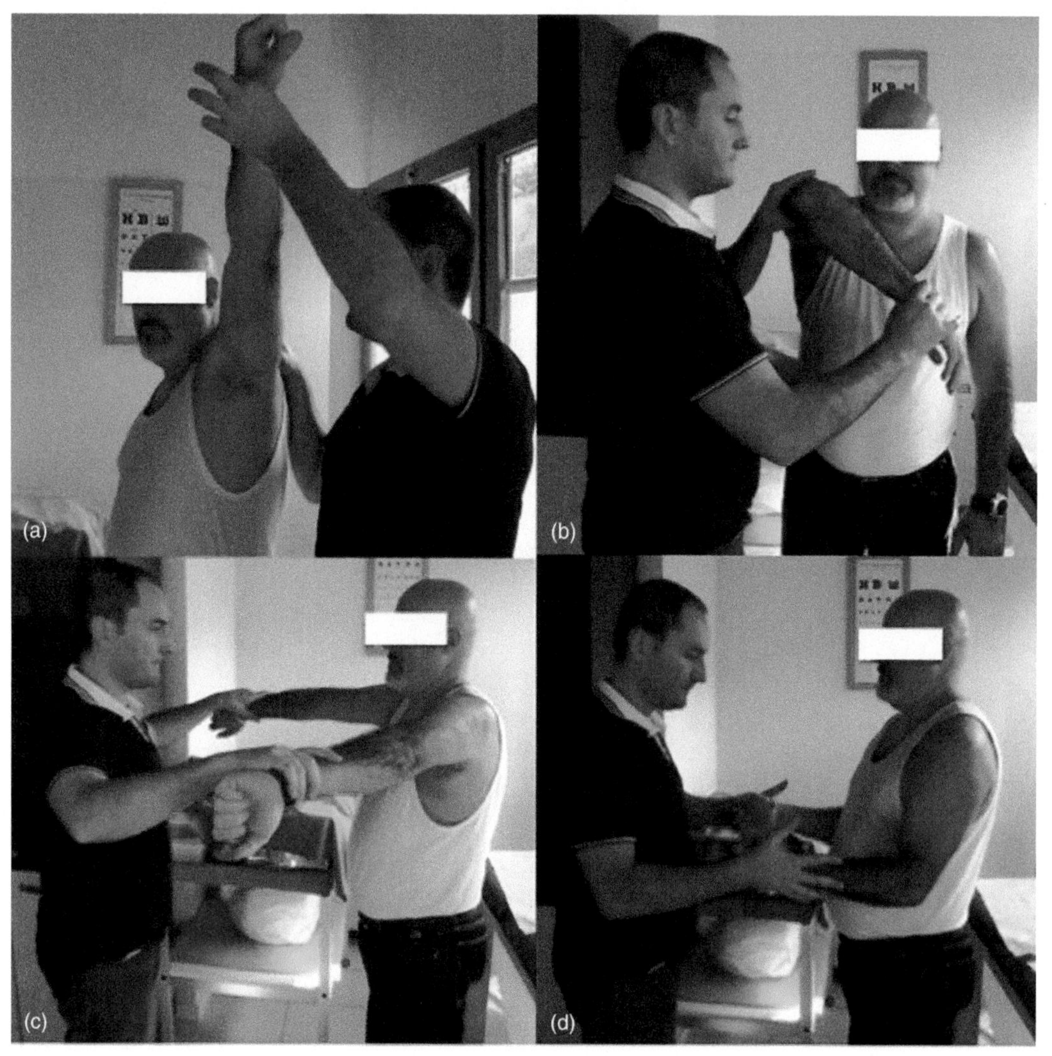

FIGURE 20.6 **Clinical tests applied to assess tendon status (Park et al., 2005).** (a) Neer impingement test; (b) Hawkins test; (c) Jobe test in empty can position; (d) infraspinatus strength test.

encouraging, since the treated group shows progressive and significantly increased tendon elasticity and significantly improved pain and clinical test scores compared with the control group.

Nutritional supplements can provide significant benefits to patients with tendon injuries managed conservatively and to those treated by surgical repair. Their judicious use can enhance pain relief, reducing the requirement for standard antiinflammatory medications. DSs are increasingly being prescribed to patients with upper limb tendinopathy, especially RC injuries. New prospective controlled trials are needed to confirm their clinical efficacy in muscle, ligament, and tendon disorders.

References

Aggarwal, B. B., Kumar, A., & Bharti, A. C. (n.d.). Anticancer potential of curcumin: preclinical and clinical studies. *Anticancer Research, 23*(1A), 363–398.

Aley, K. O., Messing, R. O., Mochly-Rosen, D., & Levine, J. D. (2000). Chronic hypersensitivity for inflammatory nociceptor sensitization mediated by the epsilon isozyme of protein kinase C. *The Journal of Neuroscience: The Official Journal of the Society for Neuroscience, 20*(12), 4680–4685.

Allampallam, K., Chakraborty, J., & Robinson, J. (2000). Effect of ascorbic acid and growth factors on collagen metabolism of flexor retinaculum cells from individuals with and without carpal tunnel syndrome. *Journal of Occupational and Environmental Medicine/ American College of Occupational and Environmental Medicine, 42*(3), 251–259.

Allison, D. J., & Ditor, D. S. (2015). Immune dysfunction and chronic inflammation following spinal cord injury. *Spinal Cord, 53*(1), 14–18.

Almekinders, L. C. (1999). Anti-inflammatory treatment of muscular injuries in sport. An update of recent studies. *Sports Medicine (Auckland, N. Z.), 28*(6), 383–388.

Ammon, H. P., Safayhi, H., Mack, T., & Sabieraj, J. (1993). Mechanism of antiinflammatory actions of curcumine and boswellic acids. *Journal of Ethnopharmacology, 38*(2–3), 113–119.

Andarawis-Puri, N., Flatow, E. L., & Soslowsky, L. J. (2015). Tendon basic science: development, repair, regeneration, and healing. *Journal of Orthopaedic Research: Official Publication of the Orthopaedic Research Society, 33*(6), 780–784.

Arafa, N. M., Hamuda, H. M., Melek, S. T., & Darwish, S. K. (2013). The effectiveness of *Echinacea* extract or composite glucosamine, chondroitin and methyl sulfonyl methane supplements on acute and chronic rheumatoid arthritis rat model. *Toxicology and Industrial Health, 29*(2), 187–201.

Archambault, J., Tsuzaki, M., Herzog, W., & Banes, A. J. (2002). Stretch and interleukin-1beta induce matrix metalloproteinases in rabbit tendon cells in vitro. *Journal of Orthopaedic Research: Official Publication of the Orthopaedic Research Society, 20*(1), 36–39.

Barnes, P. J., & Karin, M. (1997). Nuclear factor-kappaB: a pivotal transcription factor in chronic inflammatory diseases. *The New England Journal of Medicine, 336*(15), 1066–1071.

Bernard-Beaubois, K., Hecquet, C., Houcine, O., Hayem, G., & Adolphe, M. (1997). Culture and characterization of juvenile rabbit tenocytes. *Cell Biology and Toxicology, 13*(2), 103–113.

Bharti, A. C., Donato, N., Singh, S., & Aggarwal, B. B. (2003). Curcumin (diferuloylmethane) down-regulates the constitutive activation of nuclear factor-kappa B and IkappaBalpha kinase in human multiple myeloma cells, leading to suppression of proliferation and induction of apoptosis. *Blood, 101*(3), 1053–1062.

Bishnoi, M., Patil, C. S., Kumar, A., & Kulkarni, S. K. (2006). Potentiation of antinociceptive effect of NSAIDs by a specific lipooxygenase inhibitor, acetyl 11-keto-beta boswellic acid. *Indian Journal of Experimental Biology, 44*(2), 128–132.

Boden, S. E., Schweizer, S., Bertsche, T., Düfer, M., Drews, G., & Safayhi, H. (2001). Stimulation of leukotriene synthesis in intact polymorphonuclear cells by the 5-lipoxygenase inhibitor 3-oxo-tirucallic acid. *Molecular Pharmacology, 60*(2), 267–273.

Brandt, K. D., & Palmoski, M. J. (1984). Effects of salicylates and other nonsteroidal anti-inflammatory drugs on articular cartilage. *The American Journal of Medicine, 77*(1A), 65–69.

Buhrmann, C., Mobasheri, A., Busch, F., Aldinger, C., Stahlmann, R., Montaseri, A., & Shakibaei, M. (2011). Curcumin modulates nuclear factor kappaB (NF-kappaB)-mediated inflammation in human tenocytes in vitro: role of the phosphatidylinositol 3-kinase/Akt pathway. *The Journal of Biological Chemistry, 286*(32), 28556–28566.

Buhrmann, C., Mobasheri, A., Matis, U., & Shakibaei, M. (2010). Curcumin mediated suppression of nuclear factor-κB promotes chondrogenic differentiation of mesenchymal stem cells in a high-density co-culture microenvironment. *Arthritis Research & Therapy, 12*(4), R127.

Burkhead, W. Z. (2011). A history of the rotator cuff before Codman. *Journal of Shoulder and Elbow Surgery/American Shoulder and Elbow Surgeons ... [et al.], 20*(3), 358–362.

Butler, D. L., Juncosa, N., & Dressler, M. R. (2004). Functional efficacy of tendon repair processes. *Annual Review of Biomedical Engineering, 6*, 303–329.

Calve, S., Dennis, R. G., Kosnik, P. E., Baar, K., Grosh, K., & Arruda, E. M. (n.d.). Engineering of functional tendon. *Tissue Engineering, 10*(5–6), 755–761.

Chan, W. -H., Wu, H. -Y., & Chang, W. H. (2006). Dosage effects of curcumin on cell death types in a human osteoblast cell line. *Food and Chemical Toxicology: An International Journal Published for the British Industrial Biological Research Association, 44*(8), 1362–1371.

Codman, E. A. (1934). *The shoulder: rupture of the supraspinatus tendon and other lesions in or about the subacromial bursa*. Boston, MA: Thomas Todd Co.

Farrell, C. M., Sperling, J. W., & Cofield, R. H. (n.d.). Manipulation for frozen shoulder: long-term results. *Journal of Shoulder and Elbow Surgery/ American Shoulder and Elbow Surgeons ... [et al.], 14*(5), 480–484.

Fisher-Wellman, K., & Bloomer, R. J. (2009). Acute exercise and oxidative stress: a 30 year history. *Dynamic Medicine: DM, 8*, 1.

Fitzgerald, G. A. (2004). Coxibs and cardiovascular disease. *The New England Journal of Medicine, 351*(17), 1709–1711.

Gayathri, B., Manjula, N., Vinaykumar, K. S., Lakshmi, B. S., & Balakrishnan, A. (2007). Pure compound from *Boswellia serrata* extract exhibits anti-inflammatory property in human PBMCs and mouse macrophages through inhibition of TNFalpha, IL-1beta, NO and MAP kinases. *International Immunopharmacology, 7*(4), 473–482.

Gotoh, M., Hamada, K., Yamakawa, H., Nakamura, M., Yamazaki, H., Ueyama, Y., & Fukuda, H. (2000). Perforation of rotator cuff increases interleukin 1beta production in the synovium of glenohumeral joint in rotator cuff diseases. *The Journal of Rheumatology, 27*(12), 2886–2892.

Gotoh, M., Hamada, K., Yamakawa, H., Yanagisawa, K., Nakamura, M., Yamazaki, H., & Fukuda, H. (2002). Interleukin-1-induced glenohumeral synovitis and shoulder pain in rotator cuff diseases. *Journal of Orthopaedic Research: Official Publication of the Orthopaedic Research Society, 20*(6), 1365–1371.

Gumina, S., Passaretti, D., Gurzì, M. D., & Candela, V. (2012). Arginine L-alpha-ketoglutarate, methylsulfonylmethane, hydrolyzed type I collagen and bromelain in rotator cuff tear repair: a prospective randomized study. *Current Medical Research and Opinion, 28*(11), 1767–1774.

Harris, W. S., & Von Schacky, C. (2004). The Omega-3 Index: a new risk factor for death from coronary heart disease? *Preventive Medicine, 39*(1), 212–220.

Harvie, P., Ostlere, S. J., Teh, J., McNally, E. G., Clipsham, K., Burston, B. J., & Carr, A. J. (2004). Genetic influences in the aetiology of tears of the rotator cuff. Sibling risk of a full-thickness tear. *The Journal of Bone and Joint Surgery. British Volume, 86*(5), 696–700.

Hashimoto, T., Nobuhara, K., & Hamada, T. (2003). Pathologic evidence of degeneration as a primary cause of rotator cuff tear. *Clinical Orthopaedics and Related Research*(415), 111–120.

Hasvold, T., & Johnsen, R. (1993). Headache and neck or shoulder pain—frequent and disabling complaints in the general population. *Scandinavian Journal of Primary Health Care, 11*(3), 219–224.

Hatcher, H., Planalp, R., Cho, J., Torti, F. M., & Torti, S. V. (2008). Curcumin: from ancient medicine to current clinical trials. *Cellular and Molecular Life Sciences: CMLS, 65*(11), 1631–1652.

Hostanska, K., Daum, G., & Saller, R. (n.d.). Cytostatic and apoptosis-inducing activity of boswellic acids toward malignant cell lines in vitro. *Anticancer Research, 22*(5), 2853–2862.

James, R., Kesturu, G., Balian, G., & Chhabra, A. B. (2008). Tendon: biology, biomechanics, repair, growth factors, and evolving treatment options. *The Journal of Hand Surgery, 33*(1), 102–112.

Kaergaard, A., & Andersen, J. H. (2000). Musculoskeletal disorders of the neck and shoulders in female sewing machine operators: prevalence, incidence, and prognosis. *Occupational and Environmental Medicine, 57*(8), 528–534.

Keener, J. D., Steger-May, K., Stobbs, G., & Yamaguchi, K. (2010). Asymptomatic rotator cuff tears: patient demographics and baseline shoulder function. *Journal of Shoulder and Elbow Surgery/American Shoulder and Elbow Surgeons ... [et al.], 19*(8), 1191–1198.

Khan, I. A., & Abourashed, I. A. (n.d.). *Leung's encyclopedia of common natural ingredients: Used in food, drugs and cosmetics.* (3rd ed.). New York: Wiley. Retrieved from http://eu.wiley.com/WileyCDA/WileyTitle/productCd-047146743X.html (accessed April 8, 2016).

Kim, L. S., Axelrod, L. J., Howard, P., Buratovich, N., & Waters, R. F. (2006). Efficacy of methylsulfonylmethane (MSM) in osteoarthritis pain of the knee: a pilot clinical trial. *Osteoarthritis and Cartilage/OARS, Osteoarthritis Research Society, 14*(3), 286–294.

Kim, C. -W., Kim, J. -H., & Kim, D. -G. (2014). The factors affecting pain pattern after arthroscopic rotator cuff repair. *Clinics in Orthopedic Surgery, 6*(4), 392–400.

Kumar, A., Takada, Y., Boriek, A. M., & Aggarwal, B. B. (2004). Nuclear factor-kappaB: its role in health and disease. *Journal of Molecular Medicine (Berlin, Germany), 82*(7), 434–448.

Lake, S. P., Miller, K. S., Elliott, D. M., & Soslowsky, L. J. (2010). Tensile properties and fiber alignment of human supraspinatus tendon in the transverse direction demonstrate inhomogeneity, nonlinearity, and regional isotropy. *Journal of Biomechanics, 43*(4), 727–732.

Largo, R., Alvarez-Soria, M. A., Díez-Ortego, I., Calvo, E., Sánchez-Pernaute, O., Egido, J., & Herrero-Beaumont, G. (2003). Glucosamine inhibits IL-1beta-induced NFkappaB activation in human osteoarthritic chondrocytes. *Osteoarthritis and Cartilage/OARS, Osteoarthritis Research Society, 11*(4), 290–298.

Maroon, J. C., Bost, J. W., Borden, M. K., Lorenz, K. M., & Ross, N. A. (2006). Natural antiinflammatory agents for pain relief in athletes. *Neurosurgical Focus, 21*(4), E11.

Maroon, J. C., Bost, J. W., & Maroon, A. (2010). Natural anti-inflammatory agents for pain relief. *Surgical Neurology International, 1*, 80.

Merolla, G., Dellabiancia, F., Ingardia, A., Paladini, P., & Porcellini, G. (2015). Co-analgesic therapy for arthroscopic supraspinatus tendon repair pain using a dietary supplement containing *Boswellia serrata* and *Curcuma longa*: a prospective randomized placebo-controlled study. *Musculoskeletal Surgery, 99*(suppl. 1), S43–S52.

Meyer, A. W. (1924). Further evidences of attrition in the human body. *American Journal of Anatomy, 34*(1), 241–267.

Miller, M. J. S., Ahmed, S., Bobrowski, P., & Haqqi, T. M. (2006). The chrondoprotective actions of a natural product are associated with the activation of IGF-1 production by human chondrocytes despite the presence of IL-1beta. *BMC Complementary and Alternative Medicine, 6*, 13.

Millett, P. J., & Warth, R. J. (2014). Posterosuperior rotator cuff tears: classification, pattern recognition, and treatment. *The Journal of the American Academy of Orthopaedic Surgeons, 22*(8), 521–534.

Morillas-Ruiz, J., Zafrilla, P., Almar, M., Cuevas, M. J., López, F. J., Abellán, P., & González-Gallego, J. (2005). The effects of an antioxidant-supplemented beverage on exercise-induced oxidative stress: results from a placebo-controlled double-blind study in cyclists. *European Journal of Applied Physiology, 95*(5–6), 543–549.

Moussaieff, A., Shohami, E., Kashman, Y., Fride, E., Schmitz, M. L., Renner, F., & Mechoulam, R. (2007). Incensole acetate, a novel anti-inflammatory compound isolated from *Boswellia* resin, inhibits nuclear factor-kappa B activation. *Molecular Pharmacology, 72*(6), 1657–1664.

Neer, C. S. (2005). Anterior acromioplasty for the chronic impingement syndrome in the shoulder. 1972. *The Journal of Bone and Joint Surgery. American Volume, 87*(6), 1399.

Notarnicola, A., Pesce, V., Vicenti, G., Tafuri, S., Forcignanò, M., & Moretti, B. (2012). SWAAT study: extracorporeal shock wave therapy and arginine supplementation and other nutraceuticals for insertional Achilles tendinopathy. *Advances in Therapy, 29*(9), 799–814.

Park, H. B., Yokota, A., Gill, H. S., El Rassi, G., & McFarland, E. G. (2005). Diagnostic accuracy of clinical tests for the different degrees of subacromial impingement syndrome. *The Journal of Bone and Joint Surgery. American Volume, 87*(7), 1446–1455.

Picavet, H. S. J., & Schouten, J. S. A. G. (2003). Musculoskeletal pain in the Netherlands: prevalences, consequences and risk groups, the DMC(3)-study. *Pain, 102*(1–2), 167–178.

Rees, S. G., Flannery, C. R., Little, C. B., Hughes, C. E., Caterson, B., & Dent, C. M. (2000). Catabolism of aggrecan, decorin and biglycan in tendon. *The Biochemical Journal, 350*(pt 1), 181–188.

Rehman, Q., & Sack, K. E. (1999). When to try COX-2-specific inhibitors. Safer than standard NSAIDs in some situations. *Postgraduate Medicine, 106*(4), 95–97101–102, 105–106.

Seitz, A. L., McClure, P. W., Finucane, S., Boardman, N. D., & Michener, L. A. (2011). Mechanisms of rotator cuff tendinopathy: intrinsic, extrinsic, or both? *Clinical Biomechanics (Bristol, Avon), 26*(1), 1–12.

Shakibaei, M., John, T., Schulze-Tanzil, G., Lehmann, I., & Mobasheri, A. (2007). Suppression of NF-kappaB activation by curcumin leads to inhibition of expression of cyclo-oxygenase-2 and matrix metalloproteinase-9 in human articular chondrocytes: implications for the treatment of osteoarthritis. *Biochemical Pharmacology, 73*(9), 1434–1445.

Sharma, P., & Maffulli, N. (n.d.). Biology of tendon injury: healing, modeling and remodeling. *Journal of Musculoskeletal & Neuronal Interactions, 6*(2), 181–190.

Sharma, R. A., McLelland, H. R., Hill, K. A., Ireson, C. R., Euden, S. A., Manson, M. M., & Steward, W. P. (2001). Pharmacodynamic and pharmacokinetic study of oral *Curcuma* extract in patients with colorectal cancer. *Clinical Cancer Research: An Official Journal of the American Association for Cancer Research, 7*(7), 1894–1900.

Silverstein, B. A., Viikari-Juntura, E., Fan, Z. J., Bonauto, D. K., Bao, S., & Smith, C. (2006). Natural course of nontraumatic rotator cuff tendinitis and shoulder symptoms in a working population. *Scandinavian Journal of Work, Environment & Health, 32*(2), 99–108.

Singh, G. B., & Atal, C. K. (1986). Pharmacology of an extract of salai guggal ex-*Boswellia serrata*, a new non-steroidal anti-inflammatory agent. *Agents and Actions, 18*(3–4), 407–412.

Smith, J. G. (2010). The classic: pathological appearances of seven cases of injury of the shoulder-joint: with remarks. 1834. *Clinical Orthopaedics and Related Research, 468*(6), 1471–1475.

Sugaya, H., Maeda, K., Matsuki, K., & Moriishi, J. (2007). Repair integrity and functional outcome after arthroscopic double-row rotator cuff repair. A prospective outcome study. *The Journal of Bone and Joint Surgery. American Volume, 89*(5), 953–960.

Sung, B., Pandey, M. K., Ahn, K. S., Yi, T., Chaturvedi, M. M., Liu, M., & Aggarwal, B. B. (2008). Anacardic acid (6-nonadecyl salicylic acid), an inhibitor of histone acetyltransferase, suppresses expression of nuclear factor-kappaB-regulated gene products involved in cell survival, proliferation, invasion, and inflammation through inhibition of the inhibitory subunit of nuclear factor-kappaBalpha kinase, leading to potentiation of apoptosis. *Blood, 111*(10), 4880–4891.

Talalay, P. (2001). The importance of using scientific principles in the development of medicinal agents from plants. *Academic Medicine: Journal of the Association of American Medical Colleges, 76*(3), 238–247.

Tsuzaki, M., Bynum, D., Almekinders, L., Yang, X., Faber, J., & Banes, A. J. (2003a). ATP modulates load-inducible IL-1beta, COX 2, and MMP-3 gene expression in human tendon cells. *Journal of Cellular Biochemistry, 89*(3), 556–562.

Tsuzaki, M., Guyton, G., Garrett, W., Archambault, J. M., Herzog, W., Almekinders, L., & Banes, A. J. (2003b). IL-1 beta induces COX2, MMP-1, -3 and -13, ADAMTS-4, IL-1 beta and IL-6 in human tendon cells. *Journal of Orthopaedic Research: Official Publication of the Orthopaedic Research Society, 21*(2), 256–264.

Vishal, A. A., Mishra, A., & Raychaudhuri, S. P. (2011). A double blind, randomized, placebo controlled clinical study evaluates the early efficacy of Aflapin in subjects with osteoarthritis of knee. *International Journal of Medical Sciences, 8*(7), 615–622.

Wang, J. H. -C., Iosifidis, M. I., & Fu, F. H. (2006). Biomechanical basis for tendinopathy. *Clinical Orthopaedics and Related Research, 443*, 320–332.

Webster, B. S., & Snook, S. H. (1994). The cost of compensable upper extremity cumulative trauma disorders. *Journal of Occupational Medicine: Official Publication of the Industrial Medical Association, 36*(7), 713–717.

Yamaguchi, K., Ditsios, K., Middleton, W. D., Hildebolt, C. F., Galatz, L. M., & Teefey, S. A. (2006). The demographic and morphological features of rotator cuff disease. A comparison of asymptomatic and symptomatic shoulders. *The Journal of Bone and Joint Surgery. American Volume, 88*(8), 1699–1704.

Yamaguchi, K., Tetro, A. M., Blam, O., Evanoff, B. A., Teefey, S. A., & Middleton, W. D. (n.d.). Natural history of asymptomatic rotator cuff tears: a longitudinal analysis of asymptomatic tears detected sonographically. *Journal of Shoulder and Elbow Surgery/American Shoulder and Elbow Surgeons ... [et al.], 10*(3), 199–203.

CHAPTER

21

Folic Acid in Pain: An Epigenetic Link

N. Sharma, A.B. Gaikwad*, Y.A. Kulkarni***

*Department of Pharmacy, Birla Institute of Technology and Science, Pilani Campus, Pilani, Rajasthan, India; **Shobhaben Pratapbhai Patel School of Pharmacy & Technology Management, SVKM's NMIMS, Vile Parle (West), Mumbai, Maharashtra, India

INTRODUCTION

Pain is the topmost reason patients consult a healthcare provider in the United States, with at least one in every three emergency room patients and more than 60% of all primary care patients listing pain as their major complaint (Simon, 2012). According to the International Association for the Study of Pain (IASP), "Pain is an unpleasant sensory and emotional experience associated with actual or potential tissue damage, or described in terms of such damage" (Loeser & Melzack, 1999). Pain is a discomforting feeling often caused by intense or damaging stimuli, such as stubbing a toe, burning a finger, putting alcohol on a cut, and striking the "funny bones" (Descalzi et al., 2015). Defining pain has been a challenge as it is a composite, subjective phenomenon. IASP classified pain according to specific characteristics such as (1) area of the body involved (e.g., upper limbs, abdomen), (2) system whose impairment may be causing the pain (e.g., cardiovascular, gastrointestinal), (3) duration and pattern of occurrence, (4) intensity and time since onset, and (5) etiology (Merskey, 1986). But according to Woolf (2010), pain is classified into three categories: (1) nociceptive pain; (2) inflammatory pain, associated with tissue damage and the infiltration of immune cells; and (3) pathological pain. Pain, however, remains a poorly understood symptom. No one experiences pain like any other and even the same person may encounter pain in different ways, at different times, and under different circumstances, challenging both assessment and treatment. Without a clear comprehension of the mechanisms underlying these differences, healthcare providers are limited in their ability to build an evidence-based intervention science in order to guide symptom management (Lessans & Dorsey, 2013). Where most pain research has focused on griping the underlying genomics and pharmacogenetics of injury, inflammation, and pain, epigenetics furnishes a new paradigm in order to explore the plasticity of the nervous system (Buchheit, Van de Ven, & Shaw, 2012; Doehring, Geisslinger, & Lötsch, 2011; Seo et al., 2013). Epigenetic mechanisms underlying nutrition (nutrition epigenetics) are crucial in understanding human health. Nutritional supplements, such as folic acid that is a cofactor in one-carbon metabolism, balance epigenetic alterations and may play a crucial role in the maintenance of neuronal integrity. Folic acid also improves hyperhomocysteinemia (Hhcy), a consequence of elevated levels of homocysteine (Kalani et al., 2014). Homocysteine is an intermediate sulfhydryl-containing amino acid derived from methionine. It has two providences: remethylation to methionine (with methionine synthase enzyme) or transsulfuration to cysteine (Huang et al., 2007). The elevated levels of homocysteine are linked with a higher risk of neurovascular diseases (Beard, Reynolds, & Bearden, 2011; Dayal & Lentz, 2008; Selhub, 1999). The causes of Hhcy are mainly genetic deficiencies in the enzymes [cystathionine-β-synthase (CBS) and methylene tetrahydrofolate reductase (MTHFR)] responsible for the remethylation or transsulfuration of homocysteine and nutritional (B_6, B_{12}, and folate) deficiencies of vitamins serving as cofactors for the enzymes. Hhcy produces oxidative stress that may epigenetically conciliate cerebrovascular remodeling and leads to neurodegeneration; nevertheless, the mechanisms behind such alterations remain unclear (Kalani et al., 2014). The dietary nutrients—B_6, B_{12}, choline, and folate—are

Nutritional Modulators of Pain in the Aging Population. http://dx.doi.org/10.1016/B978-0-12-805186-3.00021-7
Copyright © 2017 Elsevier Inc. All rights reserved.

the best sources to affect the supply of methyl (–CH_3) groups and further control the biochemical pathways for methylation processes. Folic acid, or folate, is a powerful nutritional and pharmacological determinant of plasma homocysteine levels (Kalani et al., 2014). Folate plays an important role in generating *S*-adenosylmethionine (SAM) for deoxyribonucleic acid (DNA) methylation. DNA methylation (DNAme) leads to the control of gene and, eventually, protein expression (McNeil, Beattie, Gordon, Pirie, & Duthie, 2011). Thus, modification in DNAme by folate deficiency or Hhcy may alter this function. However, mechanisms remain unclear. Sulfhydryl group of homocysteine elevates oxidation, which could also affect DNAme by changing the DNA methyltransferase (DNMT) activity that might further influence the "methionine–homocysteine metabolism pathway" (Kalani, Kamat, Tyagi, & Tyagi, 2013). DNMTs are well known as genomic methylation agents and classified into three types: DNMT 3a (DNMT-3a), DNMT 3b (DNMT-3b), and DNMT 1 (DNMT-1) (Gnyszka, Jastrzebski, & Flis, 2013). These epigenetic changes may lead to alteration of the physiological and pathological processes of homocysteine-mediated vasculopathies that leads to impairment in endothelial function, loss of extracellular matrix collagen, and damage to the blood–brain barrier (BBB) (Beard et al., 2011). Elevated levels of homocysteine result in increased cerebrovascular permeability and neurodegeneration. Moreover, dietary folate supplementation has been proven to be a possible prophylactic approach in order to revert back to the biochemical, molecular, physiological, and epigenetic alterations in the nervous system (Bourre, 2006; Kalani et al., 2014; Li et al., 2015).

VITAMINS

Although all of the vitamins are essential for functioning of the brain, few of them are much important in maintaining a proper functioning of neurons and other brain cells. Vitamins can be assigned according to their specific efficacy for definite actions in the cognitive domain. It has been proved that vitamins A, B_6, B_{12}, and E fortify a better visuospatial memory and improve abstraction test results; vitamin C boosts visuospatial performance (La Rue et al., 1997), although vitamins B_1, B_2, B_3, and the folates enhance the level of intellectual thinking and lead to a more favorable biochemical status. As per concern to pregnant women and infants, the major sources of mental abnormality in the world are iron and iodine deficiencies and protein–energy malnutrition (Wasantwisut, 1996). It has also been postulated that during aging, daily vitamin intakes equal to 3 mg for vitamin B_6 [French recommended dietary allowances (RDAs), 5], 3 mg for riboflavin (RDA, 1.6), and 150 mg for vitamin C (RDA, 110) shielded cognitive levels (Dror, Stern, Nemesh, Hart, & Grinblat, 1996). Progressive deterioration of memory and aging are due to peroxidation, which is protected by antioxidants (Wang, Wen, Huang, Chen, & Ku, 2006). Due to the fact that appreciative effects on cognitive performance are not totally explained by fruit, vegetables, and vitamin E intake (Masaki et al., 2000), other antioxidants (e.g., polyphenols) are being considered.

FOLIC ACID

Folic acid (folate) basically is a "B vitamin." It is also known by several other names: vitamin B_c (or folacin), vitamin M, vitamin B_9, pteroyl-L-glutamic acid, and pteroyl-L-glutamate. Folic acid or folate names are derived from the Latin word *folium*, meaning "leaf." Folate is necessary for various body functions. As human body is unable to synthesize folates de novo, in order to meet its daily requirements, folic acid has to be provided through the diet. In humans, folic acid contributes in synthesis of DNA and repair of DNA and methylate DNA and also acts as a cofactor in certain biological reactions (Weinstein et al., 2003). Basically, it is essential in abetting rapid cell division and growth, likewise in infancy and pregnancy. In childhood and adulthood, folate is important to produce healthy red blood cells and also prevent anemia (Smith, Kim, & Refsum, 2008). During pregnancy, folic acid deficiency leads to a large number of anomalies during the development of the nervous system in the infant. However, it has been reported that this problem can be minimized by ~85% with systematic folate supplementation, few weeks before starting of pregnancy (Moyers & Bailey, 2001). Geriatric patients have shown marked reduction in intellectual capacity (Gottfries, Blennow, Lehmann, Regland, & Gottfries, 2001) and impairment in memory (Agarwal, 2011). Vitamin B_9 serves as a safeguard for brain during its development and memory during aging. Folic acid exists in many fruits and vegetables, especially in dark green leafy vegetables (asparagus, broccoli, cauliflower, cress, leeks, lentils, spinach) (National Institutes of Health, 2009), and other sources are liver, eggs, maize, chickpeas, almonds, and chestnuts (Bourre, 2006).

EPIGENETICS

Epigenetics is rising to eminence in biology as a study of changes in gene expression without a change in underlying DNA sequence of the genome and is mitotically, and sometimes meiotically, heritable. An individual's epigenotype is entrenched during his or her development and is sustained to a degree throughout the lifetime.

The complexes that initiate and maintain the epigenetic state of DNA, and finally a person's epigenotype, involve histone posttranslational modifications (PTMs), cytosine methylation of DNA (DNAme), and RNA-associated silencing. All of these gravitate to interact and stabilize each other (Fraga et al., 2005; Frigola et al., 2006; Ting, Schuebel, Herman, & Baylin, 2005). Epigenetics plays pivotal roles in cell identity and development, lyonization, genomic imprinting, and differential disease susceptibility between monozygotic twins (Reddy & Natarajan, 2015). Histones are composed of globular proteins, around which DNA is reeled to form chromatin. Tail-like projections get extended from the globular domains of histone, which further undergo PTMs: methylation, acetylation, ubiquitination, phosphorylation, sumoylation, ADP ribosylation, and glycosylation. This modified histone tail further acts as a code, which is identified by proteins that regulate chromatin structure and gene expression (Becker, 2006; Nightingale, O'Neill, & Turner, 2006). For example, heterochromatin protein 1 (HP1) is associated with the methylated lysine 9 of histone H3 (H3K9me). The combination of H3K9me and overall histone underacetylation acts as critical marker of epigenetic silencing (Zeng, Ball, & Yokomori, 2010). Conversely, the nucleosome remodeling factor, chromodomain helicase DNA-binding protein 1 (CHD1), binds to the di- or trimethylated histone H3 at lysine 4 (H3K4me2/3), leading to local loosening of chromatin. H3K4me3, together with overall histone hyperacetylation, is a characteristic of active genes (Flanagan et al., 2005). Gene silencing can be actuated by regulating chromatin structure with noncoding RNAs (ncRNAs) (Goodrich & Kugel, 2006). ncRNAs are composed of short interfering RNA (siRNA), PIWI-interacting RNAs (piRNAs), small nucleolar RNAs (snoRNAs), microRNA (miRNA), transcribed ultraconserved regions (T-UCRs), and large intergenic noncoding RNA (lincRNAs) molecules, which are appearing as major elements of cellular homeostasis (Esteller, 2011).

DNAme is another process to attain epigenetic gene silencing. About 80% of all cytosine phosphate guanine (CpG) dinucleotides undergo methylation in mammalian DNA. Methyl groups are attached to CpG dinucleotides by DNMTs. Methylation recruits methyl CpG-binding protein 2 (MeCP2)–like proteins, which can hamper the gene expression. Methylation can also inhibit the binding of transcriptional activators such as myelocytomatosis viral oncogene homolog (Myc) (Moore, Le, & Fan, 2013).

FOLIC ACID AND DNA METHYLATION

It has already been discussed previously that folic acid is one of the essential vitamins among all nutrients. The folate (B_9) is a water-soluble vitamin that plays an important role in mediating the transfer of one-carbon moiety. In folate cycle, methyl groups get synthesized, which are crucial for many genomic and nongenomic methylation reactions, through SAM, and are also essential for the de novo biosynthesis of purines and thymidine and, further, of nucleotides, RNA, and DNA (Reynolds, 2006). It is involved in the synthesis of methionine from homocysteine by methionine synthase, in which 5-methyltetrahydrofolate acts as a cofactor (Fig. 21.1). 5,10-Methylenetetrahydrofolate is an intracellular coenzymatic form of folate, which is required for conversion of deoxyuridylate to thymidylate and can be oxidized to 10-formyltetrahydrofolate for de novo purine synthesis. Therefore, folate is crucial in DNA synthesis, stability and integrity, and repair (Fig. 21.1). Evidence from in vitro animal and human studies stipulates that folate deficiency is related to DNA strand breaks, DNA repair impairment, and development of mutations and that folate supplementation could work in ameliorating these defects instigated by folate deficiency. DNAme occurs on cytosines that antecede a guanine nucleotide (CpG sites). Methylation at cytosine residues in the CpG sequences is heritable, tissue as well as species specific (Jones & Baylin, 2002; Jones & Laird, 1999). Thus, DNAme is a crucial epigenetic determinant in gene expression, which is actually an inverse relationship, preserving DNA integrity and stability, chromatin modifications, and increased mutations (Jones & Baylin, 2002; Jones & Laird, 1999).

FOLIC ACID AND RHEUMATOID ARTHRITIS

Rheumatic arthritis (RA) is a chronic, ongoing, and inflammatory autoimmune disease linked with articular, systemic effects and further characterized by swelling, tenderness, and destruction of synovial joints, leading to severe disability and premature mortality (Firestein, 2003; Isomäki, 1992; McInnes & Schett, 2011; Scott, Coulton, Symmons, & Popert, 1987). Despite the fact that the exact cause of RA remains unknown (Smolen & Steiner, 2003), new findings propose a genetic basis for disease development. The pathophysiology of RA involves the role of B cells and T cells, and the interaction of proinflammatory cytokines (Smolen, Aletaha, Koeller, Weisman, & Emery, 2007). IL-1 and IL-17 may play important roles in the disease process, but TNF-α and IL-6 cytokines are most directly implicated in this process (Smolen & Steiner, 2003). Native T cells are differentiated into Th 17 (TH17) cells, which lead to the production of a potent cytokine (IL-17) that further promotes synovitis. Dendritic cells, macrophages, and activated B cells are antigen-presenting cells, which present arthritis-associated antigens to T cells. B cells also

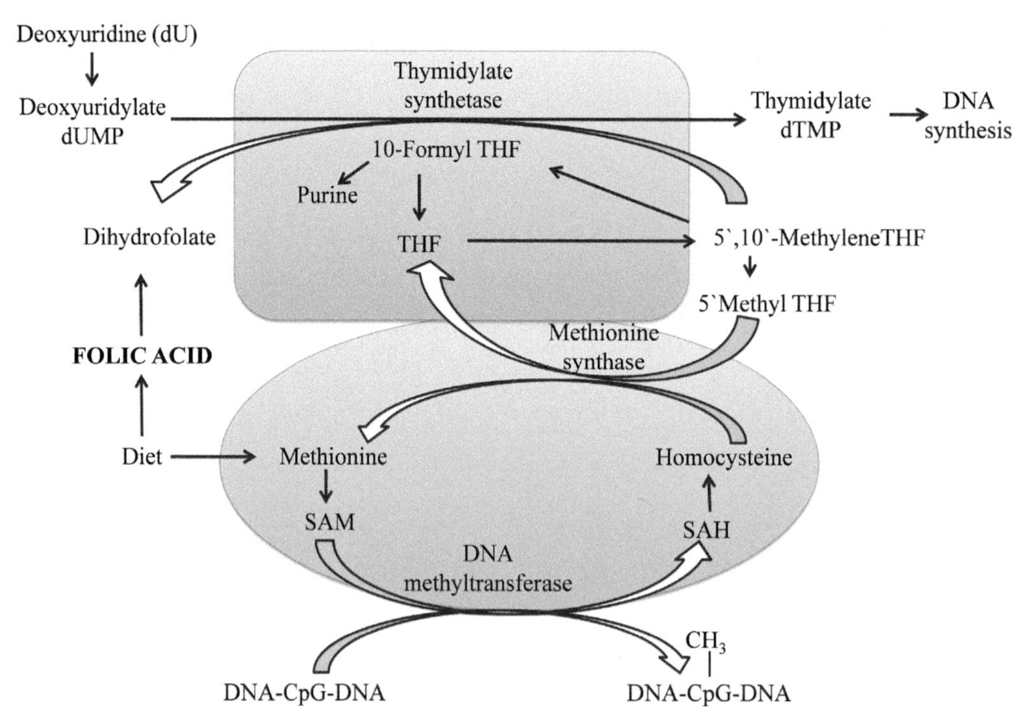

FIGURE 21.1 **Folate metabolism including DNA synthesis and methylation.** *SAM*, *S*-Adenosylmethionine; *THF*, tetrahydrofolate.

help in the production of antibodies, autoantibodies, and cytokines (Smolen et al., 2007). Joint damage starts from synovial membrane, where an arrival and/or local activation of mononuclear cells and new blood vessel formation cause synovitis. The major cause of bone erosion is the pannus, which is osteoclast-rich portion of the synovial membrane, found at the interface with cartilage and bone (Paleolog, 2002). The release of cytokines causes synovial inflammation. Furthermore, the immune response is magnified through antigen-activated CD4+ T cells by stimulating other mononuclear cells, synovial fibroblasts, and osteoclasts. Articular effects result in production of C-reactive proteins, cardiovascular diseases (CVD), anemia of chronic disease, and osteoporosis (Combe et al., 2001; Kaplan, 2006; McInnes & Schett, 2011; Nikolaisen, Figenschau, & Nossent, 2008). They also affect the hypothalamic–pituitary–adrenal axis, resulting in fatigue and depression (Kojima et al., 2009; Rupp, Boshuizen, Jacobi, Dinant, & van den Bos, 2004).

The classification of drugs used for the treatment of RA involves antiinflammatory and disease-modifying antirheumatic drug (DMARD). Methotrexate (MTX) is one of the most commonly used DMARDs, which is used in other inflammatory conditions as well (Cronstein, 1996). It acts by inhibiting the enzyme dihydrofolate reductase (DHFR), as a result of which it depletes the pool of reduced folates. Folate actually acts as a donor of one-carbon moiety during several metabolic intermediate formation, involving purines, methionine, and deoxythymidylate monophosphate, which further leads to a state of effective folate deficiency (Cronstein, 1996). Because of this, several side effects such as gastrointestinal intolerance, cytopenias, and alopecia occur. Moreover, folate deficiency is recognized as a risk factor for MTX toxicity (Ortiz et al., 1998). Theoretically, folic acid supplementation may decrease the efficacy of MTX in treating RA. But in reality, folic acid supplementation reduces MTX-related toxicity such as liver function test abnormalities, GI intolerance, and stomatitis (Morgan, Baggott, Alarcón, & Koopman, 2002; Van Ede et al., 2001). MTX also causes vascular endothelial dysfunction by producing Hhcy, which occurs by directly affecting endothelium or by increasing the oxidative stress (raising levels of 7,8-dihydrobiopterin). Hhcy is found as an independent cardiovascular risk factor (Ganguly & Alam, 2015). It is to be noted that folate antagonism by MTX leads to elevated plasma homocysteine levels by hindering with the remethylation of homocysteine to methionine by means of methyltetrahydrofolate (Blom & Smulders, 2011; Van Ede et al., 2002). MTX and sulfasalazine, used as a combined therapy, may also change folate absorption or metabolism and might lead to an elevated plasma homocysteine than treatment with MTX alone (Haagsma et al., 1999). The addition of folic acid, in doses ranging from 5 to 27.5 mg/week, in patients treated with MTX has been demonstrated to completely abolish the MTX-induced elevation in plasma homocysteine (Whittle & Hughes, 2004).

ROLE OF FOLIC ACID IN COLORECTAL ADENOMAS

Most of the cancer patients experience both somatic and visceral pain. Neuropathic pain is reported only by 15–20% of all cancer patients, as different types of pain respond divergently to the various pain management therapies. The relative causes of pain in cancer patients might be direct tumor involvement, diagnostic/therapeutic methods, side effects, or toxicities of cancer treatment. The major problem with cancer patients is uncontrolled pain, which can affect every aspect of a patient's quality of life leading to suffering, improper sleep, lower appetite, and reduced physical and social activity (Brawley, Smith, & Kirch, 2009).Various reports have suggested that DNA hypomethylation is an early and consistent event in colorectal carcinogenesis (Jones & Baylin, 2002). Multistep process of colorectal adenoma (CRA) includes accumulation of mutations in oncogenes and tumor suppressor genes in colonic mucosa cells, which further suggests that the epigenetic modifications of several genes occur in CRA genome (Lao & Grady, 2011). Large-scale DNAme studies demonstrated that according to frequency of DNAme and mutations in key CRA genes, CRA might be divided into three/four subtypes. DNAme process highly depends on one-carbon metabolism related to a metabolic pathway needed for SAM (major intracellular methylating agent) production. Actually, 5-methyltetrahydrofolate form of folic acid is involved in remethylation of homocysteine to methionine, which is a precursor of SAM. The mechanism by which folate deficiency amplifies colorectal carcinogenesis might be through an induction of genomic DNA hypomethylation based on the biochemical function of folate in mediating one-carbon transfer and evidence was given from animal experiments that demonstrated methyl group donor deficiency-induced DNA hypomethylation (Cravo et al., 1992). Moreover, folic acid supplementation has been found to improve colorectal cancer (Antonakoloulos & Karamanolis, 2007; Coppede, 2014). Although folic acid does not have a direct action on pain relief, it reduces the risk of colorectal cancer and provides a link between nutrients, DNAme, and cancer. As it has been proven that folic acid shows a protective role in CRA, more research has to be done in this aspect.

ROLE OF FOLIC ACID IN MYOFASCIAL PAIN

Myofascial pain is a remarkable health problem affecting about 85% of the general population sometime in their lifetime while the overall prevalence is as much as 46% (Fleckenstein et al., 2010; Simons, 1996). The definition of myofascial pain syndrome (MPS) is specified by regional pain originating from hyperirritable spots located within taut bands of skeletal muscle, studied as myofascial trigger points (MTrps) (Leite et al., 2009). Myofascial pain and dysfunction occurs from direct or indirect trauma, spine pathology, subjection to cumulative and repetitive strain, postural dysfunction, and physical deconditioning (Simons, Travell, & Simons, 1999). It is important to differentiate between myofascial pain and neuropathic pain. Myofascial pain originates at the muscle, while consequences related to neuropathic pain result from an injury to or malfunction of the peripheral or central nervous system (Baron, 2000). Patients suffering with this disorder not only suffer from reduced functional status associated with musculoskeletal pain and loss of function but also encounter impaired mood as well as poor quality of life (Gerber et al., 2013). Medical factors responsible for neurological functional impairment involve iron insufficiency, chronic infections, such as Lyme disease, thyroid deficiency states, recurrent *Candida albicans* infections in women, and folic acid, vitamin B_{12}, and other vitamin insufficiency states (Gerwin, 2005). Vitamin B_{12} and folic acid play their role in synthesis of DNA; both are necessary for normal growth and tissue repair. Folic acid deficiency impairs the DNA synthesis resulting in megaloblastosis in all duplicating cells (mostly in bone marrow cells) of the body (Chanarin, Mollin, & Anderson, 1958). Folic acid is crucial for the appropriate development and functioning of the brain. Folic acid deficiency is the most common vitamin insufficiency and among those inadequacies likely to perpetuate MTrps. It should be taken into consideration that symptoms experienced by patients with myofascial pain having marginally low serum folate levels are very much analogous to, but less intense than, many symptoms described by patients with neurological disorders responsive to folic acid therapy. Patients with low folic acid levels reported showing high susceptibility to MTrPs and also reported fatigue, sleep disturbances, and depression. Moreover, these patients also have a reduced basal temperature, like patients having thyroid hypofunction, and usually their symptoms are relieved by multivitamin therapy involving folic acid. Therefore, vitamin B_{12} and folic acid inadequacy should be pinpointed in the management of MTrPs (Okumus et al., 2010; Simons, 1983).

LIST OF ABBREVIATIONS

CpG	Cytosine phosphate guanine
CRA	Colorectal adenoma
DNA	Deoxyribonucleic acid
DNMT	DNA methyltransferase
MTrps	Myofascial trigger point
MTX	Methotrexate
RA	Rheumatic arthritis

References

Agarwal, R. (2011). Vitamin B12 deficiency & cognitive impairment in elderly population. *The Indian Journal of Medical Research*, *134*(4), 410.

Antonakoloulos, N., & Karamanolis, D. (2007). Folic acid and colorectal cancer. *Annals of Gastroenterology*, *17*(1), 13–14.

Baron, R. (2000). Peripheral neuropathic pain: from mechanisms to symptoms. *The Clinical Journal of Pain*, *16*(2), S12–S20.

Beard, R. S., Reynolds, J. J., & Bearden, S. E. (2011). Hyperhomocysteinemia increases permeability of the blood–brain barrier by NMDA receptor-dependent regulation of adherens and tight junctions. *Blood*, *118*(7), 2007–2014.

Becker, P. B. (2006). Gene regulation: a finger on the mark. *Nature*, *442*(7098), 31–32.

Blom, H. J., & Smulders, Y. (2011). Overview of homocysteine and folate metabolism. With special references to cardiovascular disease and neural tube defects. *Journal of Inherited Metabolic Disease*, *34*(1), 75–81.

Bourre, J. -M. (2006). Effects of nutrients (in food) on the structure and function of the nervous system: update on dietary requirements for brain. Part 1: micronutrients. *Journal of Nutrition Health and Aging*, *10*(5), 377.

Brawley, O. W., Smith, D. E., & Kirch, R. A. (2009). Taking action to ease suffering: advancing cancer pain control as a health care priority. *CA: A Cancer Journal for Clinicians*, *59*(5), 285–289.

Buchheit, T., Van de Ven, T., & Shaw, A. (2012). Epigenetics and the transition from acute to chronic pain. *Pain Medicine*, *13*(11), 1474–1490.

Chanarin, I., Mollin, D., & Anderson, B. (1958). Folic acid deficiency and the megaloblastic anaemias. *Proceedings of the Royal Society of Medicine*, *51*(9), 757.

Combe, B., Dougados, M., Goupille, P., Cantagrel, A., Eliaou, J., Sibilia, J., …, Dubois, A. (2001). Prognostic factors for radiographic damage in early rheumatoid arthritis: a multiparameter prospective study. *Arthritis & Rheumatism*, *44*(8), 1736–1743.

Coppede, F. (2014). Epigenetic biomarkers of colorectal cancer: focus on DNA methylation. *Cancer Letters*, *342*(2), 238–247.

Cravo, M. L., Mason, J. B., Dayal, Y., Hutchinson, M., Smith, D., Selhub, J., & Rosenberg, I. H. (1992). Folate deficiency enhances the development of colonic neoplasia in dimethylhydrazine-treated rats. *Cancer Research*, *52*(18), 5002–5006.

Cronstein, B. N. (1996). Molecular therapeutics. Methotrexate and its mechanism of action. *Arthritis & Rheumatism*, *39*(12), 1951–1960.

Dayal, S., & Lentz, S. R. (2008). Murine models of hyperhomocysteinemia and their vascular phenotypes. *Arteriosclerosis, Thrombosis, and Vascular Biology*, *28*(9), 1596–1605.

Descalzi, G., Ikegami, D., Ushijima, T., Nestler, E. J., Zachariou, V., & Narita, M. (2015). Epigenetic mechanisms of chronic pain. *Trends in Neurosciences*, *38*(4), 237–246.

Doehring, A., Geisslinger, G., & Lötsch, J. (2011). Epigenetics in pain and analgesia: an imminent research field. *European Journal of Pain*, *15*(1), 11–16.

Dror, Y., Stern, F., Nemesh, L., Hart, J., & Grinblat, J. (1996). Estimation of vitamin needs—riboflavin, vitamin B6 and ascorbic acid—according to blood parameters and functional-cognitive and emotional indices in a selected well-established group of elderly in a home for the aged in Israel. *Journal of the American College of Nutrition*, *15*(5), 481–488.

Esteller, M. (2011). Non-coding RNAs in human disease. *Nature Reviews. Genetics*, *12*(12), 861–874.

Firestein, G. S. (2003). Evolving concepts of rheumatoid arthritis. *Nature*, *423*(6937), 356–361.

Flanagan, J. F., Mi, L.-Z., Chruszcz, M., Cymborowski, M., Clines, K. L., Kim, Y., …, Khorasanizadeh, S. (2005). Double chromodomains cooperate to recognize the methylated histone H3 tail. *Nature*, *438*(7071), 1181–1185.

Fleckenstein, J., Zaps, D., Rüger, L. J., Lehmeyer, L., Freiberg, F., Lang, P. M., & Irnich, D. (2010). Discrepancy between prevalence and perceived effectiveness of treatment methods in myofascial pain syndrome: results of a cross-sectional, nationwide survey. *BMC Musculoskeletal Disorders*, *11*(1), 32.

Fraga, M. F., Ballestar, E., Villar-Garea, A., Boix-Chornet, M., Espada, J., Schotta, G., …, Esteller, M. (2005). Loss of acetylation at Lys16 and trimethylation at Lys20 of histone H4 is a common hallmark of human cancer. *Nature Genetics*, *37*(4), 391–400.

Frigola, J., Song, J., Stirzaker, C., Hinshelwood, R. A., Peinado, M. A., & Clark, S. J. (2006). Epigenetic remodeling in colorectal cancer results in coordinate gene suppression across an entire chromosome band. *Nature Genetics*, *38*(5), 540–549.

Ganguly, P., & Alam, S. F. (2015). Role of homocysteine in the development of cardiovascular disease. *Nutrition Journal*, *14*(1), 6.

Gerber, L. H., Sikdar, S., Armstrong, K., Diao, G., Heimur, J., Kopecky, J., …, Shah, J. (2013). A systematic comparison between subjects with no pain and pain associated with active myofascial trigger points. *PM&R*, *5*(11), 931–938.

Gerwin, R. D. (2005). A review of myofascial pain and fibromyalgia—factors that promote their persistence. *Acupuncture in Medicine*, *23*(3), 121–134.

Gnyszka, A., Jastrzebski, Z., & Flis, S. (2013). DNA methyltransferase inhibitors and their emerging role in epigenetic therapy of cancer. *Anticancer Research*, *33*(8), 2989–2996.

Goodrich, J. A., & Kugel, J. F. (2006). Non-coding-RNA regulators of RNA polymerase II transcription. *Nature Reviews. Molecular Cell Biology*, *7*(8), 612–616.

Gottfries, J., Blennow, K., Lehmann, M. W., Regland, B., & Gottfries, C. -G. (2001). One-carbon metabolism and other biochemical correlates of cognitive impairment as visualized by principal component analysis. *Journal of Geriatric Psychiatry and Neurology*, *14*(3), 109–114.

Haagsma, C. J., Blom, H. J., van Riel, P. L., van't Hof, M. A., Giesendorf, B. A., van Oppenraaij-Emmerzaal, D., & van de Putte, L. B. (1999). Influence of sulphasalazine, methotrexate, and the combination of both on plasma homocysteine concentrations in patients with rheumatoid arthritis. *Annals of the Rheumatic Diseases*, *58*(2), 79–84.

Huang, C., Chen, T., Lin, H., Tseng, Y., Lai, S., Chen, W., …, Liu, J. (2007). The relation between plasma homocysteine levels and cardiovascular risk factors in cerebral ischemia. *Acta Neurologica Taiwanica*, *16*(2), 81.

Isomäki, H. (1992). Long-term outcome of rheumatoid arthritis. *Scandinavian Journal of Rheumatology*, *21*(S95), 3–8.

Jones, P. A., & Baylin, S. B. (2002). The fundamental role of epigenetic events in cancer. *Nature Reviews. Genetics*, *3*(6), 415–428.

Jones, P. A., & Laird, P. W. (1999). Cancer-epigenetics comes of age. *Nature Genetics*, *21*(2), 163–167.

Kalani, A., Kamat, P. K., Givvimani, S., Brown, K., Metreveli, N., Tyagi, S. C., & Tyagi, N. (2014). Nutri-epigenetics ameliorates blood–brain barrier damage and neurodegeneration in hyperhomocysteinemia: role of folic acid. *Journal of Molecular Neuroscience*, *52*(2), 202–215.

Kalani, A., Kamat, P. K., Tyagi, S. C., & Tyagi, N. (2013). Synergy of homocysteine, microRNA, and epigenetics: a novel therapeutic approach for stroke. *Molecular Neurobiology*, *48*(1), 157–168.

Kaplan, M. J. (2006). Cardiovascular disease in rheumatoid arthritis. *Current Opinion in Rheumatology*, *18*(3), 289–297.

Kojima, M., Kojima, T., Suzuki, S., Oguchi, T., Oba, M., Tsuchiya, H., …, Tokudome, S. (2009). Depression, inflammation, and pain in patients with rheumatoid arthritis. *Arthritis Care & Research*, *61*(8), 1018–1024.

La Rue, A., Koehler, K. M., Wayne, S. J., Chiulli, S. J., Haaland, K. Y., & Garry, P. J. (1997). Nutritional status and cognitive functioning in a normally aging sample: a 6-y reassessment. *The American Journal of Clinical Nutrition*, *65*(1), 20–29.

Lao, V. V., & Grady, W. M. (2011). Epigenetics and colorectal cancer. *Nature Reviews. Gastroenterology and Hepatology, 8*(12), 686–700.

Leite, F., Atallah, A., El Dib, R., Grossmann, E., Januzzi, E., Andriolo, R. B., & da Silva, E. (2009). Cyclobenzaprine for the treatment of myofascial pain in adults. *Cochrane Database of Systematic Reviews*(3), CD006830.

Lessans, S., & Dorsey, S. G. (2013). The role for epigenetic modifications in pain and analgesia response. *Nursing Research and Practice, 2013*, 961493.

Li, W., Jiang, M., Zhao, S., Liu, H., Zhang, X., Wilson, J. X., & Huang, G. (2015). Folic acid inhibits amyloid β-peptide production through modulating DNA methyltransferase activity in N2a-APP cells. *International Journal of Molecular Sciences, 16*(10), 25002–25013.

Loeser, J. D., & Melzack, R. (1999). Pain: an overview. *The Lancet, 353*(9164), 1607–1609.

Masaki, K., Losonczy, K., Izmirlian, G., Foley, D., Ross, G., Petrovitch, H., ..., White, L. (2000). Association of vitamin E and C supplement use with cognitive function and dementia in elderly men. *Neurology, 54*(6), 1265–1272.

McInnes, I. B., & Schett, G. (2011). The pathogenesis of rheumatoid arthritis. *The New England Journal of Medicine, 365*(23), 2205–2219.

McNeil, C. J., Beattie, J. H., Gordon, M., Pirie, L. P., & Duthie, S. J. (2011). Differential effects of nutritional folic acid deficiency and moderate hyperhomocysteinemia on aortic plaque formation and genome-wide DNA methylation in vascular tissue from ApoE−/− mice. *Clinical Epigenetics, 2*(2), 361–368.

Merskey, H. E. (1986). Classification of chronic pain: Descriptions of chronic pain syndromes and definitions of pain terms. Pain. Supplement 3. pp. 209–214. Elsevier, Amsterdam.

Moore, L. D., Le, T., & Fan, G. (2013). DNA methylation and its basic function. *Neuropsychopharmacology, 38*(1), 23–38.

Morgan, S. L., Baggott, J. E., Alarcón, G. S., & Koopman, W. J. (2002). Folic acid and folinic acid supplementation during low-dose methotrexate therapy for rheumatoid arthritis: comment on the article by van Ede et al. *Arthritis & Rheumatism, 46*(5), 1413–1414.

Moyers, S., & Bailey, L. B. (2001). Fetal malformations and folate metabolism: review of recent evidence. *Nutrition Reviews, 59*(7), 215–224.

National Institutes of Health. (2009). *Dietary supplement fact sheet: Vitamin E.* Bethesda, MD: National Institutes of Health, Office of Dietary Supplements. Available at: http://ods.od.nih.gov/factsheets/vitamine/ [accessed February 2011).

Nightingale, K. P., O'Neill, L. P., & Turner, B. M. (2006). Histone modifications: signalling receptors and potential elements of a heritable epigenetic code. *Current Opinion in Genetics & Development, 16*(2), 125–136.

Nikolaisen, C., Figenschau, Y., & Nossent, J. C. (2008). Anemia in early rheumatoid arthritis is associated with interleukin 6-mediated bone marrow suppression, but has no effect on disease course or mortality. *The Journal of Rheumatology, 35*(3), 380–386.

Okumus, M., Ceceli, E., Tuncay, F., Kocaoglu, S., Palulu, N., & Yorgancioglu, Z. (2010). The relationship between serum trace elements, vitamin B. *Journal of Back and Musculoskeletal Rehabilitation, 23*, 187–191.

Ortiz, Z., Shea, B., Suarez-Almazor, M., Moher, D., Wells, G., & Tugwell, P. (1998). The efficacy of folic acid and folinic acid in reducing methotrexate gastrointestinal toxicity in rheumatoid arthritis. A metaanalysis of randomized controlled trials. *The Journal of Rheumatology, 25*(1), 36–43.

Paleolog, E. M. (2002). Angiogenesis in rheumatoid arthritis. *Arthritis Research, 4*(suppl. 3), S81–S90.

Reddy, M. A., & Natarajan, R. (2015). Recent developments in epigenetics of acute and chronic kidney diseases. *Kidney International, 88*(2), 250–261(review).

Reynolds, E. (2006). Vitamin B12, folic acid, and the nervous system. *The Lancet Neurology, 5*(11), 949–960.

Rupp, I., Boshuizen, H. C., Jacobi, C. E., Dinant, H. J., & van den Bos, G. A. (2004). Impact of fatigue on health-related quality of life in rheumatoid arthritis. *Arthritis Care & Research, 51*(4), 578–585.

Scott, D., Coulton, B., Symmons, D., & Popert, A. (1987). Long-term outcome of treating rheumatoid arthritis: results after 20 years. *The Lancet, 329*(8542), 1108–1111.

Selhub, J. (1999). Homocysteine metabolism. *Annual Review of Nutrition, 19*(1), 217–246.

Seo, S., Grzenda, A., Lomberk, G., Ou, X. -M., Cruciani, R. A., & Urrutia, R. (2013). Epigenetics: a promising paradigm for better understanding and managing pain. *The Journal of Pain, 14*(6), 549–557.

Simons, D. G. (1983). *Myofascial pain syndrome due to trigger points*. Ohio: Rademaker.

Simons, D. G. (1996). Clinical and etiological update of myofascial pain from trigger points. *Journal of Musculoskelatal Pain, 4*(1–2), 93–122.

Simons, D. G., Travell, J. G., & Simons, L. S. (1999). *Travell & Simons' myofascial pain and dysfunction: Upper half of body* (vol. 1). Netherlands: Lippincott Williams & Wilkins.

Simon, L. S. (2012). Relieving pain in America: A blueprint for transforming prevention, care, education, and research. *Journal of Pain & Palliative Care Pharmacotherapy, 26*(2), 197–198.

Smith, A. D., Kim, Y. -I., & Refsum, H. (2008). Is folic acid good for everyone? *The American Journal of Clinical Nutrition, 87*(3), 517–533.

Smolen, J. S., Aletaha, D., Koeller, M., Weisman, M. H., & Emery, P. (2007). New therapies for treatment of rheumatoid arthritis. *The Lancet, 370*(9602), 1861–1874.

Smolen, J. S., & Steiner, G. (2003). Therapeutic strategies for rheumatoid arthritis. *Nature Reviews. Drug Discovery, 2*(6), 473–488.

Ting, A. H., Schuebel, K. E., Herman, J. G., & Baylin, S. B. (2005). Short dsRNA induces transcriptional gene silencing in human cancer cells in the absence of DNA methylation. *Nature Genetics, 37*(8), 906–910.

Van Ede, A., Laan, R., Blom, H., Boers, G., Haagsma, C., Thomas, C., ..., Van de Putte, L. (2002). Homocysteine and folate status in methotrexate-treated patients with rheumatoid arthritis. *Rheumatology, 41*(6), 658–665.

Van Ede, A. E., Laan, R. F., Rood, M. J., Huizinga, T. W., Van De Laar, M. A., Denderen, C. J. V., ..., Jacobs, M. J. (2001). Effect of folic or folinic acid supplementation on the toxicity and efficacy of methotrexate in rheumatoid arthritis: A forty-eight-week, multicenter, randomized, double-blind, placebo-controlled study. *Arthritis & Rheumatism, 44*(7), 1515–1524.

Wang, J. -Y., Wen, L. -L., Huang, Y. -N., Chen, Y. -T., & Ku, M. -C. (2006). Dual effects of antioxidants in neurodegeneration: direct neuroprotection against oxidative stress and indirect protection via suppression of glia-mediated inflammation. *Current Pharmaceutical Design, 12*(27), 3521–3533.

Wasantwisut, E. (1996). Nutrition and development: other micronutrients' effect on growth and cognition. *The Southeast Asian Journal of Tropical Medicine and Public Health, 28*, 78–82.

Weinstein, S. J., Hartman, T. J., Stolzenberg-Solomon, R., Pietinen, P., Barrett, M. J., Taylor, P. R., ..., Albanes, D. (2003). Null association between prostate cancer and serum folate, vitamin B6, vitamin B12, and homocysteine. *Cancer Epidemiology Biomarkers & Prevention, 12*(11), 1271–1272.

Whittle, S., & Hughes, R. (2004). Folate supplementation and methotrexate treatment in rheumatoid arthritis: a review. *Rheumatology, 43*(3), 267–271.

Woolf, C. J. (2010). What is this thing called pain? *The Journal of Clinical Investigation, 120*(11), 3742.

Zeng, W., Ball, A. R., & Yokomori, K. (2010). HP1: heterochromatin binding proteins working the genome. *Epigenetics: Official Journal of the DNA Methylation Society, 5*(4), 287–292.

S E C T I O N F

ANIMAL MODELS FOR PAIN: FOOD AND PLANT EXTRACT

CHAPTER

22

Analgesic and Neuroprotective Effects of B Vitamins

X.-J. Song*,**

*Section of Basic Science Research, Parker University Research Institute, Dallas, TX, United States; Center for Pain Medicine and Cancer Hospital, Peking University, Beijing, China; **Center for Pain Medicine and Cancer Hospital, Peking University, Beijing, China

The B vitamins serve as important cofactors for numerous cellular metabolic pathways. They include eight water-soluble vitamins: thiamine (vitamin B1), riboflavin (vitamin B2), niacin (vitamin B3), pantothen (vitamin B5), pyridoxine (vitamin B6), biotin (vitamin H), folic acid (vitamin M), and cyanocobalamin (vitamin B12). Adequate B vitamin intake is a general requirement for nucleic acid synthesis and healthy growth of all cells. These B vitamins were once considered to comprise a single vitamin, like vitamin C and vitamin D, but then found to include a variety of different vitamin. It has been well established that deficiencies in certain B vitamins can cause severe symptoms and diseases. For instance, vitamin B1 is essential for carbohydrate metabolism and normal function of the nervous system. Deficiency of B1 can cause serophthisis perniciosa endemica involving several systems including respiratory, cardiovascular, muscular, gastrointestinal, and nervous systems. It has been hypothesized that B vitamin deficiencies are etiological factors in the development of various neuropathies including those associated with diabetes and alcoholism, which likely result from the metabolic disturbances common in these diseases (Fennelly, Frank, Baker, & Leevy, 1964; Mader et al., 1988; Parry, 1994).

In addition, deficiency of B1 and B6 can cause many severe neuropathies including neuropathic pain (Metz, 1992; Weir & Scott, 1995; Kril, 1996; Scalabrino, 2009; National Academy of Sciences Institute of Medicine, Food and Nutrition Board, 1998. Certain neuropathies and neuropathic pain after nerve injury can be prevented or alleviated by supplying additional B vitamins (Wang, Gan, Rupert, Zeng, & Song, 2005; Song, Ultenius, Meyerson, & Linderoth, 2009b; Yu et al., 2014). Early indications of the analgesic properties of B vitamins came from studies in the 1950s investigating therapies for herpetic and trigeminal neuralgias (Leitch, 1953; Surtees & Hughes, 1954) and diabetic neuropathy (Davidson, 1954). Later studies continued to investigate B vitamin therapy for diabetic neuropathy (Yamauchi, 1970; Goto, 1979) and for other painful conditions, including carpal tunnel syndrome (McCann & Davis, 1978; Kasdan & Janes, 1987; Bernstein, 1990; Talebi et al., 2013), lumboischialgia (Marcolongo et al., 1988), and various other neuropathies (Eckert & Schejbal, 1992). However, some of these effects have been disputed, owing to the relatively low quality of many human studies, as well as negative findings in some human studies (Levin et al., 1981; Bromm, Herrmann, & Schulz, 1995; Simeonov, Pavlova, Mitkov, Mincheva, & Troev, 1997; Woelk, Lehrl, Bitsch, & Kopcke, 1998) and animal studies (Eschalier, Aumaitre, Decamps, & Dordain, 1983; Reyes-Garcia, Medina-Santillan, Teran-Rosales, Mateos-Garcia, & Castillo-Henkel, 1999).

ANALGESIC EFFECTS OF B VITAMINS ON ACUTE PAIN

The analgesic effects of vitamins B1, B6, and B12 have been tested a couple of decades ago in experimental animals with acute, transient pain evoked by electrical, chemical, or thermal stimulation. These studies showed that vitamin B1, B6, and B12 can inhibit chemical- or heat-stimulation induced acute pain (Bartoszyk & Wild, 1989; Franca et al., 2001), as well as noxious heat-evoked responses of the dorsal horn neurons of the spinal cord

Nutritional Modulators of Pain in the Aging Population. http://dx.doi.org/10.1016/B978-0-12-805186-3.00022-9
Copyright © 2017 Elsevier Inc. All rights reserved.

(Fu, Carstens, Stelzer, & Zimmermann, 1988). These observations suggest that these B vitamins may possess antinociceptive efficacy, although documentation of this efficacy was incomplete.

Several clinical trials have shown that B vitamins may facilitate analgesic effect of diclofenac for the treatment of certain acute pain. Brüggemann and coworkers compared the clinical efficacy of diclofenac (25 mg) and a combination preparation with diclofenac (25 mg) plus vitamins B1 (thiamine nitrate 50 mg), B6 (pyridoxine hydrochloride 50 mg), and B12 (cyanocobalamin 0.25 mg) in a multicentric randomized double-blind study including 418 patients with painful vertebral syndromes. They observed significantly better treatment outcomes for the combination of diclofenac and B vitamins. The analgesic effect of B-vitamin-diclofenac-combination was particularly large in patients with severe pain at the beginning of therapy, but these vitamins alone did not produce significant analgesic effects (Bruggemann, Koehler, & Koch, 1990). A recent clinical trial has also shown that a complex of B vitamins containing B1, B6, and B12 can facilitate the analgesic effect of diclofenac for the treatment of acute pain originating from lower-limb fracture and surgery in 122 patients (Ha et al., 2012). These clinical trials provide evidence that the combination therapy with diclofenac plus B vitamins is more effective than diclofenac alone for the treatment of acute pain. As indicated by these reviews and reports, however, while numerous encouraging outcomes have been independently reported over decades of research, a general lack of consistency and methodological rigor within the literature makes it difficult to draw firm conclusions about the overall efficacy of B vitamins in reducing pain in clinic.

ANALGESIC EFFECT OF B VITAMINS ON PAINFUL DIABETIC NEUROPATHY

Diabetic neuropathy is a prevalent and disabling disorder. Painful diabetic neuropathy, a common sequel of diabetic peripheral neuropathy, is severe and intractable, and affects 10–20% of the millions of patients with diabetes (Alge-Priglinger et al., 2011; DiBonaventura, Cappelleri, & Joshi, 2011; de Salas-Cansado et al., 2012; Sandercock, Cramer, Biton, & Cowles, 2012). Despite decades of studies and numerous processes that have been implicated, the specific cellular and molecular mechanisms underlying the pathogenesis of diabetic neuropathic pain remain elusive. The possible etiologies that underlie the pathogenesis of diabetic neuropathic pain may include the following: (1) hyperglycemia-induced damage to nerve cells, including the reduced conduction failure of the main axon of polymodal nociceptive C-fibers (Sun et al., 2012) and a decrease in neurovascular flow (Edwards, Vincent, Cheng, & Feldman, 2008); (2) production of proinflammatory cytokines including tumor necrosis factor-α (TNF-α), interleukin-1β, and interleukin-6; (3) perturbations in growth factors, such as insulin-like growth factor, nerve growth factor, and neurotrophin 3; (4) immune dysfunction; (5) diabetes-related oxidant stresses, such as mitochondrial oxidant stress, and other cellular stresses including endoplasmic reticulum stress; and (6) multifocal loss of myelinated and unmyelinated fibers (Obrosova et al., 2004; Brownlee, 2005; Obrosova, 2009). Because of the complexities of pathogenesis, painful diabetic neuropathy is still a common and challenging complication of diabetes mellitus, and the clinical approaches for its treatment are very limited. It is often resistant to treatment with the available modalities. Currently, the most effective treatment available to patients with diabetic neuropathy is likely pain management, in addition to critical glucose control. B vitamins, however, have been demonstrated to be effective in treating painful diabetic neuropathy.

Several clinical trials and observations have shown the efficacy of B vitamins (B1 and B12) and its combination with analgesics, such as gabapentin in treating painful diabetic neuropathy. Benfotiamine, a lipid-soluble vitamin B1 prodrug with high bioavailability, may extend the treatment option for patients with diabetic polyneuropathy based on its influence on impaired glucose metabolism (Stracke, Gaus, Achenbach, Federlin, & Bretzel, 2008). It was observed that the most pronounced effect of benfotiamine was a reported decrease in pain, and no side effects were observed in patients with diabetic pain (Haupt, Ledermann, & Kopcke, 2005). A recent study shows that benfotiamine acts on μ-opioid receptor mediated antinociception in experimental diabetes (Nacitarhan, Minareci, & Sadan, 2014). This study determined the effects of benfotiamine on the antinociception produced by μ-opioid receptor agonist fentanyl in diabetic mice. It was found that μ-opioid agonist fentanyl in the benfotiamine-treated diabetic group caused more potent antinociceptive effects than in the diabetic group without benfotiamine treatment. A brief benfotiamine dietary supplement did not show an antinociceptive effect, but during the development of streptozotocin-induced diabetes, benfotiamine replacement increased the antinociceptive effect of fentanyl in mice based on the tail-flick test. This study suggests that benfotiamine replacement therapy may be useful in ameliorating the analgesic effect of μ-opioid agonists on neuropathic pain in diabetics.

Vitamin B12 has also been shown to be effective in treating diabetic neuropathy (Kuwabara et al., 1999). A very recent study shows that gabapentin plus the B1/B12 combination is as effective as gabapentin by itself. Moreover, the combination therapy reduced pain intensity with a gabapentin dose at 50% of the minimum dose required when gabapentin was used alone (800 vs. 1600 mg/day). Decreased occurrence of vertigo and dizziness was also observed with the combination treatment (Alvarado, 2016). These observations support an extended use of vitamins B1 and B12 for painful diabetic neuropathy in the clinic. In addition, deficiency of vitamins B1 and B6 was thought to contribute to the diabetic peripheral neuropathy in Dar es Salaam (Abbas & Swai, 1997).

ANALGESIC EFFECT OF B VITAMINS ON NEUROPATHIC PAIN AFTER PERIPHERAL NERVE INJURY AND DORSAL ROOT GANGLION COMPRESSION

Neuropathic pain, often caused by peripheral nerve injury, is a severe and intractable pain. Current drugs, including opioids and nondrug therapies, offer substantial pain relief to no more than half of affected patients (Hansson, 2003). Although the concept that B vitamins can produce analgesic effects in several painful conditions has been supported by experimental and some clinical evidence for decades, there has been no direct experimental evidence of the use of B vitamins to treat neuropathic pain until an article published in 2005 (Wang et al., 2005). In recent decades, researchers have developed animal models of painful sequelae in humans after primary sensory neuron injury, such as loose ligation of the sciatic nerve (Bennett & Xie, 1988), segmental spinal nerve ligation (Kim & Chung, 1992), chronic compression of DRG (Hu & Xing, 1998; Song, Hu, Greenquist, Zhang, & LaMotte, 1999), partial dorsal rhizotomy (Song, Vizcarra, Xu, Rupert, & Wong, 2003a), etc. Nerve-injured animals exhibit behavioral symptoms of neuropathic pain manifested as hypersensitivity to thermal and mechanical stimulation, termed as thermal hyperalgesia and mechanical allodynia, respectively. Cellularly, nerve injury induces long-term hyperexcitability of dorsal root ganglion (DRG) neurons (Rizzo, Kocsis, & Waxman, 1995; Waxman, 1999; Baccei & Kocsis, 2000; Abdulla & Smith, 2001; Abdulla, Stebbing, & Smith, 2001; Song et al., 2003a; Song, Zhang, Hu, & LaMotte, 2003c) and the DRG somata become more sensitive to norepinephrine (Birder & Perl, 1999), inflammatory mediators (Song, Xu, Vizcarra, & Rupert, 2003b), tumor necrosis factor (Schafers, Lee, Brors, Yaksh, & Sorkin, 2003), and brain-derived neurotrophic factor (Obata et al., 2003). Nerve injury also alters synaptic plasticity in spinal dorsal horn neurons (Ikeda, Heinke, Ruscheweyh, & Sandkuhler, 2003; Kohno, Moore, Baba, & Woolf, 2003), promotes a selective loss of GABAergic inhibition (Moore et al., 2002), and causes phenotypic switches in the primary afferent terminals of the spinal dorsal horn (Neumann, Doubell, Leslie, & Woolf, 1996). These studies have provided promising models that are useful for understanding the mechanisms of neuropathic pain and exploring new approaches to therapy.

We investigated the analgesic effects of vitamins B1, B6, and B12 on neuropathic pain caused by primary sensory neuron injury using CCI and CCD models (Wang et al., 2005). We found that systematic application of high doses of vitamins B1, B6, and B12 produces immediate, transient, and dose-dependent inhibition on thermal hyperalgesia in nerve-injured rats. Intraperitoneal injection of vitamin B1 (5, 10, 33, and 100 mg/kg), B6 (33 and 100 mg/kg), or B12 (0.5 and 2 mg/kg) alone significantly alleviated the thermal hyperalgesia. Combinations of B1, B6, and B12 synergistically inhibit thermal hyperalgesia. Repetitive intraperitoneal injection of a vitamin B complex containing 33 mg/kg of B1, 33 mg/kg of B6, and 0.5 mg/kg of B12, daily for 7–14 consecutive days, produced long-lasting inhibition of thermal hyperalgesia, particularly at the very beginning of DRG compression in animals with CCD treatment. Meanwhile, this combination treatment affects neither mechanical allodynia nor normal pain sensation including mechanical and thermal sensitivity. This study demonstrates, for the first time, that vitamins B1, B6, and B12 and their combination can significantly alleviate neuropathic pain due to peripheral nerve injury or sensory neuron somata compression. This finding serves as experimental evidence supporting the utility of B vitamins in treating neuropathic pain, as well as inflammatory pain in humans with similar conditions. It is known that inflammation is inevitably induced during nerve injury, DRG compression, or other available nerve injury models used for research. The idea of analgesic effect of B vitamins on neuropathic pain is also supported by certain clinical observations in patients with lumboischialgia (Misra, Vadlamani, & Pontani, 1977), neuritis (Small, 1978), chronic cephalgia (Mader et al., 1988), diabetic polyneuropathy (Stracke, Lindemann, & Federlin, 1996), and rheumatoid arthritis (Chiang, Bagley, Selhub, Nadeau, & Roubenoff, 2003; Yxfeldt, Wallberg-Jonsson, Hultdin, & Rantapaa-Dahlqvist, 2003).

It should be emphasized that the vitamins B1, B6, and B12 exhibit significant dose-related inhibitory effects on neuropathic thermal hyperalgesia intraperitoneally injected at high doses in experimental animals with DRG compression or peripheral nerve injury (Wang et al., 2005). This result is consistent with clinical reports that indicate that only high doses of B vitamins exhibit antinociceptive effects in human patients (Mader et al., 1988) and in animals with acute pain (Zimmerman, Bartoszyk, Bonke, Jurna, & Wild, 1990; Leuschner, 1992). B vitamins in low doses similar to the recommended average daily doses for humans evidently have no effect, or only very weak effects, on the behavior pain in patients (Mader et al., 1988). In a single treatment, the minimum doses required of B1, B6, and B12 vitamins needed to produce significant analgesic effect were 5, 33, and 0.5 mg/kg, respectively (Wang et al., 2005). These doses are crudely 33, 800, and 10,000 times the recommended daily doses for humans, which are 0.15, 0.04, and 5×10^{-5} mg/kg for B1, B6, and B12 vitamins, respectively. The doses effective in producing analgesic effects are also approximately 1, 20, and 4700 times the recommended maximum daily doses for humans, which are 8.3, 1.7, and 2.1×10^{-5} mg/kg for B1, B6, and B12, respectively (assuming an average body weight of 60 kg). The analgesic doses of B1 and B6 for the rats in the study (Wang et al., 2005) are much higher than the recommended average daily doses for humans, but the same as or close to the recommended maximum daily doses, as well as similar to the doses that have been given in clinical studies on analgesia (5 and 10 mg/kg·day) (Bromm et al., 1995). In addition, the blood concentrations of the B vitamins in healthy humans and rats are within similar ranges, that is, B1=0.8–2.8 g/L, B6=5–24 g/L, and B12=0.2–1.2 g/L (Groziak & Kirksey, 1987; Terasawa, Nakahara, Tsukada, Sugawara, & Itokawa, 1999; Choi et al., 2004). Therefore, the doses of B1 and B6 presented by Wang et al. appear reasonable for clinical use. B12 showed analgesic effects only when the dose reached 5,000–10,000 times the recommended daily supplementary doses for humans. It is worth noting that rats treated with high doses of B vitamins did not show any toxic-related abnormal behavior. This supports the clinical observations that no toxic effects are observed in humans for B1, B6, and B12 given alone or in combination up to an oral dose of 5000 mg/kg body weight (Leuschner, 1992), and that 100–150 mg/day of vitamin B6 shows minimal or no toxicity in adults in a study that lasted 5–10 years, although doses at 500–1000 mg/day shows peripheral neuropathy within 1–3 years (Bernstein, 1990).

In addition, we showed that combinations of B1, B6, and B12 could synergistically inhibit thermal hyperalgesia, providing the possibility of reducing the dose of individual vitamins. Furthermore, repetitive administrations of a combination of the B vitamins produce long-lasting inhibition, persisting after termination of the treatment, suggesting an accumulated analgesic efficacy and/or fasting recovery of the previously injured nerves (Wang et al., 2005). Since virtually no adverse side effects were reported for any of the dosages and regimens used in any of the examined studies, relative high dose B complex vitamin therapy should be considered as a viable conservative primary or adjunctive therapy for patients with neuropathic pain or other similar painful disorders. This is especially true for patients whose pain is refractory to treatment with standard analgesic therapy, which is unfortunately a nearly ubiquitous feature of neuropathic pain (Woolf, 2011). Moreover, there is a need for more treatment options even for subsets of patients that respond to mainstay treatments for neuropathic pain (e.g., anticonvulsants, tricyclic antidepressants), since these treatments often have serious and debilitating side effects that limit patient tolerability (Backonja & Serra, 2004a; 2004b).

ANALGESIC AND NEUROPROTECTIVE EFFECTS OF B VITAMINS FOLLOWING TEMPORARY SPINAL CORD ISCHEMIA

Central nervous system injury, such as that caused by spinal cord ischemia may cause long-lasting neuropathic pain in addition to other disorders. Studies have shown that 65–85% of patients develop clinically significant pain following spinal cord injury (Bonica, 1991; Levi, Hultling, Nash, & Seiger, 1995; Siddall, McClelland, Rutkowski, & Cousins, 2003) Following ischemia or other forms of injury to the spinal cord, certain molecules and cells that may contribute to the development of pain are activated, accompanied by apoptosis of certain types of neurons, particularly γ-aminobutyric acid (GABA)ergic inhibitory interneurons (Schwartz-Bloom & Sah, 2001). Mechanisms underlying neuropathic pain following spinal cord ischemia remain elusive. It has been demonstrated that B vitamins are capable of protecting and reducing neurons from certain injuries. For example, vitamin B6 attenuates glutamate-induced neurotoxicity (Kaneda et al., 1997) and counteracts ischemia (Wang et al., 2002) or glucose deprivation-induced neuronal death (Geng, Saito, & Nishiyama, 1997). B12 could protect neurons from glutamate-induced neurotoxicity in cortical and retinal neurons in vitro (Hung, Wang, Huang, & Wang, 2009). These neuroprotective effects of B vitamins may contribute to their analgesic effects, probably through reducing the loss of the inhibitory GABA interneurons.

We have recently shown that systematic administration of the vitamin B complex containing B1, B6, and B12 can significantly attenuate neuropathic hyperalgesia and greatly reducing ischemia-induced loss of GABAergic neurons in the spinal cord following temporary spinal cord ischemia in a rat model of spinal cord ischemia-reperfusion injury (SCII) (Yu et al., 2014). SCII produced by transiently blocking the unilateral lumbar arteries caused behaviorally expressed thermal hyperalgesia and mechanical allodynia, along with neurochemical alterations of neuropathic pain including increased expression of the vanilloid receptor 1 (VR1) and induction of c-Fos, as well as activation of astrocytes and microglial cells in the spinal cord. Daily repetitive systemic administration of the vitamin B complex containing B1, B6, and B12 at 33 and 0.5 mg/kg, respectively, for 7–14 consecutive days, significantly reduced behavioral hyperalgesia and reversed the neurochemical alterations of neuropathic pain. In addition, SCII caused a dramatic decrease of expression of the rate-limiting enzyme glutamic aciddecarboxylase-65 (GAD65), which synthesizes GABA in the axonal terminals, and β-III-tubulin, and also caused loss of Nissl bodies in the spinal cord. These cell toxicity alterations following SCII were significantly prevented or reduced by the vitamin B complex treatment. Rescuing the loss of inhibitory GABAergic tone may reduce spinal central sensitization and contribute to B vitamin-induced analgesia. This study demonstrates the antinociceptive effect and neuroprotective capacity of B vitamins following spinal cord injury due to temporary ischemia and reperfusion. The neuroprotective capacity of the B vitamin, particularly its ability to rescue spinal GABA inhibitory neurons, may contribute to its analgesic effect after SCII. This study strongly suggests a clinical use of B vitamins in protecting spinal neurons from injury during the performance of certain surgeries in which temporary loss of blood supply would be required or inevitable, and its use in treating the associated neuropathic pain.

MECHANISMS UNDERLYING ANALGESIC EFFECTS OF B VITAMINS

Despite growing evidence of the benefits of B vitamin therapy for treating the general acute and chronic pain, experimental studies and human clinical literature provide limited insight into the basic mechanisms for putative analgesic and neuroprotective effects. It remains unclear from human studies as to whether and to what extent these benefits result from alleviation of nutritional deficiencies, or whether they can be attributed to other metabolic effects or the general analgesic properties of B vitamins at high dosages. However, several lines of studies have provided evidence for possible explanations. The general effects of the B vitamins on axonal conduction may contribute to the immediate analgesic effect. Studies have indicated that vitamin B1 may play an important biophysiological role in nerve conduction and excitation (Itokawa & Cooper, 1970; Sun et al., 2012) and B12 can selectively block conduction in sensory nerve (Takeshige, Ando, & Ando, 1971; Leishear et al., 2012).

The potential interactions of B vitamins at intra- or supraspinal receptors either with tonically released endogenous opiates or with nonopioid inhibitory neurotransmitters systems, such as serotonergic and GABAergic systems (Misra et al., 1977; Plaitakis, Nicklas, & Berl, 1978; Brennan et al., 1980; Bernstein, 1990; Yu et al., 2014) have been thought to contribute to the prolonged inhibitory effect of B vitamins. There is GABAergic tone lost in certain kinds of pathological condition, such as peripheral nerve injury, spinal cord injury, and spinal cord ischemia (Zhang et al., 1994). GABA is the major endogenous inhibitory neurotransmitter in the spinal cord. GABAergic tone loss occurs in about 24–33% of the interneurons in laminae I–IV of the dorsal horn of the spinal cord following spinal cord injury (Price et al., 1987; Meisner, Marsh, & Marsh, 2010) Such a loss of GABAergic tone may increase the excitability of the nociceptive neurons and cause spinal cord central sensitization (Ji & Woolf, 2001). Thus, exogenous B vitamin treatment that releases the shortage of B vitamins for GABA synthesis induced by SCII may be a mechanism underlying the antinociceptive effect of B vitamins, since vitamin B1 and B6 are coenzymes of enzymes responsible for GABA synthesis. Pharmacological treatments that could enhance GABAergic function attenuate central neuropathic pain behavior and neuronal hyperexcitability following spinal cord injury (Liu et al., 2004; Liu et al., 2008). Administration of bicuculline, a $GABA_A$ receptor antagonist, produces neuronal hyperexcitability and behaviorally expressed pain in naive rats (Drew, Siddall, & Duggan, 2004). Hypofunction of GABAergic tone has been demonstrated to be a substrate for neuropathic pain following spinal cord injury by pharmacological and molecular approaches. GABA is synthesized by the rate-limiting enzyme glutamic acid decarboxylase (GAD), which exists as two different isoforms—GAD65 and GAD67 (Erlander, Tillakaratne, Feldblum, Patel, & Tobin, 1991). GAD65 and GAD67 are widely distributed in the superficial layers, especially in lamina II of the dorsal horn, of the spinal cord (Mackie, Hughes, Maxwell, Tillakaratne, & Todd, 2003). GAD65 primarily synthesizes GABA in the axonal terminal, where GAD67 synthesizes GABA in the cytoplasm of the cell body. After spinal cord injury, GAD expression in the spinal dorsal horn is demonstrated to decrease in correlation with central neuropathic pain behavior (Zhang et al., 1994; Meisner et al., 2010). In addition, it is demonstrated that transplantation of herpes simplex virus-mediated GAD65 and GAD67, produces a gene vector that transfers human foamy virus-mediated GAD67 gene, attenuated central neuropathic pain following spinal cord injury (Liu et al., 2004, 2008). These studies indicate that the decreased GABAergic tone following spinal cord injury may be due to a loss of GABAergic neurons and/or a decrease in the level of GAD proteins. Thus, B vitamin treatment can successfully prevent SCII-induced downregulation of GAD65 and the loss of Nissl body, suggesting that the B vitamin treatment may rescue the function of GABAergic neurons (Yu et al., 2014).

The cGMP signaling pathway may also be involved in B vitamin-induced analgesia. It is known that the B vitamins can potently activate the soluble guanylyl cyclase (GC) and enhance cyclic guanosine monophosphate (cGMP) synthesis in a wide variety of tissues (Vesely, 1985). The cGMP plays an antinociceptive role in nociceptive processing (Vocci, Petty, & Dewey, 1978; Song, Chen, & Zhou, 2002). The B vitamins may produce antinociception through the activation of GC mediated by cGMP in the *p*-benzoquinone-induced mouse writhing model (Abacioglu, Demir, Cakici, Tunctan, & Kanzik, 2000). Glutamate and calcium channels are important in neurotransmission and may contribute in some way to vitamin B6-induced inhibition of hyperalgesia, since B6 can alter levels of intracellular glutamate and cell surface calcium channels (Dakshinamurti, Sharma, & Geiger, 2003).

Recently, it has been demonstrated in our study that vitamin B1 may modulate neuronal excitability of the compressed DRG by correcting or rebalancing the ectopic activity of sodium channels Nav1.7 and Nav1.8, in addition to alleviating neuropathic hyperalgesia (Song, Huang, & Song, 2009a). Nav1.7 and Nav1.8 are critical ion channels responsible for DRG neuron hyperexcitability (Cox et al., 2006; Waxman, 2006; Mannes & Iadarola, 2007). Through intracellular and patch-clamp recordings made in vitro from intact and dissociated DRG neurons from the nerve-injured or DRG compressed rats, we examined the effects of vitamin B1 on the altered DRG neuron excitability and the sodium channel activity. They found that repetitive in vivo intraperitoneal administration of B1 significantly inhibited DRG neuron hyperexcitability, while in vitro treatment of B1 inhibited neural hyperexcitability in a dose-dependent manner. The small and medium-sized nociceptive neurons exhibited higher sensitivity than the large neurons to B1 treatment. B1 treatment partially reversed injury-induced alterations of densities and inactivation properties of tetrodotoxin-resistant (TTX-R) and TTX-sensitive (TTX-S) sodium currents and ramp currents in small DRG neurons. These findings demonstrate, for the first time, that vitamin B1 can modulate neural excitability and sodium channel activity in injured DRG neurons, in addition to suppressing thermal hyperalgesia. This study begins to address mechanisms in these neurons that may contribute to the analgesic effects of B1 in neuropathic pain. This important study supports the promise that B vitamins show for treating painful neuropathic conditions following injury, inflammation, degeneration, or other disorders in the human nervous system.

Injury to the peripheral axons and/or somata of DRG neurons can cause severe hyperalgesia and allodynia associated with neural hyperexcitability (Bennett & Xie, 1988; Zimmermann, 2001; Song et al., 2003a, 2003b, 2003c; Rogers, Tang, Madge, & Stevens, 2006; Song, Wang, Gan, & Walters, 2006b; Song, Gan, Cao, Wang, & Rupert, 2006a; Huang & Song, 2008). DRG neuron hyperexcitability is thought to underlie neuropathic pain by causing central sensitization. Voltage-gated sodium channels (VGSCs), which are necessary for electrogenesis and nerve impulse conduction, can be dynamically regulated after nerve injury, DRG compression, or peripheral inflammation, and play important roles in modulating neural excitability (Tan, Donnelly, & LaMotte, 2006; Cummins, Sheets, & Waxman, 2007; Huang & Song, 2008). In DRG neurons, these VGSCs include Nav1.8 and Nav1.9, which conduct TTX-R currents, and Nav1.3, Nav1.6, and Nav1.7, which conduct TTX-S currents. Several reports have shown that TTX-R currents, Nav1.8 mRNA, and Nav1.8 protein are significantly decreased in nociceptive DRG neurons after nerve injury in animals (Tan et al., 2006; Huang & Song, 2008), as well as in patients (Coward et al., 2000). TTX-S currents and channels are also altered in models of nerve injury or inflammation (Cummins et al., 2007) and downregulation of Nav1.7 appears to play an important role in neuropathic pain sensation in erythromelalgia (Cox et al., 2006; Harty et al., 2006; Waxman, 2006; Mannes & Iadarola, 2007). Conversely, interference with Nav1.8 expression can inhibit neuropathic pain (Gaida, Klinder, Arndt, & Weiser, 2005; Mikami & Yang, 2005; Joshi et al., 2006; Dong et al., 2007). Since vitamin B1 can effectively modulate and correct the ectopic neural excitability of DRG neurons and activity of the sodium channels Nav1.7 and Nav1.8 altered by nerve compression, while suppressing the neuropathic thermal hyperalgesia (Huang, Cai, Chen, & Hong, 2009), it is convincing that B1 may suppress hyperalgesia by modulating abnormal sodium channel activity and inhibiting DRG neuron hyperexcitability after nerve injury.

Another interesting result found in our study (Song et al., 2009a, 2009b) is that the large DRG neurons exhibit significantly less sensitivity to the B1 treatment than medium-sized and small neurons. This finding may provide an explanation for the behavioral observation that in vivo administration of B vitamins inhibits thermal hyperalgesia, but not mechanical allodynia, in rats with chronic constriction injury of the sciatic nerve or DRG compression (Wang et al., 2005), because spontaneously active Aβ-fibers and the hyperexcitability of large DRG neurons have been considered to contribute to mechanical allodynia after nerve injury (Zimmermann, 2001). It is interesting to further investigate the possible mechanisms underlying the differential effects of B vitamins on thermal and mechanical hypersensitivity. In addition to the fact that B1 can reverse hyperexcitability and alterations of sodium currents after neuronal injury, recent studies have implicated B1-dependent processes in oxidative stress, protein processing, peroxisomal function, and gene expression (Karuppagounder et al., 2009). These processes are all important after nerve injury, which can alter properties of diverse types of neurons and trigger a myriad of changes in gene expression that affect many proteins including ion channels, receptors, and other membrane proteins (Wang et al., 2002; Xiao et al., 2002). These observations encourage further clinical investigation of the utility of the B vitamins in treating chronic pain and related disorders after nerve injury or disease.

Finally, reconstructive activity of B vitamins for degenerated nerves (Fujii, Matsumoto, & Yamamoto, 1996) may also contribute to the recovery of nerve function and therefore shorten the duration of hyperalgesia. Elucidation of such therapeutic mechanisms of B vitamins is essential for advancing their use in human clinical applications. The continued need to address such fundamental mechanisms of action should be apparent, for example, in order to determine which subsets of neuropathic patients are most likely to benefit from B vitamin therapy. This may be especially true in light of the fact that, as has often been pointed out, part of the challenge in advancing treatment options for neuropathic pain management involves ameliorating an inadequate understanding of the fundamental science of neuropathic pain. Moreover, owing to the numerous etiologies of human neuropathic pain, successful treatment is impeded by substantive heterogeneity among neuropathic patients, often leading to more of a trial and error clinical strategy rather than a targeted approach.

In summary, B vitamins have been demonstrated to be effective in analgesia and neuroprotection in certain disorders and thus are a good option for chronic pain treatment, especially for patients whose pain is refractory to treatment with standard analgesic therapy, which is an unfortunately nearly ubiquitous feature of neuropathic pain, as well as for subsets of patients who respond well to mainstay treatments for neuropathic pain in order to minimize the serious and debilitating side effects often caused by the mainstay treatments for neuropathic pain.

Acknowledgment

The author thanks Angela A. Song at University of Pennsylvanian Medical School for stimulating discussion and help editing English.

References

Abacioglu, N., Demir, S., Cakici, I., Tunctan, B., & Kanzik, I. (2000). Role of guanylyl cyclase activation via thiamine in suppressing chemically-induced writhing in mouse. *Arzneimittelforschung, 50*, 554–558.

Abbas, Z. G., & Swai, A. B. (1997). Evaluation of the efficacy of thiamine and pyridoxine in the treatment of symptomatic diabetic peripheral neuropathy. *East African Medicine Journal, 74*, 803–808.

Abdulla, F. A., & Smith, P. A. (2001). Axotomy—and autotomy-induced changes in the excitability of rat dorsal root ganglion neurons. *Journal of Neurophysiology, 85*, 630–643.

Abdulla, F. A., Stebbing, M. J., & Smith, P. A. (2001). Effects of substance P on excitability and ionic currents of normal and axotomized rat dorsal root ganglion neurons. *European Journal of Neuroscience, 13*, 545–552.

Alge-Priglinger, C. S., Andre, S., Schoeffl, H., Kampik, A., Strauss, R. W., Kernt, M., Gabius, H. J., & Priglinger, S. G. (2011). Negative regulation of RPE cell attachment by carbohydrate-dependent cell surface binding of galectin-3 and inhibition of the ERK-MAPK pathway. *Biochimie, 93*, 477–488.

Alvarado, L. (2016). Adherence to treatment in chronic diseases and the patient's experience. *Review Medicine of Chile, 144*, 269–270.

Baccei, M. L., & Kocsis, J. D. (2000). Voltage-gated calcium currents in axotomized adult rat cutaneous afferent neurons. *Journal of Neurophysiology, 83*, 2227–2238.

Backonja, M. M., & Serra, J. (2004a). Pharmacologic management part 1: better-studied neuropathic pain diseases. *Pain Medicine, 5*(Suppl. 1), S28–S47.

Backonja, M. M., & Serra, J. (2004b). Pharmacologic management part 2: lesser-studied neuropathic pain diseases. *Pain Medicine, 5*(Suppl. 1), S48–S59.

Bartoszyk, G. D., & Wild, A. (1989). B-vitamins potentiate the antinociceptive effect of diclofenac in carrageenin-induced hyperalgesia in the rat tail pressure test. *Neuroscience Letters, 101*, 95–100.

Bennett, G. J., & Xie, Y. K. (1988). A peripheral mononeuropathy in rat that produces disorders of pain sensation like those seen in man. *Pain, 33*, 87–107.

Bernstein, A. L. (1990). Vitamin B6 in clinical neurology. *Annals of the New York Academy of Sciences, 585*, 250–260.

Birder, L. A., & Perl, E. R. (1999). Expression of alpha2-adrenergic receptors in rat primary afferent neurones after peripheral nerve injury or inflammation. *The Journal of Physiology, 515*(Pt 2), 533–542.

Bonica, J. J. (1991). History of pain concepts and pain therapy. *The Mount Sinai Journal of Medicine, 58*, 191–202.

Brennan, M. J., Cantrill, R. C., Warner, S. J., van der Westhuyzen, J., Fernandes-Costa, F., Kramer, S., & Metz, J. (1980). Amino acid transmitter transport in nerve endings from normal and vitamin B12 deficient fruit bats. *Brain Research, 200*, 213–215.

Bromm, K., Herrmann, W. M., & Schulz, H. (1995). Do the B-vitamins exhibit antinociceptive efficacy in men? Results of a placebo-controlled repeated-measures double-blind study. *Neuropsychobiology, 31*, 156–165.

Brownlee, M. (2005). The pathobiology of diabetic complications: a unifying mechanism. *Diabetes, 54*, 1615–1625.

Bruggemann, G., Koehler, C. O., & Koch, E. M. (1990). Results of a double-blind study of diclofenac + vitamin B1, B6, B12 versus diclofenac in patients with acute pain of the lumbar vertebrae. A multicenter study. *Klinische Wochenschrift, 68*, 116–120.

Chiang, E. P., Bagley, P. J., Selhub, J., Nadeau, M., & Roubenoff, R. (2003). Abnormal vitamin B(6) status is associated with severity of symptoms in patients with rheumatoid arthritis. *The American Journal of Medicine, 114*, 283–287.

Choi, S. W., Friso, S., Ghandour, H., Bagley, P. J., Selhub, J., & Mason, J. B. (2004). Vitamin B-12 deficiency induces anomalies of base substitution and methylation in the DNA of rat colonic epithelium. *Journal of Nutrition, 134*, 750–755.

Coward, K., Plumpton, C., Facer, P., Birch, R., Carlstedt, T., Tate, S., Bountra, C., & Anand, P. (2000). Immunolocalization of SNS/PN3 and NaN/SNS2 sodium channels in human pain states. *Pain, 85*, 41–50.

Cox, J. J., Reimann, F., Nicholas, A. K., Thornton, G., Roberts, E., Springell, K., Karbani, G., Jafri, H., Mannan, J., Raashid, Y., Al-Gazali, L., Hamamy, H., Valente, E. M., Gorman, S., Williams, R., McHale, D. P., Wood, J. N., Gribble, F. M., & Woods, C. G. (2006). An SCN9A channelopathy causes congenital inability to experience pain. *Nature, 444*, 894–898.

Cummins, T. R., Sheets, P. L., & Waxman, S. G. (2007). The roles of sodium channels in nociception: implications for mechanisms of pain. *Pain, 131*, 243–257.

Dakshinamurti, K., Sharma, S. K., & Geiger, J. D. (2003). Neuroprotective actions of pyridoxine. *Biochimica et Biophysica Acta, 1647*, 225–229.

Davidson, S. (1954). The use of vitamin B12 in the treatment of diabetic neuropathy. *Journal of Florida Medicine Association, 40*, 717–721.

de Salas-Cansado, M., Perez, C., Saldana, M. T., Navarro, A., Gonzalez-Gomez, F. J., Ruiz, L., & Rejas, J. (2012). An economic evaluation of pregabalin versus usual care in the management of community-treated patients with refractory painful diabetic peripheral neuropathy in primary care settings. *Primary Care Diabetes, 6*, 303–312.

DiBonaventura, M. D., Cappelleri, J. C., & Joshi, A. V. (2011). Association between pain severity and health care resource use, health status, productivity and related costs in painful diabetic peripheral neuropathy patients. *Pain Medicine, 12*, 799–807.

Dong, X. W., Goregoaker, S., Engler, H., Zhou, X., Mark, L., Crona, J., Terry, R., Hunter, J., & Priestley, T. (2007). Small interfering RNA-mediated selective knockdown of Na(V)1.8 tetrodotoxin-resistant sodium channel reverses mechanical allodynia in neuropathic rats. *Neuroscience, 146*, 812–821.

Drew, G. M., Siddall, P. J., & Duggan, A. W. (2004). Mechanical allodynia following contusion injury of the rat spinal cord is associated with loss of GABAergic inhibition in the dorsal horn. *Pain, 109*, 379–388.

Eckert, M., & Schejbal, P. (1992). Therapy of neuropathies with a vitamin B combination. Symptomatic treatment of painful diseases of the peripheral nervous system with a combination preparation of thiamine, pyridoxine and cyanocobalamin. *Fortschritte Medicine, 110*, 544–548.

Edwards, J. L., Vincent, A. M., Cheng, H. T., & Feldman, E. L. (2008). Diabetic neuropathy: mechanisms to management. *Pharmacology and Therapeutics, 120*, 1–34.

Erlander, M. G., Tillakaratne, N. J., Feldblum, S., Patel, N., & Tobin, A. J. (1991). Two genes encode distinct glutamate decarboxylases. *Neuron, 7*, 91–100.

Eschalier, A., Aumaitre, O., Decamps, A., & Dordain, G. (1983). A comparison of the effects of vitamin B12 and aspirin in three experimental pain models in rats and mice. *Psychopharmacology, 81*, 228–231.

Fennelly, J., Frank, O., Baker, H., & Leevy, C. M. (1964). Peripheral neuropathy of the alcoholic: i, aetiological role of aneurin and other B-complex vitamins. *British Medicine Journal, 2*, 1290–1292.

Franca, D. S., Souza, A. L., Almeida, K. R., Dolabella, S. S., Martinelli, C., & Coelho, M. M. (2001). B vitamins induce an antinociceptive effect in the acetic acid and formaldehyde models of nociception in mice. *European Journal of Pharmacology, 421*, 157–164.

Fu, Q. G., Carstens, E., Stelzer, B., & Zimmermann, M. (1988). B vitamins suppress spinal dorsal horn nociceptive neurons in the cat. *Neuroscience Letters, 95*, 192–197.

Fujii, A., Matsumoto, H., & Yamamoto, H. (1996). Effect of vitamin B complex on neurotransmission and neurite outgrowth. *General Pharmacology, 27*, 995–1000.

Gaida, W., Klinder, K., Arndt, K., & Weiser, T. (2005). Ambroxol, a Nav1.8-preferring Na(+) channel blocker, effectively suppresses pain symptoms in animal models of chronic, neuropathic and inflammatory pain. *Neuropharmacology, 49*, 1220–1227.

Geng, M. Y., Saito, H., & Nishiyama, N. (1997). Protective effects of pyridoxal phosphate against glucose deprivation-induced damage in cultured hippocampal neurons. *Journal of Neurochemistry, 68*, 2500–2506.

Goto, Y. (1979). Pathophysiology and treatment of diabetes mellitus. *Masui, 28*, 1625–1633.

Groziak, S. M., & Kirksey, A. (1987). Effects of maternal dietary restriction in vitamin B-6 on neocortex development in rats: B-6 vitamer concentrations, volume and cell estimates. *Journal Nutrition, 117*, 1045–1052.

Ha, P. M., Ortiz, M. I., Garza-Hernández, A. F., Monroy-Maya, R., Soto-Ríos, M., Carrillo-Alarcón, L., Reyes-García, G., & Fernández-Martínez, E. (2012). Effect of diclofenac with B vitamins on the treatment of acute pain originated by lower-limb fractureand surgery. *Pain Research Treatment, 2012*, 104782.

Hansson, P. (2003). Difficulties in stratifying neuropathic pain by mechanisms. *European Journal of Pain, 7*, 353–357.

Harty, T. P., Dib-Hajj, S. D., Tyrrell, L., Blackman, R., Hisama, F. M., Rose, J. B., & Waxman, S. G. (2006). Na(V)1.7 mutant A863P in erythromelalgia: effects of altered activation and steady-state inactivation on excitability of nociceptive dorsal root ganglion neurons. *Journal of Neuroscience, 26*, 12566–12575.

Haupt, E., Ledermann, H., & Kopcke, W. (2005). Benfotiamine in the treatment of diabetic polyneuropathy—a three-week randomized, controlled pilot study (BEDIP study). *International Journal of Clinical Pharmacology and Therapeutics, 43*, 71–77.

Hu, S. J., & Xing, J. L. (1998). An experimental model for chronic compression of dorsal root ganglion produced by intervertebral foramen stenosis in the rat. *Pain, 77*, 15–23.

Huang, J., Cai, Q., Chen, Y., & Hong, Y. (2009). Treatment with ketanserin produces opioid-mediated hypoalgesia in the late phase of carrageenan-induced inflammatory hyperalgesia in rats. *Brain Research, 1303*, 39–47.

Huang, Z. J., & Song, X. J. (2008). Differing alterations of sodium currents in small dorsal root ganglion neurons after ganglion compression and peripheral nerve injury. *Molecular Pain, 4*, 20.

Hung, K. L., Wang, C. C., Huang, C. Y., & Wang, S. J. (2009). Cyanocobalamin, vitamin B12, depresses glutamate release through inhibition of voltage-dependent Ca^{2+} influx in rat cerebrocortical nerve terminals (synaptosomes). *European Journal of Pharmacology, 602*, 230–237.

Ikeda, H., Heinke, B., Ruscheweyh, R., & Sandkuhler, J. (2003). Synaptic plasticity in spinal lamina I projection neurons that mediate hyperalgesia. *Science, 299*, 1237–1240.

Itokawa, Y., & Cooper, J. R. (1970). Ion movements and thiamine. II. The release of the vitamin from membrane fragments. *Biochimica et Biophysica Acta, 196*, 274–284.

Ji, R. R., & Woolf, C. J. (2001). Neuronal plasticity and signal transduction in nociceptive neurons: implications for the initiation and maintenance of pathological pain. *Neurobiology of Disease, 8*, 1–10.

Joshi, S. K., Mikusa, J. P., Hernandez, G., Baker, S., Shieh, C. C., Neelands, T., Zhang, X. F., Niforatos, W., Kage, K., Han, P., Krafte, D., Faltynek, C., Sullivan, J. P., Jarvis, M. F., & Honore, P. (2006). Involvement of the TTX-resistant sodium channel Nav 1.8 in inflammatory and neuropathic, but not post-operative, pain states. *Pain, 123*, 75–82.

Kaneda, K., Kikuchi, M., Kashii, S., Honda, Y., Maeda, T., Kaneko, S., & Akaike, A. (1997). Effects of B vitamins on glutamate-induced neurotoxicity in retinal cultures. *European Journal of Pharmacology, 322*, 259–264.

Karuppagounder, S. S., Xu, H., Shi, Q., Chen, L. H., Pedrini, S., Pechman, D., Baker, H., Beal, M. F., Gandy, S. E., & Gibson, G. E. (2009). Thiamine deficiency induces oxidative stress and exacerbates the plaque pathology in Alzheimer's mouse model. *Neurobiology Aging, 30*, 1587–1600.

Kasdan, M. L., & Janes, C. (1987). Carpal tunnel syndrome and vitamin B6. *Plastic and Reconstructive Surgery, 79*, 456–462.

Kim, S. H., & Chung, J. M. (1992). An experimental model for peripheral neuropathy produced by segmental spinal nerve ligation in the rat. *Pain, 50*, 355–363.

Kohno, T., Moore, K. A., Baba, H., & Woolf, C. J. (2003). Peripheral nerve injury alters excitatory synaptic transmission in lamina II of the rat dorsal horn. *Journal of Physiology, 548*, 131–138.

Kril, J. J. (1996). Neuropathology of thiamine deficiency disorders. *Metabolic Brain Disease, 11*, 9–17.

Kuwabara, S., Nakazawa, R., Azuma, N., Suzuki, M., Miyajima, K., Fukutake, T., & Hattori, T. (1999). Intravenous methylcobalamin treatment for uremic and diabetic neuropathy in chronic hemodialysis patients. *Internal Medicine, 38*, 472–475.

Leishear, K., Boudreau, R. M., Studenski, S. A., Ferrucci, L., Rosano, C., de Rekeneire, N., Houston, D. K., Kritchevsky, S. B., Schwartz, A. V., Vinik, A. I., Hogervorst, E., Yaffe, K., Harris, T. B., Newman, A. B., & Strotmeyer, E. S. (2012). Relationship between vitamin B12 and sensory and motor peripheral nerve function in older adults. *Journal of the American Geriatrics Society, 60*(6), 1057–1063.

Leitch, G. B. (1953). Vitamin B12 in massive dosages for herpetic lesions. *Northwest Medicine, 52*, 291–292.

Leuschner, J. (1992). Antinociceptive properties of thiamine, pyridoxine and cyanocobalamin following repeated oral administration to mice. *Arzneimittelforschung, 42*, 114–115.

Levi, R., Hultling, C., Nash, M. S., & Seiger, A. (1995). The Stockholm spinal cord injury study: 1. Medical problems in a regional SCI population. *Paraplegia, 33*, 308–315.

Levin, E. R., Hanscom, T. A., Fisher, M., Lauvstad, W. A., Lui, A., Ryan, A., Glockner, D., & Levin, S. R. (1981). The influence of pyridoxine in diabetic peripheral neuropathy. *Diabetes Care, 4*, 606–609.

Liu, W., Liu, Z., Liu, L., Xiao, Z., Cao, X., Cao, Z., Xue, L., Miao, L., He, X., & Li, W. (2008). A novel human foamy virus mediated gene transfer of GAD67 reduces neuropathic pain following spinal cord injury. *Neuroscience Letters, 432*, 13–18.

Liu, J., Wolfe, D., Hao, S., Huang, S., Glorioso, J. C., Mata, M., & Fink, D. J. (2004). Peripherally delivered glutamic acid decarboxylase gene therapy for spinal cord injury pain. *Molecular Therapy, 10*, 57–66.

Mackie, M., Hughes, D. I., Maxwell, D. J., Tillakaratne, N. J., & Todd, A. J. (2003). Distribution and colocalisation of glutamate decarboxylase isoforms in the rat spinal cord. *Neuroscience, 119*, 461–472.

Mader, R., Deutsch, H., Siebert, G. K., Gerbershagen, H. U., Gruhn, E., Behl, M., & Kubler, W. (1988). Vitamin status of inpatients with chronic cephalgia and dysfunction pain syndrome and effects of a vitamin supplementation. *International Journal for Vitamin and Nutrition Research.*, *58*, 436–441.

Mannes, A., & Iadarola, M. (2007). Potential downsides of perfect pain relief. *Nature, 446*, 24.

Marcolongo, R., Mathieu, A., Pala, R., Giordano, N., Fioravanti, A., & Panzarasa, R. (1988). The efficacy and safety of auranofin in the treatment of juvenile rheumatoid arthritis. A long-term open study. *Arthritis and Rheumatism, 31*, 979–983.

McCann, V. J., & Davis, R. E. (1978). Carpal tunnel syndrome, diabetes and pyridoxal. *The Australian and New Zealand Journal of Medicine, 8*, 638–640.

Meisner, J. G., Marsh, A. D., & Marsh, D. R. (2010). Loss of GABAergic interneurons in laminae I–III of the spinal cord dorsal horn contributes to reduced GABAergic tone and neuropathic pain after spinal cord injury. *Journal of Neurotrauma, 27*, 729–737.

Metz, J. (1992). Cobalamin deficiency and the pathogenesis of nervous system disease. *Annual Review of Nutrition, 12*, 59–79.

Mikami, M., & Yang, J. (2005). Short hairpin RNA-mediated selective knockdown of NaV1.8 tetrodotoxin-resistant voltage-gated sodium channel in dorsal root ganglion neurons. *Anesthesiology, 103*, 828–836.

Misra, A. L., Vadlamani, N. L., & Pontani, R. B. (1977). Differential effects of opiates on the incorporation of [14C] thiamine in the central nervous system of the rat. *Experientia, 33*, 372–374.

Moore, K. A., Kohno, T., Karchewski, L. A., Scholz, J., Baba, H., & Woolf, C. J. (2002). Partial peripheral nerve injury promotes a selective loss of GABAergic inhibition in the superficial dorsal horn of the spinal cord. *Journal of Neuroscience, 22*, 6724–6731.

Nacitarhan, C., Minareci, E., & Sadan, G. (2014). The effect of benfotiamine on mu-opioid receptor mediated antinociception in experimental diabetes. *Experimental and Clinical Endocrinology and Diabetes, 122*, 173–178.

Neumann, S., Doubell, T. P., Leslie, T., & Woolf, C. J. (1996). Inflammatory pain hypersensitivity mediated by phenotypic switch in myelinated primary sensory neurons. *Nature, 384*, 360–364.

Obata, K., Yamanaka, H., Dai, Y., Tachibana, T., Fukuoka, T., Tokunaga, A., Yoshikawa, H., & Noguchi, K. (2003). Differential activation of extracellular signal-regulated protein kinase in primary afferent neurons regulates brain-derived neurotrophic factor expression after peripheral inflammation and nerve injury. *Journal of Neuroscience, 23*, 4117–4126.

Obrosova, I. G. (2009). Diabetic painful and insensate neuropathy: pathogenesis and potential treatments. *Neurotherapeutics, 6*, 638–647.

Obrosova, I. G., Li, F., Abatan, O. I., Forsell, M. A., Komjati, K., Pacher, P., Szabo, C., & Stevens, M. J. (2004). Role of poly(ADP-ribose) polymerase activation in diabetic neuropathy. *Diabetes, 53*, 711–720.

Parry, T. E. (1994). Folate responsive neuropathy. *Presse Medicale, 23*, 131–137.

Plaitakis, A., Nicklas, W. J., & Berl, S. (1978). Thiamine deficiency: selective impairment of the cerebellar serotonergic system. *Neurology, 28*, 691–698.

Price, D. L., Cork, L. C., Struble, R. G., Kitt, C. A., Walker, L. C., Powers, R. E., Whitehouse, P. J., & Griffin, J. W. (1987). Dysfunction and death of neurons in human degenerative neurological diseases and in animal models. *Ciba Found Symposium, 126*, 30–48.

Reyes-Garcia, G., Medina-Santillan, R., Teran-Rosales, F., Mateos-Garcia, E., & Castillo-Henkel, C. (1999). Characterization of the potentiation of the antinociceptive effect of diclofenac by vitamin B complex in the rat. *Journal of Pharmacology Toxicology Methods, 42*, 73–77.

Rizzo, M. A., Kocsis, J. D., & Waxman, S. G. (1995). Selective loss of slow and enhancement of fast Na^+ currents in cutaneous afferent dorsal root ganglion neurones following axotomy. *Neurobiology Disease, 2*, 87–96.

Rogers, M., Tang, L., Madge, D. J., & Stevens, E. B. (2006). The role of sodium channels in neuropathic pain. *Seminars in Cell and Developmental Biology, 17*, 571–581.

Sandercock, D., Cramer, M., Biton, V., & Cowles, V. E. (2012). A gastroretentive gabapentin formulation for the treatment of painful diabetic peripheral neuropathy: efficacy and tolerability in a double-blind, randomized, controlled clinical trial. *Diabetes Research and Clinical Practice, 97*, 438–445.

Scalabrino, G. (2009). The multi-faceted basis of vitamin B12 (cobalamin) neurotrophism in adult central nervous system: lessons learned from its deficiency. *Progress in Neurobiology, 88*, 203–220.

Schafers, M., Lee, D. H., Brors, D., Yaksh, T. L., & Sorkin, L. S. (2003). Increased sensitivity of injured and adjacent uninjured rat primary sensory neurons to exogenous tumor necrosis factor-alpha after spinal nerve ligation. *Journal of Neuroscience, 23*, 3028–3038.

Schwartz-Bloom, R. D., & Sah, R. (2001). Gamma-aminobutyric acid(A) neurotransmission and cerebral ischemia. *Journal of Neurochemistry, 77*, 353–371.

Siddall, P. J., McClelland, J. M., Rutkowski, S. B., & Cousins, M. J. (2003). A longitudinal study of the prevalence and characteristics of pain in the first 5 years following spinal cord injury. *Pain, 103*, 249–257.

Simeonov, S., Pavlova, M., Mitkov, M., Mincheva, L., & Troev, D. (1997). Therapeutic efficacy of "Milgamma" in patients with painful diabetic neuropathy. *Folia Medica (Plovdiv), 39*, 5–10.

Small, F. B. (1978). Relief of pain by infiltration of autonomic ganglia with steroids. *Canada Medicine Association Journal, 119*, 217–218.

Song, X. J., Gan, Q., Cao, J. L., Wang, Z. B., & Rupert, R. L. (2006a). Spinal manipulation reduces pain and hyperalgesia after lumbar intervertebral foramen inflammation in the rat. *Journal of Manipulative and Physiological Therapeutics, 29*, 5–13.

Song, X. J., Hu, S. J., Greenquist, K. W., Zhang, J. M., & LaMotte, R. H. (1999). Mechanical and thermal hyperalgesia and ectopic neuronal discharge after chronic compression of dorsal root ganglia. *Journal of Neurophysiology, 82*, 3347–3358.

Song, X. J., Vizcarra, C., Xu, D. S., Rupert, R. L., & Wong, Z. N. (2003a). Hyperalgesia and neural excitability following injuries to central and peripheral branches of axons and somata of dorsal root ganglion neurons. *Journal of Neurophysiology, 89*, 2185–2193.

Song, X. J., Wang, Z. B., Gan, Q., & Walters, E. T. (2006b). cAMP and cGMP contribute to sensory neuron hyperexcitability and hyperalgesia in rats with dorsal root ganglia compression. *Journal of Neurophysiology, 95*, 479–492.

Song, X. J., Xu, D. S., Vizcarra, C., & Rupert, R. L. (2003b). Onset and recovery of hyperalgesia and hyperexcitability of sensory neurons following intervertebral foramen volume reduction and restoration. *Journal of Manipulative and Physiological Therapeutics, 26*, 426–436.

Song, X. J., Zhang, J. M., Hu, S. J., & LaMotte, R. H. (2003c). Somata of nerve-injured sensory neurons exhibit enhanced responses to inflammatory mediators. *Pain, 104*, 701–709.

Song, X. S., Huang, Z. J., & Song, X. J. (2009a). Thiamine suppresses thermal hyperalgesia, inhibits hyperexcitability, and lessens alterations of sodium currents in injured, dorsal root ganglion neurons in rats. *Anesthesiology, 110*, 387–400.

Song, Y. H., Chen, J. Q., & Zhou, H. L. (2002). Cyclic nucleotides phosphodiesterase activity in a rat lung model of asthma. *Zhejiang Da Xue Xue Bao Yi Xue Ban, 31*, 127–130.

Song, Z., Ultenius, C., Meyerson, B. A., & Linderoth, B. (2009b). Pain relief by spinal cord stimulation involves serotonergic mechanisms: an experimental study in a rat model of mononeuropathy. *Pain, 147*, 241–248.

Stracke, H., Gaus, W., Achenbach, U., Federlin, K., & Bretzel, R. G. (2008). Benfotiamine in diabetic polyneuropathy (BENDIP): results of a randomised, double blind, placebo-controlled clinical study. *Experimental and Clinical Endocrinology and Diabetes, 116*, 600–605.

Stracke, H., Lindemann, A., & Federlin, K. (1996). A benfotiamine-vitamin B combination in treatment of diabetic polyneuropathy. *Experimental and Clinical Endocrinology and Diabetes, 104*, 311–316.

Sun, W., Miao, B., Wang, X. C., Duan, J. H., Wang, W. T., Kuang, F., Xie, R. G., Xing, J. L., Xu, H., Song, X. J., Luo, C., & Hu, S. J. (2012). Reduced conduction failure of the main axon of polymodal nociceptive C-fibres contributes to painful diabetic neuropathy in rats. *Brain, 135*, 359–375.

Surtees, S. J., & Hughes, R. R. (1954). Treatment of trigeminal neuralgia with vitamin B12. *Lancet, 266*, 439–441.

Takeshige, C., Ando, Y., & Ando, M. (1971). Effects of vitamin B12 and aldosterone on the conduction of sensory and motor nerve impulse. *Vitamins, 44*, 10.

Talebi, M., Andalib, S., Bakhti, S., Ayromlou, H., Aghili, A., & Talebi, A. (2013). Effect of vitamin b6 on clinical symptoms and electrodiagnostic results of patients with carpal tunnel syndrome. *Advanced Pharmacy Bullentin, 3*, 283–288.

Tan, Z. Y., Donnelly, D. F., & LaMotte, R. H. (2006). Effects of a chronic compression of the dorsal root ganglion on voltage-gated Na+ and K+ currents in cutaneous afferent neurons. *Journal of Neurophysiology, 95*, 1115–1123.

Terasawa, M., Nakahara, T., Tsukada, N., Sugawara, A., & Itokawa, Y. (1999). The relationship between thiamine deficiency and performance of a learning task in rats. *Metabolic Brain Disease, 14*, 137–148.

Vesely, D. L. (1985). B complex vitamins activate rat guanylate cyclase and increase cyclic GMP levels. *European Journal of Clinical Investigation, 15*, 258–262.

Vocci, F. J., Petty, S. K., & Dewey, W. L. (1978). Antinociceptive action of the butyryl derivatives of cyclic guanosine 3′:5′-monophosphate. *The Journal of Pharmacology and Experimental Therapeutics, 207*, 892–898.

Wang, X. D., Kashii, S., Zhao, L., Tonchev, A. B., Katsuki, H., Akaike, A., Honda, Y., Yamashita, J., & Yamashima, T. (2002). Vitamin B6 protects primate retinal neurons from ischemic injury. *Brain Research, 940*, 36–43.

Wang, Z. B., Gan, Q., Rupert, R. L., Zeng, Y. M., & Song, X. J. (2005). Thiamine, pyridoxine, cyanocobalamin and their combination inhibit thermal, but not mechanical hyperalgesia in rats with primary sensory neuron injury. *Pain, 114*, 266–277.

Waxman, S. G. (1999). The molecular pathophysiology of pain: abnormal expression of sodium channel genes and its contributions to hyperexcitability of primary sensory neurons. *Pain Supplement, 6*, S133–140.

Waxman, S. G. (2006). Neurobiology: a channel sets the gain on pain. *Nature, 444*, 831–832.

Weir, D. G., & Scott, J. M. (1995). The biochemical basis of the neuropathy in cobalamin deficiency. *Baillieres Clinical Haematology, 8*(3), 479–497.

Woelk, H., Lehrl, S., Bitsch, R., & Kopcke, W. (1998). Benfotiamine in treatment of alcoholic polyneuropathy: an 8-week randomized controlled study (BAP I Study). *Alcohol Alcohol, 33*, 631–638.

Woolf, C. J. (2011). Central sensitization: implications for the diagnosis and treatment of pain. *Pain, 152*, S2–S15.

Xiao, H. S., Huang, Q. H., Zhang, F. X., Bao, L., Lu, Y. J., Guo, C., Yang, L., Huang, W. J., Fu, G., Xu, S. H., Cheng, X. P., Yan, Q., Zhu, Z. D., Zhang, X., Chen, Z., Han, Z. G., & Zhang, X. (2002). Identification of gene expression profile of dorsal root ganglion in the rat peripheral axotomy model of neuropathic pain. *Proceedings of the National Academy of Sciences of the United States of America, 99*, 8360–8365.

Yamauchi, Y. (1970). Diabetes mellitus and neuropathies. *Kango Gijutsu, 16*, 56–64.

Yu, C. Z., Liu, Y. P., Liu, S., Yan, M., Hu, S. J., & Song, X. J. (2014). Systematic administration of B vitamins attenuates neuropathic hyperalgesia and reduces spinal neuron injury following temporary spinal cord ischaemia in rats. *European Journal of Pain, 18*, 76–85.

Yxfeldt, A., Wallberg-Jonsson, S., Hultdin, J., & Rantapaa-Dahlqvist, S. (2003). Homocysteine in patients with rheumatoid arthritis in relation to inflammation and B-vitamin treatment. *Scandinavian Journal of Rheumatology, 32*, 205–210.

Zhang, A. L., Hao, J. X., Seiger, A., Xu, X. J., Wiesenfeld-Hallin, Z., Grant, G., & Aldskogius, H. (1994). Decreased GABA immunoreactivity in spinal cord dorsal horn neurons after transient spinal cord ischemia in the rat. *Brain Research, 656*, 187–190.

Zimmermann, M. (2001). Pathobiology of neuropathic pain. *European Journal of Pharmacology, 429*, 23–37.

Zimmerman, M., Bartoszyk, G. D., Bonke, D., Jurna, I., & Wild, A. (1990). Antinociceptive properties of pyridoxine. Neurophysiological and behavioral findings. *Annals of the New York Academy of Sciences, 585*, 219–230.

C H A P T E R

23

Pain Relief in Chronic Pancreatitis—Role of Nutritional Antioxidants

P. Bhardwaj[*,**], *R.K. Yadav*[†], *P.K. Garg*[*]

[*]Department of Gastroenterology, All India Institute of Medical Sciences, New Delhi, India; [**]Tata Consultancy Services, Noida, Uttar Pradesh, India; [†]Department of Physiology, All India Institute of Medical Sciences, New Delhi, India

INTRODUCTION

Chronic pancreatitis (CP) is a pathologic chronic inflammatory disease of the pancreas resulting in progressive parenchymal injury and fibrosis that occurs due to genetic and/or environmental risk factors. The disease manifests itself as a variably progressive glandular dysfunction presenting with abdominal pain and functional impairment in the form of diabetes and steatorrhea (Tandon, Sato, & Garg, 2002). The common causes of CP are hereditary, alcohol abuse, smoking, genetic mutations, metabolic derangements, such as hyperlipidemia and hypercalcemia, and idiopathic.

Abdominal pain is the most common symptom in patients with CP, which may be intermittent or chronic. Pain is often unrelenting, and significant affecting patient's quality of life (QoL). It is a therapeutic challenge to treat pain effectively in patients with CP. The main reason for the difficulty in treating pain is limited understanding of its pathophysiology. Acinar cells of the exocrine pancreas synthesize and secrete pancreatic enzymes, and it is believed that the initiating events in the pathogenesis of pancreatitis start in the acinar cells. Activated digestive enzymes due to several reasons, such as mutations in cationic trypsinogen gene or mutations in genes encoding for antiproteases, such as *SPINK1* and *CTRC* may cause intracellular perturbations that initiate inflammation. The intracellular events include endoplasmic reticulum (ER) stress and electrophilic stress [oxidative stress (OS)] due to free radical (FR) generation. ER stress and OS may lead to inflammation through activation of nuclear factor (NF)κB activation. NFκB, a nuclear transcription factor, is considered to be a master regulator of inflammation. Several theories have been put forwards to explain the pain of pancreatic origin. These include pancreatic ductal hypertension due to ductal obstruction by stones/stricture, pancreatic inflammation, interstitial hypertension, perineural infiltration by immune cells, and neuropathic pain. Pancreatic inflammation is the most likely mechanism to cause pain because most patients in the first few years of illness do not have ductal obstruction and neuropathic pain is seen in late advanced form of the disease. OS seems to play an important role in pancreatic inflammation. Deficiency of micronutrient antioxidants exacerbates OS. Research in the past decade has brought more evidence to support the role of OS in the pathophysiology of CP (Tandon & Garg, 2011; Grigsby, Rodriguez-Rilo, & Khan, 2012). OS is a result of an imbalance between the levels of FR and antioxidants in cells. In the context of CP, this may be attributed to diverse reasons including but not limited to intracellular generation of FR due to ER stress, alcohol and tobacco abuse, suboptimal dietary intake of micronutrients, and environmental factors, which promote the OS and inflammatory reactions.

FREE RADICALS IN CELLULAR PHYSIOLOGY AND PATHOPHYSIOLOGY

FRs play a key role in intracellular physiology, as these can act as second messengers contemplating physiological redox, and regulate intracellular signaling (Droge, 2002). A regulated increase in FR production causes a temporary imbalance, which is called physiological redox, and is responsible for normal cellular

Nutritional Modulators of Pain in the Aging Population. http://dx.doi.org/10.1016/B978-0-12-805186-3.00023-0
Copyright © 2017 Elsevier Inc. All rights reserved.

physiology. This type of OS is generally mild and is physiological rather than pathological.

Endogenous Sources of Free Radicals

The key sources of FRs in normal cellular physiology are electron transport chain and tricarboxylic acid cycle in mitochondria. Though only a small proportion (2–5%) of the electrons that pass through this cycle are converted to FR, this contributes to the overall physiological production of FR since this cycle processes at least 95% of all the oxygen used by the body. The continual flux of single electrons to oxygen generates an endogenous OS. Another key source of FR is detoxification system, which metabolizes xenobiotics. During phase I of detoxification, enzymes break the parent molecule rendering these more or less toxic while an endogenous molecule is attached to the phase I biotransformed compound so to excrete it, that is, glucuronidation and glutathione conjugation. During increased xenobiotic load, there may be overinduction of phase I enzymes, that is, CYP450 oxidase system and hydrolyzing enzymes (Anzenbacher & Anzenbacherová, 2001). The CYP2E1 overinduction is especially pertinent, as it is known to generate FR from alcohol itself. The over-induction of CYP2E1 develops metabolic tolerance to alcohol in chronic alcoholics. At times, the detoxification acts as a double-edged sword as it may increase the toxicity of biotransformed compounds. This means an increased enzymatic activity may upset the homeostasis and may alter the capacity of this system in handling toxic compounds and their metabolites.

Erythrocytes are also key players in the production of FR and generation of OS by virtue of auto-oxidation of oxy-hemoglobin into met-hemoglobin, and interaction of hemoglobin with redox drugs and xenobiotics (Freeman & Crapo, 1982). This is important as the erythrocyte membranes are largely made up of polyunsaturated fatty acids, which make them highly susceptible to OS injury. Though erythrocytes are rich in antioxidant enzymes, which efficiently handle FR (Toth, Clifford, Berger, White, & Repine, 1984; van Asbeck et al., 1985), but an overwhelming production of FR may go undefended and result in OS.

Another source of FR is the scavenging cells, such as macrophages and neutrophils. These generate large quantities of FR that participate in an antimicrobial and tumoricidal milieu, commonly called as "oxidative burst," and play an important role in immunity against viruses and bacteria.

Exogenous Sources of Free Radicals

There are multiple exogenous sources of FR, such as smoke, industrial pollutants, UV rays, environmental factors, but alcohol and cigarette are key sources as far as CP is concerned. Alcohol metabolism is associated with FR production (Di Luzio, 1966), and commences through alcohol dehydrogenase, microsomal ethanol oxidation system (MEOS), and catalase. Each of these pathways could produce FR, which compromises the antioxidant system. The resultant lipid peroxidation products may be highly toxic to the body (Shaw, 1989). Similarly, cigarette smoke contains a range of xenobiotics, including oxidants and FR that can increase lipid peroxidation. Cigarette smoke may contain up to 10^{14} FR/inhalation (Church & Pryor, 1985), and significantly impacts the micronutrient antioxidant defense of the body.

FREE RADICALS IN PANCREATIC PATHOPHYSIOLOGY

Many causes have been identified for the pathophysiological state in CP, which are based on OS theory. This may include induction of cytochrome (CYP) P450 induction by alcohol and cigarette smoke, chronic exposure to occupational volatile petrochemical products, and habitually lower intake of nutritional antioxidants (Bhardwaj & Yadav, 2013). In addition, increased intracellular generation of FR may be due to increased ER stress induced by misfolded proteins. An overview of the same is presented in Fig. 23.1.

Pancreas has a quiescent xenobiotics metabolism system, and may be over-induced during xenobiotic overload. This may results in an increased OS in acinar cell CYP over-induction, resulting in bioactivation and an undefended FR burden causing glutathione (GSH) deficit (Gómez-Cambronero et al., 2000). Inhaled toxins, for example, from cigarette smoke may cause CYP over-induction in islet cells. Besides, there may be an endogenous OS, which may be due to PRSS1, SPINK1, and CTRC gene mutations that elicit an unfolded protein response and endoplasmic stress resulting in increased production of FR. Recent epidemiological studies suggested the role of genetic factors, cigarette smoking, high physical activity at work, occupational exposure to hydrocarbons, high protein/fat diet, and malnutrition in the development of CP (Pitchumoni & Bordalo, 1996; McNamee et al., 1994; Matsumoto et al., 1996; Breuer-Katschinski, Bracht, Tietjen-Harms, & Goebell, 1996).

Sources of Free Radicals in Pancreas

Exogenous sources of FR in the pancreas include alcohol and cigarette smoke, which is known to be independently associated with alcoholic CP, and may promote calcification in CP (Talamini et al., 1996; Imoto & DiMagno, 2000; Yen, Hsieh, & MacMahon, 1982; Bourliere, Barthet, Berthezene, Durbec, & Sarles, 1991; Cavallini

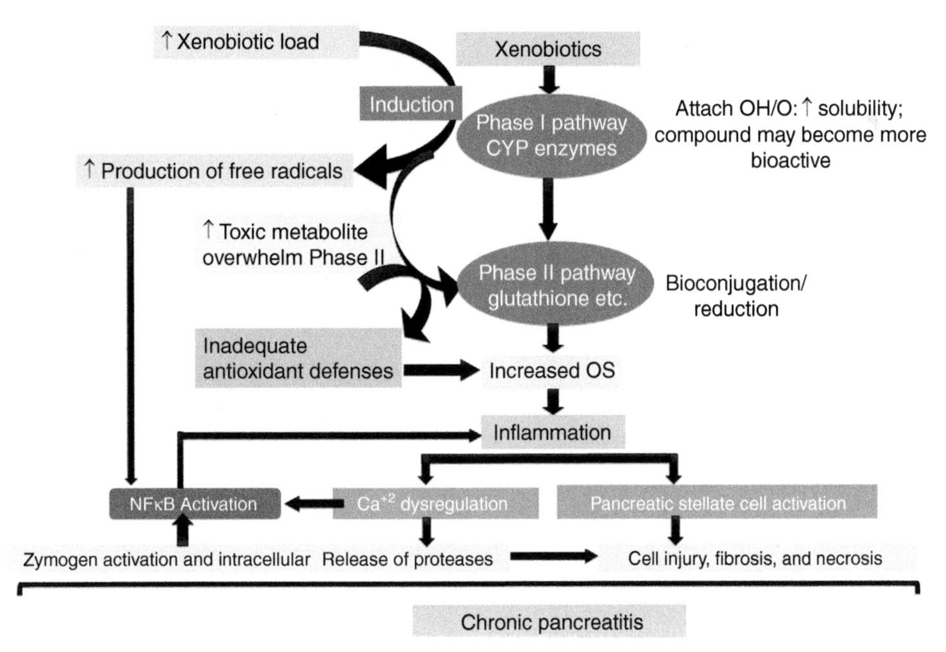

FIGURE 23.1 **Oxidative stress mediated pancreatic acinar cell injury.**

et al., 1994). Nicotine adversely affects the pancreatic acinar cell function (Dubick, Palmer, Lau, Morrill, & Geokas, 1988). Levels of serum vitamin C are generally lower in smokers (Pelletier, 1970). Pancreatic stellate cells (PSCs) are activated early in the course of pancreatic injury, and are the predominant source of collagen in the fibrotic pancreas (Haber et al., 1999). The data show that serum and duodenal bile have a high concentration of FR, and also their peroxidation products during asymptomatic period between pancreatitis attacks, which substantiate the prevailing OS in patients with CP (Guyan, Uden, & Braganza, 1990; Bhardwaj et al., 2009; Tandon & Garg, 2011).

Oxidative Stress and Inflammation in Pancreas

The OS-mediated injury promotes inflammation by increased production of interleukin-6, tumor necrosis factor-α, and monocyte chemoattractant protein-1. Additionally, stress-sensitive kinases, such as c-Jun N-terminal kinases, protein kinase (PK)-C isoforms, mitogen-activated protein kinases, and inhibitor of kappa B kinase are activated. These together trigger the oxidative-inflammation cascade and propagate the injury (Yu & Kim, 2014). OS seems to block exocytosis, which is compensated by enhanced crinophagy and autophagy to dispense the zymogens causing autodigestion. FRs trigger the production of stress and inflammatory pathways (Tamura et al., 1992). Importantly, the release and activation of pancreatic enzymes is controlled by a fluctuation in Ca^{+2} levels. Excessive production of FR disrupts intracellular Ca^{+2} homeostasis, releasing Ca^{+2} from ER and mitochondria (Pariente, Camello, Camello, & Salido, 2001; González, Schmid, Salido, Camello, & Pariente, 2002). A continued disruption of Ca^{+2} homeostasis adversely affects ATP synthesis and triggers fibrosis-necrosis along with other functional and morphological alterations (Leist, Single, & Castoldi, 1997; Niederau, Schultz, & Letko, 1991; Klonowski-Stumpe et al., 1997).

PAIN IN CHRONIC PANCREATITIS

The pathophysiology of pain in CP remains poorly understood, though several mechanisms of pain have been implicated. Increased intrapancreatic pressure due to obstruction of pancreatic duct by stones and/or stricture may cause pain in some patients with CP. However, endoscopic or surgical therapy to decrease ductal pressure does not always result in pain relief. Recent data suggest that neuroimmune interactions and chronic inflammation could be the key mechanism for pain in majority of patients with CP (Di Sebastiano, di Mola, Bockman, Friess, & Büchler, 2003; Viggiano et al., 2005). Increased OS and resulting inflammation may increase pancreatic nociception where, damaged perineurium is surrounded by inflammatory cells (Fig. 23.2). The intensity of pain correlated with eosinophils in perineural inflammatory cell infiltrates (Keith, Keshavjee, & Kerenyi, 1985). This may be further aggravated and sustained by pancreatic enzymes soaking the exposed nerves (Büchler et al., 1992). There may be an upregulation of neuropeptides within the enlarged nerves, thereby changing the intrinsic and extrinsic innervation of the pancreas, playing an important role in the transmission of pain stimuli. The enlargement of pancreatic nerves appears to be mediated by overexpression of nerve growth factor and one of its receptors, tyrosine

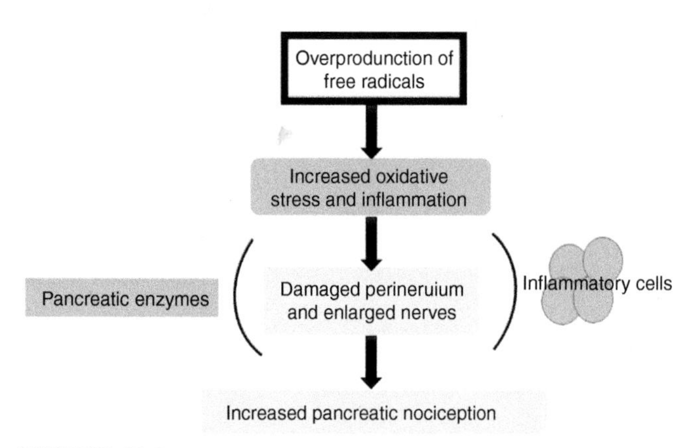

FIGURE 23.2 **A mechanistic model of how oxidative stress could contribute to inflammation and pain in chronic pancreatitis (CP).**

kinase A (Friess et al., 1999). Modulation of PKC and ion channels, such as transient receptor potential vanilloid 1 (TRPV1), and alterations in glutamatergic neurotransmission and neuroinflammation, substance P and calcitonin gene-related peptide (CGRP); and the crucial mediator of central pain, brain-derived neurotrophic factor also contribute toward acute and chronic inflammatory neuropathic pain (Miyamoto, Dubin, Petrus, & Patapoutian, 2009; Zhu et al., 2011, 2012). FRs have been shown to induce NFkB, which in turn leads to cytokine production and may cause alteration in signal transduction and induce cell injury (Kabe, Ando, Hirao, Yoshida, & Handa, 2005; Shiva et al., 2004; Levonen et al., 2004). Transient receptor potential A1 (TRPA1), an excitatory ion channel, is present on the primary afferent somatosensory neurons that contain substance P and CGRP and mediates peripheral nociception (Bautista et al., 2006). It has been shown that 4-hydroxy-2-nonenal (HNE), a by-product of FR injury stimulated release of substance P and CGRP from spinal cord and peripheral nerve endings. When HNE was injected in the rodent hind paw, it elicited pain-related behaviors, which could be inhibited by TRPA1 antagonist (Trevisani et al., 2007). It is thus likely that a reduction in OS by antioxidants might decrease perineural inflammation, attenuate stimulation of the neurogenic nociceptive receptors, and relieve pain.

ANTIOXIDANT DEFENSE IN CELLULAR PHYSIOLOGY

An antioxidant is "any substance that, when present in low concentration compared to those of an oxidizable substrate, significantly delays or inhibits oxidation of that substrate" (Halliwell & Gutteridge, 1989). These may include enzymes, such as superoxide dismutase (SOD), glutathione peroxidase (GPx), and CAT, nonenzyme protein systems, such as glutathione, free amino acids, peptides, and proteins, and importantly, dietary antioxidants, such as α-tocopherol (vitamin E), β-carotene, and ascorbate (vitamin C). The antioxidants circulating in body are important, as most of the amino acids are highly sensitive to FR attack (Davies, Delsignore, & Lin, 1987a; Davies, Lin, & Pacifici, 1987b). The antioxidant defenses are summarized in Table 23.1.

NUTRITIONAL ANTIOXIDANTS

The role of various nutritional antioxidants has been evaluated to relive the pain in patients with CP. These include micronutrient antioxidants, such as vitamin C (ascorbate), vitamin E (α-tocopherol), β-carotene, methionine, and selenium. The proposed mechanism of pain relief is by reducing the OS and related inflammation. A brief mechanism of action of these dietary antioxidants is presented here.

Vitamin C

Vitamin C (ascorbic acid) has a broad spectrum of antioxidant activities due to its ability to react with numerous aqueous FR. It provides the first line of defense, particularly against cigarette smoke (Frei & Ames, 1988).

TABLE 23.1 The Antioxidant Defenses

Endogenous		Exogenous
Enzymatic	**Nonenzymatic**	**Nutritional**
Superoxide dismutase	Glutathione	Vitamin E (mainly α-tocopherol)
Glutathione peroxidase	Uric acid	Vitamin A (β-carotene)
Catalase	Melatonin	Vitamin C (ascorbate)
Peroxiredoxin I	Thioredoxin	Selenium
Thioredoxin reductase	Amino acids	Lycopene
		Flavonoids
		Omega-3 and omega-6 fatty acids

It has antiinflammatory activity also (Wannamethee, Lowe, Rumley, Bruckdorfer, & Whincup, 2006). Since it is water-soluble, it protects other antioxidants, such as vitamins A and E, and essential fatty acids (Frei, Stocker, England, & Ames, 1990). Plasma is completely saturated at doses of 400 mg/day or more, producing a steady-state plasma concentration of approximately 80 μM (Padayatty et al., 2003). At a dose of 500 mg and above, the entire absorbed vitamin C is excreted.

Vitamin E

Vitamin E is by far the most abundant lipid soluble antioxidant in human beings and plays a key role in saving cell membranes from FR induced injury. It circulates in the lipoproteins and chylomicron. Unlike other fat- soluble vitamins, it has no specific plasma carrier proteins (Granot, Tamir, & Deckelbaum, 1988) and the molar ratio to cholesterol is a good index of vitamin E status (Ford, Farr, Morris, & Berg, 2006). It may also potentiate the immune response (Meydani, Han, & Wu, 2005; Bergman et al., 2004), prevent oxidation of DNA, and influence cellular functions, such as proliferation, platelet aggregation, cytokine production, and adhesion molecule expression (Samandari, Visarius, Zingg, & Azzi, 2006; Singh & Jialal, 2004). Vitamin E supplementation (400–1200 IU/day) increases plasma alpha-tocopherol concentrations to the normal. The animal model of CP shows that vitamin E supplementation had antiinflammatory effects on the pancreatic gene expression of some inflammatory genes, which suggests its role in antiinflammatory pathways in the pancreas (Monteiro, Silva, Cordeiro Simões Ambrosio, Zucoloto, & Vannucchi, 2012). Similar results were noted in other studies where vitamin E supplementation improved pancreatic inflammation and fibrosis (Jiang et al., 2011; Li, Lu, & Chen, 2011).

Carotenoids and Vitamin A

Carotenoids have long been considered as antioxidants because of their capacity to scavenge FR (Krinsky & Deneke, 1982; Edge, McGarvey, & Truscott, 1997). Carotenoids protect against lipid peroxidation by quenching FR and display an efficient FR trapping antioxidant activity (Cantrell, McGarvey, Truscott, Rancan, & Bohm, 2003). Compared with α-tocopherol, however, β-carotene is a relatively weak antioxidant. Retinol is circulated in a combined state with retinol-binding protein (RBP). Patients with CP have lower levels of vitamin A and RBP (Nakamura et al., 1995), which is also attributed by lower intake and absorption of vitamin A. However, increasing protein intake may improve the levels of both RBP and vitamin A (Smith et al., 1975). The available data show that patients with CP may be deficient in carotenoids and supplementation with natural carotenoids may be helpful (Quilliot, Forbes, Dubois, Gueant, & Ziegler, 2011).

Methionine

Methionine is an antioxidant by contributing sulfur atom in the synthesis of cysteine. Inadequate intake of methionine can adversely impact the synthesis of cysteine and hence GSH, one of the key endogenous antioxidant. In liver, methionine is adenosylated and is then converted to s-adenosyl methionine (SAM). SAM is then converted to s-adenosyl homocysteine (SAH). In the presence of vitamin B6, SAH is converted to cystathione and then cysteine (Stipanuk, 1986). This cysteine is then used in biosynthesis of glutathione along with serine.

Selenium

Selenium (Se) is an integral part of GPx and Se-dependent enzyme thioredoxin reductase, which may be implicated in inflammation associated with CP. This enzyme is decreased to 25-fold in Se-deficient animals, although with very little change in hepatic GSH levels. Selenium is affected by malabsorption (Kellener, 1981). The dietary intake of these trace elements could be low in patients with CP because of reduced fat intake (Vaona et al., 1997) and may also be modulated by the withdrawal of alcohol (Lecomte et al., 1994).

DIETARY ANTIOXIDANTS AS MODULATORS OF PAIN AND OXIDATIVE STRESS

The data available clearly support the role of antioxidants in ameliorating pancreatic acinar cell OS. Micronutrient antioxidants interact with glutathione in tissues to facilitate the disposal of FR and xenobiotic metabolites derived via cytochrome P450. The requirement of nutritional antioxidants in the pancreas is therefore twofold. First, there is a requirement of cystine/cysteine for synthesis of pancreatic enzymes, which is provided by GSH. Second, there is a high xenobiotic load on pancreas, causing an induction of CYP450 enzymes in pancreatic acinar cells (Foster et al., 1993). If there is a dietary deficiency of cystine/cysteine, there is a direct impact on both, the enzyme synthesis, as well as detoxification. Another important nutritional antioxidant is methionine, the deficiency of which impacts glutathione synthesis as methionine participates in the trans-sulfuration pathway affecting cysteine and glutathione synthesis. This renders the pancreatic acinar cell a highly vulnerable target for FR effects (Braganza, 1996). The evidence shows that patients with CP have a poor nutritional antioxidant status (Rose, Fraine, Hunt, Acheson, & Braganza, 1986;

Braganza, Schofield, Snehlatha, & Mohan, 1993; Bhardwaj, Thareja, Prakash, & Saraya, 2004). Patients with idiopathic CP had significantly lower levels of plasma selenium, plasma copper, plasma zinc, serum Vitamin E, serum vitamin A, and plasma vitamin C versus controls (Uden et al., 1988; Segal, Gut, Schofield, Shiel, & Braganza, 1995; van Gossum, Closset, Noel, Cremer, & Neve, 1996; Vaona et al., 2005; Sajewicz, Milnerowicz, & Nabzdyk, 2006). Nevertheless, the levels of endogenous antioxidants may also be altered due to genetic factors in some patients posing a significant threat from OS in the pancreas (Cullen, Mitros, & Oberley, 2003).

It has been over 2 decades when the role of micronutrient antioxidants was first explored and evaluated in CP, especially for ameliorating pain. In this regard, the study at the Royal Infirmary, Manchester, UK was the pioneer study (Uden et al., 1992), which specifically used a combination of dietary antioxidants for supplementation. The cocktail included 600 μg organic selenium, 9000 IU β-carotene, 0.54 g vitamin C, 270 IU vitamin E, and 2 g methionine. The results showed notable pain relief in patients with pancreatitis, both recurrent acute and chronic. Similar results were shown in another study later (Kirk et al., 2006). In a large, randomized, placebo-controlled trial, we showed that pain was significantly reduced during 6-month therapy and the benefit was evident as early as 3 months. The reduction in pain was accompanied by reduction in OS and improved levels of antioxidants in blood. The antioxidants used in our study were same as that used in the Manchester study (Bhardwaj et al., 2009).

A recent systematic review and metaanalysis showed that antioxidants can help ameliorate pain in patients with CP (Talukdar, Murthy, & Reddy, 2015). This analysis included 9 RCTs with 390 patients (Cai et al., 2013). A combination of antioxidants (selenium, β-carotene, vitamin C, vitamin E, and methionine) showed significant pain relief while studies with single antioxidant therapy showed no significant pain relief. Two other recent systematic reviews and metaanalyses evaluated antioxidants in CP; one of these showed that there was no significant reduction in pain in patients with CP (Gooshe, Abdolghaffari, Nikfar, Mahdaviani, & Abdollahi, 2015) and the other showed a significant reduction in pain (Zhou, Wang, Cheng, Wei, & Zheng, 2015). The QoL also showed a significant improvement in patients with CP who received antioxidant therapy for pain (Shah, Makin, Sheen, & Siriwardena, 2010). A recent randomized trial from United Kingdom, however, did not document any reduction in pain (Siriwardena, Mason, Sheen, Makin, & Shah, 2012). There have been some limitations of that study, such as improper patient selection with predominantly alcohol induced CP, continued alcohol intake and smoking, opiate dependence, failed endoscopic/surgical therapy, and so on (Garg, 2013; Braganza, 2013). The latest RCT has shown that a combination of pregabalin and antioxidants for 2 months followed by only antioxidants for 4 months resulted in significant pain relief in patients with CP who had recurrence of pain after ductal clearance by endotherapy or surgery (Talukdar, Lakhtakia, Rebala, Rao, & Reddy, 2016).

The mechanism of action behind pain relief is likely to be due to reduction in OS and pancreatic inflammation possibly through TRPV1, which is upregulated and mediates hyperalgesia in experimental CP or TRPA1, which is involved in peripheral mechanisms controlling pain hypersensitivity (Bautista et al., 2006; Yu, Lim, Namkung, Kim, & Kim, 2002; Vaquero, Gukovsk, Zaninovic, Gukovskaya, & Pandol, 2001; Xu et al., 2007). It should be noted that FR products stimulate painful sensations in central and peripheral nerve endings, and could be inhibited by TRPA1 antagonist (Trevisani et al., 2007). The reduction in pain could also be attributed to reduction in fibrosis (Dhingra, Singh, Sachdev, Upadhyay, & Saraya, 2013).

WAY FORWARD

Although a substantial body of evidence supports the use of micronutrient antioxidants in ameliorating pain in patients with CP, more studies are required to understand the pathophysiological basis of OS in acinar cells, mechanism of action of antioxidants and their long-term effect. Whether or not OS plays a primary role in the pathogenesis of CP or more of a modifier role also needs to be studied. The role of OS and antioxidants in the early form of CP or even in idiopathic recurrent acute pancreatitis (probably even an earlier form of CP) also needs to be explored to understand if OS could be important during the progression of early to advanced CP.

References

Anzenbacher, P., & Anzenbacherová, E. (2001). Cytochromes P450 and metabolism of xenobiotics. *Cellular and Molecular Life Sciences, 58*, 737–747.

Bautista, D. M., Jordt, S. E., Nikai, T., Tsuruda, P. R., Read, A. J., Poblete, J., Yamoah, E. N., Basbaum, A. I., & Julius, D. (2006). TRPA1 mediates the inflammatory actions of environmental irritants and proalgesic agents. *Cell, 124*, 1269–1282.

Bergman, M., Salman, H., Djaldetti, M., Fish, L., Punsky, I., & Bessler, H. (2004). In vitro immune response of human peripheral blood cells to vitamins C and E. *The Journal of Nutritional Biochemistry, 15*, 45–50.

Bhardwaj, P., Thareja, S., Prakash, S., & Saraya, A. (2004). Micronutrient antioxidant intake in patients with chronic pancreatitis. *Tropical Gastroenterology, 25*, 69–72.

Bhardwaj, P., Garg, P. K., Maulik, S. K., Saraya, A., Tandon, R. K., & Acharya, S. K. (2009). A randomized controlled trial of antioxidant supplementation for pain relief in patients with chronic pancreatitis. *Gastroenterology, 136*, 149–159.

Bhardwaj, P., & Yadav, R. K. (2013). Chronic pancreatitis: role of oxidative stress and antioxidants. *Free Radical Research, 47*, 941–949.

Bourliere, M., Barthet, M., Berthezene, P., Durbec, J. P., & Sarles, H. (1991). Is tobacco a risk factor for chronic pancreatitis and alcoholic cirrhosis? *Gut, 32*, 1392–1395.

Braganza, J. M. (1996). The pathogenesis of chronic pancreatitis. *QJM, 89*, 243–250.

Braganza, J. M. (2013). Limitations of patient selection and other issues in chronic pancreatitis antioxidant trial. *Gastroenterology, 144*, e17–e18.

Braganza, J. M., Schofield, D., Snehlatha, C., & Mohan, V. (1993). Micronutrient stasis in tropical compared to temperate zone pancreatitis. *Scandinavian Journal of Gastroenterology, 28*, 1098–1104.

Breuer-Katschinski, B. D., Bracht, J., Tietjen-Harms, S., & Goebell, H. (1996). Physical activity at work and the risk of chronic pancreatitis. *European Journal of Gastroenterology and Hepatology, 8*, 399–402.

Büchler, M., Weihe, E., Friess, H., Malfertheiner, P., Bockman, E., Müller, S., Nohr, D., & Beger, H. G. (1992). Changes in peptidergic innervation in chronic pancreatitis. *Pancreas, 7*, 183–192.

Cai, G. H., Huang, J., Zhao, Y., Chen, J., Wu, H. H., Dong, Y. L., Smith, H. S., Li, Y. Q., Wang, W., & Wu, S. X. (2013). Antioxidant therapy for pain relief in patients with chronic pancreatitis: systematic review and meta-analysis. *Pain Physician, 16*, 521–532.

Cantrell, A., McGarvey, D. J., Truscott, T. G., Rancan, F., & Bohm, F. (2003). Singlet oxygen quenching by dietary carotenoids in a model membrane environment. *Archives of Biochemistry and Biophysics, 412*, 47–54.

Cavallini, G., Talamini, G., Vaona, B., Bovo, P., Filippini, M., Rigo, L., Angelini, G., Vantini, I., Riela, A., Frulloni, L., Di Francesco, V., Brunori, M. P., Bassi, C., & Pederzoli, P. (1994). Effect of alcohol and smoking on pancreatic lithogenesis in the course of chronic pancreatitis. *Pancreas, 9*, 42–46.

Church, D. F., & Pryor, W. A. (1985). Free-radical chemistry of cigarette smoke and its toxicological implications. *Environmental Health Perspectives, 64*, 111–126.

Cullen, J. J., Mitros, F. A., & Oberley, L. W. (2003). Expression of antioxidant enzymes in diseases of the human pancreas: another link between chronic pancreatitis and pancreatic cancer. *Pancreas, 26*, 23–27.

Davies, K. J. A., Delsignore, M. E., & Lin, S. W. (1987a). Protein damage and degradation by oxygen radicals. II. Modification of amino acids. *The Journal of Biological Chemistry, 262*, 9902–9907.

Davies, K. J. A., Lin, S. W., & Pacifici, R. E. (1987b). Protein damage and degradation by oxygen radicals. IV. Degradation of denatured protein. *The Journal of Biological Chemistry, 262*, 9914–9920.

Dhingra, R., Singh, N., Sachdev, V., Upadhyay, A. D., & Saraya, A. (2013). Effect of antioxidant supplementation on surrogate markers of fibrosis in chronic pancreatitis: a randomized, placebo-controlled trial. *Pancreas, 42*, 589–595.

Di Luzio, N. R. (1966). A mechanism of the acute ethanol-induced fatty liver and the modification of liver injury by antioxidants. *American Journal of Pharmaceutical Sciences Support Public Health, 15*, 50–63.

Di Sebastiano, P., di Mola, F. F., Bockman, D. E., Friess, H., & Büchler, M. W. (2003). Chronic pancreatitis: the perspective of pain generation by neuroimmune interaction. *Gut, 52*, 907–911.

Droge, W. (2002). Free radicals in the physiological control of cell function. *Physiological Reviews, 82*, 47–95.

Dubick, M. A., Palmer, R., Lau, P. P., Morrill, P. R., & Geokas, M. C. (1988). Altered exocrine pancreatic function in rats treated with nicotine. *Toxicology and Applied Pharmacology, 96*, 132–139.

Edge, R., McGarvey, D. J., & Truscott, T. G. (1997). The carotenoids as anti-oxidants—a review. *Journal of Photochemistry and Photobiology B, 41*, 189–200.

Ford, L., Farr, J., Morris, P., & Berg, J. (2006). The value of measuring serum cholesterol-adjusted vitamin E in routine practice. *Annals of Clinical Biochemistry, 43*, 130–134.

Foster, J. R., Idle, J. R., Hardwick, J. P., Bars, R., Scott, P., & Braganza, J. M. (1993). Induction of drug-metabolizing enzymes in human pancreatic cancer and chronic pancreatitis. *Journal of Pathology, 169*, 457–463.

Freeman, B. A., & Crapo, J. D. (1982). Biology of disease: free radicals and tissue injury. *Lab Invest, 47*(5), 412–426.

Frei, B., & Ames, B. N. (1988). Antioxidant defenses and lipid peroxidation in human blood plasma. *Proceedings of the National Academy of Sciences of the United States of America, 85*, 9748–9752.

Frei, B., Stocker, R., England, L., & Ames, B. N. (1990). Ascorbate: the most effective antioxidant in human blood plasma. *Advances in Experimental Medicine and Biology, 264*, 155–163.

Friess, H., Zhu, Z. W., di Mola, F. F., Kulli, C., Graber, H. U., Andren-Sandberg, A., Zimmermann, A., Korc, M., Reinshagen, M., & Büchler, M. W. (1999). Nerve growth factor and its high affinity receptor in chronic pancreatitis. *Annals of Surgery, 230*, 615–624.

Garg, P. K. (2013). Antioxidants for chronic pancreatitis: reasons for disappointing results despite sound principles. *Gastroenterology, 144*, e19–e20.

Gómez-Cambronero, L., Camps, B., de La Asunción, J. G., Cerdá, M., Pellín, A., Pallardó, F. V., Calvete, J., Sweiry, J. H., Mann, G. E., Viña, J., & Sastre, J. (2000). Pentoxifylline ameliorates cerulein-induced pancreatitis in rats: role of glutathione and nitric oxide. *The Journal of Pharmacology and Experimental Therapeutics, 293*, 670–676.

González, A., Schmid, A., Salido, G. M., Camello, P. J., & Pariente, J. A. (2002). XOD-catalyzed ROS generation mobilizes calcium from intracellular stores in mouse pancreatic acinar cells. *Cellular Signalling, 14*, 153–159.

Gooshe, M., Abdolghaffari, A. H., Nikfar, S., Mahdaviani, P., & Abdollahi, M. (2015). Antioxidant therapy in acute, chronic and post-endoscopic retrograde cholangiopancreatography pancreatitis: an updated systematic review and meta-analysis. *World Journal of Gastroenterology, 21*, 9189–9208.

Granot, E., Tamir, I., & Deckelbaum, R. J. (1988). Neutral lipid transfer protein does not regulate alpha-tocopherol transfer between human plasma lipoproteins. *Lipids, 23*, 17–21.

Grigsby, B., Rodriguez-Rilo, H., & Khan, K. (2012). Antioxidants and chronic pancreatitis: theory of oxidative stress and trials of antioxidant therapy. *Digestive Diseases and Sciences, 57*, 835–841.

Guyan, P. M., Uden, S., & Braganza, J. M. (1990). Heightened free radical activity in pancreatitis. *Free Radical Biology and Medicine, 8*, 347–354.

Haber, P. S., Keogh, G. W., Apte, M. V., Moran, C. S., Stewart, N. L., Crawford, D. H., Pirola, R. C., McCaughan, G. W., Ramm, G. A., & Wilson, J. S. (1999). Activation of pancreatic stellate cells in human and experimental pancreatic fibrosis. *The American Journal of Pathology, 155*, 1087–1095.

Halliwell, B., & Gutteridge, J. M. C. (1989). *Free radicals in biology and medicine* (2nd ed.). UK: Oxford.

Imoto, M., & DiMagno, E. P. (2000). Cigarette smoking increases the risk of pancreatic calcification in late-onset but not early-onset idiopathic chronic pancreatitis. *Pancreas, 21*, 115–119.

Jiang, F., Liao, Z., Hu, L. H., Du, Y. Q., Man, X. H., Gu, J. J., Gao, J., Gong, Y. F., & Li, Z. S. (2011). Comparison of antioxidative and antifibrotic effects of α-tocopherol with those of tocotrienol-rich fraction in a rat model of chronic pancreatitis. *Pancreas, 40*, 1091–1096.

Kabe, Y., Ando, K., Hirao, S., Yoshida, M., & Handa, H. (2005). Redox regulation of NF-kappa B activation: distinct redox regulation between the cytoplasm and the nucleus. *Antioxidants and Redox Signaling, 7*, 395–403.

Keith, R. G., Keshavjee, S. H., & Kerenyi, N. R. (1985). Neuropathology of chronic pancreatitis in humans. *Canadian Journal of SurgeryV 28*, 207–211.

Kellener, J. (1981). Nutritional status in chronic pancreatic steatorrhea. In Mitchell, C.J., Kellener, J., (Eds.), *Pancreatic disease in clinical practice* (pp. 257–266). London.

Kirk, G. R., White, J. S., McKie, L., Stevenson, M., Young, I., Clements, W. D., & Rowlands, B. J. (2006). Combined antioxidant therapy reduces pain and improves quality of life in chronic pancreatitis. *Journal of Gastrointestinal Surgery*, *10*, 499–503.

Klonowski-Stumpe, H., Schreiber, R., Grolik, M., Schulz, H. U., Häussinger, D., & Niederau, C. (1997). Effect of oxidative stress on cellular functions and cytosolic free calcium of rat pancreatic acinar cells. *American Journal of Physiology*, *272*, G1489–G1498.

Krinsky, N. I., & Deneke, S. M. (1982). Interaction of oxygen and oxy-radicals with carotenoids. *Journal of the National Cancer Institute*, *69*, 205–210.

Lecomte, E., Herbeth, B., Pirollet, P., Chancerelle, Y., Arnaud, J., Musse, N., Paille, F., Siest, G., & Artur, Y. (1994). Effect of alcohol consumption on blood antioxidant nutrients and oxidative stress indicators. *American Journal of Clinical Nutrition*, *60*, 255–261.

Leist, M., Single, B., & Castoldi, A. F. (1997). Intracellular adenosine triphosphate (ATP) concentration: a switch in the decision between apoptosis and necrosis. *Journal of Experimental Medicine*, *185*, 1481–1486.

Levonen, A. L., Landar, A., Ramachandran, A., Ceaser, E. K., Dickinson, D. A., Zanoni, G., Morrow, J. D., & Darley-Usmar, V. M. (2004). Cellular mechanisms of redox cell signalling: role of cysteine modification in controlling antioxidant defences in response to electrophilic lipid oxidation products. *Biochemical Journal*, *378*, 373–382.

Li, X. C., Lu, X. L., & Chen, H. H. (2011). α-Tocopherol treatment ameliorates chronic pancreatitis in an experimental rat model induced by trinitrobenzene sulfonic acid. *Pancreatology*, *11*, 5–11.

Matsumoto, M., Takahashi, H., Maruyama, K., Higuchi, S., Matsushita, S., Muramatsu, T., Okuyama, K., Yokoyama, A., Nakano, M., & Ishii, H. (1996). Genotypes of alcohol-metabolizing enzymes and the risk for alcoholic chronic pancreatitis in Japanese alcoholics. *Alcoholism, Clinical and Experimental Research*, *20*, 289A–292A.

McNamee, R., Braganza, J. M., Hogg, J., Leck, I., Rose, P., & Cherry, N. M. (1994). Occupational exposure to hydrocarbons and chronic pancreatitis: a case-referent study. *Occupational Environmental Medicine*, *51*, 631–637.

Meydani, S. N., Han, S. N., & Wu, D. (2005). Vitamin E and immune response in the aged: molecular mechanisms and clinical implications. *Immunology Review*, *205*, 269–284.

Miyamoto, T., Dubin, A. E., Petrus, M. J., & Patapoutian, A. (2009). TRPV1 and TRPA1 mediate peripheral nitric oxide-induced nociception in mice. *PLoS One*, *4910*, e7596.

Monteiro, T. H., Silva, C. S., Cordeiro Simões Ambrosio, L. M., Zucoloto, S., & Vannucchi, H. (2012). Vitamin E alters inflammatory gene expression in alcoholic chronic pancreatitis. *Journal of Nutrigenetics and Nutrigenomics*, *5*, 94–105.

Nakamura, T., Takebe, K., Imamura, K., Arai, Y., Kudoh, K., Terada, A., Ishii, M., Yamada, N., Tandoh, Y., Machida, K., & Kikuchi, H. (1995). Changes in plasma fatty acid profile in Japanese patients with chronic pancreatitis. *The Journal of International Medical Research*, *23*, 27–36.

Niederau, C., Schultz, H. U., & Letko, G. (1991). Involvement of free radicals in the pathophysiology of chronic pancreatitis: potential of treatment with antioxidant and scavenger substances. *Klinische Wochenschrift*, *69*, 1018–1024.

Padayatty, S. J., Katz, A., Wang, Y., Eck, P., Kwon, O., Lee, J. H., Chen, S., Corpe, C., Dutta, A., Dutta, S. K., & Levine, M. (2003). Vitamin C as an antioxidant: evaluation of its role in disease prevention. *Journal of the American College of Nutrition*, *22*, 18–35.

Pariente, J. A., Camello, C., Camello, P. J., & Salido, G. M. (2001). Release of calcium from mitochondrial and nonmitochondrial intracellular stores in mouse pancreatic acinar cells by hydrogen peroxide. *The Journal of Membrane biology*, *179*, 27–35.

Pelletier, O. (1970). Vitamin C status of cigarette smokers and non-smokers. *American Journal of Clinical Nutrition*, *23*, 520–524.

Pitchumoni, C. S., & Bordalo, O. (1996). Evaluation of hypotheses on pathogenesis of alcoholic pancreatitis. *Ameraican Journal of Gastroenterology*, *91*, 637–647.

Quilliot, D., Forbes, A., Dubois, F., Gueant, J. L., & Ziegler, O. (2011). Carotenoid deficiency in chronic pancreatitis: the effect of an increase in tomato consumption. *European Journal of Clinical Nutrition*, *65*, 262–268.

Rose, P., Fraine, E., Hunt, L. P., Acheson, W. K., & Braganza, J. M. (1986). Dietary antioxidants and chronic pancreatitis. *Human Nutrition and Clinical Nutrition*, *40*, 151–164.

Sajewicz, W., Milnerowicz, S., & Nabzdyk, S. (2006). Blood plasma antioxidant defense in patients with pancreatitis. *Pancreas*, *32*, 139–144.

Samandari, E., Visarius, T., Zingg, J. M., & Azzi, A. (2006). The effect of gamma-tocopherol on proliferation, integrin expression, adhesion, and migration of human glioma cells. *Biochemical and Biophysical Research Communications*, *342*, 1329–1333.

Segal, I., Gut, A., Schofield, D., Shiel, N., & Braganza, J. M. (1995). Micronutrient antioxidant status in black South Africans with chronic pancreatitis: opportunity for prophylaxis. *Clinica Chimica Acta*, *239*, 71–79.

Shah, N. S., Makin, A. J., Sheen, A. J., & Siriwardena, A. K. (2010). Quality of life assessment in patients with chronic pancreatitis receiving antioxidant therapy. *World Journal of Gastroenterology*, *16*, 4066–4071.

Shaw, S. (1989). Lipid peroxidation, iron mobilization and radical generation induced by alcohol. *Free Radical Biology and Medicine*, *7*, 541–547.

Shiva, S., Moellering, D., Ramachandran, A., Levonen, A. L., Landar, A., Venkatraman, A., Ceaser, E., Ulasova, E., Crawford, J. H., Brookes, P. S., Patel, R. P., & Darley-Usmar, V. M. (2004). Redox signalling: from nitric oxide to oxidized lipids. *Biochemical Society Symposium*, *71*, 107–120.

Singh, U., & Jialal, I. (2004). Anti-inflammatory effects of alpha-tocopherol. **A***nnals of the New York Academy of Sciences*, *031*, 195–203.

Siriwardena, A. K., Mason, J. M., Sheen, A. J., Makin, A. J., & Shah, N. S. (2012). Antioxidant therapy does not reduce pain in patients with chronic pancreatitis: the ANTICIPATE study. *Gastroenterology*, *143*, 655–663.

Smith, F. R., Suskind, R., Thanangkul, O., Leitzmann, C., Goodman, D. S., & Olson, R. E. (1975). Plasma vitamin A, retinol-binding protein and prealbumin concentrations in protein-calorie malnutrition. III. Response to varying dietary treatments. *American Journal of Clinical Nutrition*, *28*, 732–738.

Stipanuk, M. H. (1986). Metabolism of sulfur-containing amino acids. *Annual Review of Nutrition*, *6*, 179–209.

Talamini, G., Bassi, C., Falconi, M., Frulloni, L., Di Francesco, V., Vaona, B., Bovo, P., Rigo, L., Castagnini, A., Angelini, G., Vantini, I., Pederzoli, P., & Cavallini, G. (1996). Cigarette smoking: an independent risk factor in alcoholic pancreatitis. *Pancreas*, *12*, 131–137.

Talukdar, R., Murthy, H. V., & Reddy, D. N. (2015). Role of methionine containing antioxidant combination in the management of pain in chronic pancreatitis: a systematic review and meta-analysis. *Pancreatology*, *15*, 136–144.

Talukdar, R., Lakhtakia, S., Rebala, P., Rao, G. V., & Reddy, D. N. (2016). Antioxidant cocktail and pregabalin combination ameliorates pain recurrence after ductal clearance in chronic pancreatitis: results of a randomized, double blind, placebo-controlled trial. *Journal of Gastroenterology and Hepatology*. [Epub ahead of print].

Tamura, K., Manabe, T., Imanishi, K., Nishikawa, H., Ohshio, G., & Tobe, T. (1992). Toxic effects of oxygen derived free radicals on rat pancreatic acini; an in vitro study. *Hepatogastroenterology*, *39*, 536–539.

Tandon, R. K., & Garg, P. K. (2011). Oxidative stress in chronic pancreatitis: pathophysiological relevance and management. *Antioxidants and Redox Signaling*, *15*, 2757–2766.

Tandon, R. K., Sato, N., & Garg, P. K. (2002). Chronic pancreatitis: Asia-Pacific consensus report. *Journal of Gastroenterology and Hepatology*, *17*, 508–518.

Toth, K. M., Clifford, D. P., Berger, E. M., White, C. W., & Repine, J. E. (1984). Intact human erythrocytes prevent hydrogen peroxide-mediated damage to isolated perfused rat lungs and cultured bovine pulmonary endothelial cells. *Journal of Clinical Investigation, 74*, 292–295.

Trevisani, M., Siemens, S., Bautista, D. M., Nassini, R., Campi, B., Imamachi, N., Andrè, E., Patacchini, R., Cottrell, G. S., Gatti, R., Basbaum, A. I., Bunnett, N. W., Julius, D., & Geppetti, P. (2007). 4-Hydroxynonenal, an endogenous aldehyde, causes pain and neurogenic inflammation through activation of the irritant receptor TRPA1. *Proceedings of the National Academy of Sciences of the United States of America, 104*, 13519–13524.

Uden, S., Acheson, D. W., Reeves, J., Worthington, H. V., Hunt, L. P., Brown, S., & Braganza, J. M. (1988). Antioxidants, enzyme induction, and chronic pancreatitis: a reappraisal following studies in patients on anticonvulsants. *European Journal of Clinical Nutrition, 42*, 561–569.

Uden, S., Schofield, D., Miller, P. F., Day, J. P., Bottiglier, T., & Braganza, J. M. (1992). Antioxidant therapy for recurrent pancreatitis: biochemical profiles in a placebo-controlled trial. *Aliment Pharmacology and Therapeutics, 6*, 229–240.

van Asbeck, B. S., Hoidal, J., Vercelotti, G. M., Schwartz, B. A., Moldow, C. F., & Jacob, H. S. (1985). Protection against lethal hyperoxia by tracheal insufflation of erythrocytes: role of red cell glutathione. *Science, 227*, 756–759.

van Gossum, A., Closset, P., Noel, E., Cremer, M., & Neve, J. (1996). Deficiency in antioxidant factors in patients with alcohol related chronic pancreatitis. *Digestive Disease and Sciences, 41*, 1225–1231.

Vaona, B., Armellini, F., Bovo, P., Rigo, L., Zamboni, M., Brunori, M. P., Dall'O, E., Filippini, M., Talamini, G., Di Francesco, V., Frulloni, L., Micciolo, R., & Cavallini, G. (1997). Food intake of patients with chronic pancreatitis after onset of the disease. *American Jounal of Clinical Nutrition, 65*, 851–854.

Vaona, B., Stanzial, A. M., Talamini, P., Bovo, P., Corrocher, R., & Cavallini, G. (2005). Serum selenium concentrations in chronic pancreatitis and controls. *Digestive and Liver Disease, 37*, 522–525.

Vaquero, E., Gukovsk, I., Zaninovic, V., Gukovskaya, A. S., & Pandol, S. J. (2001). Localized pancreatic NF-kappaB activation and inflammatory response in taurocholate-induced pancreatitis. *American Journal of Physiology Gastrointestinal and Liver Physiology, 280*, G1197–G1208.

Viggiano, A., Monda, M., Viggiano, A., Viggiano, D., Viggiano, E., Chiefari, M., Aurilio, C., & De Luca, B. (2005). Trigeminal pain transmission requires reactive oxygen species production. *Brain Research, 1050*, 72–78.

Wannamethee, S. G., Lowe, G. D., Rumley, A., Bruckdorfer, K. R., & Whincup, P. H. (2006). Associations of vitamin C status, fruit and vegetable intakes, and markers of inflammation and hemostasis. *American Journal of Clinical Nutrition, 83*, 567–574.

Xu, G. Y., Winston, J. H., Shenoy, M., Yin, H., Pendyala, S., & Pasricha, P. J. (2007). Transient receptor potential vanilloid 1 mediates hyperalgesia and is up-regulated in rats with chronic pancreatitis. *Gastroenterology, 133*, 1282–1292.

Yen, S., Hsieh, C. C., & MacMahon, B. (1982). Consumption of alcohol and tobacco and other risk factors for pancreatitis. *American Journal of Epidemiology, 116*, 407–414.

Yu, J. H., & Kim, H. (2014). Oxidative stress and inflammatory signaling in cerulein pancreatitis. *World Journal of Gastroenterology, 20*, 17324–17329.

Yu, J. H., Lim, J. W., Namkung, W., Kim, H., & Kim, K. H. (2002). Suppression of cerulein-induced cytokine expression by antioxidants in pancreatic acinar cells. *Laboratory Investigation, 82*, 1359–1368.

Zhou, D., Wang, W., Cheng, X., Wei, J., & Zheng, S. (2015). Antioxidant therapy for patients with chronic pancreatitis: a systematic review and meta-analysis. *Clinical Nutrition, 34*, 627–634.

Zhu, Y., Colak, T., Shenoy, M., Liu, L., Mehta, K., Pai, R., Zou, B., Xie, X. S., & Pasricha, P. J. (2012). Transforming growth factor beta induces sensory neuronal hyperexcitability, and contributes to pancreatic pain and hyperalgesia in rats with chronic pancreatitis. *Molecular Pain, 8*, 65.

Zhu, Y., Colak, T., Shenoy, M., Liu, L., Pai, R., Li, C., Mehta, K., & Pasricha, P. J. (2011). Nerve growth factor modulates TRPV1 expression and function and mediates pain in chronic pancreatitis. *Gastroenterology, 141*, 370–377.

CHAPTER

24

Vitamin D and Disc Herniation Associated Pain

M. *Sedighi*

Shiraz Medical School, Shiraz University of Medical Sciences (Shiraz Branch), Shiraz, Iran

The history of human affliction with back pain dates back to the era of Hippocrates. It is one of the most common conditions with a lifetime prevalence that ranges between 49% and 80% (Maniadakis & Gray, 2000). It is considered a socio-economic problem, since it has many costs in the form of medical and surgical or loss of productivity time and affecting quality of life of patients. Among various causes for low back pain, lumbar disc herniation (LDH) is the most common cause (Hansson & Hansson, 2007). The risk factors attributed to the development of LDH are genetics, gender, smoking, and repetitive vibrations. Not all cases with disc herniation on imaging studies report discogenic pain, as evidenced from reports that show a rate of 20–70% of asymptomatic cases with disc herniation detected by Magnetic resonance imaging (MRI). Symptoms of LDH may include back pain, lower extremity radicular pain, and lower extremity sensory complaints, such as numbness, tingling, foot weakness, or cauda equine syndrome. Diagnosis is made based on history, physical examination, and imaging studies. Taking into account the cost of surgery and its intraoperative and immediate and late complications, surgery is indicated for cauda equina syndrome, morphine-resistant hyperalgesic sciatica, paralyzing sciatica, and residual disabling pain despite 6–8 weeks of receiving full medical treatment (Blamoutier, 2013). Other than those who require surgical decompression, the first step in the management of cases with symptomatic lumbar disc herniation, is medical treatment that includes short-term bed rest, physiotherapy, and different kinds of medication from various drug classes, such as analgesics, corticosteroids, antiepileptics, antidepressants and muscle relaxants, and epidural injections (Green, 1975; Legrand, Bouvard, Audran, Fournier, & Valat, 2007; Levin, 2007; Pinto et al., 2012; Smeal, Tyburski, Alleva, Prather, & Hunt, 2004; Stafford, Peng, & Hill, 2007; Valat, Genevay, Marty, Rozenberg, & Koes, 2010). Almost 90% of sciatica attacks respond to conservative treatment. One of the major targets to alleviate disc herniation related pain is the inflammation factor. Nucleous polposus initiates an inflammatory response in the nerve roots, dorsal root ganglia, and surrounding muscles either through its innate immunogenic properties or induction of inflammation. This inflammatory reaction involves immune cell activation and infiltration with subsequent production of various inflammatory cytokines and pain modulators (Anzai, Hamba, Onda, Konno, & Kikuchi, 2002; Burke, Watson, McCormack, Dowling, Walsh, & Fitzpatrick, 2002a, 2002b; Cuellar, Montesano, & Carstens, 2004; Doita, Kanatani, Harada, & Mizuno, 1996; Grönblad et al., 1994; Kobayashi, Yoshizawa, & Yamada, 2004; Mulleman, Mammou, Griffoul, Watier, & Goupille, 2006; Murai et al., 2010; Ohtori et al., 2013; Olmarker et al., 1995; Olmarker & Larsson, 1998; Olmarker & Rydevik, 2001; Omoigui, 2007; Onda, Hamba, Yabuki, & Kikuchi, 2002; Park, Chang, & Kim, 2002; Rand, Reichert, Floman, & Rotshenker, 1997; Rothman, Huang, Lee, Weisshaar, & Winkelstein, 2009; Saal, 1995; Shamji et al., 2010; Specchia, Pagnotta, Toesca, & Greco, 2002; Takahashi et al., 1996; Xu, Xin, Zang, Wu, & Liu, 2006; Yoshida et al., 2005). A brief role description of cytokines and pain mediators involved in disc herniation is discussed here:

1. Interferon-gamma (INF-γ) is a proinflammatory cytokine with neurotoxic properties that is produced from Th1 lymphocytes. Its serum level has been correlated with intensity of low back pain (Mulleman et al., 2006; Olmarker et al., 1995; Olmarker & Larsson, 1998).
2. Interleukin-1 (IL-1) a proinflammatory cytokine that upregulates leukocyte migration. It may also play

Nutritional Modulators of Pain in the Aging Population. http://dx.doi.org/10.1016/B978-0-12-805186-3.00024-2
Copyright © 2017 Elsevier Inc. All rights reserved.

a role in producing discogenic pain. IL-1 stimulates production of matrix metalloproteinases, nitric oxide (NO), Cyclooxygenase-2 (COX-2), and prostaglandin E2 (PGE2) (Ahn et al., 2002; Goupille, Jayson, Valat, & Freemont, 1998; Le Maitre, Hoyland, & Freemont, 2007).

a. IL-6 has effects on mediating inflammation and modulating pain (Gadient & Otten, 1997; Kang et al., 1996; Shamash, Reichert, & Rotshenker, 2002; Shamji et al., 2010; Specchia et al., 2002).

b. IL-8 has chemotactic and activation properties for neutrophils and T-cells. Furthermore, it has been shown that IL-8 has effects on angiogenesis. Furthermore, its association with radicular pain has been investigated (Ahn et al., 2002; Burke et al., 2002b).

c. IL-10 downregulates the synthesis of many inflammatory cytokines, namely it suppresses macrophage activity in releasing TNF-α. It also reduces the genesis of interleukin-1 beta and inducible nitric oxide synthetase. IL-10 has also been shown to play a role in attenuation of hyperalgesia (Chen, Shen, Zhang, & Zhang, 2015).

d. IL-12 activates T lymphocytes into differentiating to Th1 and also stimulates Th1 lymphocytes to produce INFγ. This activation pattern could be suggestive of Th1 cells activation in disc herniation (Shamji et al., 2010).

e. IL-17 is a cytokine with pro-inflammatory properties that can potentiate the inflammation cascade by activating cells and increasing the synthesis of NO, PGE2, COX-2, and IL-6, therefore influences pain as well (Shamji et al., 2010).

f. Monocyte chemoattractant protein (MCP) is a chemokine that belongs to beta chemokine family. It has chemotactic and activation properties for macrophage. Production of MCP is induced by IL-1 beta and tumor necrosis factor alpha (TNF-α) (Kikuchi, Nakamura, Ikeda, Ogata, & Takagi, 1998; Yoshida et al., 2005).

g. Matrix metalloproteinase (MMP) is an enzyme that degrades proteoglycan and collagen. MMP production is stimulated by Tumor Necrosis Factor (TNF and IL-1. TNF is a proinflammatory cytokine that contributes to the development of discogenic pain. Anti-TNF drugs have been tested to alleviate sciatica and discogenic pain. Likewise, IL-1 has effects on producing discogenic pain. Furthermore, it degrades disc proteoglycans (Bachmeier et al., 2009; Benoist, 2002).

h. Nitric oxide (NO) has inflammatory mediatory properties and is released by macrophages. NO is induced by release of Tumor Necrosis factor-α (TNF-α). It plays different roles either through production of free oxygen radicals that is implicated in disc degeneration, or its role in the pain produced in nerve roots. It alters cellular metabolism and inhibits proteoglycan synthesis. Inhibition of nitric oxidase synthetase has been shown to decrease the swelling caused by herniated nucleous polposus in spinal nerve roots (Anderson & Tannoury, 2005; Brisby et al., 2000; Kawakami, Tamaki, Hayashi, Hashizume, & Nishi, 1998; Watkins & Maier, 2002).

i. Glutamate is produced from aggrecan protein degradation that is released from joints undergoing degeneration. Free glutamate with its receptors located on dorsal root ganglia could be a pain mediator. Glutamate release is induced when Prostaglandin is released in large amounts (Harrington, Messier, Bereiter, Barnes, & Epstein, 2000; Harrington et al., 2005).

j. Prostaglandin (PG) is an inflammatory mediator that appears to be important in genesis and maintenance of neuropathic pain. It is induced by IL-1. PG decrease firing thresholds of sensory neurons. Phospholipase A2 which is the catalytic enzyme in genesis of PG has been identified in herniated disc materials (Benoist, 2002; Kang et al., 1996).

k. Substance P is a neurotransmitter that besides its function in transmitting pain, it also acts with other inflammatory cytokines, such as TNF-α to recruit and activate immune cells (Peng et al., 2005; Sameshima, 1995).

l. Transforming Growth Factor-beta (TGF-beta) is a cytokine that has anti-inflammatory properties. Interferon-gamma (INF-γ), IL-1, IL-2 ad TNF-α activity is suppressed by TGF-beta 1. In herniated disc, extracellular proteolysis is stimulated by this cytokine (Tolonen et al., 2001).

Vitamin D roles have gone beyond its classic role in bone health. We have taken a long journey to reach an understanding on how it affects many nonskeletal diseases. Focusing on nervous system, it has been considered a neurosteorid with its neuroprotective roles mediating its actions through detoxification pathways. Zooming in more, receptors for vitamin D are present in spinal cord, nerve roots, dorsal root ganglia, and glial cells. With further focus on intervertebral discs, vitamin D receptor gene polymorphism has been linked with development of disc degeneration and herniation. As mentioned before, once nucleus polpusus herniates , it initiates a chemical reaction in form of producing cytokine, neurotransmitter and pain mediators in its surrounding structures. Vitamin D, with its immunoregulatory properties, could modulate many of the involved substances in the cascade of inflammation, either by downregulating pro-inflammatory cytokines or upregulating antiinflammtory cytokines (Sedighi & Haghnegahdar, 2014). Below is a brief review of how vitamin D exerts its immunologic properties on these substances:

1. INF-γ, IL-1, IL-4, IL-6, IL-12, and IL-17 expression are downregulated by vitamin D (Kalueff et al., 2006; Nagpal, Na, & Rathnachalam, 2005).
2. Expression of immunosuppressive cytokines IL-4 and IL-10 is upregulated by vitamin D (Baeke, Takiishi, Korf, Gysemans, & Mathieu, 2010; Garcion, Wion-Barbot, Montero-Menei, Berger, & Wion, 2002; Guillot, Semerano, Saidenberg-Kermanac'h, Falgarone, & Boissier, 2010; McKelvey, Shorten, & O'Keeffe, 2013; Szodoray et al., 2008).
3. NO synthase is inhibited by vitamin D (Deluca & Cantorna, 2001; Marchand, Perretti, & McMahon, 2005).
4. PG genesis is inhibited by vitamin D through vitamin D actions on inhibiting COX-2 or inducing its degrading enzyme (15-prostaglandin dehydrogenase). Furthermore, vitamin D directs actions on PG by inhibition of PGE2 receptors (Feldman et al., 2007).
5. MCP and MMP genesis is inhibited by vitamin D (Gruber et al., 2008; Maeda, Dean, Sylvia, Boyan, & Schwartz, 2001).
6. Glutamate production is inhibited by vitamin D (Ibi et al., 2001; Taniura et al., 2006).
7. Substance P is inhibited by vitamin D (Moalem & Tracey, 2006).
8. TGF-beta- an anti-inflammatory cytokine-expression is upregulated by vitamin D (Garcion et al., 2002).

Increased expression of IL-4, IL-6, IL-12, and IFN-γ guides us toward the shift in T helper-1 activity that occurs during disc herniation (Burke et al., 2002b; Kang et al., 1996; Murai et al., 2010; Park et al., 2002; Shamji et al., 2010). Interestingly, Vitamin D decreases the number and the function of T helper-1 (Cantorna & Mahon, 2004; Guillot et al., 2010; Lemire & Archer, 1991; Szodoray et al., 2008; Turner et al., 2008). Besides the immunomodulatory effects of vitamin D on pain mediators, this neurosteroid hormone acts on pain processes, such as pain modulation in sensory neurons, neuron excitability, pain perception, and pain sensitivity (Bazzani, Arletti, & Bertolini, 1984; Fernandes de Abreu, Eyles, & Feron, 2009; Garcion et al., 2002; Moalem & Tracey, 2006; Stumpf, Clark, O'Brien, & Reid, 1988; Stumpf & O'Brien, 1987; von Kanel, Muller-Hartmannsgruber, Kokinogenis, & Egloff, 2014).

Muscles are the other structures that could act as pain producers in disc herniation. The changes that occur in the paraspinal muscles in patients with lumbar disc herniation, are thought to be caused partly by denervation. Denervation will subsequently result in muscular atrophy, changes in muscle fibers and intracellular fat infiltration on histochemical basis. Although other histochemical changes in the paraspinal muscles could be attributed to ischemia and the effect of pain that alters the use of back muscles. Muscles are affected by the release of inflammatory cytokines since motor nerves that innervate muscles are activated by these mediators and this activation produces muscular pain, tension, and spasm. Tension and spasm of muscles will result in genesis of more pain. On the other hand, tension and muscular spams will cause inactivity and disuse. Also the herniated or degenerated disc would change the paraspinal muscles in a biodynamic way as well. Breaking the vicious cycle of pain and altered muscular function is desirable. Functional or imaging studies could demonstrate the changes in the paraspinal muscles after disc herniation (Epker & Block, 2001; Franke et al., 2009; Hodges, Holm, Hansson, & Holm, 2006; Hyun, Lee, Lee, & Jeon, 2007; Kader, Wardlaw, & Smith, 2000; Yoshihara, Shirai, Nakayama, & Uesaka, 2001; Zhao, Kawaguchi, Matsui, Kanamori, & Kimura, 2000; Zhu, Parnianpour, Nordin, & Kahanovitz, 1989). On histochemical basis, changes that are seen in the muscles of patients with vitamin D deficiency demonstrate resemblance to those seen in muscles affected by disc herniation, such as atrophy of type 2 muscle fibers (Boland, 1986; Ceglia, 2008), and enlarged interfibrillar spaces, and fat infiltration and glycogen granules (Anglin, Samaan, Walter, & McDonald, 2013; Ceglia, 2008; Tagliafico et al., 2010). Receptors of vitamin D have been identified on different tissues including muscles. Vitamin D improves muscle function (Bischoff et al., 2001; Simpson, Thomas, & Arnold, 1985), muscle growth and proliferation (Buitrago, Boland, & de Boland, 2001; Buitrago, Pardo, de Boland, & Boland, 2003; Buitrago, Gonzalez Pardo, & de Boland, 2002) and also considering its anti-inflammatory properties, it could be beneficial for muscles that are affected by inflammation and pain.

Finally, the interrelation between pain, mood, and vitamin D, in patients with disc herniation is of interest. There are links between experience and perception of increased pain and depressed mood. Since depressed cases with disc herniation have lower pain threshold and greater functional impairment (Epker & Block, 2001), vitamin D could not only affect pain threshold as outlined earlier, but could also be efficient in improving depression (Anglin et al., 2013).

DEDICATION

This chapter is dedicated to my mom, for her endless love, patience, and support.

References

Ahn, S. H., Cho, Y. W., Ahn, M. W., Jang, S. H., Sohn, Y. K., & Kim, H. S. (2002). mRNA expression of cytokines and chemokines in herniated lumbar intervertebral discs. *Spine*, *27*(9), 911–917.

Anderson, D. G., & Tannoury, C. (2005). Molecular pathogenic factors in symptomatic disc degeneration. *Spine Journal, 5*(6 Suppl), 260S–266S.

Anglin, R. E., Samaan, Z., Walter, S. D., & McDonald, S. D. (2013). Vitamin D deficiency and depression in adults: systematic review and meta-analysis. *The British Journal of Psychiatry, 202*, 100–107.

Anzai, H., Hamba, M., Onda, A., Konno, S., & Kikuchi, S. (2002). Epidural application of nucleus pulposus enhances nociresponses of rat dorsal horn neurons. *Spine, 27*(3), E50–E55.

Bachmeier, B. E., Nerlich, A., Mittermaier, N., Weiler, C., Lumenta, C., Wuertz, K., & Boos, N. (2009). Matrix metalloproteinase expression levels suggest distinct enzyme roles during lumbar disc herniation and degeneration. *European Spine Journal, 18*(11), 1573–1586.

Baeke, F., Takiishi, T., Korf, H., Gysemans, C., & Mathieu, C. (2010). Vitamin D: modulator of the immune system. *Current Opinion in Pharmacology, 10*(4), 482–496.

Bazzani, C., Arletti, R., & Bertolini, A. (1984). Pain threshold and morphine activity in vitamin D-deficient rats. *Life Science, 34*(5), 461–466.

Benoist, M. (2002). The natural history of lumbar disc herniation and radiculopathy. *Joint Bone Spine, 69*(2), 155–160.

Bischoff, H. A., Borchers, M., Gudat, F., Duermueller, U., Theiler, R., Stahelin, H. B., & Dick, W. (2001). In situ detection of 1,25-dihydroxyvitamin D3 receptor in human skeletal muscle tissue. *Histochemistry Journal, 33*(1), 19–24.

Blamoutier, A. (2013). Surgical discectomy for lumbar disc herniation: surgical techniques. *Orthop Traumatol Surg Res, 99*(Suppl. 1), S187–S196.

Boland, R. (1986). Role of vitamin D in skeletal muscle function. *Endocrine Reviews, 7*(4), 434–448.

Brisby, H., Byrod, G., Olmarker, K., Miller, V. M., Aoki, Y., & Rydevik, B. (2000). Nitric oxide as a mediator of nucleus pulposus-induced effects on spinal nerve roots. *Journal of Orthopaedic Research, 18*(5), 815–820.

Buitrago, C., Boland, R., & de Boland, A. R. (2001). The tyrosine kinase c-Src is required for 1,25$(OH)_2$-vitamin D3 signalling to the nucleus in muscle cells. *Biochimica et Biophysica Acta, 1541*(3), 179–187.

Buitrago, C., Gonzalez Pardo, V., & de Boland, A. R. (2002). Nongenomic action of 1 alpha,25(OH)(2)-vitamin D3. Activation of muscle cell PLC gamma through the tyrosine kinase c-Src and PtdIns 3-kinase. *European Journal of Biochemistry, 269*(10), 2506–2515.

Buitrago, C. G., Pardo, V. G., de Boland, A. R., & Boland, R. (2003). Activation of RAF-1 through Ras and protein kinase Calpha mediates 1alpha,25(OH)2-vitamin D3 regulation of the mitogen-activated protein kinase pathway in muscle cells. *Journal of Biological Chemistry, 278*(4), 2199–2205.

Burke, J. G., Watson, R. W., McCormack, D., Dowling, F. E., Walsh, M. G., & Fitzpatrick, J. M. (2002a). Intervertebral discs which cause low back pain secrete high levels of proinflammatory mediators. *The Journal of Bone and Joint Surgery, 84*(2), 196–201.

Burke, J. G., Watson, R. W., McCormack, D., Dowling, F. E., Walsh, M. G., & Fitzpatrick, J. M. (2002b). Spontaneous production of monocyte chemoattractant protein-1 and interleukin-8 by the human lumbar intervertebral disc. *Spine, 27*(13), 1402–1407.

Cantorna, M. T., & Mahon, B. D. (2004). Mounting evidence for vitamin D as an environmental factor affecting autoimmune disease prevalence. *Experimental Biology and Medicine, 229*(11), 1136–1142.

Ceglia, L. (2008). Vitamin D and skeletal muscle tissue and function. *Molecular Aspects of Medicine, 29*(6), 407–414.

Chen, Yu-Ming, Shen, Ruo-Wu, Zhang, Bei, & Zhang, Wei-Ning (2015). Regional tissue immune responses after sciatic nerve injury in rats. *International Journal of Clinical and Experimental Medicine, 8*(8), 13408.

Cuellar, J. M., Montesano, P. X., & Carstens, E. (2004). Role of TNF-alpha in sensitization of nociceptive dorsal horn neurons induced by application of nucleus pulposus to L5 dorsal root ganglion in rats. *Pain, 110*(3), 578–587.

Deluca, H. F., & Cantorna, M. T. (2001). Vitamin D: its role and uses in immunology. *FASEB Journal, 15*(14), 2579–2585.

Doita, M., Kanatani, T., Harada, T., & Mizuno, K. (1996). Immunohistologic study of the ruptured intervertebral disc of the lumbar spine. *Spine, 21*(2), 235–241.

Epker, J., & Block, A. R. (2001). Presurgical psychological screening in back pain patients: a review. *Clinical Journal of Pain, 17*(3), 200–205.

Feldman, D., Krishnan, A., Moreno, J., Swami, S., Peehl, D. M., & Srinivas, S. (2007). Vitamin D inhibition of the prostaglandin pathway as therapy for prostate cancer. *Nutrition Reviews, 65*(8 Pt 2), S113–S115.

Fernandes de Abreu, D. A., Eyles, D., & Feron, F. (2009). Vitamin D, a neuro-immunomodulator: implications for neurodegenerative and autoimmune diseases. *Psychoneuroendocrinology, 34*(Suppl. 1), S265–S277.

Franke, J., Hesse, T., Tournier, C., Schuberth, W., Mawrin, C., LeHuec, J. C., & Grasshoff, H. (2009). Morphological changes of the multifidus muscle in patients with symptomatic lumbar disc herniation. *Journal Neurosurgery Spine, 11*(6), 710–714.

Gadient, R. A., & Otten, U. H. (1997). Interleukin-6 (IL-6)—a molecule with both beneficial and destructive potentials. *Progress in Neurobiology, 52*(5), 379–390.

Garcion, E., Wion-Barbot, N., Montero-Menei, C. N., Berger, F., & Wion, D. (2002). New clues about vitamin D functions in the nervous system. *Trends in Endocrinology and Metabolism, 13*(3), 100–105.

Goupille, P., Jayson, M. I., Valat, J. P., & Freemont, A. J. (1998). The role of inflammation in disk herniation-associated radiculopathy. *Seminars in Arthritis and Rheumatism, 28*(1), 60–71.

Green, L. N. (1975). Dexamethasone in the management of symptoms due to herniated lumbar disc. *Journal of Neurology, Neurosurgery and Psychiatry, 38*(12), 1211–1217.

Grönblad, M., Virri, J., Tolonen, J., Seitsalo, S., Kääpä, E., Kankare, J., ... Karaharju, E. O., (1994). A controlled immunohistochemical study of inflammatory cells in disc herniation tissue. Spine, 19(24), 2744–2751

Gruber, H. E., Hoelscher, G., Ingram, J. A., Chow, Y., Loeffler, B., & Hanley, E. N., Jr. (2008). 1,25$(OH)_2$-vitamin D3 inhibits proliferation and decreases production of monocyte chemoattractant protein-1, thrombopoietin, VEGF, and angiogenin by human annulus cells in vitro. *Spine, 33*(7), 755–765.

Guillot, X., Semerano, L., Saidenberg-Kermanac'h, N., Falgarone, G., & Boissier, M. C. (2010). Vitamin D and inflammation. *Joint Bone Spine, 77*(6), 552–557.

Hansson, E., & Hansson, T. (2007). The cost-utility of lumbar disc herniation surgery. *Eur Spine J, 16*(3), 329–337.

Harrington, J. F., Messier, A. A., Bereiter, D., Barnes, B., & Epstein, M. H. (2000). Herniated lumbar disc material as a source of free glutamate available to affect pain signals through the dorsal root ganglion. *Spine, 25*(8), 929–936.

Harrington, J. F., Messier, A. A., Hoffman, L., Yu, E., Dykhuizen, M., & Barker, K. (2005). Physiological and behavioral evidence for focal nociception induced by epidural glutamate infusion in rats. *Spine, 30*(6), 606–612.

Hodges, P., Holm, A. K., Hansson, T., & Holm, S. (2006). Rapid atrophy of the lumbar multifidus follows experimental disc or nerve root injury. *Spine, 31*(25), 2926–2933.

Hyun, J. K., Lee, J. Y., Lee, S. J., & Jeon, J. Y. (2007). Asymmetric atrophy of multifidus muscle in patients with unilateral lumbosacral radiculopathy. *Spine, 32*(21), E598–E602.

Ibi, M., Sawada, H., Nakanishi, M., Kume, T., Katsuki, Hiroshi, Kaneko, S., ... Akaike, A. (2001). Protective effects of 1α, 25-(OH) 2 D 3 against the neurotoxicity of glutamate and reactive oxygen species in mesencephalic culture. *Neuropharmacology*, 40(6), 761–771.

Kader, D. F., Wardlaw, D., & Smith, F. W. (2000). Correlation between the MRI changes in the lumbar multifidus muscles and leg pain. *Clinical Radiology, 55*(2), 145–149.

Kalueff, A. V., Minasyan, A., Keisala, T., Kuuslahti, M., Miettinen, S., & Tuohimaa, P. (2006). The vitamin D neuroendocrine system as a target for novel neurotropic drugs. *CNS and Neurological Disorders Drug Targets*, *5*(3), 363–371.

Kang, J. D., Georgescu, H. I., McIntyre-Larkin, L., Stefanovic-Racic, M., Donaldson, W. F., 3rd, & Evans, C. H. (1996). Herniated lumbar intervertebral discs spontaneously produce matrix metalloproteinases, nitric oxide, interleukin-6, and prostaglandin E2. *Spine*, *21*(3), 271–277.

Kawakami, M., Tamaki, T., Hayashi, N., Hashizume, H., & Nishi, H. (1998). Possible mechanism of painful radiculopathy in lumbar disc herniation. *Clinical Orthopaedics and Related Research*, *351*, 241–251.

Kikuchi, T., Nakamura, T., Ikeda, T., Ogata, H., & Takagi, K. (1998). Monocyte chemoattractant protein-1 in the intervertebral disc. A histologic experimental model. *Spine*, *23*(10), 1091–1099.

Kobayashi, Shigeru, Yoshizawa, Hidezo, & Yamada, Shuuichi (2004). Pathology of lumbar nerve root compression Part 1: intraradicular inflammatory changes induced by mechanical compression. *Journal of Orthopaedic Research*, *22*(1), 170–179.

Le Maitre, C. L., Hoyland, J. A., & Freemont, A. J. (2007). Catabolic cytokine expression in degenerate and herniated human intervertebral discs: IL-1beta and TNFalpha expression profile. *Arthritis Research and Therapy*, *9*(4), R77.

Legrand, E., Bouvard, B., Audran, M., Fournier, D., & Valat, J. P. (2007). Sciatica from disk herniation: medical treatment or surgery? *Joint Bone Spine*, *74*(6), 530–535.

Lemire, J. M., & Archer, D. C. (1991). 1,25-dihydroxyvitamin D3 prevents the in vivo induction of murine experimental autoimmune encephalomyelitis. *Journal of Clinical Investigation*, *87*(3), 1103–1107.

Levin, K. H. (2007). Nonsurgical interventions for spine pain. *Neurologic Clinics*, *25*(2), 495–505.

Maeda, S., Dean, D. D., Sylvia, V. L., Boyan, B. D., & Schwartz, Z. (2001). Metalloproteinase activity in growth plate chondrocyte cultures is regulated by 1,25-(OH)(2)D(3) and 24,25-(OH)(2)D(3) and mediated through protein kinase C. *Matrix Biology*, *20*(2), 87–97.

Maniadakis, N., & Gray, A. (2000). The economic burden of back pain in the UK. *Pain*, *84*(1), 95–103.

Marchand, F., Perretti, M., & McMahon, S. B. (2005). Role of the immune system in chronic pain. *Nature Reviews Neuroscience*, *6*(7), 521–532.

McKelvey, Laura, Shorten, George D., & O'Keeffe, Gerard W. (2013). Nerve growth factor-mediated regulation of pain signalling and proposed new intervention strategies in clinical pain management. *Journal of Neurochemistry*, *124*(3), .

Moalem, G., & Tracey, D. J. (2006). Immune and inflammatory mechanisms in neuropathic pain. *Brain Research Reviews*, *51*(2), 240–264.

Mulleman, D., Mammou, S., Griffoul, I., Watier, H., & Goupille, P. (2006). Pathophysiology of disk-related sciatica. I.—Evidence supporting a chemical component. *Joint Bone Spine*, *73*(2), 151–158.

Murai, K., Sakai, D., Nakamura, Y., Nakai, T., Igarashi, T., Seo, N., ... Mochida, J. (2010). Primary immune system responders to nucleus pulposus cells: evidence for immune response in disc herniation. *European Cells and Materials*, 19, 13–21.

Nagpal, S., Na, S., & Rathnachalam, R. (2005). Noncalcemic actions of vitamin D receptor ligands. *Endocrine Reviews*, *26*(5), 662–687.

Ohtori, S., Inoue, G., Eguchi, Y., Orita, S., Takaso, M., Ochiai, N., ... Takahashi, K. (2013). Tumor necrosis factor-alpha-immunoreactive cells in nucleus pulposus in adolescent patients with lumbar disc herniation. *Spine*, 38(6), 459–462.

Olmarker, K., & Larsson, K. (1998). Tumor necrosis factor alpha and nucleus-pulposus-induced nerve root injury. *Spine*, *23*(23), 2538–2544.

Olmarker, K., & Rydevik, B. (2001). Selective inhibition of tumor necrosis factor-alpha prevents nucleus pulposus-induced thrombus formation, intraneural edema, and reduction of nerve conduction velocity: possible implications for future pharmacologic treatment strategies of sciatica. *Spine*, *26*(8), 863–869.

Olmarker, K., Blomquist, J., Stromberg, J., Nannmark, U., Thomsen, P., & Rydevik, B. (1995). Inflammatogenic properties of nucleus pulposus. *Spine*, *20*(6), 665–669.

Omoigui, S. (2007). The biochemical origin of pain: the origin of all pain is inflammation and the inflammatory response. Part 2 of 3—inflammatory profile of pain syndromes. *Med Hypotheses*, *69*(6), 1169–1178.

Onda, A., Hamba, M., Yabuki, S., & Kikuchi, S. (2002). Exogenous tumor necrosis factor-alpha induces abnormal discharges in rat dorsal horn neurons. *Spine*, *27*(15), 1618–1624discussion 1624.

Park, J. B., Chang, H., & Kim, Y. S. (2002). The pattern of interleukin-12 and T-helper types 1 and 2 cytokine expression in herniated lumbar disc tissue. *Spine*, *27*(19), 2125–2128.

Peng, B., Wu, W., Hou, S., Li, P., Zhang, C., & Yang, Y. (2005). The pathogenesis of discogenic low back pain. *Journal of Bone and Joint Surg. British Volume*, *87*(1), 62–67.

Pinto, R. Z., Maher, C. G., Ferreira, M. L., Ferreira, P. H., Hancock, M., Oliveira, V. C., ... Koes, B. (2012). Drugs for relief of pain in patients with sciatica: systematic review and meta-analysis. *British Medical Journal*, 344, e497.

Rand, N., Reichert, F., Floman, Y., & Rotshenker, S. (1997). Murine nucleus pulposus-derived cells secrete interleukins-1-beta, -6, and -10 and granulocyte-macrophage colony-stimulating factor in cell culture. *Spine*, *22*(22), 2598–2601discussion 2602.

Rothman, S. M., Huang, Z., Lee, K. E., Weisshaar, C. L., & Winkelstein, B. A. (2009). Cytokine mRNA expression in painful radiculopathy. *Journal of Pain*, *10*(1), 90–99.

Saal, J. S. (1995). The role of inflammation in lumbar pain. *Spine*, *20*(16), 1821–1827.

Sameshima, K. (1995). Substance P-like immunoreactivity in cerebrospinal fluid in lumbar disc herniation. *Nihon Seikeigeka Gakkai Zasshi*, *69*(4), 191–197.

Sedighi, M., & Haghnegahdar, A. (2014). Role of vitamin D3 in treatment of lumbar disc herniation--pain and sensory aspects: study protocol for a randomized controlled trial. *Trials*, *15*, 373.

Shamash, Shlomit, Reichert, Fanny, & Rotshenker, Shlomo (2002). The cytokine network of Wallerian degeneration: tumor necrosis factor-α, interleukin-1α, and interleukin-1β. *The Journal of Neuroscience*, *22*(8), 3052–3306.

Shamji, M. F., Setton, L. A., Jarvis, W., So, S., Chen, J., Jing, L., ... Richardson, W. J. (2010). Proinflammatory cytokine expression profile in degenerated and herniated human intervertebral disc tissues. *Arthritis Rheumatism*, 62(7), 1974–1982.

Simpson, R. U., Thomas, G. A., & Arnold, A. J. (1985). Identification of 1,25-dihydroxyvitamin D3 receptors and activities in muscle. *Journal of Biological Chemistry*, *260*(15), 8882–8891.

Smeal, W. L., Tyburski, M., Alleva, J., Prather, H., & Hunt, D. (2004). Conservative management of low back pain, part I. Discogenic/radicular pain. *Disease-a-Month*, *50*(12), 636–669.

Specchia, N., Pagnotta, A., Toesca, A., & Greco, F. (2002). Cytokines and growth factors in the protruded intervertebral disc of the lumbar spine. *European Spine Journal*, *11*(2), 145–151.

Stafford, M. A., Peng, P., & Hill, D. A. (2007). Sciatica: a review of history, epidemiology, pathogenesis, and the role of epidural steroid injection in management. *British Journal of Anaesthesia*, *99*(4), 461–473.

Stumpf, W. E., Clark, S. A., O'Brien, L. P., & Reid, F. A. (1988). 1,25(OH)2 vitamin D3 sites of action in spinal cord and sensory ganglion. *Anatomy and Embryology (Berl)*, *177*(4), 307–310.

Stumpf, W. E., & O'Brien, L. P. (1987). 1,25 $(OH)_2$ vitamin D3 sites of action in the brain. An autoradiographic study. *Histochemistry*, *87*(5), 393–406.

Szodoray, P., Nakken, B., Gaal, J., Jonsson, R., Szegedi, A., Zold, E., ... Bodolay, E. (2008). The complex role of vitamin D in autoimmune diseases. *Scandinavian Journal of Immunology*, 68(3), 261–269.

Tagliafico, A. S., Ameri, P., Bovio, M., Puntoni, M., Capaccio, E., Murialdo, G., & Martinoli, C. (2010). Relationship between fatty degeneration of thigh muscles and vitamin D status in the elderly: a preliminary MRI study. *American Journal of Roentgenology*, *194*(3), 728–734.

Takahashi, H., Suguro, T., Okazima, Y., Motegi, M., Okada, Y., & Kakiuchi, T. (1996). Inflammatory cytokines in the herniated disc of the lumbar spine. *Spine*, *21*(2), 218–224.

Taniura, H., Ito, M., Sanada, N., Kuramoto, N., Ohno, Y., Nakamichi, N., & Yoneda, Y. (2006). Chronic vitamin D3 treatment protects against neurotoxicity by glutamate in association with upregulation of vitamin D receptor mRNA expression in cultured rat cortical neurons. *Journal of Neuroscience Research*, *83*(7), 1179–1189.

Tolonen, J., Gronblad, M., Virri, J., Seitsalo, S., Rytomaa, T., & Karaharju, E. (2001). Transforming growth factor beta receptor induction in herniated intervertebral disc tissue: an immunohistochemical study. *European Spine Journal*, *10*(2), 172–176.

Turner, M. K., Hooten, W. M., Schmidt, J. E., Kerkvliet, J. L., Townsend, C. O., & Bruce, B. K. (2008). Prevalence and clinical correlates of vitamin D inadequacy among patients with chronic pain. *Pain Medicine*, *9*(8), 979–984.

Valat, J. P., Genevay, S., Marty, M., Rozenberg, S., & Koes, B. (2010). Sciatica. *Best Practice and Research. Clinical Rheumatology*, *24*(2), 241–252.

von Kanel, R., Muller-Hartmannsgruber, V., Kokinogenis, G., & Egloff, N. (2014). Vitamin D and central hypersensitivity in patients with chronic pain. *Pain Medicine*, *15*(9), 1609–1618.

Watkins, L. R., & Maier, S. F. (2002). Beyond neurons: evidence that immune and glial cells contribute to pathological pain states. *Physiological Reviews*, *82*(4), 981–1011.

Xu, J. T., Xin, W. J., Zang, Y., Wu, C. Y., & Liu, X. G. (2006). The role of tumor necrosis factor-alpha in the neuropathic pain induced by Lumbar 5 ventral root transection in rat. *Pain*, *123*(3), 306–321.

Yoshida, M., Nakamura, T., Sei, A., Kikuchi, T., Takagi, K., & Matsukawa, A. (2005). Intervertebral disc cells produce tumor necrosis factor alpha, interleukin-1beta, and monocyte chemoattractant protein-1 immediately after herniation: an experimental study using a new hernia model. *Spine*, *30*(1), 55–61.

Yoshihara, K., Shirai, Y., Nakayama, Y., & Uesaka, S. (2001). Histochemical changes in the multifidus muscle in patients with lumbar intervertebral disc herniation. *Spine*, *26*(6), 622–626.

Zhao, W. P., Kawaguchi, Y., Matsui, H., Kanamori, M., & Kimura, T. (2000). Histochemistry and morphology of the multifidus muscle in lumbar disc herniation: comparative study between diseased and normal sides. *Spine*, *25*(17), 2191–2199.

Zhu, X. Z., Parnianpour, M., Nordin, M., & Kahanovitz, N. (1989). Histochemistry and morphology of erector spinae muscle in lumbar disc herniation. *Spine*, *14*(4), 391–397.

CHAPTER

25

Review of Fortified Foods and Natural Medicinal Products in Companion Animals Afflicted by Naturally Occurring Osteoarthritis

*M. Moreau**,**, E. Troncy**,**

*Research Group in Animal Pharmacology of Quebec (GREPAQ), Department of Veterinary Biomedical Sciences, Faculty of Veterinary Medicine, Université de Montréal, Saint-Hyacinthe, QC, Canada; **Osteoarthritis Research Unit, University of Montreal Hospital Research Centre (CRCHUM), Montreal, QC, Canada

INTRODUCTION

Osteoarthritis (OA) is a highly prevalent musculoskeletal disorder in companion animals (i.e., dogs and cats) (Johnston, 1997; Slingerland, Hazewinkel, Meij, Picavet, & Voorhout, 2011). As in humans, the proportion of animals afflicted with OA increases with age, affecting approximately one in five adult (over 1-year old) dogs and cats (Shearer, 2011). Geriatric animals are therefore more prone to be subjected to OA pain, leading to loss of physical function and consequently to a poor quality of life. OA is thereby consequential for the owners, representing a strong emotional and financial burden.

Because the pathological process cannot be limited or reversed, there is currently no cure for OA. The abnormal changes (mostly damages) to the joint structures, particularly cartilage and subchondral bone evolve progressively. To control the pain and to improve function, the management of OA involves a multimodal approach (Fox, 2013) throughout the entire remaining life of the animal. The foundations of this approach are pharmacological (either medicinal or nutritional) substances together with the preservation of an optimal body condition. The clinical benefits of the latter are more intuitive, being associated with an overall well-being. Thus, companion animals must maintain a lean body weight, eat appropriate amounts of a balanced diet, and be physically active on a daily basis to ensure appropriate muscular strength (Budsberg & Bartges, 2006; Laflamme & Gunn-Moore, 2014; Larsen & Farcas, 2014). Counteracting muscular weakness/atrophy and excess weight (Marshall, Bockstahler, Hulse, & Carmichael, 2009) are considered highly valuable in OA regardless of the degree of improvement that may be expected with such programs. Owners of animals with certain conditions predisposing to OA, such as skeletal malformation or cranial cruciate ligament rupture should be particularly careful, avoiding high-impact activity. Ultimately, surgery is usually required in such conditions.

There is a need for consensus on the pharmacological substances and their potential benefits for OA animals. By pharmacological substances, the present authors mean any active entity, which exerts a beneficial biochemical and/or physiological effect on the cell, tissue, or organ. An active entity can be formulated as a medicinal product [or "medicament," or "drug," such as nonsteroidal antiinflammatory drugs (NSAIDs)], a fortified food, or as a natural medicinal (health) product (NMP).

In the context of OA, the goals of pharmacological substances are simple: to reduce joint pain and to restore normal function with an overall improvement in the quality of life of afflicted animals. Most importantly, claims regarding a potential delay in the progression of disease have not been reported in naturally occurring OA in animals.

Nutritional Modulators of Pain in the Aging Population. http://dx.doi.org/10.1016/B978-0-12-805186-3.00025-4
Copyright © 2017 Elsevier Inc. All rights reserved.

Therefore, the term chondroprotective, disease modifying or structuromodulator is not currently sustained in companion animals for any of the therapeutic approaches.

In the arsenal of pharmacological substances resides the well prescribed NSAID class of therapeutics. NSAIDs have been proved effective for dogs and cats although the clinical evidence is still limited for the effect of long-term management on longevity and quality of life. It is suggested that the observed clinical effects of NSAIDs occur through limiting the end product of the COX enzyme pathway, mainly prostaglandin E2. Hence, exhaustive summaries of current literature (Aragon, Hofmeister, & Budsberg, 2007; Sanderson et al., 2009) regarding the use of NSAIDs in OA-afflicted companion animal (mostly dogs), found strong evidences of clinical potential. As there is a constant quest for clinicians to provide the best possible care, such reviews are of an utmost importance. The process of systematically reviewing, appraising, and using clinical research findings to aid in the delivery of optimal clinical care is referred as evidence-based medicine (EBM) (Rosenberg & Donald, 1995). EBM is a valuable approach to determine therapeutic potential, offering strong evidence to improve clinical decision making.

This brief review presents key requirements of the good clinical practice aligned with EBM (Belsey, 2009), along with a listing of published clinical trials of fortified foods and NMPs in companion animals. A previous systematic review revealed a disappointingly low quantity and quality of scientific evidence regarding NMPs in companion animals (Vandeweerd et al., 2012). The present authors wish to address recommendations to support future studies in determining which approach purported to improve the clinical signs of OA may represent a therapeutic potential and to what extent. The authors are aware that there also exist in vitro and experimental evidences of NMP efficacy [such as avocado/soybean unsaponifiables and dietary vitamin E in a canine surgical model of OA (Boileau et al., 2009; Rhouma, de Oliveira El Warrak, Troncy, Beaudry, & Chorfi, 2013)] but this review has been limited to natural OA disease conditions.

According to Health Canada (*Standards of Evidence for Evaluating Foods with Health Claims*, 2000) and a recent publication (Aronson, 2016), the terms NMPs, fortified or functional foods, and nutraceuticals are defined as follows:

> *Natural medicinal products*, which are often called "complementary" or "alternative" medicines, are naturally occurring substances that are used to restore or maintain health. They include components extracted or purified from plants, products ground, dried, powdered, or pressed from plant materials (herbal medicinal products), and products produced, extracted, or purified from animals or microorganisms (e.g., elk velvet, essential fatty acids, vitamin, and mineral supplements) (nutritional medicinal products). Any medicinal product that exclusively contains as active (i.e., with proven pharmacological and beneficial therapeutic effect) ingredients one or more herbal/nutritional substances or one or more herbal/nutritional preparations, or a combination of both. They come in a wide variety of forms, such as tablets, capsules, tinctures, solutions, creams, ointments, and drops.
> *Herbal/nutritional substance*, a substance that consists of mainly whole, fragmented or cut plants, plant parts, algae, fungi, or lichen/animals, animal parts, microorganisms, in an unprocessed, usually dried form, but sometimes fresh.
> *Herbal/nutritional preparation*, a preparation that is obtained by subjecting herbal/nutritional substances to treatments, such as extraction, distillation, expression, fractionation, purification, concentration, or fermentation.
> *Fortified foods* are foods to which compounds of potential therapeutic or preventive efficacy have been added.
> *Functional foods* are foods (or treats) enhanced with bioactive ingredients and which have demonstrated health benefits. Because of the unsatisfactory definition (Aronson, 2016) and the intricability between functional foods and nutraceuticals, this expression will be not used in this review.
> *Nutraceuticals* are products that have been isolated or purified from foods and generally sold in medicinal forms not usually associated with food. Nutraceuticals have been shown to exhibit a physiological benefit or provide protection against chronic disease. Thus, nutraceuticals are defined by Health Canada as NMPs. That is why we used the term NMPs in this review. Because of the unsatisfactory definition (Aronson, 2016) and the intricability between functional foods and nutraceuticals, this expression will be not used in this review.

Quality standard for designing, conducting, recording, and reporting trials that involve the participation of human subjects have been published (*Guidance for Industry E6 Good Clinical Practice: Consolidated Guidance*, 1996). This guidance document should be followed when generating clinical trial data that are intended to be submitted to regulatory authorities. From this chapter, the following sections summarize key methodological requirements to conduct a clinical trial.

CLINICAL TRIAL OBJECTIVE AND PURPOSES

Clinical trials are prospective experiments conducted to provide strong scientific evidences regarding efficacy of an intervention. The trial methodology should include rationale and objectives. The trial can be done to explore an avenue providing proof of concept or can be used to confirm previous findings. The hypothesis should be clearly stated (Gonzalez, Bolanos, & de Sereday, 2009). Most of the time, they are aimed to establish the therapeutic efficacy of an intervention (Christensen, 2007). A therapeutic efficacy can be established when an intervention demonstrates superiority compared to a negative control (placebo), superiority (or similitude = noninferiority) compared to a positive control (reference treatment), or when a dose–response relationship is observed. The efficacy of the reference treatment should have been clearly established in a manner to ensure similar findings when used as a positive comparator (*ICH Harmonised Tripartite Guideline Statistical Principles for Clinical Trials E9*, 1998). The negative controls are most of the time the final formulation preparations without the active ingredients (i.e., the excipient) or inert compounds, such as cornstarch. For NMP trials, the negative control is often produced to mimic the appearance, taste, and overall appetence of the tested substance. For fortified foods, regular or experimental diets deprived of the active ingredient(s) are frequently used.

DESIGN AND RECRUITMENT

The study design should have sufficient details to be reproduced. An estimate of the sample size is required to support the hypotheses with enough statistical power and appropriate effect size should be provided. A description of the inclusion and exclusion criteria is required. The studied subjects should permit precise estimation of treatment effects as close as possible with the population for which the intervention may eventually be indicated. A description of the subject's initial condition must be possible before the introduction of the control and tested substances. For regular or experimental diets deprived of the active ingredient, it is highly recommended to perform a test–retest evaluation to ensure that change in condition did not occurs following the introduction of a new diet and feeding habits. The duration of the study follow-up must be adapted to the expected benefits (antiinflammatory, structural, and so on).

Inclusion criteria would require subjects to avoid concomitant or rescue pain medication during the trial. Such stringent protocol may be put forward to maximize the treatment effect and minimize the required sample size. However this may impair the recruitment and increase withdrawal and lost to follow-up (McAlindon et al., 2015). Actually, little is known about the relationship between a therapeutic response and the level of either the functional impairment or the structural changes of OA. Similarly, to what extent the number and localization of the afflicted joint(s) may affect the response or the sensitivity of the outcome measurement to detect a response is unknown. Until these issues are addressed, criteria should be as restrictive as possible, making sure that the included subjects show the same pattern of OA affliction.

Clinical trials in companion animals may have safety aspects (monitoring adverse effects, blood work). However, the primary goal is to determine efficacy. Nevertheless, the method for the analysis of safety parameters and time of recording should be specified.

OUTCOMES

An outcome (also called an end point) is defined as a specific key measurement used to describe the effect of an exposure to a proposed treatment. In OA clinical trials, such studies evaluate improvement, similitude, or exacerbation of the outcome of interest in animals that have a previous diagnosis of OA. There are two types of outcome: The primary outcome (s) is (are) the one(s) of greatest importance. This (these) outcome(s) is (are) used to support clinical trial objectives, hypothesis, and will be the focus of planned statistical analyses. The primary outcome should reflect the accepted norms and standards in the field thus permitting comparison of results across different trials and metaanalysis. Of upmost importance, the primary outcome should be clinically significant, meaning the detection of a change that is clinically meaningful (*ICH Harmonised Tripartite Guideline Statistical Principles for Clinical Trials E9*, 1998). The primary outcome should be used to estimate the study sample size. The follow-up schedule and time of outcome measurement should be clearly defined. Again a rationale supporting the measurement time point should be specified. Data on secondary outcomes are used to evaluate additional effects of the treatment (Schulz, Altman, Moher, & Group, 2010).

In dogs and cats with naturally occurring OA, the outcomes (either primary or secondary) are in most of the time among the functional (e.g., gait/lameness, activity performance, joint stiffness reflecting indirectly pain), behavioral (e.g., self-grooming, mood, pain), or structural (e.g., cartilage volume, osteophyte growth) domains. Since quality of life and functional impairments are the major clinical signs of OA in companion animals, collecting data on these aspects before undergoing the clinical trial, as well as at follow-up visits, is critical.

A clinical trial should use validated outcomes to measure a therapeutic benefit for a specific context of use. The outcome must have proven to be valid; meaning the precise measurement of what it is intended to measure is reliable, accurate, and comprehensive (Velentgas et al., 2013). The outcome should be well in line with the construct (e.g., a daily life activity impairment in the presence of OA) and responsive toward clinically meaningful changes in an individual over time. As validation is an ongoing process, any additional work will strengthen accuracy and effectiveness of the outcome in a particular population for a specific purpose (Rothrock, Kaiser, & Cella, 2011).

Several outcome measures have been developed to help standardize the evaluation of pain-related clinical signs of OA in companion animals. Therefore, the clinicalist has access to plenty of metrological tools or devices to describe the effectiveness of a therapeutic approach. These include collar-mounted activity monitoring and force platform gait analysis. Scaling and scoring systems are also frequently used. Hence, a trained professional can report the outcome after a thorough observation of the animal's condition. Such assessments involve a clinical judgment or interpretation of the observable signs, behaviors, or other physical manifestations thought to be related to a disease condition. The outcome can also be reported by the owner. This proxy measurement is often required to stand for variables that cannot be directly measured or expressed by the subject, such as in joint pain. Subjective outcome measures are an attractive method to interpret changes in the condition of OA afflicted animals. This is due in part to the convenient use and low cost of those instruments. However, according to EBM, objective measurements (which typically defy interpretation) provide a standardized means for clinical evaluation of therapeutic efficacy and are preferable (Vandeweerd et al., 2012).

Regarding the structural changes of OA, imaging techniques are of the greatest importance since most of the macroscopic abnormalities, such as damages or abnormalities, can be revealed and interpreted by experts in the field (Galindo-Zamora et al., 2016). However, it would be preferable to further validate a scoring system to evaluate changes in the cartilage surface and osteoarthritic damage in dogs and cats. Advances have been made using computerized technique to determine cartilage volume loss, but use in naturally occurring OA in animals is limited. Overall, claims regarding disease-modifying properties cannot be supported in naturally occurring OA due to technical limitations. In addition, whether or not the use of fortified foods or NMPs may reduce the incidence of OA has been poorly explored. To demonstrate an effect on incidence, a study model, such as done brilliantly in a longitudinal study on feeding habits (Kealy et al., 1997) could potentially provide sufficient evidence.

CONTROL AND TESTED SUBSTANCES

Beside the subjects receiving the test substance(s), a controlled study involves another group that receives the comparator, which can be negative or positive. The regiment of the tested product should be clearly stated. Ideally, a rationale supporting the dosing chart should be provided. Animal equivalent dose calculations using allometric scaling or previous investigations done in similar conditions are suggested. It is important to keep in mind that the incorporation of NMPs into fortified food requires special care and processing techniques to avoid destroying any bioactivity of the final product (Bierer & Bui, 2002). For fortified foods, the dosing chart becomes the feeding guidelines and should be carefully respected by the owner to limit the introduction of bias from subjects receiving suboptimal amounts of the test substance. Owner compliance needs to be monitored and documented, otherwise study bias may occur.

Dose calculations (either from allometric calculation or previous experiments) are usually performed using the animal's body weight determined at study enrollment. Due to the inactivity associated to OA, afflicted animals are often overweight and sometimes obese. Therefore a trial subject may receive more than what a lean dog would potentially receive. For this reason, it is recommended to determine whether the tested group and its comparator are homogeneous regarding body weight at the beginning of a clinical trial. However, this doesn't necessarily indicate similar body conditions among individuals. The substances may therefore be administered at a level that does not represent normal conditions. In geriatric animals, potential alterations in nutrient intake due to appetite variation should also be considered. Such situation may alter the amount of NMPs received and thus be a source of bias.

BLINDING AND RANDOMIZATION

To preserve the ability to draw valid conclusions, clinical trials are designed to limit any systematic deviation of the treatment effect from its true value (i.e., bias) and to maximize the potential inference applicable to the target population. Important techniques to limit bias are blinding and randomization.

A blinded clinical trial implies that no one involved in the conduct of the trial is aware of the treatment allocated, not even as a code letter (*ICH Harmonised Tripartite Guideline Statistical Principles for Clinical Trials E9*, 1998). Trialists should be kept unaware of the treatment identification until study completion and release of data for analysis. Blinding requires undistinguishable treatment appearance, taste, and similar administration schedule.

The randomization process takes place to make sure that the results are not biased against a particular treatment group. Hence, patients should not be allocated to a specific treatment group according to the perception of the investigator (e.g., to maximize the chance of observing specific clinical effects) or to the condition of the patient (e.g., to avoid side effect in predisposed patient). Randomization also helps to achieve comparability between groups regarding all individual characteristics. This is to ensure that any difference between groups will be related to a change in condition and not to initial group heterogeneity.

Many techniques exist for the random assignment of participants to treatment groups in clinical trials (Suresh, 2011). The most intuitive is the simple randomization where a single sequence of randomly assigned treatment is produced by, for example, flipping a coin. This technique is completely unpredictable. However, when an unrestricted simple randomization is used, unequal number of participants among groups could happen. Use of a restricted method may improve the similitude between groups regarding sample size or predefined characteristics.

Animals can be allocated using a block randomization. With this restricted method, for every block of specified size, there is a predefined ratio of allocated treatment. For example, a block of four with a ratio of 1:1 would contain two treatments A and two treatments B. Possible sequences of treatment are then ABAB, AABB, BBAA, BABA, BAAB, and ABBA. To control for important factors measured at study entrance, such as the severity of disease or age, the stratified randomization technique can be used. In this method, the subjects' initial characteristics are established, and then a randomization technique is used within each of the subsets.

Concealing the allocation sequence is another strategy to avoid bias in clinical trials. Allocation concealment means that trialists are not aware of the sequence of treatment and therefore cannot deduct the treatment allocated to a given subject. Sequentially numbered, opaque, sealed envelopes are often used for this purpose. In addition, knowing that a given subject receives treatment A and another treatment B may predispose to additional bias. For this reason, the use of individual codes instead of A versus B is preferred.

DATA ANALYSIS

A data analysis plan to support the hypotheses (Messier, Callahan, Golightly, & Keefe, 2015), including timing of any planned interim analysis, should be provided. Outcome analysis should consider the nature of the data and be modelized accordingly. Most of the clinical trials imply, either ordinal (e.g., mild, moderate, severe), dichotomous (e.g., improvement/no improvement), or continuous (e.g., percentage of body weight) data. Baseline characteristics potentially related to the outcome measure, such as pain level should be similar between groups, otherwise included as a covariable in an appropriate statistical data management (*Guidance for Industry E6 Good Clinical Practice: Consolidated Guidance*, 1996).

In essence, a clinical trial infers research objectives obtained from a cohort of the general population. Trialists often have to deal with dropout, loss to follow-up, and withdrawal. Incomplete data sets may disrupt the balance between groups in terms of sample size and characteristics and therefore be a potential bias against treatment effect and main conclusions while weakening the predefined statistical power. There is no universal method for handling missing data. To limit the impact, missing data can be ignored, analyzing only available data. It is also possible to impute the missing data with replacement values, and analyze the data as if they were obtained. Missing data can be replaced by the last observation obtained or by the baseline observation (Little et al., 2012). It is also possible to input the missing data differently (replacing by either the best or worst data) and test the impact of this scenario on the statistical findings. Analyses can also be modelized to allow for missing data.

Publication in a peer-reviewed journal remains the gold standard for disclosing clinical trial results. A nonexhaustive list of clinical trials in OA companion animals is presented in Table 25.1 (fortified foods) and Table 25.2 (natural medicinal products).

CRITICAL ANALYSIS

The authors wish to specify that the scope of this review wasn't to assess the quality and strength of each trial. The main clinical finding and related time point was extracted from the published articles without criticism about the credibility of such statement. The quality of the conducted trials on fortified foods and NMPs was considered as a whole.

As summarized in Tables 25.1 and 25.2, scientific evidence suggests that fortified foods (either with green-lipped mussel or omega-3 fatty acids, or both) and several NMPs have the potential to improve the pain-related clinical signs of OA in companion animals. Several clinical trials listed herein reported improvement and only a few (7 on 39 assessments) did not conclude to potential benefits. The benefit looks clear with the tested fortified foods. However, for the numerous NMPs tested, we have classified them in three categories from the most to the least optimistic:

1. *High interest in managing companion animal OA*: Medicinal multiherbal preparation (Moreau et al., 2014), Zeel homeopathic combination preparation (Hielm-Bjorkman et al., 2009a), green-lipped mussel, type-II glycosylated undenatured chicken sternum cartilage (collagen), elk velvet antler (Moreau et al., 2004), and the Chinese plant *Brachystemma calycinum* D. don (Moreau et al., 2012a).

TABLE 25.1 Clinical Trials in Companion Animals With Naturally Occurring Osteoarthritis: Efficacy of Fortified Foods

Fortified foods	Species; main clinical finding (time point): outcome (O: objective; S: subjective)
COMMERCIAL DIETS	
Green-lipped mussel, omega-3 fatty acids, glucosamine hydrochloride, and chondroitin sulfate (Rialland et al., 2013)	Dogs; improvement (60 days): O and S
Green-lipped mussel (Servet, Biourge, & Marniquet, 2006)	Dogs; improvement (45 days): S
Omega-3 fatty acids (Fritsch et al., 2010b)	Dogs; no improvement (90 days): S
Omega-3 fatty acids (Fritsch et al., 2010a)	Dogs; improvement (12 weeks): (S)
Omega-3 fatty acids (Moreau et al., 2012b)	Dogs; improvement (7, 13 weeks): O and S
Omega-3 fatty acids (Roush et al., 2010a)	Dogs; improvement (90 days): O and (S)
Omega-3 fatty acids (Roush et al., 2010b)	Dogs; improvement (6, 12, 24 weeks): (S)
EXPERIMENTAL DIETS	
Green-lipped mussel (Bui & Bierer, 2001)	Dogs; improvement (6 weeks): (S)
Omega-3 fatty acids (Fritsch et al., 2010b)	Dogs; improvement (90 days): (S)
Green-lipped mussel, omega-3 fatty acids, glucosamine hydrochloride, and chondroitin sulfate (Lascelles et al., 2010)	Cats; improvement (9 weeks): O, not with S

Objective outcomes include kinetic gait analysis, and/or telemetered motor activity.
Subjective outcomes include proxy-filled in multifactorial behavioral pain/quality of life scaling either client-specific or standardized outcome measures.
If put in parenthesis, the letter indicates that the improvement was classified as modest.

However, for the two latter, safety of the product and quality of production must be verified before anticipating commercialization.

2. *Moderate interest*: Beta-1.3/1.6-glucans (Beynen & Legerstee, 2010), herbal preparation with *Boswellia serrata* (Reichling et al., 2004), and curcumin (Innes et al., 2003) alone, gelatin hydrolysate (Beynen et al., 2010) and serum milk protein concentrate (Gingerich & Strobel, 2003) would require scientific confirmation before considering further expansion. Particularly for any herbal preparation, the formulation is essential to promote interesting absorption and pharmacokinetics (Comblain, Serisier, Barthelemy, Balligand, & Henrotin, 2016).
3. *Low interest*: Curiously, the most popular compound at this time, Glucosamine and Chondroitin, presents the lowest evidence of efficacy. This could be related to differences in dosing, nature/source/quality of compounds, and corresponding pharmacokinetics. Finally, the single assessment of S-adenosyl L-methionine (Imhoff et al., 2011) has been disappointing.

Interestingly, the time to significant improvement ranged from 1 to 150 days. However, the 1-day positive assessment with Zeel (Neumann et al., 2011) is surprising and may be more anecdotal than real. The average study follow-up is around 3 months for fortified foods and 2 months for NMPs.

A unique randomized-controlled trial may not be sufficiently informative to contribute to dissemination of the findings to clinicians and researchers to make informed clinical decisions. The value of the scientific evidence can be ranked according to pyramidal hierarchy having metaanalysis as the highest level of evidence, follow by systematic review and randomized controlled trial. Assessing systematically all published clinical trials was brilliantly done elsewhere (Vandeweerd et al., 2012). However, a metaanalysis of randomized-controlled trials is highly requested for the pharmaceutical approaches of OA in companion animals. More precisely, such method allows comparisons among therapeutics according to their relative efficacy. Statistical analysis determines individual effect size and then a pooled effect size is generated to estimate the overall effect. Actually, the lack of standardized and throughout method to conduct a clinical trial in companion animals, especially regarding the outcome measurement, compromises metaanalyses. More specifically, there is no definitive and proven relationship between the improvement denoted using common outcome measurements (including force platform gait analysis) and the satisfying response expected from owners and clinicians. What a "clinical responder" is remains unknown in companion animals.

The origin and preparation methods may also be a source of uncertainty. Can we translate the benefits observed from Canadian elk velvet antler to other

TABLE 25.2 Clinical Trials in Companion Animals With Naturally Occurring Osteoarthritis: Efficacy of Natural Medicinal Products

Natural medicinal products	Specie; main clinical finding (time point): outcome (O: objective; S: subjective)
Beta-1.3/1.6-glucans (Beynen & Legerstee, 2010)	Dogs; improvement (8 weeks): (S)
Boswellia serrata (Reichling, Schmokel, Fitzi, Bucher, & Saller, 2004)	Dogs; improvement (2, 4, 6 weeks): (S)
Brachystemma calycinum D. Don (Moreau et al., 2012a)	Dogs; improvement (3, 6 weeks): O, not with S
Chondroitin sulfate (22 mg/kg/day) (Dobenecker, Beetz, & Kienzle, 2002)	Dogs; no improvement (12 weeks): S
Curcuma domestica and *Curcuma zanthorrhiza* (Innes, Fuller, Grover, Kelly, & Burn, 2003)	Dogs; improvement (8 weeks): (S), not with O
Elk velvet antler (Moreau, Dupuis, Bonneau, & Lecuyer, 2004)	Dogs; improvement (60 days): O and S
Gelatin hydrolysate (Beynen, Van Geene, Grim, Jacobs, & Van der Vlerk, 2010)	Dogs; improvement (8 weeks): S
Glucosamine hydrochloride (≈50 mg/kg/12 h) and chondroitin sulfate (≈38.5 mg/kg/12 h) (Sul, Chase, Parkin, & Bennett, 2014)	Cats; no improvement (70 days): S
Glucosamine hydrochloride (≈57.5 mg/kg/day) and chondroitin sulfate (≈42.5 mg/kg/day) (McCarthy et al., 2007)	Dogs; improvement (70 days): S
Glucosamine hydrochloride (≈62.5 mg/kg/day) and chondroitin sulfate (≈50 mg/kg/day) (D'Altilio et al., 2007)	Dogs; no improvement (30, 60, 90, 120 days): S
Glucosamine hydrochloride (≈62.5 mg/kg/day) and chondroitin sulfate (≈50 mg/kg/day) (Gupta et al., 2012)	Dogs; improvement (90, 120, 150 days): S, not with O
Glucosamine hydrochloride (≈50 mg/kg/day), chondroitin sulfate (≈40 mg/kg/day), and manganese ascorbate (Moreau, Dupuis, Bonneau, & Desnoyers, 2003)	Dogs; no improvement (30, 60 days): O and S
Green-lipped mussel (Hielm-Bjorkman, Tulamo, Salonen, & Raekallio, 2009b)	Dogs; improvement (8 weeks): S, not with O
Green-lipped mussel (Bierer & Bui, 2002)	Dogs; improvement (6 weeks): S
Green-lipped mussel (Pollard, Guilford, Ankenbauer-Perkins, & Hedderley, 2006)	Dogs; improvement (28, 56 days): S
Greenshell mussel (Dobenecker et al., 2002)	Dogs; no improvement (12 weeks): S
Homeopathic combination preparation (Hielm-Bjorkman, Tulamo, Salonen, & Raekallio, 2009a)	Dogs; improvement (8 weeks): O and S
Homeopathic combination preparation (Neumann, Stolt, Braun, Hellmann, & Reinhart, 2011)	Dogs; improvement (1, 28, 56 days): S
Medicinal multiherbal preparation (*Harpagophytum p.*, *Boswellia s.*, *Ribes n.*, *Salix a.*, *Tanacetum p.*, *Ananas* c., *Curcuma i.*), omega-3 fatty acids, glucosamine sulfate, methylsulfonylmethane, chondroitin sulfate, L-glutamine, and hyaluronic acid (Moreau et al., 2014)	Dogs; improvement (4, 8 weeks); O, not with S
Milk protein concentrate (Gingerich & Strobel, 2003)	Dogs; improvement (4, 8 weeks): S
Omega-3 fatty acids (Corbee, Barnier, van de Lest, & Hazewinkel, 2013)	Cats; improvement (10 weeks): S
Omega-3 fatty acids (Hielm-Bjorkman et al., 2012)	Dogs; improvement (16 weeks): (O) and (S)
S-adenosyl L-methionine (Imhoff et al., 2011)	Dogs; no improvement (3, 6 weeks): O and S
Type-II glycosylated undenatured chicken sternum cartilage (D'Altilio et al., 2007)	Dogs; improvement (30, 60, 90, 120 days): S
Type-II glycosylated undenatured chicken sternum cartilage (Deparle et al., 2005)	Dogs; improvement (90 days): S
Type-II glycosylated undenatured chicken sternum cartilage (Gupta et al., 2012)	Dogs; improvement (60, 90, 120, 150 days): O and S
Type-II glycosylated undenatured chicken sternum cartilage (Peal et al., 2007)	Dogs; improvement (30 days): S
Type-II glycosylated undenatured chicken sternum cartilage, glucosamine hydrochloride, and chondroitin sulfate (Gupta et al., 2012)	Dogs; improvement (60, 90, 120, 150 days): S, not with O
Type-II glycosylated undenatured chicken sternum cartilage, glucosamine hydrochloride, and chondroitin sulfate (D'Altilio et al., 2007)	Dogs; improvement (30, 60, 90, 120 days): S

Objective outcomes include kinetic gait analysis, and/or telemetered motor activity.
Subjective outcomes include proxy-filled in multifactorial behavioral pain/quality of life scaling either client-specific or standardized outcome measures.
If put in parenthesis, the letter indicates that the improvement was classified as modest.

taxonomically related species? Perhaps elk environment and feeding protocols, season of harvesting, age of the animal influence the concentration of active compounds? Similarly, if an animal receives a specified amount of anchovy oil, will it be similar to that provided by a diet rich in rainbow trout? Although both supply omega-3 fatty acids, there may be variability of eicosapentaenoic and docosahexaenoic acids content. These two examples highlight the requirement for standardized origin, extraction and preparation methods, quality control and assessment of effective dose of active compounds. Active ingredient content and synergistic effects with other components of the formulation may also be a source of variability of expected results.

The relationship between the dose of NMPs and the response should be further addressed, particularly for exploratory trials. Such trial may be used to determine a dosing regimen beyond which no more benefits can be expected or to titrate down to the minimal effective dose. Therefore, what dose of a given NMP (alone or within fortified food) would provide the optimal efficacy is unknown. Until such issue is resolved, the use of NMPs cannot be recommended with certainty. More confusion among the NMPs resides on the product itself. The question about Curcumin formulation has been presented (Comblain et al., 2016). Hence, what about an exclusive and/or patented low molecular weight chondroitin sulfate versus regular chondroitin sulfate? What about a raw freeze-dried mussel (*Perna canaliculus*) powder versus an extract from a patented stabilized process? Again, unresolved issues exist that impair the potential for overall conclusions or consensus on fortified food and NMP efficacy in companion animals.

POSITIONING OF FORTIFIED FOODS AND NATURAL MEDICINAL PRODUCTS

Actually, in contrast to human medicine (McAlindon et al., 2014), there are no consensus guidelines for the treatment of OA in companion animals and consequently no standards of care. Textbooks refer to the management of OA as a multimodal approach (Fox, 2013). However, without guidelines supported by strong scientific evidence and expert panel consensus, a multimodal approach is deprived of its full sense. The actual multimodal approach is a step forward but remains (largely) imprecise. Little is known on the hierarchy of potency, sequence of use, combination and possible synergetic effect among the proposed pharmacological approaches. In addition, the use of words, such as "chondroprotective" is considered misleading by the present authors.

Some clinicians reserve the use of fortified foods and NMPs to individuals who do not tolerate NSAIDs. Others consider fortified foods and NMPs to animals having only mild and intermittent clinical signs of OA. While fortified foods and NMPs are often considered as a complementary approach, there is no evidence to support that they should be considered as a first or second line of treatment. Only few head-to-head clinical trials exist. Veterinary medicine is currently deprived of outcome measurements, which reflect with certainty the clinical benefits that can be expected from a pharmacological approach of OA.

CONCLUDING REMARKS AND FUTURE RECOMMENDATIONS

Typical features of OA are loss of joint integrity and poor functionality. To date, there is no curative treatment for OA and the current approach can only alleviate the clinical signs. Natural products are still the most important source of drugs and lead compounds (Helmstadter & Staiger, 2014) and have a valuable impact on veterinary medicine. Several studies that highlighted the effectiveness of fortified food and NMPs in companion animals were listed herein. In most of the studies, the trial involved previously untreated animals randomly allocated to different groups evolving over time, using a negative control as the comparator. Unfortunately, even in well-designed studies, outcome measures may not accurately reflect ongoing long-term benefits and improvements in overall OA management and quality of life. This is true of most treatments, including those generally accepted, such as NSAIDs.

These studies are relevant for academic and industrial scientists. For clinicians, there are many unresolved issues, such as demonstrated efficacy in the target population, quality control and regimen of administration, which makes it difficult to inform pet owners on the clinical potential of many fortified foods and NMPs. We also observed highly variable country-specific regulatory requirements for the development and manufacturing of NMPs and fortified foods. Additionally, within a given country, these requirements may be different for the commercialization of NMPs and of fortified foods. With this lack of consistency, extrapolation of study results to another formulation of the same compound is challenging.

Animal models of naturally occurring OA are relevant preclinical tools for studying the effects of pharmaceutical approaches and perhaps represent a final step before initiating clinical trials in humans (Mevel et al., 2014). Consensus-based standardization of clinical trial procedures is therefore highly recommended.

For future clinical trials testing the potential of fortified foods and natural medicinal products in companion animals, we recommend the following:

- Combine proxy measurement (owner's opinion) with objective outcome measures,

- Standardize the evaluation of the owner's opinion using validated scales (either multifactorial standardized scales or client specific outcome),
- Define a priori the primary and secondary outcomes,
- Use outcome measures with known measurement error,
- Use outcome measures with defined minimal clinically important changes,
- Randomize and ensure strict concealment,
- Define the maximal time until a clinical improvement can be denoted,
- Define the time necessary to conclude to a sustained relief,
- Determine a precise dosage instead of doses for large weight bands,
- Develop universally accepted data management from objective instruments (e.g., collar-mounted activity monitoring, force platform kinetic gait analysis),
- Document imputation methods for missing data,
- Determine the margin of safety for tested compounds,
- Consider large scale field trials.

We believe that veterinary medicine would benefit from clinical investigations addressing the potential of fortified foods and NMPs to delay or even prevent the development of OA in animals prone to joint damage due to developmental or acquired arthropathy. We also believe that triple therapy involving the use of NMPs, fortified food and NSAIDs might prove to be a promising approach for alleviating the clinical signs of OA in companion animals. Despite this belief, more thorough evaluation is needed.

Acknowledgments

The authors wish to thank Dr. Stéphanie Keroack, DMV for her support in the revision of the manuscript.

References

Aragon, C. L., Hofmeister, E. H., & Budsberg, S. C. (2007). Systematic review of clinical trials of treatments for osteoarthritis in dogs. *Journal of the American Veterinary Medical Association, 230*, 514–521.

Aronson, J. K. (2016). Defining "nutraceuticals": neither nutritious nor pharmaceutical. *British Journal of Clinical Pharmacology.*

Belsey, J. (2009). What is evidence-based medicine? In *What is..? series*: Hayward Medical Communications.

Beynen, A. C., & Legerstee, E. (2010). Influence of dietary beta-1,3/1,6-glucans on clinical signs of canine osteoarthritis in a double-blind, placebo-controlled trial. *American Journal of Animal and Veterinary Sciences, 5*, 97–101.

Beynen, A. C., Van Geene, H. W., Grim, H. V., Jacobs, P., & Van der Vlerk, T. (2010). Oral administration of gelatin hydrolysate reduces clinical signs of canine osteoarthritis in a double-blind, placebo-controlled trial. *American Journal of Animal and Veterinary Sciences, 5*, 102–106.

Bierer, T. L., & Bui, L. M. (2002). Improvement of arthritic signs in dogs fed green-lipped mussel (*Perna canaliculus*). *Journal of Nutrition, 132*, 1634S–1636S.

Boileau, C., Martel-Pelletier, J., Caron, J., Msika, P., Guillou, G. B., Baudouin, C., & Pelletier, J. P. (2009). Protective effects of total fraction of avocado/soybean unsaponifiables on the structural changes in experimental dog osteoarthritis: inhibition of nitric oxide synthase and matrix metalloproteinase-13. *Arthritis Research and Therapy, 11*, R41.

Budsberg, S. C., & Bartges, J. W. (2006). Nutrition and osteoarthritis in dogs: does it help? *Veterinary Clinics of North America Small Animal Practice, 36*, 1307–1323.

Bui, L. M., & Bierer, R. L. (2001). Influence of green lipped mussels (*Perna canaliculus*) in alleviating signs of arthritis in dogs. *Veterinary Therapeutics: Research in Applied Veterinary Medicine, 2*, 101–111.

Christensen, E. (2007). Methodology of superiority vs. equivalence trials and non-inferiority trials. *Journal of Hepatology, 46*, 947–954.

Comblain, F., Serisier, S., Barthelemy, N., Balligand, M., & Henrotin, Y. (2016). Review of dietary supplements for the management of osteoarthritis in dogs in studies from 2004 to 2014. *Journal of Veterinary Pharmacology and Therapeutics, 39*, 1–15.

Corbee, R. J., Barnier, M. M., van de Lest, C. H., & Hazewinkel, H. A. (2013). The effect of dietary long-chain omega-3 fatty acid supplementation on owner's perception of behaviour and locomotion in cats with naturally occurring osteoarthritis. *Journal of Animal Physiology and Animal Nutrition, 97*, 846–853.

D'Altilio, M., Peal, A., Alvey, M., Simms, C., Curtsinger, A., Gupta, R. C., Canerdy, T. D., Goad, J. T., Bagchi, M., & Bagchi, D. (2007). Therapeutic efficacy and safety of undenatured type ii collagen singly or in combination with glucosamine and chondroitin in arthritic dogs. *Toxicology Mechanisms and Methods, 17*, 189–196.

Deparle, L. A., Gupta, R. C., Canerdy, T. D., Goad, J. T., D'Altilio, M., Bagchi, M., & Bagchi, D. (2005). Efficacy and safety of glycosylated undenatured type-II collagen (UC-II) in therapy of arthritic dogs. *Journal of Veterinary Pharmacology and Therapeutics, 28*, 385–390.

Dobenecker, B., Beetz, Y., & Kienzle, E. (2002). A placebo-controlled double-blind study on the effect of nutraceuticals (chondroitin sulfate and mussel extract) in dogs with joint diseases as perceived by their owners. *Journal of Nutrition, 132*, 1690S–1691S.

Fox, S. M. (2013). *Pain Management in Small Animal Medicine* (1st ed.). Florida: CRC Press.

Fritsch, D. A., Allen, T. A., Dodd, C. E., Jewell, D. E., Sixby, K. A., Leventhal, P. S., Brejda, J., & Hahn, K. A. (2010a). A multicenter study of the effect of dietary supplementation with fish oil omega-3 fatty acids on carprofen dosage in dogs with osteoarthritis. *Journal of the American Veterinary Medical Association, 236*, 535–539.

Fritsch, D. A., Allen, T. A., Dodd, C. E., Jewell, D. E., Sixby, K. A., Leventhal, P. S., & Hahn, K. A. (2010b). Dose-titration effects of fish oil in osteoarthritic dogs. *Journal of Veterinary Internal Medicine, 24*, 1020–1026.

Galindo-Zamora, V., von Babo, V., Eberle, N., Betz, D., Nolte, I., & Wefstaedt, P. (2016). Kinetic, kinematic, magnetic resonance and owner evaluation of dogs before and after the amputation of a hind limb. *BMC Veterinary Research, 12*, 20.

Gingerich, D. A., & Strobel, J. D. (2003). Use of client-specific outcome measures to assess treatment effects in geriatric, arthritic dogs: controlled clinical evaluation of a nutraceutical. *Veterinary Therapeutics : Research in Applied Veterinary Medicine, 4*, 56–66.

Gonzalez, C. D., Bolanos, R., & de Sereday, M. (2009). Editorial on hypothesis and objectives in clinical trials: superiority, equivalence and non-inferiority. *Thrombosis Journal, 7*, 3.

Guidance for Industry E6 Good Clinical Practice: Consolidated Guidance. (1996). International Conference on Harmonization of Technical Requirements for the Registration of Pharmaceuticals for Human Use (ICH).

Gupta, R. C., Canerdy, T. D., Lindley, J., Konemann, M., Minniear, J., Carroll, B. A., Hendrick, C., Goad, J. T., Rohde, K., Doss, R., Bagchi, M.,

& Bagchi, D. (2012). Comparative therapeutic efficacy and safety of type-II collagen (UC-II), glucosamine and chondroitin in arthritic dogs: pain evaluation by ground force plate. *Journal of Animal Physiology and Animal Nutrition, 96*, 770–777.

Helmstadter, A., & Staiger, C. (2014). Traditional use of medicinal agents: a valid source of evidence. *Drug Discovery Today, 19*, 4–7.

Hielm-Bjorkman, A., Roine, J., Elo, K., Lappalainen, A., Junnila, J., & Laitinen-Vapaavuori, O. (2012). An un-commissioned randomized, placebo-controlled double-blind study to test the effect of deep sea fish oil as a pain reliever for dogs suffering from canine OA. *BMC Veterinary Research, 8*, 157.

Hielm-Bjorkman, A., Tulamo, R. M., Salonen, H., & Raekallio, M. (2009a). Evaluating complementary therapies for canine osteoarthritis—part II: a homeopathic combination preparation (Zeel). *Evidence-based Complementary and Alternative Medicine : eCAM, 6*, 465–471.

Hielm-Bjorkman, A., Tulamo, R. M., Salonen, H., & Raekallio, M. (2009b). Evaluating complementary therapies for canine osteoarthritis part I: green-lipped mussel (*Perna canaliculus*). *Evidence-based Complementary and Alternative Medicine : eCAM, 6*, 365–373.

ICH Harmonised Tripartite Guideline Statistical Principles for Clinical Trials E9. (1998). International Council for Harmonisation of Technical Requirements for Pharmaceuticals for Human Use (ICH).

Imhoff, D. J., Gordon-Evans, W. J., Evans, R. B., Johnson, A. L., Griffon, D. J., & Swanson, K. S. (2011). Evaluation of S-adenosyl l-methionine in a double-blinded, randomized, placebo-controlled, clinical trial for treatment of presumptive osteoarthritis in the dog. *Veterinary Surgery, 40*, 228–232.

Innes, J. F., Fuller, C. J., Grover, E. R., Kelly, A. L., & Burn, J. F. (2003). Randomised, double-blind, placebo-controlled parallel group study of P54FP for the treatment of dogs with osteoarthritis. *Veterinary Record, 152*, 457–460.

Johnston, S. A. (1997). Osteoarthritis. Joint anatomy, physiology, and pathobiology. *Veterinary Clinics of North America. Small Animal Practice, 27*, 699–723.

Kealy, R. D., Lawler, D. F., Ballam, J. M., Lust, G., Smith, G. K., Biery, D. N., & Olsson, S. E. (1997). Five-year longitudinal study on limited food consumption and development of osteoarthritis in coxofemoral joints of dogs. *Journal of the American Veterinary Medical Association, 210*, 222–225.

Laflamme, D., & Gunn-Moore, D. (2014). Nutrition of aging cats. *Veterinary Clinics of North America. Small Animal Practice, 44*, 761–774.

Larsen, J. A., & Farcas, A. (2014). Nutrition of aging dogs. *Veterinary Clinics of North America. Small Animal Practice, 44*, 741–759.

Lascelles, B. D., DePuy, V., Thomson, A., Hansen, B., Marcellin-Little, D. J., Biourge, V., & Bauer, J. E. (2010). Evaluation of a therapeutic diet for feline degenerative joint disease. *Journal of Veterinary Internal Medicine, 24*, 487–495.

Little, R. J., D'Agostino, R., Cohen, M. L., Dickersin, K., Emerson, S. S., Farrar, J. T., Frangakis, C., Hogan, J. W., Molenberghs, G., Murphy, S. A., Neaton, J. D., Rotnitzky, A., Scharfstein, D., Shih, W. J., Siegel, J. P., & Stern, H. (2012). The prevention and treatment of missing data in clinical trials. *New England Journal of Medicine, 367*, 1355–1360.

Marshall, W., Bockstahler, B., Hulse, D., & Carmichael, S. (2009). A review of osteoarthritis and obesity: current understanding of the relationship and benefit of obesity treatment and prevention in the dog. *Veterinary and Comparative Orthopaedics and Traumatology, 22*, 339–345.

McAlindon, T. E., Bannuru, R. R., Sullivan, M. C., Arden, N. K., Berenbaum, F., Bierma-Zeinstra, S. M., Hawker, G. A., Henrotin, Y., Hunter, D. J., Kawaguchi, H., Kwoh, K., Lohmander, S., Rannou, F., Roos, E. M., & Underwood, M. (2014). OARSI guidelines for the non-surgical management of knee osteoarthritis. *Osteoarthritis and Cartilage, 22*, 363–388.

McAlindon, T. E., Driban, J. B., Henrotin, Y., Hunter, D. J., Jiang, G. L., Skou, S. T., Wang, S., & Schnitzer, T. (2015). OARSI clinical trials recommendations: design, conduct, and reporting of clinical trials for knee osteoarthritis. *Osteoarthritis and Cartilage, 23*, 747–760.

McCarthy, G., O'Donovan, J., Jones, B., McAllister, H., Seed, M., & Mooney, C. (2007). Randomised double-blind, positive-controlled trial to assess the efficacy of glucosamine/chondroitin sulfate for the treatment of dogs with osteoarthritis. *Veterinary Journal, 174*, 54–61.

Messier, S. P., Callahan, L. F., Golightly, Y. M., & Keefe, F. J. (2015). OARSI clinical trials recommendations: design and conduct of clinical trials of lifestyle diet and exercise interventions for osteoarthritis. *Osteoarthritis and Cartilage, 23*, 787–797.

Mevel, E., Monfoulet, L. E., Merceron, C., Coxam, V., Wittrant, Y., Beck, L., & Guicheux, J. (2014). Nutraceuticals in joint health: animal models as instrumental tools. *Drug Discovery Today, 19*, 1649–1658.

Moreau, M., Dupuis, J., Bonneau, N. H., & Desnoyers, M. (2003). Clinical evaluation of a nutraceutical, carprofen and meloxicam for the treatment of dogs with osteoarthritis. *Veterinary Record, 152*, 323–329.

Moreau, M., Dupuis, J., Bonneau, N. H., & Lecuyer, M. (2004). Clinical evaluation of a powder of quality elk velvet antler for the treatment of osteoarthrosis in dogs. *Canadian Veterinary Journal, 45*, 133–139.

Moreau, M., Lussier, B., Pelletier, J. P., Martel-Pelletier, J., Bedard, C., Gauvin, D., & Troncy, E. (2012a). *Brachystemma calycinum* D. Don effectively reduces the locomotor disability in dogs with naturally occurring osteoarthritis: a randomized placebo-controlled trial. *Evidence-Based Complementary and Alternative Medicine : eCAM, 2012*, 646191.

Moreau, M., Lussier, B., Pelletier, J. P., Martel-Pelletier, J., Bedard, C., Gauvin, D., & Troncy, E. (2014). A medicinal herb-based natural health product improves the condition of a canine natural osteoarthritis model: a randomized placebo-controlled trial. *Research in Veterinary Science, 97*, 574–581.

Moreau, M., Troncy, E., Del Castillo, J. R., Bedard, C., Gauvin, D., & Lussier, B. (2012b). Effects of feeding a high omega-3 fatty acids diet in dogs with naturally occurring osteoarthritis. *Journal of Animal Physiology and Animal Nutrition, 97*, 830–837.

Neumann, S., Stolt, P., Braun, G., Hellmann, K., & Reinhart, E. (2011). Effectiveness of the homeopathic preparation Zeel compared with carprofen in dogs with osteoarthritis. *Journal of the American Animal Hospital Association, 47*, 12–20.

Peal, A., D'Altilio, M., Simms, C., Alvey, M., Gupta, R. C., Goad, J. T., Canerdy, T. D., Bagchi, M., & Bagchi, D. (2007). Therapeutic efficacy and safety of undenatured type-II collagen (UC-II) alone or in combination with (-)-hydroxycitric acid and chromemate in arthritic dogs. *Journal of Veterinary Pharmacology and Therapeutics, 30*, 275–278.

Pollard, B., Guilford, W. G., Ankenbauer-Perkins, K. L., & Hedderley, D. (2006). Clinical efficacy and tolerance of an extract of green-lipped mussel (*Perna canaliculus*) in dogs presumptively diagnosed with degenerative joint disease. *New Zealand Veterinary Journal, 54*, 114–118.

Reichling, J., Schmokel, H., Fitzi, J., Bucher, S., & Saller, R. (2004). Dietary support with Boswellia resin in canine inflammatory joint and spinal disease. *Schweizer Archiv fur Tierheilkunde, 146*, 71–79.

Rhouma, M., de Oliveira El Warrak, A., Troncy, E., Beaudry, F., & Chorfi, Y. (2013). Anti-inflammatory response of dietary vitamin E and its effects on pain and joint structures during early stages of surgically induced osteoarthritis in dogs. *Canadian Journal of Veterinary Research, 77*, 191–198.

Rialland, P., Bichot, S., Lussier, B., Moreau, M., Beaudry, F., del Castillo, J. R., Gauvin, D., & Troncy, E. (2013). Effect of a diet enriched with green-lipped mussel on pain behavior and functioning in dogs with clinical osteoarthritis. *Canadian Journal of Veterinary Research, 77*, 66–74.

Rosenberg, W., & Donald, A. (1995). Evidence based medicine: an approach to clinical problem-solving. *British Medical Journal, 310*, 1122–1126.

Rothrock, N. E., Kaiser, K. A., & Cella, D. (2011). Developing a valid patient-reported outcome measure. *Clinical Pharmacology and Therapeutics, 90*, 737–742.

Roush, J. K., Cross, A. R., Renberg, W. C., Dodd, C. E., Sixby, K. A., Fritsch, D. A., Allen, T. A., Jewell, D. E., Richardson, D. C., Leventhal, P. S., & Hahn, K. A. (2010a). Evaluation of the effects of dietary supplementation with fish oil omega-3 fatty acids on weight bearing in dogs with osteoarthritis. *Journal of the American Veterinary Medical Association, 236*, 67–73.

Roush, J. K., Dodd, C. E., Fritsch, D. A., Allen, T. A., Jewell, D. E., Schoenherr, W. D., Richardson, D. C., Leventhal, P. S., & Hahn, K. A. (2010b). Multicenter veterinary practice assessment of the effects of omega-3 fatty acids on osteoarthritis in dogs. *Journal of the American Veterinary Medical Association, 236*, 59–66.

Sanderson, R. O., Beata, C., Flipo, R. M., Genevois, J. P., Macias, C., Tacke, S., Vezzoni, A., & Innes, J. F. (2009). Systematic review of the management of canine osteoarthritis. *Veterinary Record, 164*, 418–424.

Schulz, K. F., Altman, D. G., Moher, D., & Group, C. (2010). CONSORT 2010 statement: updated guidelines for reporting parallel group randomized trials. *Annals of Internal Medicine, 152*, 726–732.

Servet, E., Biourge, V., & Marniquet, P. (2006). Dietary intervention can improve clinical signs in osteoarthritic dogs. *Journal of Nutrition, 136*, 1995S–1997S.

Shearer, P. (2011). Epidemiology of orthopedic disease. *Veterinary Focus, 21*, 24–25.

Slingerland, L. I., Hazewinkel, H. A., Meij, B. P., Picavet, P., & Voorhout, G. (2011). Cross-sectional study of the prevalence and clinical features of osteoarthritis in 100 cats. *Veterinary Journal, 187*, 304–309.

Standards of Evidence for Evaluating Foods with Health Claims, (2000). Health Canada.

Sul, R. M., Chase, D., Parkin, T., & Bennett, D. (2014). Comparison of meloxicam and a glucosamine-chondroitin supplement in management of feline osteoarthritis. A double-blind randomised, placebo-controlled, prospective trial. *Veterinary and Comparative Orthopaedics and Traumatology, 27*, 20–26.

Suresh, K. (2011). An overview of randomization techniques: an unbiased assessment of outcome in clinical research. *Journal of Human Reproductive Sciences, 4*, 8–11.

Vandeweerd, J. M., Coisnon, C., Clegg, P., Cambier, C., Pierson, A., Hontoir, F., Saegerman, C., Gustin, P., & Buczinski, S. (2012). Systematic review of efficacy of nutraceuticals to alleviate clinical signs of osteoarthritis. *Journal of Veterinary Internal Medicine, 26*, 448–456.

Velentgas, P., Dreyer, N. A., Nourjah, P., Smith, S. R., Torchia, M. M., & Quality, A. H. C. R. (2013). *Developing a Protocol for Observational Comparative Effectiveness Research: A User's Guide* (1st ed.). Rockville: Agency for Healthcare Research and Quality.

Index